CAROLINA GARCIA·DE·ALBA

# ENDOCRINOLOGY OF THE LUNG

# CONTEMPORARY ENDOCRINOLOGY

P. Michael Conn, SERIES EDITOR

# ENDOCRINOLOGY OF THE LUNG

## DEVELOPMENT AND SURFACTANT SYNTHESIS

*Edited by*

## CAROLE R. MENDELSON, PhD

*University of Texas Southwestern Medical Center
at Dallas, Dallas, TX*

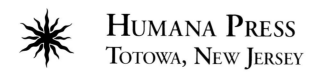

© 2000 Humana Press Inc.
999 Riverview Drive, Suite 208
Totowa, New Jersey 07512

For additional copies, pricing for bulk purchases, and/or information about other Humana titles, contact Humana at the above address or at any of the following numbers: Tel: 973-256-1699; Fax: 973-256-8341; E-mail: humana@humanapr.com; Website: http://humanapress.com

Due diligence has been taken by the publishers, editors, and authors of this book to assure the accuracy of the information published and to describe generally accepted practices. The contributors herein have carefully checked to ensure that the drug selections and dosages set forth in this text are accurate and in accord with the standards accepted at the time of publication. Notwithstanding, as new research, changes in government regulations, and knowledge from clinical experience relating to drug therapy and drug reactions constantly occurs, the reader is advised to check the product information provided by the manufacturer of each drug for any change in dosages or for additional warnings and contraindications. This is of utmost importance when the recommended drug herein is a new or infrequently used drug. It is the responsibility of the treating physician to determine dosages and treatment strategies for individual patients. Further it is the responsibility of the health care provider to ascertain the Food and Drug Administration status of each drug or device used in their clinical practice. The publisher, editors, and authors are not responsible for errors or omissions or for any consequences from the application of the information presented in this book and make no warranty, express or implied, with respect to the contents in this publication.

This publication is printed on acid-free paper. ∞

ANSI Z39.48-1984 (American National Standards Institute)
Permanence of Paper for Printed Library Materials.

Cover design by Patricia F. Cleary

Cover art: Figure 8E from Chapter 6, The Genetics of Glucocorticoid-Regulated Embryonic Lung Morphogenesis: *A First Approximation of the Epigenetic Rules*, by Tina Jaskoll and Michael Melnick.

**Photocopy Authorization Policy:**

Printed in the United States of America.   10  9  8  7  6  5  4  3  2  1

Library of Congress Cataloging-in-Publication Data

Endocrinology of the lung : development and surfactant synthesis / edited by Carole R. Mendelson.
       p. cm. -- (Contemporary endocrinology)
  Includes bibliographical references and index.
  ISBN 0-89603-676-6 (alk. paper)
    1. Lungs--Growth. 2. Lungs--Diseases--Endocrine aspects.  I. Mendelson, Carole R. II.
  Contemporary endocrinology (Totowa, N.J.)

RC756 .E48 2000
612.2--dc21
                                               99-052787

# PREFACE

The seminal observation by Liggins in 1969 that glucocorticoid treatment of fetal lambs resulted in enhanced lung maturation initiated the concept that the fetal lung is a hormonally responsive organ. During the past thirty years, great progress has been made in defining the roles of steroid, peptide, and polypeptide hormones in lung branching morphogenesis, differentiation of specialized cell types, and surfactant synthesis. In addition to glucocorticoids, it is apparent that the sex steroids, retinoids, catecholamines, prostaglandins, and peptide and polypeptide hormones, including a number of growth factors and cytokines, influence lung growth and differentiation as well as surfactant synthesis. Whereas the steroids and certain polypeptide hormones are delivered to lung through the systemic circulation, growth factors are produced locally by mesenchymal cells surrounding the developing lung buds, by type II epithelial cells, or by their precursors. Additionally, a variety of bioactive peptides are produced by innervated clusters of neuroendocrine cells that lie within the primitive airway epithelium.

*Endocrinology of the Lung: Development and Surfactant Synthesis* contains contributions from investigators studying the actions of the various classes of endocrine, paracrine, and neuroendocrine factors on lung development and surfactant synthesis. The model systems used in their studies range from whole animals to organ and cell culture and to transgenic, genetically altered, and gene-targeted mice. The first seven chapters are devoted to the actions of glucocorticoids on lung development and on the synthesis of surfactant glycerophospholipids and the surfactant proteins—SP-A, SP-B, and SP-C. Included in this group is a chapter on the role of the major histocompatibility complex (MHC) locus in glucocorticoid responsiveness, as well as one that addresses the role of corticotropin-releasing hormone (CRH) and glucocorticoids in lung development and surfactant synthesis using CRH gene-targeted mice. Two chapters address the actions of hormones that bind to other members of the nuclear receptor family; one is concerned with mechanisms that underlie the sexual dimorphism of fetal lung maturation and sex differences in responsiveness to perinatal glucocorticoid administration, while the other is concerned with the roles of retinoids and their receptors in lung development, surfactant synthesis, and the repair of lung injury in human premature newborns. Another chapter deals with fetal lung maturation and surfactant synthesis in the diabetic pregnancy and the effects of insulin on the synthesis of surfactant lipids and proteins. The remaining six chapters review the importance of cell–cell interactions and elaborate on various growth factors and bioactive peptides in lung branching morphogenesis, cell differentiation, gene expression, and pulmonary pathophysiology. The use of transgenic and gene-targeted mice to define the roles of members of a number of growth-factor families and their receptors in the regulation of lung morphogenesis and cellular differentiation also is addressed.

It is therefore apparent that lung growth, differentiation, and surfactant production are controlled by a variety of circulating and locally produced hormones and growth factors that exert their effects via endocrine, paracrine, autocrine, neuroendocrine, and possibly intracrine mechanisms. In light of the importance of circulating hormones and of growth factor-mediated cellular interactions in lung growth, cell differentiation, function, and pathophysiology, it is my hope that *Endocrinology of the Lung: Development and Surfactant Synthesis* will have appeal, not only to pulmonary biologists, but also to those working in the areas of hormone action, and developmental and cell biology of other organ systems.

I would like to express my sincere appreciation to the contributors who have collaborated to make this a comprehensive review of the lung as an endocrine-responsive organ.

*Carole R. Mendelson*

# CONTENTS

# CONTRIBUTORS

JOSEPH L. ALCORN, PhD, *Department of Pediatrics, Division of Neonatology, University of Texas Medical School at Houston, Houston, TX*

PHILIP L. BALLARD, MD, PhD, *Neonatology, Department of Pediatrics, University of Pennsylvania, Children's Hospital of Philadelphia, Philadelphia, PA*

VIJAYAKUMAR BOGGARAM, PhD, *Department of Molecular Biology, University of Texas Health Science Center at Tyler, Tyler, TX*

NICHOLAS J. CARTEL MSc, *Programme in Lung Biology Research, The Hospital for Sick Children Research Institute, Department of Laboratory Medicine and Pathobiology, University of Toronto, Toronto, Canada*

ERNEST CUTZ, MD, *Department of Pathology, Hospital for Sick Children, Toronto, Canada*

THOMAS N. GEORGE, MD, *Division of Neonatology, Department of Pediatrics, University of Iowa, Iowa City, IA*

MARY A. GRUMMER, PhD, *Department of Pediatrics, University of Wisconsin, Madison, WI*

MACHIKO IKEGAMI, MD, PhD, *Pulmonary Biology/Neonatology, Children's Hospital Medical Center, University of Cincinnati, Cincinnati, OH*

TINA JASKOLL, PhD, *Laboratory for Developmental Genetics, University of Southern California, Los Angeles, CA*

ALAN H. JOBE, MD, PhD, *Pulmonary Biology/Neonatology, Children's Hospital Medical Center, University of Cincinnati, Cincinnati, OH*

THOMAS R. KORFHAGEN, MD, PhD, *Pulmonary Biology/Neonatology, Children's Hospital Medical Center, University of Cincinnati, Cincinnati, OH*

JINXING LI, MD, PhD, *Department of Internal Medicine, New Hanover Regional Medical Center, Wilmington, NC*

JOSEPH A. MAJZOUB, MD, *Division of Endocrinology, Department of Medicine, Children's Hospital, Harvard Medical School, Boston, MA*

MICHAEL MELNICK, DDS, PhD, *Laboratory for Developmental Genetics, University of Southern California, Los Angeles, CA*

CAROLE R. MENDELSON, PhD, *Department of Biochemistry and Obstetrics-Gynecology, University of Texas Southwestern Medical Center at Dallas, Dallas, TX*

OLGA L. MIAKOTINA, PhD, *Department of Anatomy and Cell Biology, University of Iowa, Iowa City, IA*

LAURA F. MICHAEL, PhD, *Department of Cancer Biology, Dana Farber Cancer Institute, Boston, MA*

LOUIS J. MUGLIA, MD, PhD, *Division of Endocrinology, Departments of Pediatrics and Molecular Biology and Pharmacology, Washington University School of Medicine, St. Louis, MO*

HEBER C. NIELSEN, *Department of Pediatrics, Tufts-New England Medical Center, and Tufts University School of Medicine, Boston, MA*

MARTIN POST, PhD, *Programme in Lung Biology Research, The Hospital for Sick Children Research Institute, Departments of Pediatrics, Physiology and Laboratory Medicine and Pathobiology, University of Toronto, Toronto, Canada*

WAYNE A. PRICE, MD, *Department of Pediatrics, University of North Carolina at Chapel Hill, Chapel Hill, NC*

SEAMUS A. ROONEY, PhD, ScD, *Division of Perinatal Medicine, Department of Pediatrics, Yale University School of Medicine, New Haven, CT*

LEWIS P. RUBIN, MD, *Department of Pediatrics, Women and Infants Hospital of Rhode Island, Brown University School of Medicine. Providence, RI*

JEANNE M. SNYDER, PhD, *Department of Anatomy and Cell Biology, University of Iowa, Iowa City, IA*

ALAN D. STILES, MD, *Department of Pediatrics, University of North Carolina at Chapel Hill, Chapel Hill, NC*

MARY E. SUNDAY, MD, PhD, *Department of Pathology, Children's Hospital, Brigham and Women's Hospital, Harvard Medical School, Boston, MA*

JOHN S. TORDAY, PhD, *Departments of Pediatrics and Obstetrics and Gynecology, Harbor-UCLA Research and Education Institute, UCLA School of Medicine, Torrance, CA*

MARIA VENIHAKI, PhD, *Division of Endocrinology, Department of Medicine, Children's Hospital, Harvard Medical School, Boston, MA*

JEFFREY A. WHITSETT, MD, *Pulmonary Biology/Neonatology, Children's Hospital Medical Center, University of Cincinnati, Cincinnati, OH*

PAMPEE P. YOUNG, MD, PhD, *Department of Pathology, Division of Laboratory Medicine, Washington University Medical Center, St. Louis, MO*

RICHARD D. ZACHMAN, MD, PhD, *Department of Pediatrics and Nutritional Sciences, University of Wisconsin, Madison, WI*

YUN ZHAO, MD, PhD, *Department of Medicine, Duke University Medical Center, Durham, NC*

# ENDOCRINOLOGY OF THE LUNG

# 1

# The Glucocorticoid Domain in the Lung and Mechanisms of Action

*Philip L. Ballard, MD, PHD*

CONTENTS

## INTRODUCTION

The lung, like most mammalian organs, is a target tissue for glucocorticoids. Responses have been observed in a variety of pulmonary cell types, with most attention directed toward epithelial cells of airways and alveoli, mesenchymal fibroblasts, and vascular endothelial cells. Both negative and positive regulation of target genes occur paralleling the pattern of responses in other tissues. The role of glucocorticoid changes during development in many tissues, from a modulator of cellular differentiation and organogenesis in fetal life to a major regulator of metabolic homeostasis after birth, and this dichotomy of function is also well documented in the lung. The primary mechanism of glucocorticoid action during pulmonary development switches from direct modulation of gene expression to antagonism of cytokine effects via interaction with $NF\kappa_B$. This chapter reviews the identified target genes for glucocorticoids in their role as a stimulatory hormone for fetal lung maturation and as a major antiinflammatory hormone in the postnatal lung in response to injury or infection. The later part of the chapter focuses on glucocorticoid regulation of the surfactant proteins that are critical for normal respiratory function. While glucocorticoids induce a coordinated upregulation of each of the surfactant components, mechanisms of action differ among the target genes.

## GLUCOCORTICOIDS AND LUNG DEVELOPMENT

Although a variety of hormones, growth factors, cytokines, and other agents affect various aspects of lung development—in particular, the surfactant system of type II alveolar cells—glucocorticoids have wide-ranging effects in the developing lung and are

From: *Contemporary Endocrinology: Endocrinology of the Lung: Development and Surfactant Synthesis*
Edited by: C. R. Mendelson © Humana Press Inc., Totowa, NJ

the most extensively studied of all regulatory agents. Rising glucocorticoid levels during the last 10–20% of gestation are coincident with a surge in surfactant synthesis in most mammalian species, and ablation studies support their in vivo relevance as the major modulator of the timing of lung development.

Liggins *(1)* was the first to recognize accelerated synthesis of surfactant in response to glucocorticoid treatment. He reported in 1969 that dexamethasone treatment of sheep before premature delivery resulted in partial lung aeration and short-term survival at a point in gestation when lambs are previable, and speculated that persistence of lung expansion in these immature animals indicated accelerated synthesis and secretion of surfactant. Subsequently, glucocorticoids have been shown in a number of different model systems, both in vivo and in vitro, to accelerate physiologic, morphologic, biochemical, and molecular indices of lung maturation. For example, Seidner et al. *(2)* found that antenatal glucocorticoid treatment of premature rabbits improved maximal lung volume and dynamic compliance, and similar improvements in lung mechanics have been reported in other species *(3,4)*. Structurally, antenatal glucocorticoid treatment produces larger air spaces, thinning of the alveolar septa, increased invasion of capillaries into airspaces, with all of these changes representing precocious maturation *(5–7)*. The ultrastructure of the alveolar epithelium also matures precociously following glucocorticoid treatment, resulting in cells that are more cuboidal, containing lamellar inclusions and less cytoplasmic glycogen. Overall, in vivo glucocorticoid treatment resulted in an acceleration of normal developmental events by approximately 1.5 d in the fetal rabbit *(6)*. Similar precocious induction of type II cell phenotype by glucocorticoid treatment occurs during explant culture of fetal lung from several species (reviewed in ref. 5), indicating direct action of glucocorticoid in the lung. Cultured fetal lung, along with pulmonary cell lines, have been used to identify glucocorticoid target genes and to investigate mechanisms. These results are a major focus of this chapter.

The acceleration of normal developmental processes in lung and other fetal tissues resulting from glucocorticoid treatment has proven to be useful for premature infants. A large number of controlled trials beginning in 1972 have shown that antenatal glucocorticoid treatment before premature birth consistently reduces the incidence of respiratory distress syndrome and results in lower neonatal mortality and morbidity (reviewed in ref. 8). The peak fetal plasma concentration of glucocorticoid after maternal betamethasone treatment is comparable to corticoid levels occurring in untreated infants with lung disease and therefore represents a physiologic stress concentration. The level of free corticoid under these conditions is estimated to result in ≥75% occupancy of glucocorticoid receptor (GR) *(9)*.

In addition to maturational effects of exogenous glucocorticoids, experimental data in a number of species support a physiological role for endogenous glucocorticoids (reviewed in ref. 5). In the sheep, free cortisol is low and unchanging until approximately day 135, then increasing at least 10-fold by the day preceding term birth (approx 145 d) *(10,11)*. Surfactant phospholipids and surfactant proteins (SP) -A and -B and their mRNAs *(12,13)* are detectable in lung tissue of fetal sheep by approx 120 d of gestation and contents increase exponentially until term, consistent with a role of endogenous cortisol in modulation, but probably not the initiation, of surfactant lipid synthesis. In the rat, mouse, and nonhuman primate, free corticosteroid concentrations also rise substantially during the last 10% of gestation at the same time that surfactant is actively synthesized and accumulates in alveolae. Blockade of adrenal glucocorticoid production by metyrapone in fetal rats has been shown to retard development of the surfactant system *(14)*. Hypophysectomy has been used to abolish adrenocortical function in fetal sheep and was found to impair the synthesis and release of surfactant as well as the structural development of the lung, and ACTH treatment improved all maturational indices *(15–17)*. Particularly persuasive evidence for an important role of endogenous corticosteroids in lung structural development is provided by the knockout mouse models for corticotrophin-releasing hormone (CRH) and GR. Homozygous pups for CRH deficiency, delivered of homozygous females, are deprived of both maternal and fetal sources of corticosterone *in utero*, and these pups die soon after birth with immature lungs *(18)* (*see* Chapter 7). A similar delay in lung structural development was observed with GR-deficient animals *(19)*. In the human, the developmental pattern of amniotic fluid corticoid conjugates, reflecting fetal cortisol levels, parallels the lecithin:sphingomyelin ratio, which is an indicator of lung maturity *(20)*. Thus, exposure to exogenous glucocorticoid appears to mimic the role of endogenous corticosteroids in modulating the rate of lung maturation.

## *Regulated Proteins in Developing Lung*

High-resolution two-dimensional polyacrylamide gel electrophoresis (2-D PAGE) has been used to survey glucocorticoid-regulated proteins in fetal lung. In a study with human tissue, fetal lung was cultured in the presence and absence of dexamethasone, and proteins were labeled by $[^{35}S]$methionine incorporation *(21)*. Dexamethasone induced or repressed a distinct set of proteins, compared to effects of interferon-$\gamma$, comprising approx 2% of the approx 1000 proteins resolved by 2-D PAGE. Consistent with these results, dexamethasone did not affect the rate of $[^{35}S]$methionine into total protein. Three induced proteins are illustrated in the fluorograms shown in Fig. 1. The level of induction of various proteins, as analyzed by densitometric scanning of the fluorograms, ranged from 2- to 22-fold vs control (Table 1). Dexamethasone also repressed four proteins, whereas inhibition was not observed with either interferon-$\gamma$ or cAMP treatment. Treatment of cultured tissue with agents that increased intracellular cAMP induced five unique proteins as well as several proteins that were also regulated by dexamethasone. One induced protein was identified only in tissue treated with both dexamethasone and cAMP. By contrast, there were no proteins identified that were consistently regulated by $T_3$ or by TGF-$\beta$ (except for SP-A), agents that enhance phospholipid synthesis and downregulate surfactant components, respectively *(22,23)*.

Among the glucocorticoid-regulated proteins resolved on 2-D PAGE, only SP-A, and possibly prepro-SP-B, were identified based on their migration coordinants and isoform pattern. Some of the proteins were enriched in either fibroblasts or type II cells isolated from the lung explants, whereas other proteins were induced in both cell types (Table 1). In earlier studies using 2-D PAGE, Phelps and Giannopoulos *(24)* and Beresini et al. *(25)* also identified a limited number of proteins induced by dexamethasone and interferon-$\gamma$, respectively, in fetal rabbit lung and human fetal lung fibroblasts.

These findings establish that, similar to other target tissues, glucocorticoids induce and repress subsets of proteins in cells of developing lung. The limited number of proteins in the glucocorticoid domain is consistent with a selective effect on cell differentiation and function without alteration of overall synthetic activity. Presumably many of these proteins are important in glucocorticoid-mediated maturational events in fetal lung, however, at present the identity and function of most of these regulated proteins are not known.

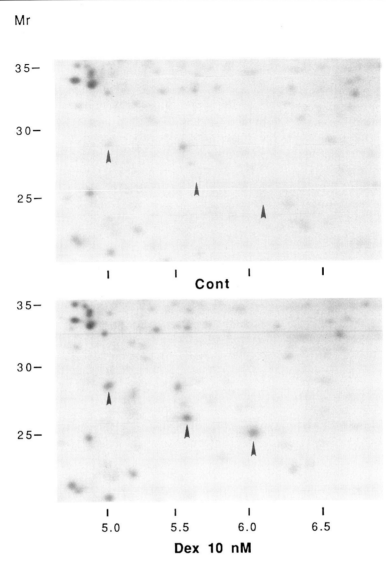

Fig. 1. Two-dimensional gel electrophoresis of fetal lung proteins. Explants of human fetal lung were cultured in the absence (**upper**) and presence (**lower**) of 10n$M$ dexamethasone, exposed to [35]S-Met, and proteins resolved on 2-D SDS PAGE. Portions of resulting fluorograms are shown illustrating induction of three proteins of $M_r$ 25–30 kDa and pI 5–6. (From ref. *21*, with permission).

## Gene Regulation in Developing Lung

While the maturational effects of glucocorticoids on both lung structural development and function, in particular lung compliance and the surfactant system, have been recognized for over 30 yr, identification and characterization of regulated genes has occurred only during the last 15 yr. A number of target genes have been identified in the developing mammalian lung. These are summarized in Table 2, which separates glucocorticoid responses as stimulatory vs inhibitory and includes information on molecular mechanisms as known for a limited number of genes.

Table 1
Proteins of Human Fetal Lung Regulated by Dexamethasone: 2-D PAGE

| Protein ($Mr \times 10^3/pI$) | Dexamethasone Effect (Fold Change vs Control) | Cell Localization |
|---|---|---|
| 18/4.8 | 5.0 | Type II |
| 25/5.9 | 18 | Both |
| 24/6.2 | 9.3 | Type II |
| 28/5.3 | 7.4 | Both |
| 28/5.6 | 6.2 | Both |
| 30/>7 | 5.5 | |
| 32/4.8 | 2.1 | Fibroblast |
| 33/6.2 | 2.7 | Both |
| 37/4.8 | 3.7 | Fibroblast |
| 38/4.8 | 6[a] | Fibroblast |
| 40/4.4 | | Type II |
| 41/5.6 | 2.1 | Both |
| 42/6.2 | (0.30) | Type II |
| 44/5.5 | (0.07 | Both |
| 44/5.6 | 3[a] | Type II |
| 51/5.7 | (0.27) | Type II |
| 53/4.4 | 5.8 | Fibroblast |
| 84/6.6 | 3.3 | Both |
| 85/>7 | (0.10) | Both |
| 109/5.6 | 9[a] | |
| 109/5.6 | 22[a] | |

Two-dimensional PAGE analysis was performed after [35]S-Met labeling of second trimester human fetal lung cultured as explants for 4 days in the presence and absence of 10nM dexamethasone. Fold change and intensity values of regulated proteins are means from 2 to 4 lungs analyzed quantitatively. Fold change values in parentheses indicate repressed proteins.
[a]Value approximate because of difficulty with spot detection or scanning resolution. Cell localization was based on 2-D PAGE studies of populations of enriched type II cells and fibroblasts isolated from explants.
Data from ref. 21.

Glucocorticoid-responsive genes in developing lung fall into four major categories: signal transduction, components of the surfactant system, structural proteins, and functions related to the process of adapting to air breathing.

1. *Signal transduction.* A number of molecules involved in signal transduction are known to be modulated by glucocorticoid treatment. This list includes proteins involved in metabolism or binding of steroid hormones (11β-hydroxysteroid dehydrogenase and retinoic acid receptor β) and growth factors (IGF-1, IGF binding proteins, TGF-β3, aminopeptidase, and fibroblast pneumonocyte factor), and at least two transcription factors (HoxB5 and C/EBPδ). In general, glucocorticoid effects on expression of these genes is stimulatory to lung maturation. The pulmonary target cells include both mesenchymal fibroblasts and differentiating epithelial cells, and some of the inducible proteins (11β-hydroxysteroid dehydrogenase, TGF-β3 and fibroblast pneumonocyte factor) participate in mesenchymal–epithelial signaling during the developmental process.

Table 2
Glucocorticoid-Regulated Genes in Developing Lung

| Gene | References[a] | Experimental System | Cell Type[b] | Response mRNA | Response Protein | Response Function | Mechanism | Mimic Developmental Change |
|---|---|---|---|---|---|---|---|---|
| **Stimulatory** | | | | | | | | |
| 11β-Hydroxysteroid dehydrogenase (reductive act.) | 26 | Fetal rat explant | | | | X | | X |
| TGF-β3 | 27 | Fetal rat cells | FB | X | | | | |
| IGFBP-6 | 28 | Fetal rat explant | FB | X | | | | X |
| Aminopeptidase N | 29 | Fetal rat organ culture | epi | X | | | | X |
| Fibroblast pneumonocyte factor | 30, 31 | Fetal rat cells and in vivo | FB | | | X | Cycloheximide and AMD block induction | |
| C/EBPδ | 32, 33 | Fetal human and mouse organ culture | epi | X | X | | | X |
| SP-A | 34–36 | Fetal human explant | Type II/Clara | X | X | | ↑ Transcription rate | X |
| | 37 | Fetal rabbit explant | | X | | | Delayed ↑ in transcription rate | |
| | 38-40 | Fetal/newborn rat in vivo | Type II/Clara | X | X | | | |
| | 41, 42 | Fetal rabbit in vivo | | | X | | | |
| | 12, 13, 43 | Fetal sheep in vivo | | X | X | | | |

| | Model | Cell type | | | Effect | |
|---|---|---|---|---|---|---|
| **SP-B** | | | | | | |
| *44–51* | Fetal human explant and isolated cells | Type II | X | X | ↑Transcription rate, mRNA stability and protein processing; Cycloheximide not block | X |
| *52–54* | Fetal rat and rabbit explant | | X | | ↑mRNA stability; No change transcription rate | |
| *55* | H820 cell line | Type II | X | X | | |
| *56* | H441 cell line | Clara | X | X | ↑ Transcription rate and mRNA stability (AMD) | |
| *12, 13, 38, 41–43, 57–59* | Fetal rat, rabbit and sheep in vivo | | X | X | | |
| **SP-C** | | | | | | |
| *45, 47, 50* | Fetal human explant | Type II | X | X | ↑Transcription rate and protein processing; No change in mRNA stability; Cycloheximide block | X |
| *60–61* | Fetal rabbit explant | | X | | ↑mRNA stability; No change transcription rate | |
| *43* | Fetal sheep in vivo | | X | X | | |
| *62* | Fetal rat explant | | X | X | | |
| **SP-D** | | | | | | |
| *63, 64* | Fetal rat and human explant | Type II | X | X | ↑ Transcription rate | X |
| *39, 52, 63* | Fetal rat in vivo | Type II/Clara | X | X | | |

Table 2 (continued)
### Glucocorticoid-Regulated Genes in Developing Lung

| Gene | References[a] | Experimental System | Cell Type[b] | Response mRNA | Protein | Function | Mechanism | Mimic Developmental Change |
|---|---|---|---|---|---|---|---|---|
| Fatty acid synthetase | 54, 65-67 | Fetal human and rat explant | epi | X | X | X | ↑mRNA stability; >increased transcription rate | X |
|  | 68 | rat and rabbit in vivo |  |  |  |  |  |  |
| Cholinephosphate cytidylyltransferase | 69 | Fetal rat explant |  |  |  | X | Secondary to ↑cofactor |  |
|  | 70 | Fetal human explant |  |  |  | X | ↑In part independent of cofactor |  |
|  | 71 | Fetal rat in vivo |  |  |  | X | Intracellular translocation |  |
| LysoPC acylCoA transferase | 72 | Fetal human explant |  |  |  | X |  |  |
| Tropoelastin | 73 | Fetal rat explant and in vivo; fetal bovine cells | FB & vascular SM | X |  |  | Functional GRE in 5' flanking sequence | X |
| Tropoelastin | 74, 75 / 76 | Fetal rat in vivo Transgenic mice in vivo | FB | X | X |  | Mediated by TGFβ$_3$ ↑Promoter activity in lung |  |
| αENaC | 77 | Fetal rat in vivo | epi | X |  |  |  | X |
| Na$^+$-K$^+$-ATPase ß1 | 78 | Fetal rat in vivo | epi | X | X |  |  | X |
| Aquaporin 1 | 79 | Fetal rat in vivo | endo | X | X |  |  | X |

| | Ref | Model | Cell type | | | | |
|---|---|---|---|---|---|---|---|
| Aquaporin 4 | 80 | Fetal rat in vivo | bronchial epi | X | | | X |
| β Adrenergic receptor | 81, 82 | Fetal rat and rabbit explant | | | X | | X |
| | 83, 84 | Fetal rabbit in vivo | alveolar epi | | X | | |
| Cu Zn SOD | 85 | Rat in vivo | | | X | | X |
| | 86 | Fetal rat explant | | | X | | |
| Catalase | 85, 87 | Rat in vivo | | X | X | ↑ Transcription rate | X |
| Glutathione peroxidase | 85 | Rat in vivo | | | X | | X |
| **Inhibitory** | | | | | | | |
| 11β-hydroxysteroid dehydrogenase (oxidative act.) | 26 | Fetal rat explant | | | X | | X |
| RARβ | 88 | Rat cell line | epi | X | | Cycloheximide block | X |
| | 89 | Fetal rat explant and in vivo | | | X | | |
| | 90 | NB rat in vivo | | | X | | |
| IGF1 | 91, 92 | Fetal human explant | FB | X | | | |
| IGFBP-2 | 28 | Fetal rat explant | | X | | | X |
| IGFBP-3 | 28 | Fetal rat explant | | X | | | |
| | 93 | Fetal rat cells | FB and epi | X | | | No |

### Table 2 (continued)
### Glucocorticoid-Regulated Genes in Developing Lung

| Gene | References[a] | Experimental System | Cell Type[b] | Response | | | Mechanism | Mimic Developmental Change |
|---|---|---|---|---|---|---|---|---|
| | | | | mRNA | Protein | Function | | |
| IGFBP-4 | 28 | Fetal rat explant | | X | X | | | No |
| IGFBP-5 | 28 | Fetal rat explant | | X | X | | | No |
| Hoxb5 | 94 | Fetal mouse organ culture | | | X | | | |
| SP-A | 35, 36, 51, 95, 96 | Fetal human and baboon explant and isolated cells | Type II | X | X | | At higher concentration and longer exposure ↓ transcription rate | No |
| | 97 | H441 cell line | Clara | X | | | | |
| SP-C | 41 | Rabbit | | X | | | | |
| β-Adrenergic receptor | 98 | Fetal human explant | | | X | | | |
| β-Galactoside-binding protein | 99, 100 | Rat in vivo | | X | | X | | No |

Abbreviations: epi, epithelial cells; FB, fibroblasts; macro, macrophages; AMD, actinomycin D; endo, endothelial; SM, smooth muscle; dex, dexamethasone; TGF, transforming growth factor; IGF, insulin-like growth factor; BP, binding protein; C/E, CAAT enhancer; PC, phosphatidylcholine; ENaC, epithelial sodium channel; SOD superoxide dismutase; RAR, retinoic acid receptor

[a]Representative references are given for genes studied by multiple investigators, with a preference for papers addressing mechanisms.

[b]The listed cell type refers to either the lung cells which express the gene in vivo or the source of cultured cells used in the studies.

[c]All responses in vitro occur with a time course and at concentrations of dexamethasone (half-maximal 1–10nM) or other corticosteroids and/or have effects blocked by RU486, consistent with GR mediation unless otherwise noted.

2. *Surfactant system.* Glucocorticoids stimulate production of pulmonary surfactant and target genes include all four surfactant proteins and at least four lipogenic enzymes. In addition, there is indirect evidence that glucocorticoids induce key, currently unidentified, enzymes for processing of pro-SP-B and pro-SP-C to the mature forms *(46,101).* Expression of surfactant proteins in fetal lung is limited to epithelial cells of developing air spaces. At least one of the lipogenic enzymes (fatty acid synthetase) is also greatly enriched in epithelial cells vs other cell types, and glucocorticoid induction of this enzyme occurs only in epithelial cells *(66).* Glucocorticoid regulation of the surfactant proteins has been investigated in some detail, and this is addressed later in the chapter.

3. *Structural proteins.* Appropriate temporal and spatial deposition of elastin in developing airways and vessels is a key component of lung structural development. Expression of the tropoelastin gene in both fibroblasts and vascular smooth muscle cells is upregulated by glucocorticoids in developing rat lung. However, the precise role of increased elastin production in glucocorticoid-stimulated structural events, such as mesenchymal condensation *(22)* and improved compliance independent of surfactant *(12)*, is not well defined. Presumably other unidentified components of the extracellular matrix and/or basement membrane are also modulated by glucocorticoids.

4. *Adaptation to air breathing.* During fetal life the lung is fluid-filled, and gas exchange is carried out by the placenta. Successful transition to air breathing requires clearance of lung fluid, secretion of surfactant, and adequate protection against oxidant damage associated with air breathing. Glucocorticoids are known to stimulate a number of proteins involved in these processes. Both ion pumps ($Na^+$-$K^+$-ATPase) and channels ($\alpha$-ENAC and the aquaporins) are precociously induced in fetal lung by glucocorticoid treatment. Induction of the $\beta$-adrenergic receptor contributes to both fluid clearance and secretion of surfactant since both processes are stimulated by $\beta$-agonists. Activities of three antioxidant enzymes are stimulated by glucocorticoids at least in lung of fetal rat.

All of the stimulatory effects of glucocorticoid treatment on gene expression in developing lung mimic normal development changes. As discussed elsewhere in the chapter, the timing of normal lung maturation is modulated by endogenous corticosteroids through developmental changes in production and metabolism of corticosteroids, levels of CBG, and distribution and levels of GR. Some of the inhibitory effects of glucocorticoid treatment also mimic the normal developmental pattern (Table 2). For example, the decrease in oxidative activity of 11$\beta$-hydroxysteroid dehydrogenase, in conjunction with increasing reductive activity, serves to precociously increase the supply of active cortisol or corticosterone to lung cells. For other genes, however, the response to glucocorticoid treatment appears to be distinct or different from the developmental changes. For example, glucocorticoid treatment decreases expression of IGF-1 and four IGF binding proteins, but only IGFBP-2 gene expression normally decreases in late gestation. Whereas lung $\beta$-adrenergic receptor function is increased by glucocorticoid treatment of fetal animals, an inhibitory response was observed in fetal human lung cultures.

Most of the studies investigating glucocorticoid responses in developing lung have utilized the fetal/newborn rat either in vivo or in explant culture. Other animal systems include the sheep for in vivo studies and fetal rabbit both in vivo and in explant culture. Explants of human fetal lung have been used extensively for studies of both surfactant proteins and lipogenic enzymes and some findings have been confirmed in human cell lines of both Clara cell and type II cell origin as well as in primary isolated cells. For most genes, responses are similar in different species. Two possible exceptions have been described for the rabbit. Although a biphasic response of SP-A to glucocorticoid treatment was observed in fetal rabbit explants, the initial response was inhibition, whereas stimulation is seen in human tissue. Also, there is one report of inhibition of SP-C gene expression by dexamethasone treatment of fetal rabbits, whereas stimulation occurs in all other species examined. The mechanism and physiologic significance of these responses in the rabbit are uncertain.

Glucocorticoid regulation of SP-A gene expression is of particular interest because of the biphasic responses that occur in some species. Expression increases in vivo during the second half of gestation in a variety of species, including the human; however, the dominant response to glucocorticoid in vitro is inhibitory. In explants of human fetal lung, content of SP-A mRNA increases transiently on exposure to lower concentrations of glucocorticoid (e.g., ≤10n$M$), whereas there is a dose-dependent decrease in SP-A on continuing exposure. A similar biphasic response was observed in explants of fetal baboon lung, and the magnitude of the inhibitory response diminished with increasing gestation. Downregulation of SP-A gene expression also occurs in the H441 cell line, which is of human Clara cell origin. Data relating to the mechanism of this biphasic response of the SP-A gene are discussed later in the chapter.

The mechanism of glucocorticoid action in the lung for most if not all examined genes occurs at the level of transcription. When comparisons have been made, there is similar induction of mRNA and protein for target genes. An apparent exception to this is glucocorticoid regulation of choline phosphate cytidylyltransferase, which is mediated at least in part by increased availability of lipid cofactor as well as by intracellular translocation of the enzyme. It is likely that increased cofactor results from the induction of fatty acid synthetase and increased de novo production of fatty acids and phospholipids. The response of choline phosphate cytidylyltransferase to glucocorticoids may represent a mechanism to amplify effects of the hormone on phospholipid production.

Transcription rate and mRNA stability have been examined for some of the genes that are upregulated by glucocorticoids. The major effect on fatty acid synthetase gene expression appears to be increased message stability, although transcription rate also increases. Upregulation of tropoelastin gene expression appears to involve transcriptional activation based on demonstration of a functional GRE in the promoter in transfection and transgenic studies. As discussed later, the glucocorticoid effects on both SP-A and SP-B gene expression include changes in both transcription rate and mRNA stability. In fetal human explant cultures, glucocorticoids increase the transcription rate of SP-C without affecting mRNA stability, whereas effects on stability but not transcription rate were observed in studies with rabbit lung. The responses of both SP-D and catalase involve increased rate of gene transcription. Inhibition of protein synthesis with cycloheximide blocked glucocorticoid induction of retinoic acid receptor β and SP-C mRNAs, consistent with a secondary mechanism of action, but did not affect induction of SP-B mRNA, suggesting a primary response. To date, however, there has been no definitive identification and characterization of a functional GRE in any glucocorticoid regulated gene of developing lung, although there is strong evidence for the presence of a GRE in the tropoelastin promoter.

## GLUCOCORTICOID-REGULATED GENES IN LUNG HOMEOSTASIS

Most of the effects of glucocorticoids that have been characterized in postnatal, mature lung relate to the response to injury and inflammation and maintenance of homeostasis. Glucocorticoid responsive genes that have been identified in resident cells of the adult

lung are described in Table 3. This listing does not include genes of neutrophils, monocytes, and other inflammatory cells that accumulate in the lung in response to a variety
of injurious stimuli.

The majority of responsive gene products listed in Table 3 have a role in lung immune
defense system and response to lung inflammation and injury, together mediating the
physiological antiinflammatory role of glucocorticoids. This response occurs through
downregulation of a number of cytokines and biosynthetic enzymes that are induced in
response to inflammatory stimuli as well as stimulated production of antiinflammatory
compounds.

There are examples of glucocorticoid effects at various steps in the inflammatory
response. Glucocorticoids decrease levels of E-selectin and endothelial–leukocyte
adhesion molecule (ELAM-1) in vascular endothelial cells and intercellular adhesion
molecule (ICAM-1) in epithelial cells, antagonizing induction by inflammatory
cytokines. E-selectin and ELAM-1 are cell-surface adhesion proteins that contribute to
the binding and extravasation of neutrophils that occurs as part of the host response to
tissue injury, infection, or allergic stimulation, and ICAM-1 is involved in interaction and
activation of T and B cells as well as intercellular adhesion. Glucocorticoids downregulate
production of the chemoattractant interleukins IL-6 and IL-8, the inflammatory cytokine
TGF-$\beta$1, the eosinophil chemoattractant chemokine eotaxin, as well as the chemokine RANTES
in various lung cell types, and production of prostaglandins is reduced through
downregulation of cytosolic phospholipase $A_2$ and cyclooxygenase (Cox-2) enzymes.
There is increased expression of IL-I $_{ra}$ and $\alpha$1-acid glycoprotein with glucocorticoid
treatment; these proteins block IL-1 action and exert various immunomodulatory effects
in the lung, respectively. Uteroglobin, a secreted protein of type II and Clara cells with
antiinflammatory properties, including inhibition of phopholipase A2 *(146)*, is also
upregulated in adult rabbit lung by in vivo glucocorticoid treatment *(119,120)*. Production of granulocyte macrophage colony stimulatory factor (GM-CSF), another
proinflammatory agent, is also reduced in airway epithelial cells by glucocorticoid
treatment. Moreover, reduction of GM-CSF secretion from lung epithelium with inhaled
glucocorticoids correlates with improved lung function and decreased airway hyper-
responsiveness, suggesting a role in the allergic etiology of asthma. There are initial
reports that dexamethasone decreases nuclear binding activity of $NF_{\kappa B}$, and induces $I_{\kappa B\alpha}$
in H441 and A549 cells, which are derived from Clara and type II cells, respectively. A
possible proinflammatory effect of glucocorticoids is the repression of vasoactive intestinal polypeptide (VIP) receptor. This presumably reduces VIP antiinflammatory effects
(inhibition of T lymphocytes and alveolar macrophages) in addition to its better known
actions as smooth muscle relaxant.

An important component of the inflammatory response by several resident lung cells
is production of nitric oxide through inducible nitric oxide synthase (NOS). Endogenous
NO reacts with superoxide to form peroxynitrite, which participates in the killing of
microorganisms within macrophages through modification of proteins, lipids, and DNA;
excessive production of peroxynitrite, for example, in hyperoxic condiions, can similarly damage constituents of lung cells producing both lung injury and the potential for
fibrosis. Glucocorticoids have been shown to downregulate iNOS and block induction by
both cytokines and LPS. In addition, the activities of two enzymes involved in the
production of intracellular glutathione, which are induced in response to oxidative stress,
are reduced by glucocorticoid treatment.

## Table 3
### Glucocorticoid Regulated Genes in Lung Homeostasis

| Gene | References[a] | Experimental System | Cell Type[b] | Response[c] | | | Mechanism |
|---|---|---|---|---|---|---|---|
| | | | | mRNA | Protein | Function | |
| E-selectin | 102 | Cultured cells | endo | | | ↓ | Block activation of promoter by IL-1β/TNF via NFκB |
| | 103 | A549 cell line | Type II | | | | |
| ICAM-1 | 104 | A549 cell line | Type II | ↓ | | | Block induction by IL-1β; only tested ≥ 1 $\mu M$ dex |
| | 105 | A292 cell line | Bronchial epi | ↓ | | | Block induction by PMA; only tested 5 $\mu M$ dex |
| ELAM-1 | 102 | Cultured cells | endo | ↓ | ↓ | ↓ | Block induction by LPS |
| IL-6 and IL-8 | | | | | | | All studies in presence of inducing cytokines or LPS Dex ≥ 0.1 $\mu M$ required |
| | 106, 107 | Cultured human cells | FB/macro | ↓ | ↓ | | |
| | 108 | 8387 cell line | FB | ↓ | ↓ | | ↓ Transcription rate of IL-8 gene; functional nGRE in proximal promoter |
| | 109 | Cultured human cells | Airway SM | ↓ | ↓ | | |
| TGF-β1 | 110 | Cultured cells | FB | ↓ | | ↓ | |
| | 111 | A549 cell line | | | | ↓ | |
| Eotaxin | 112 | A549 cell line | Type II | ↓ | | ↓ | Block cytokine induction |
| RANTES | 113 | A549 cell line | Type II | ↓ | | | Cycloheximide not block; no change in mRNA stability (AMD) |
| COX-2 | 114 | Cultured human cells | Bronchial epi | | ↓ | ↓ | Block induction by IL-1β |
| | 104, 114 | A549 cell line | Type II | ↓ | ↓ | ↓ | |

| Protein | Ref | Source | Cell type | | | | Comments |
|---|---|---|---|---|---|---|---|
| cPLA2 | *115* | A549 cell line | Type II | → | | → | Reduce basal and cytokine inducted |
| | *116* | Cultured rat cells | endo | ← | → | → | Block forskolin stimulation |
| IL-1ra | *117* | Cell line | Airway epi | ← | ← | → | |
| a1-Acid glycoprotein | *118* | Rat in vivo and cultured cells | Type II | ← | ← | | |
| Uteroglobin | *119, 120* | Rabbit in vivo | Type II/Clara | | | ← | GR required; functional nGRE in proximal promoter ↓ basal |
| VIPR$_I$ | *121* | L2 cell line | FB | → | | → | |
| GM-CSF | *122, 123* | Cultured human cells and explant | Bronchial epi | → | → | → | Block induction by IL-1β no ↓ mRNA stability |
| | *124* | BEAS-2B cell line | epi | | | | |
| NF$_{\kappa B}$ | *125* | H441 cell line | Clara | ← | ← | → | Only tested ≥ 1 μM dex |
| I$_\kappa$B$_\alpha$ | *104* | A549 cell line | Type II | → | | → | Block induction by cytokines and LPS |
| iNOS | *126* | A549 cell line | endo | → | → | → | Action involves ↓NF$_{\kappa B}$ DNA binding activity |
| | *127, 128* | A549 cell line | Type II | → | | → | |
| | *129* | J974 cell line | macro | → | → | → | |
| | *127* | Cultured human cells | bronchial epi | | | → | |
| | *130* | Rat in vivo | | | | → | |
| γ-Glutamyl synthetase | *131* | A549 cell line | Type II | | → | → | Only tested 3 μM dex |
| γ-Glutamyl transpeptidase | *131* | A549 cell line | Type II | | | → | Only tested 3 μM dex |
| Neutral endopeptidase | *132* | Human cell line | Airway epi | ← | | ← | |
| Tissue factor | *133* | Fetal human explant | | ← | ← | | |

Table 3 (continued)
Glucocorticoid Regulated Genes in Lung Homeostasis

| Gene | References[a] | Experimental System | Cell Type[b] | Response[c] mRNA | Protein | Function | Mechanism |
|---|---|---|---|---|---|---|---|
| uPlasminogen activator | 134 | Isolated rat cells | Type II | | | ↓ | Dex 0.1 μM block induction by PMA ↓ mRNA stability (AMD) |
| | 133 | Fetal human explant | | ↓ | | | |
| uPlasminogen activator | 134 | Isolated rat cells | Type II | | | ↓ | Dex 0.1 μM block induction by PMA |
| uPlasminogen activator receptor | 135 | A549 cell line | Type II | ↓ | | | Block induction by IL-1β |
| Aquaporin 1 | 79, 80 | Adult rat in vivo | endo | ↑ | ↑ | | |
| Aquaporin 3, 4, and 5 | 80, 136 | A549 cell line | Type II | ↑ | ↑ | | |
| α, β, γ ENaC | 137 | Adult rat in vivo | | ↑ | ↑ | | Cycloheximide not block; No change in mRNA stability |
| | 138 | Fetal human explant | | ↑ | | | |
| β-Adrenergic receptor | 139 | Adult human explant | | ↑ | | ↑ | ↑ Transcription rate; No effect on mRNA stability (AMD) |
| Na+-K+-ATPase β₁ | 140 | Isolated rat cells | Type II | ↑ | | ↑ | ↑ mRNA > ↑ protein |
| Glutamine synthetase | 141 | Rat in vivo | | ↑ | ↑ | ↑ | 2 GREs identified |
| | 142 | L2 cell line | epi | | | | |
| Angiotensin-converting enzyme | 143 | Rabbit cells | macro | | | ↑ | Blocked by AMD and cycloheximide |
| | 144 | Rat in vivo | | | | ↑ | |
| Cardiac ventricular myosin light chain 2 | 145 | A549 cell line | Type II | ↑ | | | Identified by differential display |
| RNA polymerase subunit hRPB33 | 145 | A549 cell line | Type II | ↓ | | | Identified by differential display |

epi, epithelial cells; FB, fibroblasts; macro, macrophages; AMD, actinomycin D; endo, endothelial; SM, smooth muscle; dex, dexamethasone; PMA, phorbol myristate acetate; ICAM, intercellular adhesion molecule; ELAM, endothelial-leukocyte adhesion molecule; IL, interleukin; TGF, transforming growth factor; COX, cyclooxygenase; ra, receptor antagonist; VIPR, vasoactive intestinal peptide receptor; GM-CSF, granulocyte macrophage colony stimulatory factor; NF, nuclear factor; I, (NF) inhibitory; NOS, nitric oxide synthase; ENaC, epithelial sodium channel; cPL, cytosolic phospholipase

[a] Representative references are given for genes studied by multiple investigators, with a preference for papers addressing mechanisms.
[b] The listed cell type refers to either the lung cells which express the gene in vivo or the source of cultured cells used in the studies.
[c] All responses in vitro occur with a time course and at concentrations of dexamethasone (half-maximal 1–10 nM) or cortisol (half-maximal 10–100 nM) consistent with GR mediation unless otherwise noted.

Glucocorticoids influence at least three components of the coagulation/fibrinolysis pathway. Formation of fibrin in the lung is part of the normal tissue repair process, serving as a hemostatic agent and a matrix for tissue repair following injury. Production of tissue factor by epithelial cells is a procoagulant stimulus, whereas production of plasmin from plasminogen through the action of plasminogen activator results in fibrinolysis. Through induction of tissue factor and by blocking cytokine-induced increases in both plasminogen activator and its receptor, glucocorticoids act to modulate the injury-induced host response related to fibrin deposition in the lung.

The second category of glucocorticoid responsive genes of adult lung is related to maintenance of fluid and electrolyte balance within the alveolar space to maintain the alveolar hypophase, clear inhaled water, and resolve pulmonary edema. Identified genes in this category include the aquaporins, each of the eNAC subunits, $\beta$-adrenergic receptor and $Na^+$-$K^+$-ATPase. Glucocorticoid treatment upregulates expression of each of these genes, presumably mimicking the role of increased endogenous cortisol in conditions of injury and stress associated with increased alveolar fluid content. These proteins are present in both endothelial and type II cells, sites of fluid movement, and it would be expected that glucocorticoids induce at least some of these genes in other airway epithelial cell types. At present, there is little information regarding the mechanism of glucocorticoid action for induction of genes related to fluid homeostasis other than evidence that regulation occurs at the level of transcription. Many of these genes are also regulated by glucocorticoids in the developing lung where they are involved in production of fetal lung fluid and its reabsorption before delivery.

At least one responsive enzyme in the lung (glutamine synthetase) is induced by glucocorticoids as a component of the catabolic response, which is observed primarily in other organs, such as the liver and skeletal muscle. This response results in increased production of glutamine and release into the circulation as a significant contribution to maintaining glutamine homeostasis.

All of the characterized antiinflammatory effects of glucocorticoids in lung cells occur at the level of transcription and involve antagonism of the inductive effects of cytokines and other agents. Recently, considerable evidence has accumulated that many of these glucocorticoid responses involve an inhibitory effect on the transactivation activity of $NF_{\kappa B}$ *(103–105, 147–149)*. $NF_{\kappa B}$ is known to up-regulate expression of many genes involved in mammalian immune and inflammatory responses, in lung as well as other tissues. Target genes include cytokines, complement-related factors, cell-adhesion molecules, and various immunoreceptors of both resident pulmonary cells and inflammatory cells from the circulation. $NF_{\kappa B}$ is a heterodimeric protein comprised of p50 and p65 subunits that are members of the rel family of transcriptional activators. In the absence of stimulatory signals, $NF_{\kappa B}$ is located in the cytoplasm in association with the inhibitory phosphoprotein $I_{\kappa B}$. Recently, it has been found that the catalytic subunit of PKA is associated with the $NF_{\kappa B}$/$I_{\kappa B\alpha}$ complex, rendering $PKA_c$ inactive and blocking the nuclear localization signal on $NF_{\kappa B}$ *(150)*. Extracellular signals, such as cytokines, oxidative stress, and viruses, result in phosphorylation of $I_{\kappa B}\alpha$, which targets the protein for ubiquitination and proteolysis, resulting in the release of $NF_{\kappa B}$ and $PKA_c$. Phosphorylation of the p65 subunit by the released, activated $PKA_c$ results in nuclear translocation and binding of p65 to specific response sequences of target genes involved in immune and inflammatory functions. Current evidence indicates that glucocorticoid downregulation of $NF_{\kappa B}$-responsive genes involves direct interaction between activated GR and the p65 subunit of $NF_{\kappa B}$. This physical interaction blocks transactivation activity of both GR and p65. For p65, interaction with GR does not interfere with nuclear translocation or DNA binding, rather appears to inhibit the transactivation function of the protein. In selected cell types, such as monocytes, lymphocytes, and the pulmonary A549 cell line, glucocorticoids also induce expression of $I_{\kappa B\alpha}$, which promotes retention of $NF_{\kappa B}$ in the cytoplasm, thereby contributing to the antiinflammatory process.

At present, there is no evidence that any of the inhibitory effects of glucocorticoids in the developing lung (Table 2) involve antagonism of $NF_{\kappa B}$ effects. Pryhuber et al. *(125)* found that TNF and phorbol ester (TPA) increased $NF_{\kappa B}$ nuclear binding activity in H441 cells in parallel with inhibition of SP-A and SP-B mRNAs. However, these inhibitory effects were not blocked in the presence of pyrrolidine dithiocarbamate, an inhibitor of $NF_{\kappa B}$ activation. Interpretation of these results is complicated by the inhibitory effect of pyrrolidine dithiocarbamate alone on the mRNAs.

## GLUCOCORTICOID RECEPTORS

High-affinity glucocorticoid binding activity has been detected in both fetal and adult lung tissue of every species that has been examined. The initial observations of glucocorticoid receptor activity in developing lung were made in 1972 with extensive characterization subsequently as reviewed in 1986 *(5)*. In studies comparing binding capacity in cytosolic preparations, lung has one of the highest concentrations of any tissue examined in rat, both fetal and adult rabbit, and fetal human. Binding affinity of various corticosteroids, in lungs of various species, displays a pattern consistent with GR activity as characterized in other target tissues.

The developmental pattern and cellular distribution of receptor activity in lung has been of particular interest with regard to the effects of glucocorticoid on lung maturation. In the rat, for example, the number of dexamethasone binding sites in lung cytosol increases from approx 4000 to 8000 per cell during the final days of gestation. After birth there is a further increase in receptor number, reaching approx 19,000 binding sites per cell in lungs of adult adrenalectomized animals. A similar developmental increase occurs in lung of fetal rabbits during late gestation, while a study in the fetal sheep found a decrease in glucocorticoid binding activity of lung during the final trimester of gestation. In the human, as in other species, glucocorticoid receptor activity was detected at the earliest point in gestation examined (approx 13 wk), and the receptors were functional based on nuclear localization of activated GR and glucocorticoid inducibility of phospholipid synthesis. Based on autoradiographic evidence, along with binding studies in isolated cell types, it is likely that most, if not all, major pulmonary cell types contain GR. The type II cells and mesenchymal fibroblasts have been of major interest with regard to glucocorticoid effects on the surfactant system of the fetus. In studies with fetal rat, for example, comparable levels of glucocorticoid binding activity and immunoreactive GR protein were found in distal airway epithelial cells and fibroblasts *(151)*. The developmental change in GR activity during late gestation in both cell types was paralleled by changes in GR mRNA content, indicating developmental effects at the level of gene transcription which may differ for lung fibroblasts and distal airway epithelial cells. Studies with cells isolated at various points in late gestation and cultured for two days indicated an earlier peak in both GR activity and mRNA content for fibroblasts (day 19) compared to epithelial cells (day 20) *(151)*.

The effect of glucocorticoids on GR gene expression and binding activity in lung is uncertain. Treatment of pregnant rats with dexamethasone was found to decrease fetal lung GR mRNA *(152)*, to have no effect on GR mRNA while increasing cytosolic GR binding activity *(151)* and to increase GR mRNA by semiquantitative *in situ* hybridization *(153)*. Although this issue is unresolved, the possible modulation of GR by increasing endogenous corticosteroid and by glucocorticoid administration is of interest with regard to understanding the mechanisms of glucocorticoid-induced lung maturation. If GR protein and/or activity is regulated by levels of endogenous corticosteroids, there is potential for a substantial effect during late gestation. Circulating concentrations of free corticoids increase in the fetus before term, and there is both cell specificity and developmental regulation of 11β-hydroxysteroid dehydrogenase activity (reviewed in ref. *5*). During gestation, the fetal lung displays increasing corticosteroid reductive activity, favoring formation of cortisol/corticosterone from cortisone/deoxycorticosterone. This developmental change, along with increasing levels of GR in the lung, serve to amplify stimulatory effects from increasing endogenous corticosteroids during late fetal development. A currently unexplored area in this regard is the possible role of GR-β; it is possible that changing levels of GR-β, which appears to act as a dominant negative receptor form *(154)*, could modulate GR activity, and therefore glucocorticoid responsiveness, during development.

## SURFACTANT PROTEINS

The surfactant-associated proteins, in particular SP-A, SP-B, and SP-C, coisolate with the surfactant fraction in lung lavage fluid and participate in surfactant structural transformations, film formation, surface activity, and metabolism (reviewed in refs. *155* and *156*). The SPs are developmentally regulated and a deficiency of SPs contributes to developmental immaturity of the lung and occurrence of respiratory distress syndrome (RDS) in infants born prematurely. The physiologic importance of SP-B and SP-C to normal lung function is underscored by their essential role in naturally derived surfactant preparations used for replacement treatment, and the observations that inherited deficiency causes respiratory failure in mice and human infants delivered at full term *(157,158)*. Among the known glucocorticoid-regulated proteins, the SPs have received the most attention with regard to studies of mechanism.

### SP-A

First identified in 1973 *(159)* with subsequent cloning of two highly homologous human genes (SP-A1, SP-A2) in 1985 and 1992 *(160–162)*, SP-A is a highly modified glycoprotein of 28–35 kDa that contains a collagenlike region plus binding sites for sugars, calcium, and lipid *(155,156)*. The native, secreted form of SP-A contains six units of triple helices, each terminating in a globular structure, and it has been proposed that a 2:1 ratio for SP-A1 and SP-A2 is required for proper oligomerization *(163)*. In vitro, SP-A inhibits secretion of surfactant from type II cells and promotes recycling of phospholipid, effects that appear to be mediated through binding of SP-A to a membrane receptor. SP-A promotes transformation of lamellar bodies into tubular myelin, reduces leakage of serum proteins into lung alveoli, decreases the inhibitory effect of serum proteins on surface activity in vitro, activates macrophages, and acts as an opsonin to enhance uptake and clearance of bacteria (reviewed in ref. *164*). Thus, it is likely that

SP-A has multiple functions in vivo related to lung immune defense, and may affect surfactant metabolism, structure, and function as well. SP-A mRNA and protein are detected and increase during late gestation in animals, reaching adult levels soon after birth. Multiple transcripts of both SP-A1 and SP-A2 occur through allelic variability and alternative splicing *(165,166)*.

## *SP-B and SP-C*

These are highly lipophilic proteins of approx8 and 3.7 kDa, respectively, that are localized within lamellar bodies of type II cells *(155,156)*. Mature SP-B is highly folded due to seven cysteines and exists as a dimer, whereas SP-C contains two palmitoyl molecules linked to cysteines and exists as a monomer in vivo. Both proteins are extracted from lung lavage fluid by organic solvents along with surfactant lipids, and the presence of at least one of the proteins is required for both rapid film formation in vitro and efficacy of surfactant in vivo. SP-B also promotes both lateral stability of the lipid monolayer and the squeeze-out of nonsurface-active lipids from the surface film *(155,156,167)*. The genes for SP-B and SP-C are expressed during the first trimester of human pregnancy ($\leq$12 wk) and content of the mRNAs increases to approx 50% and 15% of the adult level by 24 wk *(50)*. Both proteins are derived by amino and carboxy-termini processing of primary translation products (SP-B$_{42}$ and SP-C$_{21}$), and these events are developmentally regulated *(46,49,101)*. At 24 wk gestation, when human fetal lung contains appreciable amounts of both SP-B and SP-C mRNAs, little mature SP-B or SP-C protein is detected. Thus, it is likely that expression of specific endoproteases for processing of pro-SP-B and pro-SP-C is a key event in the ontogeny of these proteins.

Inherited deficiency of SP-B, which blocks formation of mature SP-C, results in fatal respiratory disease in term infants *(158,168)*. Similarly, monoclonal antibodies to SP-B produce respiratory distress when administered to animals and also inactivate preparations of surfactant that contain SP-B *(169,170)*. These observations suggest that SP-B, and perhaps SP-C, play a critical role in formation of the surface tension lowering film in vivo.

## *SP-D*

Lung lavage fluid contains a second collagenous glycoprotein originally designated CP-4 and since named surfactant protein-D. This protein is a 43-kDa glycoprotein containing a collagenous region and exhibiting both calcium and carbohydrate binding activity *(171–174)*. Although there are sequence and domain similarities between SP-D and SP-A of the rat, the highest homology occurs with members of the C-type lectin family such as conglutinin and serum mannose binding proteins. The human gene for SP-D localizes to chromosome 10q in the same region that contains the genes for SP-A *(175)*.

In studies with the rat, immunoreactive SP-D was associated with both type II cells and Clara cells of distal bronchioles, with intracellular localization to secretory compartments of both cells (but not lamellar bodies). In the alveolar space, SP-D localized to granular material but not to tubular myelin or lamellar bodies *(172,176)*. Expression of the SP-D gene was limited to pulmonary tissue where mRNA was first detected in abundance on day 21 of gestation in the rat and reached adult levels shortly after birth *(177)*. In another report, however, SP-D was detected by immunoassay on fetal day 19 and increased to adult levels by birth, differing in the postnatal pattern of expression from SP-A *(178)*. In human fetal lung, a low level of SP-D gene expression is first detected by 16 wk gestation and levels of the protein increase to approx 35% of the adult value at 24 wk gestation *(64)*.

Although designated as a surfactant protein, the possible roles of SP-D in surfactant metabolism are not well defined. In the presence of calcium SP-D binds phosphatidyl-inositol but not other lipids of surfactant, which may account for its association with surfactant *(39)*. SP-D that copurified with surfactant lipids of lung lavage reversed the inhibitory effect of SP-A on phosphatidylcholine secretion by isolated type II cells *(179)*. In transgenic mice lacking SP-D there is accumulation of surfactant in air spaces, consistent with a role of SP-D in surfactant homeostasis *(180)*. A major function of SP-D is apparently related to pulmonary antimicrobial host defense, reflecting the structural and functional similarity to SP-A, conglutinin, and mannose binding proteins, which agglutinate bacteria and activate complement (reviewed in ref. *164*).

## Glucocorticoid Regulation of SPs

Since the initial observation in 1986 of glucocorticoid regulation of SP-A *(95)*, effects on surfactant proteins have been extensively investigated using organ cultures of fetal lung, cell lines derived from human lung adenocarcinomas, and in vivo in both fetal and adult animals. It is now well established that glucocorticoids influence all four surfactant proteins, consistent with the concept that endogenous glucocorticoids are major hormonal modulators of lung development influencing both structural and cellular differentiation. Administration of glucocorticoids to fetal animals precociously induces the mRNAs for SP-A, -B, -C, and -D often increasing content by many fold. By contrast, glucocorticoid treatment in adult rat has a more modest effect on surfactant protein mRNA levels, suggesting that endogenous corticosteroids are less important regulators postnatally. Although there is a coordinated induction of the four surfactant proteins in cultured tissue, the properties of the induction process differ (e.g., time and dose response characteristics), indicating differences in the mechanisms of gene activation. The involvement of GR in the induction processes is well documented; however, details of GR interaction with the target genes have not yet been fully described. Nevertheless, the studies of SPs provide, at present, the best insight into molecular events mediating glucocorticoid-induced lung maturation. The following discussion reviews the current understanding of glucocorticoid mechanisms of action on these genes.

### SP-A GENE EXPRESSION

The initial studies of dexamethasone effects on SP-A synthesis in cultured fetal lung were conflicting with reports of both stimulation and inhibition *(95,181–183)*. Subsequently, data from two laboratories have established that glucocorticoids stimulate or inhibit production of SP-A depending on hormone concentration and time of exposure *(34,35,184–186)*.

Stimulation of SP-A by glucocorticoids has been studied in some detail in cultured human lung explants. SP-A and its mRNA are not detected or present at very low levels in second trimester fetal lung. When the tissue is placed in organ culture, the SP-A gene begins to be expressed after 2 d and there is continued accumulation of mRNA and protein for at least 7 d of culture. This response occurs in the absence of serum or exogenous hormones, and is due at least in part to increasing content of cAMP under the influence of endogenous prostaglandins *(187,188)*. There is a many fold increase in SP-A gene transcription rate during culture, paralleling accumulation of SP-A mRNA, suggesting a direct transcriptional effect of cAMP and possibly other mediators (P. L. Ballard, *unpublished data*).

Addition of relatively low concentrations of glucocorticoids to lung explant cultures (e.g., 1–10n$M$ dexamethasone) accelerates accumulation of SP-A and its mRNA by severalfold during the next 48 h of culture. This stimulatory response is completely reversed within 24–48 h after removal of glucocorticoid from the culture medium, consistent with a GR-mediated process. There are no data at present regarding possible requirement for ongoing protein synthesis for the stimulatory component. The biphasic nature of the glucocorticoid response is illustrated in Fig. 2 which shows the initial increase in content of SP-A mRNA and subsequent inhibition with 100n$M$ dexamethasone treatment. Although the duration of increased mRNA content is longer at lower concentrations of dexamethasone (e.g., 10n$M$ *(34)*, continued exposure eventually reduces mRNA below control levels. A similar but temporally delayed biphasic effect is observed for content of SP-A protein, assayed by ELISA or Western blot, consistent with regulation at the level of transcription. SP-A gene expression is also responsive in the same biphasic manner to natural glucocorticoids such as cortisol, corticosterone, and cortisone, whereas various sex steroids have no effect at 1 μ$M$ concentration. Thus, glucocorticoids not only slow the production of SP-A that occurs during culture but can rapidly repress induced SP-A gene expression. These findings indicate that the dominant response to glucocorticoids in human fetal lung in vitro is inhibition.

The complexity of glucocorticoid regulation of SP-A is also evident in other systems that have been studied. Dexamethasone has a dose-dependent biphasic effect on SP-A mRNA in fetal baboon lung cultured in the absence of 8-Br-cAMP and antagonizes the stimulatory effect of cAMP treatment. Sensitivity to dexamethasone inhibition decreased in older baboon fetuses *(96)*. In the NCI H820 cell-line dexamethasone caused a modest increase in SP-A mRNA at concentrations of 0.1–10n$M$ and was without effect or inhibitory at higher concentrations *(55)*. Similarly in the H-441 cell line, low concentrations of dexamethasone may increase SP-A mRNA content *(189)*, whereas inhibition occurs under most experimental conditions. Treatment with 10n$M$ dexamethasone, for example, reduced SP-A mRNA content by 50% within 12 h *(190)*. In explants of fetal rabbit lung, the responses to cortisol treatment were temporally reversed, with decreased SP-A mRNA content after 6 h and increased levels at 48 h *(186)*. In cultured fetal rat lung, however, SP-A mRNA content was increased at all concentrations of dexamethasone (10–200n$M$) after 48 h of exposure *(191)*. There is a preliminary report that the response of cultured adult human lung to glucocorticoid is similar to that described for fetal tissue *(192)*. Thus, in primate lung, at least, the dominant response to glucocorticoid is repression of SP-A gene expression.

The studies of SP-A mRNA content described above used cDNA probes which hybridized with transcript from both of the human SP-A genes. Recently, several groups have investigated expression and glucocorticoid regulation of SP-A$_1$ vs SP-A$_2$ genes, using approaches that distinguish between the highly homologous mRNAs. In human fetal lung, under basal conditions, SP-A$_1$ mRNA is more abundant than SP-A$_2$ mRNA (Table 4), whereas in adult lung SP-A$_2$ mRNA is more abundant *(165,195)*. This indicates that the developmental change from fetal to adult pattern of SP-A gene expressions occurs after 24 wk gestation, although the switch can be induced precociously by explant culture *(195)*. Karinch et al. *(36)* found that the ratio of SP-A$_1$ to SP-A$_2$ was quite variable between specimens. This likely reflects the extensive allelic variability in the human SP-A genes, and could also result from differential developmental expression. In three of the four studies glucocorticoid treatment of lung explants decreased SP-A$_1$ and SP-A$_2$ mRNA to a similar extent, whereas only SP-A$_2$ mRNA was significantly decreased in the McCormick study

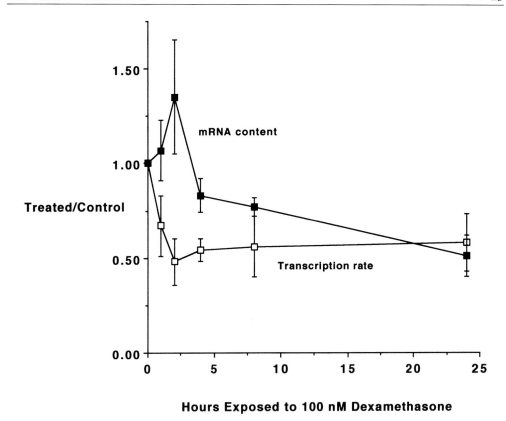

**Hours Exposed to 100 nM Dexamethasone**

Fig. 2. Time-course for dexamethasone effect on SP-A mRNA and transcription rate in cultured human fetal lung. Explants were cultured for 4 d in hormone-free medium and then exposed to 100n*M* dexamethasone for 1–24 h. mRNA content increases slightly initially and then is suppressed. Transcription rate is maximally decreased by 2 h. In the same experiments there was no effect of dexamethasone on β-actin mRNA content and transcription rate (not shown). Data are mean ± SE for 3 experiments. (From P. L. Ballard, *unpublished data*).

*(193)*. In H441 cells both SP-A$_1$ and SP-A$_2$ mRNAS were reduced by dexamethasone in one study and only SP-A$_1$ in the report by Kumar and Snyder *(194)*. These findings indicate that expression of both human SP-A genes can be repressed by glucocorticoid in vitro; apparent differences in magnitude of the effect may be due to variable times of culture and exposure to dexamethasone, or to the particular alleles present in study specimens. There is differential developmental regulation of SP-A$_1$ and SP-A$_2$ in fetal baboon lung, but at present there are no data regarding glucocorticoid effects on the two genes *(196)*.

In vivo, dexamethasone treatment increases SP-A mRNA content in fetal rats, but the degree of stimulation is modest and depends on both gestational age and duration of treatment *(40,197)*. In fetal rabbits, dexamethasone exposure for 24 h elevated SP-A mRNA levels severalfold *(41)*, whereas SP-A was inhibited by in vivo glucocorticoid treatment in the baboon *(198)*. Treatment of fetal sheep with betamethasone causes a two to threefold increase in SP-A, SP-B and SP-C mRNAs at 24–48 h which fully reverses in each case after a 7-d interval. With repetitive dosing at weekly intervals there was no evidence of an inhibitory effect on SP-A *(13)*. Thus, there may be species differences in glucocorticoid action of SP-A gene expression. Although it is likely that the usual regimen

Table 4
Glucocorticoid Regulation of the Two Human SP-A Genes

| Experimental System | Basal mRNA $SP\text{-}A_1\text{:}SP\text{-}A_2$ | Glucocorticoid Response | | Reference |
|---|---|---|---|---|
| | | *SP-A1* | *SP-A2* | |
| Cultured human fetal lung | 1.9:1 | No change[a] | ↓↓[a] | *165,193* |
| | 7.8:1 | ↓↓ | ↓ | *36* |
| | 4:1 | ↓↓ | ↓↓ | *194* |
| | 26:1 | ↓ | ↓ | *194* |
| H441 cells | 1.5:1 | ↓↓ | No change | *194* |
| | 0.9:1 | ↓↓ | ↓↓ | *195* |

Gene-specific SP-A mRNA content was determined using oligonucleotide probes for SP-A$_1$ and SP-A$_2$ and Northern analyses, RT-PCR or primer extension analysis. Glucocorticoid treatment was 100 n$M$ dexamethasone for 1–6 d.

[a] Change comparing treatment with dexamethasone and dibutyryl cAMP vs dibutyryl cAMP alone.

of prenatal betamethasone treatment for human fetuses, which transiently elevates circulating glucocorticoid activity approx threefold, stimulates SP-A production, it is possible that fetuses exposed to repeated high doses of steroids could become deficient in SP-A.

The regulation of SP-A differs from the few other examples of biphasic regulation by glucocorticoids that have been described. When mouse mammary explants were cultured with insulin and prolactin, cortisol produced an initial stimulation of α-lactalbumin followed by a decrease to baseline levels but not inhibition (199). A similar biphasic effect of dexamethasone was found for aromatase activity in fibroblasts (200). Continued treatment of cultured hepatoma cells with dexamethasone increased GR mRNA initially, followed by inhibition and then a return to control levels (201). Also in hepatoma cells, dexamethasone exerts dual regulation of tissue plasminogen activator activity by stimulating synthesis of both an activator and an inhibitor of its activity (202). Thus, glucocorticoid regulation of SP-A appears to be unique in that both stimulation and inhibition of gene expression occur simultaneously with different kinetics and sensitivity to glucocorticoid treatment.

Studies in cultured human lung have explored the mechanism of glucocorticoid regulation by determining SP-A gene transcription rate and mRNA stability. In initial studies by Boggaram et al. (185,186) there was no apparent change in transcription rate 2–24 h after adding dexamethasone (100n$M$) on day 5 of culture and an increased rate after continuous exposure during culture. Under both treatment conditions the content of SP-A mRNA was decreased. Dexamethasone did not cause premature termination of nascent transcripts as judged by nuclear run-on hybridization studies with different fragments of the SP-A gene. Subsequently, Iannuzzi et al. (35) examined the effect of glucocorticoid on transcription rate in fetal lung cultures at a time when SP-A gene expression was established; dexamethasone treatment (100n$M$) on day 4 of explant culture caused a 50% decrease in transcription rate within 4 h, preceding temporally the decline in mRNA content (Fig. 2). A similar parallel decrease in SP-A transcription rate and mRNA content was found in dexamethasone treated H441 cells (97). The apparent discrepancies between the different observations in human lung cells and further details of transcriptional regulation of the two SP-A genes remain to be explored. Nevertheless, it is clear that glucocorticoids regulate SP-A genes at the transcriptional level in a complex and possibly unique manner.

Glucocorticoids also decrease the stability of SP-A mRNA, which contributes to the inhibitory process *(35,186)*. Comparable results were obtained using actinomycin D to inhibit RNA synthesis and with a label/chase procedure *(35)*. When dexamethasone (100n$M$) was added at the beginning of the time-course study, the decay slope for glucocorticoid treated tissue was biphasic with an initial faster half-life (approx 3 h), followed by a lower decay ($t_{1/2}$ approx 8 h) similar to control (Fig. 3). The faster degradation rate occurs within approx 3 h, which is soon enough to contribute to the decrease in SP-A mRNA content. In experiments where tissue was exposed for longer times to dexamethasone before labeling, half-life values were comparable in treated and control cultures *(35)*. Thus, in these experiments dexamethasone appeared to induce a transient instability in SP-A mRNA that did not persist with continued exposure to hormone; however, Boggaram et al. *(186)* observed a persistent decrease in SP-A mRNA $t_{1/2}$ (5 vs 11 h) by dexamethasone in explants maintained in cAMP. These findings establish an effect of glucocorticoids on SP-A mRNA degradation, but at present there is no information on the mechanism or possible differential action on the two SP-A transcripts.

Inhibitors of protein synthesis have been used to assess whether glucocorticoids act in a primary or secondary fashion to repress SP-A gene expression. Results in two studies have been conflicting. Iannuzzi et al. *(35)* found that cycloheximide blocked the decrease in SP-A mRNA induced by dexamethasone within 9 h. By contrast, Boggaram et al. *(185)* found no inhibition of the dexamethasone response in cultures previously treated for 6 d with dibutyryl cAMP. It is possible that the presence of another positive regulator of SP-A (i.e., cAMP) alters the response to glucocorticoids. Additional studies are needed to address the requirement for protein synthesis in both glucocorticoid stimulation and inhibition of SP-A.

Current studies are addressing the identification of functional glucocorticoid response elements (GRE) in the SP-A gene. Putative half-site GREs have been identified in the proximal promoter of rat *(203)* rabbit *(204)* and human *(205)* SP-A genes. At present there are limited data related to functional activity of these sequences. Alcorn et al. *(206)* found that dexamethasone decreased expression of growth hormone reporter gene in rat type II cells transduced with an adenovirus construct using the rabbit SP-A promoter. Responsiveness mapped to the region –378/+20 bp, was dependent on dexamethasone dose and was competed by RU486 (Fig. 4) (*see* Chapter 3). These data provide evidence for a functional negative GRE in the rabbit SP-A gene which will require further characterization to establish its role in vivo. There are also preliminary reports of elements in the 5' flanking region of the human SP-A gene that impart negative glucocorticoid regulation *(189)*. Based on the recent evidence for interaction of regulatory elements, it is likely that the complex glucocorticoid regulation of SP-A will involve a number of different *cis-* and *trans-*acting elements.

## SP-B Gene Eexpression

Glucocorticoids increase SP-B gene expression both in vivo and in vitro. Dexamethasone treatment of pregnant rats or rabbits causes a precocious developmental increase in SP-B mRNA and protein content representing a severalfold induction *(40,41,197)*. The increase in SP-B mRNA occurs in both alveolar epithelial cells and bronchiolar Clara cells. In adult animals, dexamethasone treatment for 1 wk increased SP-B mRNA only twofold, and adrenalectomy had no effect on levels of SP-B mRNA in both whole-lung tissue and isolated type II cells *(58,197,207)*. This developmental change in glucocorti-

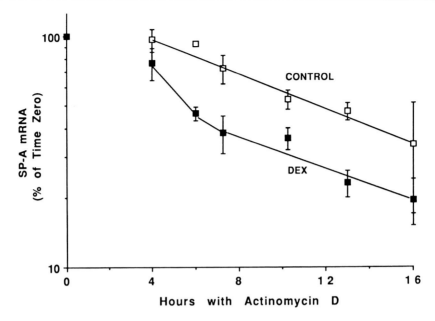

Fig. 3. Effect of dexamethasone on SP-A mRNA stability in cultured human fetal lung. After 4 d of explant culture, actinomycin D (5 μg/mL) was added 1.5 h before exposure to dexamethasone (dex, 100n$M$) or diluent (control), and SP-A mRNA content was determined at intervals. The $t1/2$ with dex was initially approx 4 h and then 7 h compared to approx 8 h in control cultures. Data are mean ± SE from 3 experiments. Similar results were obtained with a label-dose procedure. (From ref. *35*, with permission).

coid sensitivity could reflect the increased basal expression in adult lung, changes in levels of other negative or positive regulators, or developmental modifications in glucocorticoid signal transduction.

Regulation of SP-B has been further characterized in cultured lung explants and cell lines. Whereas SP-B mRNA is present in 20-wk gestation human lung at approx 15% of adult level, mature SP-B protein is essentially undetectable until tissue has been cultured for several days (without hormones) as explants *(101,208)*. The appearance of mature SP-B in explants reflects increased processing of precursor protein and the presence of multivesicular and lamellar bodies that develop during culture, with resulting stabilization of mature SP-B *(46)*.

Glucocorticoid induction of SP-B mRNA is similar in human and rat lung explant cultures with regard to sensitivity to dexamethasone (maximal increase at ≤10n$M$, (Fig. 5A) and cortisol (maximal at 1 μ$M$, [Fig. 5B]), time course of induction (maximal stimulation by approx 12 h) and an additive response in the presence of glucocorticoid and cAMP, but differs in magnitude (approx 15-fold in rat tissue vs approx fourfold in human); properties of induction are consistent with mediation by GR *(44,47,50,53,57, 208)*. Content of mature SP-B protein in human tissue is also stimulated severalfold by glucocorticoid treatment *(101)*, indicating that transcription, translation, and processing are closely linked. Levels of SP-B mRNA and protein are quite low in NCI-H441 and NCI-H820 cells and are increased many fold by dexamethasone treatment *(55,190)*. Inducibility of SP-B in these cell lines indicates that glucocorticoids act directly in type II and Clara cells of fetal lung to regulate gene expression.

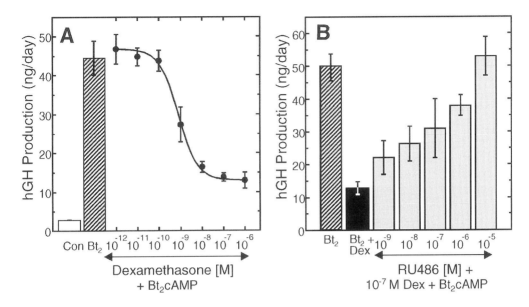

Fig. 4. Glucocorticoid responsiveness of rabbit SP-A promoter. Rat type II cells were transduced with recombinant adenovirus expressing human growth hormone (hGH) under control of rabbit SP-A DNA (−1766/+20) and cultured in dibutyryl-cAMP (1 m$M$) alone or with dexamethasone/ RU486. Dibutyryl-cAMP increased hGH secretion and dexamethasone reduced stimulated secretion. (From ref. *206*, with permission).

The glucocorticoid effect on SP-B mRNA involves both increased gene transcription rate and enhanced mRNA stability *(47,56,59)*. In a study with human lung explants, for example, dexamethasone treatment maximally increased the rate of transcription (approx threefold) within 2 h of hormone treatment (Fig. 6 and Table 5) and increased the $t_{1/2}$ of SP-B mRNA from approx 7 h (control) to approx 19 h (Table 5). The increased mRNA stability persisted for at least 48 h of hormone treatment in contrast to the transient effect of glucocorticoids on SP-A mRNA stability *(35)*. Since glucocorticoids increase SP-B mRNA content by approx fourfold, effects on both transcription and mRNA stability appear to contribute in an equivalent fashion to increased gene expression.

Similar effects of glucocorticoids on SP-B mRNA have been noted in H441 cells *(56,97)*. In these cells dexamethasone increased SP-B gene transcription by two- to fourfold and mRNA content increased ≥8-fold. SP-B mRNA stability was increased approx twofold from the basal $t_{1/2}$ of 14 h in response to cortisol treatment *(97)*.

O'Reilly and associates *(56)* found that dexamethasone induction of SP-B mRNA in H441 cells was inhibited by both cycloheximide and puromycin, suggesting that continued protein synthesis was required. By contrast, cycloheximide did not inhibit the glucocorticoid response in lung explants *(45)*. This discrepancy may reflect different inhibitor concentrations and exposure times in the two studies or indicate basic differences in glucocorticoid action in bronchiolar versus alveolar cells. The lack of a requirement for ongoing or new protein synthesis in SP-B induction in lung tissue indicates a primary mode of response and is consistent with the rapid stimulation (within 1 h) (Fig. 6) and reversibility (Table 5) of SP-B gene transcription rate by glucocorticoid. The mechanism of increased SP-B mRNA stability induced by gluco-

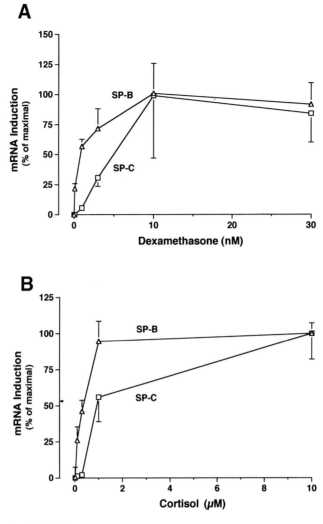

Fig. 5. Dose-dependent induction of SP-B and SP-C mRNAs in cultured human fetal lung. Explants were exposed to different concentration of dexamethasone (**A**) or cortisol (**B**) for 48 h and content of mRNAs determined. Data are mean ± SE, revised from ref. *50*

corticoids is not yet defined. This effect does not require ongoing RNA synthesis, since the $t_{1/2}$ was similar in experiments using actinomycin D versus label/chase protocol. The cycloheximide results also suggest that a labile protein is not involved in either basal or induced gene expression. This finding is in contrast to the sensitivity of SP-A gene expression to inhibition of protein synthesis in both the presence and absence of glucocorticoid *(35)*.

Current studies are attempting to define functional GREs in SP-B gene. The minimal sequence required for basal promoter activity has been determined by deletional analysis of the gene and transient transfection studies *(48,209)*. Based on the properties of glucocorticoid stimulation, it is expected that the SP-B gene is a direct target for gluco-corticoids and thus contains one or more GREs. The sequence data obtained by Pilot-Matias et al. *(210)* identified several sequences similar to the consensus GRE, but at

Table 5
Glucocorticoid Effects on Transcription Rate and mRNA Stability for SP-B and SP-C in
Cultured Human Fetal Lung

|  | *SP-B* | *SP-C* |
| --- | --- | --- |
| Transcription rate |  |  |
| (treated/control) |  |  |
| 28 h exposure to cortisol | $3.2 \pm 0.4$ | $5.6 \pm 0.7$ |
| 24 h cortisol exposure, remove for 4 h | $1.8 \pm 0.2^{*}$ | $2.9 \pm 0.8^{*}$ |
| mRNA half-life (h) |  |  |
| Control | $7.5 \pm 0.4$ | $9.3 \pm 1.7$ |
| Dexamethasone (10n$M$) | $18.8 \pm 2.9^{+}$ | $8.1 \pm 2.4$ |

Transcription rates were determined by nuclear run-on assay after exposure of human fetal lung explants to cortisol (1 μ$M$) for 28 h or for 24 h plus 4 h after media changes to remove the steroid. mRNA half-lives were calculated from time-course experiments using actinomycin D.

Data from refs. *45* and *47*.

$^{*}p < 0.05$ vs 28 h exposure; $+ p < .05$ vs control.

present there are no studies demonstrating receptor binding or glucocorticoid responsiveness mediated through these sequences. H441 cells transfected with plasmid constructs containing approx 1 kb of SP-B gene 5'-flanking sequence and downstream sequence into the second exon were not responsive to dexamethasone in both the absence and presence of cotransfected GR (Table 6). In the same experiment, constructs containing a known GRE (from the MMTV gene) were stimulated severalfold by dexamethasone treatment. These results indicate that this region of the human SP-B gene does not contain sequences sufficient for GR binding and transactivation. Comparable negative findings have been observed in vivo with transgenic mice expressing CAT activity under the same SP-B promoter region (M. Strayer and P. L. Ballard, *unpublished data*).

There are a number of possibilities for the mechanism of glucocorticoid stimulation of SP-B gene expression that will require investigation. First, a functional GRE may reside elsewhere in the SP-B gene, either upstream or downstream of the –1039/+431 bp region. There are a number of sequences resembling GRE half-sites (TGTTCT) within the published gene sequence and one or more of these sites may be functional in vivo. To date, however, there are no published data indicating binding of GR to any of these sites. Second, it is possible that glucocorticoid regulation of SP-B gene expression is indirect, reflecting glucocorticoid effects on either negative or other positive regulators of SP-B. For example, glucocorticoids could decrease production of endogenous factors such as TGF-β, TNF-α and activators of PKC, which are known negative regulators of SP-B. This possibility could be examined in H441 cells using various approaches to inhibit endogenous production or activity of these agents which should increase basal levels of SP-B. However, this mechanism seems unlikely in view of the observation that inhibition of protein synthesis with cycloheximide, which might be expected to decrease production of endogenous cytokines, did not alter basal SP-B mRNA content *(45)*. SP-B gene expression is increased by treatment of lung cells and explants with cAMP analogs and inhibitors of phosphodiesterase *(50)*, and there is evidence for a stimulatory response to increasing levels of endogenous cAMP *(187)*. Thus, it is possible that glucocorticoids increase SP-B gene expression indirectly by promoting accumulation or effects of cAMP in lung cells. This possibility is not supported by the finding that glucocorticoids are

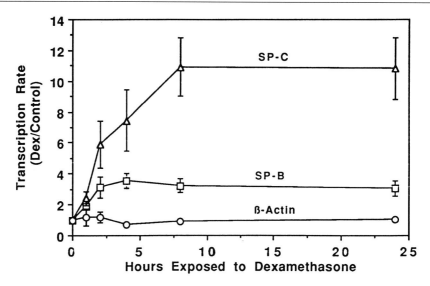

Fig. 6. Transcription rates for SP-B and SP-C: time course of dexamethasone induction. Explants of human fetal lung were treated with dexamethasone (100n*M*) for 1–24 h and tissue was collected for nuclear run-on assay. Maximal stimulation of transcription rate occurred at 2 and 8 h for SP-B and SP-C, respectively, and there was no change for β-actin. (From ref. *45*, with permission).

stimulatory in the absence of protein synthesis. Third, glucocorticoids could modify SP-B gene expression by affecting either the DNA binding or transactivation activity of transcription factors involved in SP-B promoter function. For example, glucocorticoids could release SP-B gene expression from the inhibitory influence of $NF_{\kappa B}$. Although there are putative $NF_{\kappa B}$ response elements in the SP-B gene, a recent study concluded that the $NF_{\kappa B}$ system was not involved in cytokine-induced downregulation of SP-B gene expression *(125)*. Similar scenarios could involve interactions between GR and *jun/fos* or CCAAT enhancer binding protein *(211,212)*. Finally, it is possible that glucocorticoids affect SP-B gene expression indirectly by altering levels or activity of GR. This could include either increased content of GRα and/or decreased levels of GR-β, which appears to function as a dominant negative receptor and has been detected in many mammalian tissues, including the lung *(154)*. Presumably, this potential mechanism would require a functional GRE in the SP-B gene or GR-mediated effects in other genes involved in the secondary response.

In summary, glucocorticoid regulation of the SP-B gene has been characterized but molecular details remain undefined. Responsiveness is mediated by GR as indicated by dose-response properties, specificity for steroids with glucocorticoid activity, and rapid reversibility of increased transcription rate consistent with the disassociation of steroid from GR. Induction of SP-B is a result of direct action of glucocorticoid in epithelial cells as indicated by responsiveness of H441 cells and isolated type II cells *(51)*, suggesting that mesenchymal-epithelial cell interactions in vivo are not required for glucocorticoid response. Based on both in vivo and in vitro data, induction of SP-B occurs in both type II alveolar cells and bronchiolar Clara cells. Increased levels of SP-B mRNA involves both increased transcription and mRNA stability and induction appears to be independent of new or ongoing protein synthesis. Molecular details of glucocorticoid activation of the SP-B gene remain undefined.

Table 6
Failure of Dexamethasone to Increase Promoter Activity in Transfection Studies

| Reporter Construct | Cotransfected Plasmid | CAT Activity (Dexamethasone/Control) |
|---|---|---|
| G46TCO | None | 6.7 ± 1.7* |
| G46TCO | VARO | 16.5 ± 0.9* |
| SP-B -1039/+431 CAT | VARO | 1.2 ± 0.2 |
| G46SP-B -1039/+431 CAT | VARO | 3.7 ± 0.3 |

Mean ± SE, n = 3; *$p$ <.05 vs control.

H-441 cells were transfected with the indicated plasmid construct containing CAT reporter gene in the absence or presence of VARO, a GR expression construct. After culture for 2 d without (control) or with 100n$M$ dexamethasone, CAT activity was assayed. Constructs are G46TCO, GRE from MMTV gene upstream of tk promoter and CAT; SP-B-1039/+431CAT, hSPB -1039/+431 driving CAT; G46SP-B -1039/+431 CAT, same construct with upstream GRE. From V. Venkatesh and P. L. Ballard, unpublished data.

## SP-C GENE EXPRESSION

Glucocorticoids are the only known positive regulators of human SP-C gene expression. In vivo treatment of fetal rats with dexamethasone causes a precocious increase in SP-C mRNA as for the other surfactant proteins. A 1-d exposure was sufficient to increase mRNA levels to the adult value and responsiveness was similar in both male and female pups (40). Treatment of adult animals caused a modest increase in SP-C mRNA levels (+60 to +100%) and adenalectomy did not affect SP-C gene expression (58,207). The only negative data related to glucocorticoid induction of SP-C were reported by Connelly et al. (41), who found that in vivo dexamethasone treatment of the rabbit for 24 h reduced SP-C mRNA levels to approx 40% of control, whereas both SP-B and SP-A mRNAs were increased. This unexpected finding has not yet been confirmed.

Levels of SP-C mRNA are relatively low (compared to adult) in second trimester human lung and there is little change in mRNA content during explant culture. Treatment of lung explants with dexamethasone or other glucocorticoids increases SP-C mRNA levels by 10- to 30-fold within 24 h (47,50), whereas other classes of steroids are without effects (50). The kinetics of induction are somewhat slower than for SP-B in the same tissue, with a lag period of several hours before increased content is detected. In addition, the dose response for both dexamethasone and cortisol is shifted to the right (i.e., less sensitive) compared to SP-B induction in the same explants (Fig. 5). These findings may reflect differences in the affinity and possibly type of response elements mediating glucocorticoid induction of the two SPs.

In rat tissue ex vivo (62), glucocorticoid induction is less (three- to fivefold) than for human but similar with regard to dose-response properties (maximal increase requires approx 50n$M$ dexamethasone) and relatively slow kinetics. The NCI-H820 cell line expresses SP-C and exposure to dexamethasone at ≥10n$M$ increases the content of SP-C mRNA and immunoreactive proSP-C (55).

The primary mechanism of glucocorticoid effects on the SP-C gene are transcriptional. Treatment of human explants with 100n$M$ dexamethasone increases gene transcription rate >10-fold within 8 h (Fig. 6) and this response is rapidly reversed on removal of hormone (Table 5). By contrast exposure to glucocorticoid does not affect SP-C mRNA stability (Table 5). Induction of SP-C is sensitive to cycloheximide treatment, in contrast to findings for SP-B in the same experiments *(45)*. Cycloheximide sensitivity suggests that glucocorticoid effects on SP-C gene expression involve either induced synthesis of an intermediary protein (i.e., a secondary response) or a labile transcription factor necessary for the glucocorticoid response. These two models predict different molecular sites of glucocorticoid action in SP-C gene regulation. If a newly synthesized protein is involved, glucocorticoids presumably have their primary effect at a separate gene. The product of this gene would presumably be a transcription factor that influences expression of the SP-C gene either independently or in conjunction with glucocorticoids. If the cycloheximide sensitivity reflects a labile, *noninduced* protein involved in glucocorticoid regulation, this model then predicts the presence of functional GREs in the SP-C gene that activate transcription in the presence of the labile factor. These two possibilities were examined in experiments where cultured tissue was exposed to cycloheximide which was then removed before adding glucocorticoid. Since inhibition of protein synthesis by cycloheximide is rapidly reversed on removing the agent, this experimental design should preferentially inhibit glucocorticoid induction of SP-C by a process involving a preexisting, labile factor rather than induction of an intermediary protein. The data for SP-C transcription rate in this experimental approach support a role for a labile factor in glucocorticoid induction of SP-C (Fig 7). By contrast, induction of SP-B transcription was not affected by prior cycloheximide treatment.

There is a preliminary report of a consensus GRE sequence in the distal 5'-flanking region (–1.8 kb) of the human SP-C gene *(213)*. The presence of a functional GRE is supported by data of Glasser et al. *(214)* in studies with transgenic mice. They found that both endogenous SP-C and a transgene driven by 3 kb of the human SP-C 5'-flanking sequence were induced by dexamethasone treatment of cultured fetal lung from transgenic animals.

## SP-D Gene Expression

Developmental expression of SP-D in the rat is accelerated by in vivo glucocorticoid treatment. Exposure of pregnant rats to dexamethasone (1 mg/kg) produced a severalfold increase in content of SP-D mRNA and protein in fetal lung of day-19 animals, but did not increase levels on fetal day 20 and 21 when basal expression is higher. This induction process was maximal within approx 24 h and SP-D mRNA content increased to levels comparable to those at term *(52,63)*. Similar results were obtained for SP-D gene transcription rate during both lung development and in response to *in utero* dexamethasone, suggesting that both events occur primarily at the level of transcription *(63)*. No data are available for effects of glucocorticoids on SP-D in adult lung; however, the findings in rat fetuses at term predict that glucocorticoid responsiveness is minimal or absent in postnatal animals with normal adrenal cortical function *(63)*.

Additional studies using explant culture of fetal lung have confirmed the in vivo observations and further characterized glucocorticoid induction. In explants of fetal rat lung, maximal induction of SP-D mRNA (three- to 25-fold) occurred with 1 µ*M* hydrocortisone or 0.1 µ*M* dexamethasone by 12 h. As also observed in vivo, glucocorticoid treatment of lung explants increased the amount of immunoreactive SP-D protein. In vitro glucocor-

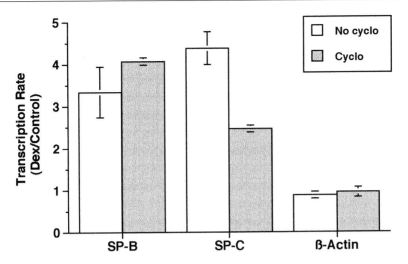

Fig. 7. Glucocorticoid induction of SP-B and SP-C transcription: effect of pretreatment with cycloheximide (cyclo). Explants of human fetal lung were treated for 1.5 h with diluent (no cyclo) or cyclo (2.5 µg/mL), cyclo was then removed by medium changes, and 100n$M$ dexamethasone was added for 4 h. Dexamethasone treatment alone (no cyclo) increased the transcription rates for both SP-B and SP-C, but not actin, and the increase for SP-C but not SP-B was partially blocked by prior exposure to cycloheximide. (From ref. *45*, with permission.

ticoid induction of SP-D, as for the other surfactant proteins, occurs on the background of increasing gene expression during explant culture in the absence of hormone.

Similar studies of SP-D have been performed in explants of second trimester human fetal lung with comparable findings *(64)*. Dexamethasone treatment produced approx twofold increase in both SP-D mRNA and protein, with maximal stimulation of mRNA occurring by ≤24 h. The response was maximal at 10n$M$ dexamethasone, which is a lower concentration that reported for rat lung, consistent with the higher affinity of human vs rat GR. Of interest, differences were found in the properties of induction for SP-D and SP-A in this culture system. SP-A is increased by low concentrations and short exposures to glucocorticoid, and inhibited by higher concentrations. By contrast, induction of SP-D mRNA was similar at both 10 and 100n$M$ dexamethasone after both 1 and 3 d of exposure. These findings emphasize the unique nature of the biphasic response that is observed with SP-A.

Rust et al. *(215)* have characterized the upstream sequence of the human SP-D gene and examined for functional GREs. Four consensus half-site GREs exist in the 5'-flanking sequence (−195 to −1583 bp) and two half-sites are present in intron 1. In transient transfection studies with H441 cells, dexamethasone increased reporter gene expression approx threefold using plasmid constructs containing 800–1700 bp of the SP-D gene 5'-flanking sequence; the smallest fragment tested (161 bp), which lacks any recognizable GRE half-sites, still gave a 2-fold increase in CAT activity with dexamethasone treatment (Fig. 8). Constructs including intron 1, which has two putative GRE half-sites, were not more responsive to dexamethasone that those without the intron. These findings are consistent with a primary mode of action of glucocorticoids on SP-D gene expression and suggest that responsiveness is mediated through the interaction of a variety of *cis*- and *trans*-acting factors as observed for other target genes.

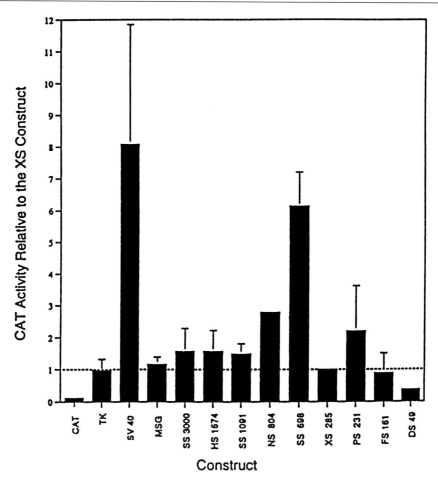

Fig. 8. Glucocorticoid responsiveness of SP-D promoter constructs. H441 cells were transfected with plasmid constructs containing restriction fragments of human SP-D 5'-flanking sequence linked to CAT, and cells were cultured 48 h in presence or absence of dexamethasone (50n$M$). All constructs except for DS 49 exhibited both basal promoter activity and dexamethasone responsiveness comparable to that observed with control plasmid MSG which contains multiple GREs. Data are mean ± SE of three experiments. (From ref. *215*, with permission).

## SUMMARY

The lung is a target tissue for glucocorticoids during both fetal and postnatal life. The level of free circulating corticoids increases in late gestation, and in some species the concentration of GR in lung also rises. These temporal associations with lung development, along with the effects of adrenal ablation and knockout of glucocorticoid-related genes, provide support for the concept that endogenous glucocorticoids are a major modulator of fetal lung maturation.

Administration of glucocorticoid in vivo or to cultured lung causes precocious maturation and changes in developmentally regulated genes. Based on high resolution gel electrophoresis, glucocorticoids regulate approx 2% of fetal lung proteins and approx 30 proteins in a variety of cell types have been identified that are either stimulated or inhibited by glucocorticoids. Most responses involve transcriptional regulation, including changes in both transcription rate and mRNA stability, and all effects appear to be mediated by GR.

Most of the effects of glucocorticoids that have been identified in postnatal lung relate to the antiinflammatory role of glucocorticoids. Glucocorticoids act in a variety of lung cells to suppress attachment and influx of circulating inflammatory cells, suppress the production of proinflammatory cytokines and immunoreceptors, and block inductive effects of cytokines and other inflammatory agents. At least 23 different proteins of postnatal lung cells are regulated by glucocorticoids. Recent evidence suggests that many of these antiinflammatory effects of glucocorticoids derive from a direct inhibitory effect of activated GR on the transactivation activity of $NF_{\kappa B}$, which is a key mediator of inflammatory signals in responsive genes.

The surfactant-associated proteins, in particular SP-B and SP-C are essential for normal function of surfactant and consequently normal respiration. All of the surfactant proteins are regulated by glucocorticoids in developing lung and the properties of induction/repression have been extensively investigated. Administration of glucocorticoids either in vivo or to cultured lung causes a precocious increase in levels of surfactant protein mRNAs and immunoreactive proteins. The induction processes involve increased transcription rate and/or mRNA stability and responses are fully reversed on removal of glucocorticoid consistent with GR-mediated enhancement of gene expression. To date, however, a functional GRE or other response elements have not been definitively identified in the surfactant protein genes. Glucocorticoid regulation of SP-A is particularly complex, at least in primates (human and baboon), where glucocorticoids either stimulate or inhibit SP-A gene expression depending on hormone concentration, duration of exposure, and gestational age. In vitro, the dominant response of both SP-A genes to glucocorticoids is inhibition; however, responsiveness has not been characterized in vivo. By contrast, glucocorticoids have only a stimulatory effect on expression of SP-D that is similar to SP-A in both structure and immune function.

Although glucocorticoids are well established as a major endocrine modulator of both differentiation and function of the lung, there remain many gaps in our understanding of regulatory mechanisms. Future challenges include identification of the functional response elements in target genes, interactions of GR with other transcription factors, and the role of glucocorticoids in the changing milieu of other hormones, cytokines, and growth factors that also regulate a number of the glucocorticoid responsive genes of lung cells. Future research on glucocorticoid action in the lung will likely have a major impact on our understanding of both fetal development and lung inflammation and should lead to improved strategies for hormonal intervention.

## REFERENCES

1. Liggins GC. Premature delivery of foetal lambs infused with glucocorticoids. J Endocrinol 1969;45:515–523.
2. Seidner S, Pettenazzo A, Ikegami M, Jobe A. Corticosteroid potentiation of surfactant dose response in preterm rabbits. J Appl Physiol 1988;64:2366–2371.
3. Platzker AC, Kitterman JA, Mescher EJ, Clements JA, Tooley WH. Surfactant in the lung and tracheal fluid of the fetal lamb and acceleration of its appearance by dexamethasone. Pediatrics 1975;56:554–561.
4. Johnson JW, Mitzner W, London WT, Palmer AE, Scott R, Kearney K. Glucocorticoids and the rhesus fetal lung. Am J Obstet Gynecol 1978;130:905–916.
5. Ballard PL. Hormones and lung maturation. Monogr Endocrinol 1986;28:1–354.
6. Kikkawa Y, Kaibara M, Motoyama EK, Orzalesi MM, Cook CD. Morphologic development of fetal rabbit lung and its acceleration with cortisol. Am J Pathol 1971;64:423–442.
7. Bunton TE, Plopper CG. Triamcinolone-induced structural alterations in the development of the lung of the fetal rhesus macaque. Am J Obstet Gynecol 1984;148:203–215.
8. Crowley P, Chalmers I, Keirse MJ. The effects of corticosteroid administration before preterm delivery: an overview of the evidence from controlled trials. Br J Obstet Gynaecol 1990;97:11–25.

9. Ballard PL, Ballard RA. Scientific basis and therapeutic regimens for use of antenatal glucocorticoids. Am J Obstet Gynecol 1995;173:254–262.

10. Fairclough RJ, Liggins GC. Protein binding of plasma cortisol in the foetal lamb near term. J Endocrinol 1975;67:333–341.

11. Ballard PL, Kitterman JA, Bland RD, Clyman RI, Gluckman PD, Platzker AC, Kaplan SL, Grumbach MM. Ontogeny and regulation of corticosteroid binding globulin capacity in plasma of fetal and newborn lambs. Endocrinology 1982;110:359–366.

12. Ballard PL, Ning Y, Polk D, Ikegami M, Jobe AH. Glucocorticoid regulation of surfactant components in immature lambs. Am J Physiol 1997;273:L1048–L1057.

13. Tan RC, Ikegami M, Jobe AH, Yao LY, Possmayer F, Ballard PL. Developmental and glucocorticoid regulation of surfactant protein mRNAs in fetal lambs. Am J Physiol 1999;277:L1142–L1148.

14. Hitchcock KR. Hormones and the lung. I. Thyroid hormones and glucocorticoids in lung development. Anat Rec 1979;194:15–39.

15. Liggins GC, Kitterman JA, Campos GA, Clements JA, Forster CS, Lee CH, Creasy RK. Pulmonary maturation in the hypophysectomised ovine fetus. Differential responses to adrenocorticotrophin and cortisol. J Dev Physiol 1981;3:1–14.

16. Kitterman JA, Liggins GC, Campos GA, Clements JA, Forster CS, Lee CH, Creasy RK. Prepartum maturation of the lung in fetal sheep: relation to cortisol. J Appl Physiol 1981;51:384–390.

17. Crone RK, Davies P, Liggins GC, Reid L. The effects of hypophysectomy, thyroidectomy, and postoperative infusion of cortisol or adrenocorticotrophin on the structure of the ovine fetal lung. J Dev Physiol 1983;5:281–288.

18. Muglia L, Jacobson L, Dikkes P, Majzoub JA. Corticotropin-releasing hormone deficiency reveals major fetal but not adult glucocorticoid need. Nature 1995;373:427–432.

19. Cole TJ, Blendy JA, Monaghan AP, Krieglstein K, Schmid W, Aguzzi A, Fantuzzi G, Hummler E, Unsicker K, Schutz G. Targeted disruption of the glucocorticoid receptor gene blocks adrenergic chromaffin cell development and severely retards lung maturation. Genes Dev 1995;9:1608–1621.

20. Murphy BE. Conjugated glucocorticoids in amniotic fluid and fetal lung maturation. J Clin Endocrinol Metab 1978;47:212–215.

21. Odom MW, Ertsey R, Ballard PL. Hormonally regulated proteins in cultured human fetal lung: analysis by two-dimensional gel electrophoresis. Am J Physiol 1990;259:L283–L293.

22. Gonzales LW, Ballard PL, Ertsey R, Williams MC. Glucocorticoids and thyroid hormones stimulate biochemical and morphological differentiation of human fetal lung in organ culture. J Clin Endocrinol Metab 1986;62:678–691.

23. Beers MF, Solarin KO, Guttentag SH, Rosenbloom J, Kormilli A, Gonzales LW, Ballard PL. TGF-beta1 inhibits surfactant component expression and epithelial cell maturation in cultured human fetal lung. Am J Physiol 1998;275:L950–L960.

24. Phelps DS, Giannopoulos G. Effect of dexamethasone on the synthesis of specific proteins in fetal rabbit lung in vivo and in organ culture. Exp Lung Res 1984;7:195–210.

25. Beresini MH, Lempert MJ, Epstein LB. Overlapping polypeptide induction in human fibroblasts in response to treatment with interferon-alpha, interferon-gamma, interleukin 1 alpha, interleukin 1 beta, and tumor necrosis factor. J Immunol 1988;140:485–493.

26. Hundertmark S, Buhler H, Ragosch V, Dinkelborg L, Arabin B, Weitzel HK. Correlation of surfactant phosphatidylcholine synthesis and 11 beta- hydroxysteroid dehydrogenase in the fetal lung. Endocrinology 1995;136:2573–2578.

27. Wang J, Kuliszewski M, Yee W, Sedlackova L, Xu J, Tseu I, Post M. Cloning and expression of glucocorticoid-induced genes in fetal rat lung fibroblasts: transforming growth factor-beta 3. J Biol Chem 1995;270:2722–2728.

28. van de Wetering JK, Elfring RH, Oosterlaken-Dijksterhuis MA, Mol JA, Haagsman HP, Batenburg JJ. Perinatal expression of IGFBPs in rat lung and its hormonal regulation in fetal lung explants. Am J Physiol 1997;273:L1174–L1181.

29. Tangada SD, Peterson RD, Funkhouser JD. Regulation of expression of aminopeptidase N in fetal rat lung by dexamethasone and epidermal growth factor. Biochim Biophys Acta 1995;1268:191–199.

30. Smith BT, Post M. Fibroblast-pneumonocyte factor. Am J Physiol 1989;257:L174–L178.

31. Floros J, Post M, Smith BT. Glucocorticoids affect the synthesis of pulmonary fibroblast-pneumonocyte factor at a pretranslational level. J Biol Chem 1985;260:2265–2267.

32. Breed DR, Margraf LR, Alcorn JL, Mendelson CR. Transcription factor C/EBPdelta in fetal lung: developmental regulation and effects of cyclic adenosine 3',5'-monophosphate and glucocorticoids. Endocrinology 1997;138:5527–5534.

33. Feinstein SI, Matlapudi A, Zgleszewski SE, Cilley RE, Chinoy MR. Developmental and hormonal regulation of mRNA for the transcription factor, C/EBPδ in mouse lung. Am J Respir Crit Care Med 1999;159:A900.

34. Liley HG, White RT, Benson BJ, Ballard PL. Glucocorticoids both stimulate and inhibit production of pulmonary surfactant protein A in fetal human lung. Proc Natl Acad Sci USA 1988;85:9096–9100.

35. Iannuzzi DM, Ertsey R, Ballard PL. Biphasic glucocorticoid regulation of pulmonary SP-A: characterization of inhibitory process. Am J Physiol 1993;264:L236–L244.

36. Karinch AM, Deiter G, Ballard PL, Floros J. Regulation of expression of human SP-A1 and SP-A2 genes in fetal lung explant culture. Biochim Biophys Acta 1998;1398:192–202.

37. Boggaram V, Mendelson CR. Transcriptional regulation of the gene encoding the major surfactant protein (SP-A) in rabbit fetal lung. J Biol Chem 1988;263:19,060–19,065.

38. Floros J, Phelps DS, Harding HP, Church S, Ware J. Postnatal stimulation of rat surfactant protein A synthesis by dexamethasone. Am J Physiol 1989;257:L137–L143.

39. Ogasawara Y, Kuroki Y, Tsuzuki A, Ueda S, Misaki H, Akino T. Pre- and postnatal stimulation of pulmonary surfactant protein D by in vivo dexamethasone treatment of rats. Life Sci 1992;50:1761–1767.

40. Schellhase DE, Shannon JM. Effects of maternal dexamethasone on expression of SP-A, SP-B, and SP-C in the fetal rat lung. Am J Respir Cell Mol Biol 1991;4:304–312.

41. Connelly IH, Hammond GL, Harding PG, Possmayer F. Levels of surfactant-associated protein messenger ribonucleic acids in rabbit lung during perinatal development and after hormonal treatment. Endocrinology 1991;129:2583–2591.

42. Durham PL, Wohlford-Lenane CL, Snyder JM. Glucocorticoid regulation of surfactant-associated proteins in rabbit fetal lung in vivo. Anat Rec 1993;237:365–377.

43. Polk DH, Ikegami M, Jobe AH, Sly P, Kohan R, Newnham J. Preterm lung function after retreatment with antenatal betamethasone in preterm lambs. Am J Obstet Gynecol 1997;176:308–315.

44. Whitsett JA, Weaver TE, Clark JC, Sawtell N, Glasser SW, Korfhagen TR, Hull WM. Glucocorticoid enhances surfactant proteolipid Phe and pVal synthesis and RNA in fetal lung. J Biol Chem 1987;262:15,618–15,623.

45. Ballard PL, Ertsey R, Gonzales LW, Gonzales J. Transcriptional regulation of human pulmonary surfactant proteins SP-B and SP-C by glucocorticoids. Am J Respir Cell Mol Biol 1996;14:599–607.

46. Guttentag SH, Beers MF, Bieler BM, Ballard PL. Surfactant protein B processing in human fetal lung. Am J Physiol 1998;275:L559–L566.

47. Venkatesh VC, Iannuzzi DM, Ertsey R, Ballard PL. Differential glucocorticoid regulation of the pulmonary hydrophobic surfactant proteins SP-B and SP-C. Am J Respir Cell Mol Biol 1993;8:222–228.

48. Venkatesh VC, Planer BC, Schwartz M, Vanderbilt JN, White RT, Ballard PL. Characterization of the promoter of human pulmonary surfactant protein B gene. Am J Physiol 1995;268:L674–L682.

49. Beers MF, Shuman H, Liley HG, Floros J, Gonzales LW, Yue N, Ballard PL. Surfactant protein B in human fetal lung: developmental and glucocorticoid regulation. Pediatr Res 1995;38:668–675.

50. Liley HG, White RT, Warr RG, Benson BJ, Hawgood S, Ballard PL. Regulation of messenger RNAs for the hydrophobic surfactant proteins in human lung. J Clin Invest 1989;83:1191–1197.

51. Alcorn JL, Smith ME, Smith JF, Margraf LR, Mendelson CR. Primary cell culture of human type II pneumonocytes: maintenance of a differentiated phenotype and transfection with recombinant adenoviruses. Am J Respir Cell Mol Biol 1997;17:672–682.

52. Deterding RR, Shimizu H, Fisher JH, Shannon JM. Regulation of surfactant protein D expression by glucocorticoids in vitro and in vivo. Am J Respir Cell Mol Biol 1994;10:30–37.

53. Floros J, Gross I, Nichols KV, Veletza SV, Dynia D, Lu HW, Wilson CM, Peterec SM. Hormonal effects on the surfactant protein B (SP-B) mRNA in cultured fetal rat lung. Am J Respir Cell Mol Biol 1991;4:449–454.

54. Xu J, Possmayer F. Exposure of rabbit fetal lung to glucocorticoids in vitro does not enhance transcription of the gene encoding pulmonary surfactant-associated protein-B (SP-B). Biochim Biophys Acta 1993;1169:146–155.

55. O'Reilly MA, Gazdar AF, Clark JC, Pilot-Matias TJ, Wert SE, Hull WM, Whitsett JA. Glucocorticoids regulate surfactant protein synthesis in a pulmonary adenocarcinoma cell line. Am J Physiol 1989;257:L385–L392.

56. O'Reilly MA, Clark JC, Whitsett JA. Glucocorticoid enhances pulmonary surfactant protein B gene transcription. Am J Physiol 1991;260:L37–L43.

57. Shimizu H, Miyamura K, Kuroki Y. Appearance of surfactant proteins, SP-A and SP-B, in developing rat lung and the effects of in vivo dexamethasone treatment. Biochim Biophys Acta 1991;1081:53–60.

58.  Fisher J, McCormack F, Park S, Stelzner T, Shannon JM, Hofmann T. In vivo regulation of surfactant proteins by glucocorticoids. Am J Resp Cell Mol Biol 1991;5:63–70.
59.  Margana RK, Boggaram V. Transcription and mRNA stability regulate developmental and hormonal expression of rabbit surfactant protein B gene. Am J Physiol 1995;268:L481–L490.
60.  Boggaram V, Margana RK. Rabbit surfactant protein C: cDNA cloning and regulation of alternatively spliced surfactant protein C mRNAs. Am J Physiol 1992;263:L634–L644.
61.  Boggaram V, Margana RK. Developmental and hormonal regulation of surfactant protein C (SP-C) gene expression in fetal lung: role of transcription and mRNA stability. J Biol Chem 1994;269:27,767–27,772.
62.  Veletza SV, Nichols KV, Gross I, Lu H, Dynia DW, Floros J. Surfactant protein C: hormonal control of SP-C mRNA levels in vitro. Am J Physiol 1992;262:L684–L687.
63.  Mariencheck W, Crouch E. Modulation of surfactant protein D expression by glucocorticoids in fetal rat lung. Am J Respir Cell Mol Biol 1994;10:419–429.
64.  Dulkerian SJ, Gonzales LW, Ning Y, Ballard PL. Regulation of surfactant protein D in human fetal lung. Am J Respir Cell Mol Biol 1996;15:781–786.
65.  Gonzales LW, Ertsey R, Ballard PL, Froh D, Goerke J, Gonzales J. Glucocorticoid stimulation of fatty acid synthesis in explants of human fetal lung. Biochim Biophys Acta 1990;1042:1–12.
66.  Wagle S, Bui R, Ballard PL, Shuman H, Gonzalcs J, Gonzales LW. IIormonal stimulation and cellular localization of fatty acid synthetase in human fetal lung. Am J Physiol 1999;277:L381–L390.
67.  Pope TS, Smart DA, Rooney SA. Hormonal effects on fatty-acid synthase in cultured fetal rat lung; induction by dexamethasone and inhibition of activity by triiodothyronine. Biochim Biophys Acta 1988;959:169–177.
68.  Maniscalco WM, Finkelstein JN, Parkhurst AB. Dexamethasone increases de novo fatty acid synthesis in fetal rabbit lung explants. Pediatr Res 1985;19:1272–1277.
69.  Rooney SA, Smart DA, Weinhold PA, Feldman DA. Dexamethasone increases the activity but not the amount of choline-phosphate cytidylyltransferase in fetal rat lung. Biochim Biophys Acta 1990;1044:385–389.
70.  Sharma A, Gonzales LW, Ballard PL. Hormonal regulation of cholinephosphate cytidylyltransferase in human fetal lung. Biochim Biophys Acta 1993;1170:237–244.
71.  Post M. Maternal administration of dexamethasone stimulates choline-phosphate cytidylyltransferase in fetal type II cells. Biochem J 1987;241:291–296.
72.  Serrato CM, Gonzales LW, Ballard PL. Hormonal stimulation of lysophosphatidylcholine acyltransferase in explants of human fetal lung. Clin Res 1991;39:109A.
73.  Pierce RA, Mariencheck WI, Sandefur S, Crouch EC, Parks WC. Glucocorticoids upregulate tropoelastin expression during late stages of fetal lung development. Am J Physiol 1995;268:L491–L500.
74.  Yee W, Wang J, Liu J, Tseu I, Kuliszewski M, Post M. Glucocorticoid-induced tropoelastin expression is mediated via transforming growth factor-beta 3. Am J Physiol 1996;270:L992–L1001.
75.  Schellenberg JC, Liggins GC, Stewart AW. Growth, elastin concentration, and collagen concentration of perinatal rat lung: effects of dexamethasone. Pediatr Res 1987;21:603–607.
76.  Ledo I, Wu M, Katchman S, Brown D, Kennedy S, Hsu-Wong S, Uitto J. Glucocorticosteroids up-regulate human elastin gene promoter activity in transgenic mice. J Invest Dermatol 1994;103:632–636.
77.  Tchepichev S, Ueda J, Canessa C, Rossier BC, O'Brodovich H. Lung epithelial Na channel subunits are differentially regulated during development and by steroids. Am J Physiol 1995;269:C805–C812.
78.  Ingbar DH, Duvick S, Savick SK, Schellhase DE, Detterding R, Jamieson JD, Shannon JM. Developmental changes of fetal rat lung Na-K-ATPase after maternal treatment with dexamethasone. Am J Physiol 1997;272:L665–L672.
79.  King LS, Nielsen S, Agre P. Aquaporin-1 water channel protein in lung: ontogeny, steroid-induced expression, and distribution in rat. J Clin Invest 1996;97:2183–2191.
80.  Yasui M, Serlachius E, Lofgren M, Belusa R, Nielsen S, Aperia A. Perinatal changes in expression of aquaporin-4 and other water and ion transporters in rat lung. J Physiol (Lond) 1997;505:3–11.
81.  Giannopoulos G, Smith SK. Hormonal regulation of beta-adrenergic receptors in fetal rabbit lung in organ culture. Life Sci 1982;31:795–802.
82.  Maniscalco WM, Shapiro DL. Effects of dexamethasone on beta-adrenergic receptors in fetal lung explants. Pediatr Res 1983;17:274–277.
83.  Cheng JB, Goldfien A, Ballard PL, Roberts JM. Glucocorticoids increase pulmonary beta-adrenergic receptors in fetal rabbit. Endocrinology 1980;107:1646–1648.
84.  Barnes P, Jacobs M, Roberts JM. Glucocorticoids preferentially increase fetal alveolar beta-adrenoreceptors: autoradiographic evidence. Pediatr Res 1984;18:1191–1194.

85. Frank L, Lewis PL, Sosenko IR. Dexamethasone stimulation of fetal rat lung antioxidant enzyme activity in parallel with surfactant stimulation. Pediatrics 1985;75:569–574.

86. Randhawa P, Hass M, Frank L, Massaro D. Dexamethasone increases superoxide dismutase activity in serum-free rat fetal lung organ cultures. Pediatr Res 1986;20:895–898.

87. Clerch LB, Iqbal J, Massaro D. Perinatal rat lung catalase gene expression: influence of corticosteroid and hyperoxia. Am J Physiol 1991;260:L428–L433.

88. Grummer MA, Zachman RD. Retinoic acid and dexamethasone affect RAR-beta and surfactant protein C mRNA in the MLE lung cell line. Am J Physiol 1998;274:L1–L7.

89. Grummer MA, Zachman RD. Postnatal rat lung retinoic acid receptor (RAR) mRNA expression and effects of dexamethasone on RAR beta mRNA. Pediatr Pulmonol 1995;20:234–240.

90. McMenamy KR, Anderson MJ, Zachman RD. Effect of dexamethasone and oxygen exposure on neonatal rat lung retinoic acid receptor proteins. Pediatr Pulmonol 1994;18:232–238.

91. Snyder JM, D'Ercole AJ. Somatomedin C/insulin-like growth factor I production by human fetal lung tissue maintained in vitro. Exp Lung Res 1987;13:449–458.

92. Clemmons DR, Underwood LE, Van Wyk JJ. Hormonal control of immunoreactive somatomedin production by cultured human fibroblasts. J Clin Invest 1981;67:10–19.

93. Price WA, Moats-Staats BM, D'Ercole AJ, Stiles AD. Insulin-like growth factor binding protein production and regulation in fetal rat lung cells. Am J Respir Cell Mol Biol 1993;8:425–432.

94. Chinoy MR, Volpe MV, Cilley RE, Zgleszewski SE, Vosatka RJ, Martin A, Nielsen HC, Krummel TM. Growth factors and dexamethasone regulate Hoxb5 protein in cultured murine fetal lungs. Am J Physiol 1998;274:L610–L620.

95. Ballard PL, Hawgood S, Liley H, Wellenstein G, Gonzales LW, Benson B, Cordell B, White RT. Regulation of pulmonary surfactant apoprotein SP 28–36 gene in fetal human lung. Proc Natl Acad Sci USA 1986;83:9527–9531.

96. Seidner SR, Smith ME, Mendelson CR. Developmental and hormonal regulation of SP-A gene expression in baboon fetal lung. Am J Physiol 1996;271:L609–L616.

97. George TN, Miakotina OL, Goss KL, Snyder JM. Mechanism of all trans-retinoic acid and glucocorticoid regulation of surfactant protein mRNA. Am J Physiol 1998;274:L560–L566.

98. Davis DJ, Jacobs MM, Ballard PL, Gonzales LK, Roberts JM. Beta-adrenergic receptors and cAMP response increase during explant culture of human fetal lung: partial inhibition by dexamethasone. Pediatr Res 1990;28:190–195.

99. Clerch LB, Whitney PL, Massaro D. Rat lung lectin synthesis, degradation and activation: developmental regulation and modulation by dexamethasone. Biochem J 1987;245:683–690.

100. Clerch LB, Whitney P, Massaro D. Rat lung lectin gene expression is regulated developmentally and by dexamethasone. Am J Physiol 1989;256:C501–C505.

101. Solarin KO, Ballard PL, Guttentag SH, Lomax CA, Beers MF. Expression and glucocorticoid regulation of surfactant protein C in human fetal lung. Pediatr Res 1997;42:356–364.

102. Cronstein BN, Kimmel SC, Levin RI, Martiniuk F, Weissmann G. A mechanism for the antiinflammatory effects of corticosteroids: the glucocorticoid receptor regulates leukocyte adhesion to endothelial cells and expression of endothelial-leukocyte adhesion molecule 1 and intercellular adhesion molecule 1. Proc Natl Acad Sci USA 1992;89:9991–9995.

103. Ray KP, Farrow S, Daly M, Talabot F, Searle N. Induction of the E-selectin promoter by interleukin 1 and tumour necrosis factor alpha, and inhibition by glucocorticoids. Biochem J 1997;328:707–715.

104. Wissink S, van Heerde EC, vand der Burg B, van der Saag PT. A dual mechanism mediates repression of NF-kappaB activity by glucocorticoids. Mol Endocrinol 1998;12:355–363.

105. van der Saag PT, Caldenhoven E, van de Stolpe A. Molecular mechanisms of steroid action: a novel type of cross-talk between glucocorticoids and NF-kappa B transcription factors. Eur Respir J Suppl 1996;22:146s–153s.

106. Monick MM, Aksamit TR, Geist LJ, Hunninghake GW. Dexamethasone inhibits IL-1 and TNF activity in human lung fibroblasts without affecting IL-1 or TNF receptors. Am J Physiol 1994;267:L33–L38.

107. Standiford TJ, Kunkel SL, Rolfe MW, Evanoff HL, Allen RM, Strieter RM. Regulation of human alveolar macrophage- and blood monocyte-derived interleukin-8 by prostaglandin E2 and dexamethasone. Am J Respir Cell Mol Biol 1992;6:75–81.

108. Mukaida N, Gussella GL, Kasahara T, Ko Y, Zachariae CO, Kawai T, Matsushima K. Molecular analysis of the inhibition of interleukin-8 production by dexamethasone in a human fibrosarcoma cell line. Immunology 1992;75:674–679.

109. John M, Au BT, Jose PJ, Lim S, Saunders M, Barnes PJ, Mitchell JA, Belvisi MG, Chung KF. Expression and release of interleukin-8 by human airway smooth muscle cells: inhibition by Th-2 cytokines and corticosteroids. Am J Respir Cell Mol Biol 1998;18:84–90.

110. Shull S, Meisler N, Absher M, Phan S, Cutroneo K. Glucocorticoid-induced down regulation of transforming growth factor- beta 1 in adult rat lung fibroblasts. Lung 1995;173:71–78.

111. Danielpour D, Kim KY, Winokur TS, Sporn MB. Differential regulation of the expression of transforming growth factor- betas 1 and 2 by retinoic acid, epidermal growth factor, and dexamethasone in NRK-49F and A549 cells. J Cell Physiol 1991;148:235–244.

112. Lilly CM, Nakamura H, Kesselman H, Nagler-Anderson C, Asano K, Garcia-Zepeda EA, Rothenberg ME, Drazen JM, Luster AD. Expression of eotaxin by human lung epithelial cells: induction by cytokines and inhibition by glucocorticoids. J Clin Invest 1997;99:1767–1773.

113. Kwon OJ, Jose PJ, Robbins RA, Schall TJ, Williams TJ, Barnes PJ. Glucocorticoid inhibition of RANTES expression in human lung epithelial cells. Am J Respir Cell Mol Biol 1995;12:488–496.

114. Mitchell JA, Belvisi MG, Akarasereenont P, Robbins RA, Kwon OJ, Croxtall J, Barnes PJ, Vane JR. Induction of cyclo-oxygenase-2 by cytokines in human pulmonary epithelial cells: regulation by dexamethasone. Br J Pharmacol 1994;113:1008–1014.

115. Newton R, Kuitert LM, Slater DM, Adcock IM, Barnes PJ. Cytokine induction of cytosolic phospholipase $A_2$ and cyclooxygenase-2 mRNA is suppressed by glucocorticoids in human epithelial cells. Life Sciences 1997;60:67–78.

116. Nakano T, Ohara O, Teraoka H, Arita H. Glucocorticoids suppress group II phospholipase $A_2$ production by blocking mRNA synthesis and post-transcriptional expression. J Biol Chem 1990;265:12,745–12,748.

117. Levine SJ, Benfield T, Shelhamer JH. Corticosteroids induce intracellular interleukin-1 receptor antagonist type I expression by a human airway epithelial cell line. Am J Respir Cell Mol Biol 1996;15:245–251.

118. Crestani B, Rolland C, Lardeux B, Fournier T, Bernuau D, Pous C, Vissuzaine C, Li L, Aubier M. Inducible expression of the alpha1–acid glycoprotein by rat and human type II alveolar epithelial cells. J Immunol 1998;160:4596–4605.

119. Torkkeli T, Krusius T, Janne O. Uterine and lung uteroglobins in the rabbit: two similar proteins with differential hormonal regulation. Biochim Biophys Acta 1978;544:578–592.

120. Lombardero M, Nieto A. Glucocorticoid and developmental regulation of uteroglobin synthesis in rabbit lung. Biochem J 1981;200:487–494.

121. Pei L. Identification of a negative glucocorticoid response element in the rat type 1 vasoactive intestinal polypeptide receptor gene. J Biol Chem 1996;271:20,879–20,884.

122. Churchill L, Friedman B, Schleimer RP, Proud D. Production of granulocyte-macrophage colony-stimulating factor by cultured human tracheal epithelial cells. Immunology 1992;75:189–195.

123. Kato M, Schleimer RP. Antiinflammatory steroids inhibit granulocyte/macrophage colony- stimulating factor production by human lung tissue. Lung 1994;172:113–124.

124. Adkins KK, Levan TD, Miesfeld RL, Bloom JW. Glucocorticoid regulation of GM-CSF: evidence for transcriptional mechanisms in airway epithelial cells. Am J Physiol 1998;275:L372–L378.

125. Pryhuber GS, Khalak R, Zhao Q. Regulation of surfactant proteins A and B by TNF-alpha and phorbol ester independent of NF-kappa B. Am J Physiol 1998;274:L289–L295.

126. Radomski MW, Palmer RM, Moncada S. Glucocorticoids inhibit the expression of an inducible, but not the constitutive, nitric oxide synthase in vascular endothelial cells. Proc Natl Acad Sci USA 1990;87:10,043–10,047.

127. Robbins RA, Barnes PJ, Springall DR, Warren JB, Kwon OJ, Buttery LD, Wilson AJ, Geller DA, Polak JM. Expression of inducible nitric oxide in human lung epithelial cells. Biochem Biophys Res Commun 1994;203:209–218.

128. Kleinert H, Euchenhofer C, Ihrig-Biedert I, Forstermann U. Glucocorticoids inhibit the induction of nitric oxide synthase II by down-regulating cytokine-induced activity of transcription factor nuclear factor-kappa B. Mol Pharmacol 1996;49:15–21.

129. Di Rosa M, Radomski M, Carnuccio R, Moncada S. Glucocorticoids inhibit the induction of nitric oxide synthase in macrophages. Biochem Biophys Res Commun 1990;172:1246–1252.

130. Knowles RG, Salter M, Brooks SL, Moncada S. Anti-inflammatory glucocorticoids inhibit the induction by endotoxin of nitric oxide synthase in the lung, liver and aorta of the rat. Biochem Biophys Res Commun 1990;172:1042–1048.

131. Rahman I, Bel A, Mulier B, Donaldson K, MacNee W. Differential regulation of glutathione by oxidants and dexamethasone in alveolar epithelial cells. Am J Physiol 1998;275:L80–L86.

132. Borson DB, Gruenert DC. Glucocorticoids induce neutral endopeptidase in transformed human tracheal epithelial cells. Am J Physiol 1991;260:L83–L89.

133. Venkatesh VC, Dong WWD, Mawji N. Urokinase-type plasminogen activator gene expression is inhibited by glucocorticoids in human fetal lung. Pediatr Res 1998;43:56A.

134. Marshall BC, Sageser DS, Rao NV, Emi M, Hoidal JR. Alveolar epithelial cell plasminogen activator: characterization and regulation. J Biol Chem 1990;265:8198–8204.

135. Hasegawa T, Sorensen L, Dohi M, Rao NV, Hoidal JR, Marshall BC. Induction of urokinase-type plasminogen activator receptor by IL-1 beta. Am J Respir Cell Mol Biol 1997;16:683–692.

136. Tanaka M, Inase N, Fushimi K, Ishibashi K, Ichioka M, Sasaki S, Marumo F. Induction of aquaporin 3 by corticosteroid in a human airway epithelial cell line. Am J Physiol 1997;273:L1090–L1095.

137. Renard S, Voilley N, Bassilana F, Lazdunski M, Barbry P. Localization and regulation by steroids of the alpha, beta and gamma subunits of the amiloride-sensitive Na+ channel in colon, lung and kidney. Pflugers Arch 1995;430:299–307.

138. Venkatesh VC, Katzberg HD. Glucocorticoid regulation of epithelial sodium channel genes in human fetal lung. Am J Physiol 1997;273:L227–L233.

139. Mak JC, Nishikawa M, Barnes PJ. Glucocorticosteroids increase beta 2–adrenergic receptor transcription in human lung. Am J Physiol 1995;268:L41–L46.

140. Barquin N, Ciccolella DE, Ridge KM, Sznajder JI. Dexamethasone upregulates the Na-K-ATPase in rat alveolar epithelial cells. Am J Physiol 1997;273:L825–L830.

141. Labow BI, Abcouwer SF, Lin CM, Souba WW. Glutamine synthetase expression in rat lung is regulated by protein stability. Am J Physiol 1998;275:L877–L886.

142. Chandrasekhar S, Souba WW, Abcouwer SF. Identification of glucocorticoid-responsive elements that control transcription of rat glutamine synthetase. Am J Physiol 1999;276:L319–L331.

143. Friedland J, Setton C, Silverstein E. Angiotensin converting enzyme: induction by steroids in rabbit alveolar macrophages in culture. Science 1977;197:64,65.

144. Mendelsohn FA, Lloyd CJ, Kachel C, Funder JW. Induction by glucocorticoids of angiotensin converting enzyme production from bovine endothelial cells in culture and rat lung in vivo. J Clin Invest 1982;70:684–692.

145. Matsuba T, Keicho N, Higashimoto Y, Granleese S, Hogg JC, Hayashi S, Bondy GP. Identification of glucocorticoid- and adenovirus E1A-regulated genes in lung epithelial cells by differential display. Am J Respir Cell Mol Biol 1998;18:243–254.

146. Guy J, Dhanireddy R, Mukherjee AB. Surfactant-producing rabbit pulmonary alveolar type II cells synthesize and secrete an antiinflammatory protein, uteroglobin. Biochem Biophys Res Commun 1992;189:662–669.

147. Ray A, LaForge KS, Sehgal PB. On the mechanism for efficient repression of the interleukin-6 promoter by glucocorticoids: enhancer, TATA box, and RNA start site (Inr motif) occlusion. Mol Cell Biol 1990;10:5736–5746.

148. LeVan TD, Behr FD, Adkins KK, Miesfeld RL, Bloom JW. Glucocorticoid receptor signaling in a bronchial epithelial cell line. Am J Physiol 1997;272:L838–L843.

149. McKay LI, Cidlowski JA. Cross-talk between nuclear factor-kappa B and the steroid hormone receptors: mechanisms of mutual antagonism. Mol Endocrinol 1998;12:45–56.

150. Chen ZJ, Parent L, Maniatis T. Site-specific phosphorylation of IkappaBalpha by a novel ubiquitination-dependent protein kinase activity. Cell 1996;84:853–862.

151. Sweezey N, Mawdsley C, Ghibu F, Song L, Buch S, Moore A, Antakly T, Post M. Differential regulation of glucocorticoid receptor expression by ligand in fetal rat lung cells. Pediatr Res 1995;38:506–512.

152. Bronnegard M, Okret S. Regulation of the glucocorticoid receptor in fetal rat lung during development. J Steroid Biochem Mol Biol 1991;39:13–17.

153. Sweezey NB, Ghibu F, Gagnon S, Schotman E, Hamid Q. Glucocorticoid receptor mRNA and protein in fetal rat lung in vivo: modulation by glucocorticoid and androgen. Am J Physiol 1998;275:L103–L109.

154. Bamberger CM, Bamberger AM, de Castro M, Chrousos GP. Glucocorticoid receptor beta, a potential endogenous inhibitor of glucocorticoid action in humans. J Clin Invest 1995;95: 2435–2441.

155. Hawgood S, Clements JA. Pulmonary surfactant and its apoproteins. J Clin Invest 1990;86:1–6.

156. Weaver T, Whitsett J. Function and regulation of expression of pulmonary surfactant-associated proteins. Biochem J 1991;273:249–264.

157. Clark JC, Weaver TE, Iwamoto HS, Ikegami M, Jobe AH, Hull WM, Whitsett JA. Decreased lung compliance and air trapping in heterozygous SP-B-deficient mice. Am J Respir Cell Molec Biol 1997;16:46–52.

158. Nogee LM, de Mello DE, Dehner LP, Colten HR. Brief report: deficiency of pulmonary surfactant protein B in congenital alveolar proteinosis. N Engl J Med 1993;328:406–410.

159. King RJ, Klass DJ, Gikas EG, Clements JA. Isolation of apoproteins from canine surface active material. Am J Physiol 1973;224:788–795.

160. Benson B, Hawgood S, Schilling J, Clements J, Damm D, Cordell B, White RT. Structure of canine pulmonary surfactant apoprotein: cDNA and complete amino acid sequence. Proc Natl Acad Sci USA 1985;82:6379–6383.

161. White RT, Damm D, Miller J, Spratt K, Schilling J, Hawgood S, Benson B, Cordell B. Isolation and characterization of the human pulmonary surfactant apoprotein gene. Nature 1985;317:361–363.

162. Katyal SL, Singh G, Locker J. Characterization of a second human pulmonary surfactant-associated protein SP-A gene. Am J Respir Cell Mol Biol 1992;6:446–452.

163. Voss T, Melchers K, Scheirle G, Schafer KP. Structural comparison of recombinant pulmonary surfactant protein SP-A derived from two human coding sequences: implications for the chain composition of natural human SP-A. Am J Respir Cell Mol Biol 1991;4:88–94.

164. Mason RJ, Greene K, Voelker DR. Surfactant protein A and surfactant protein D in health and disease. Am J Physiol 1998;275:L1–L13.

165. McCormick SM, Boggaram V, Mendelson CR. Characterization of mRNA transcripts and organization of human SP-A1 and SP-A2 genes. Am J Physiol 1994;266:L354–L366.

166. Karinch AM, Floros J. 5′ splicing and allelic variants of the human pulmonary surfactant protein A genes. Am J Respir Cell Mol Biol 1995;12:77–88.

167. Cochrane CG, Revak SD. Pulmonary surfactant protein B (SP-B): structure-function relationships. Science 1991;254:566–568.

168. Nogee LM, Garnier G, Dietz HC, Singer L, Murphy AM, deMello DE, Colten HR. A mutation in the surfactant protein B gene responsible for fatal neonatal respiratory disease in multiple kindreds. J Clin Invest 1994;93:1860–1863.

169. Robertson B, Kobayashi T, Ganzuka M, Grossmann G, Li WZ, Suzuki Y. Experimental neonatal respiratory failure induced by a monoclonal antibody to the hydrophobic surfactant-associated protein SP-B. Pediatr Res 1991;30:239–243.

170. Kobayashi T, Robertson B, Grossmann G, Nitta K, Carstedt T, Suzuki Y. Exogenous porcine surfactant (Curosurf) is inactivated by monoclonal antibody to the surfactant-associated hydrophobic protein SP-B. Acta Paediatr 1992;81:665–671.

171. Persson A, Chang D, Rust K, Moxley M, Longmore W, Crouch E. Purification and biochemical characterization of CP4 (SP-D), a collagenous surfactant-associated protein. Biochemistry 1989;28:6361–6367.

172. Crouch E, Persson A, Chang D, Parghi D. Surfactant protein D. Increased accumulation in silica-induced pulmonary lipoproteinosis. Am J Pathol 1991;139:765–776.

173. Rust K, Grosso L, Zhang V, Chang D, Persson A, Longmore W, Cai GZ, Crouch E. Human surfactant protein D: SP-D contains a C-type lectin carbohydrate recognition domain. Arch Biochem Biophys 1991;290:116–126.

174. Persson A, Chang D, Crouch E. Surfactant protein D is a divalent cation-dependent carbohydrate-binding protein. J Biol Chem 1990;265:5755–5760.

175. Crouch E, Persson A, Chang D. Accumulation of surfactant protein D in human pulmonary alveolar proteinosis. Am J Pathol 1993;142:241–248.

176. Crouch E, Parghi D, Kuan SF, Persson A. Surfactant protein D: subcellular localization in nonciliated bronchiolar epithelial cells. Am J Physiol 1992;263:L60–L66.

177. Crouch E, Rust K, Marienchek W, Parghi D, Chang D, Persson A. Developmental expression of pulmonary surfactant protein D (SP-D). Am J Respir Cell Mol Biol 1991;5:13–18.

178. Ogasawara Y, Kuroki Y, Shiratori M, Shimizu H, Miyamura K, Akino T. Ontogeny of surfactant apoprotein D, SP-D, in the rat lung. Biochim Biophys Acta 1991;1083:252–256.

179. Kuroki Y, Shiratori M, Murata Y, Akino T. Surfactant protein D (SP-D) counteracts the inhibitory effect of surfactant protein A (SP-A) on phospholipid secretion by alveolar type II cells: interaction of native SP-D with SP-A. Biochem J 1991;279:115–119.

180. Botas C, Poulain F, Akiyama J, Brown C, Allen L, Goerke J, Clements J, Carlson E, Gillespie AM, Epstein C, Hawgood S. Altered surfactant homeostasis and alveolar type II cell morphology in mice lacking surfactant protein D. Proc Natl Acad Sci USA 1998;95:11,869–11,874.

181. Liley HG, Hawgood S, Wellenstein GA, Benson, B, White RT, Ballard PL. Surfactant protein of molecular weight 28,000–36,000 in cultured human fetal lung: cellular localization and effect of dexamethasone. Mol Endocrinol 1987;1:205–215.

182. Whitsett JA, Pilot T, Clark JC, Weaver TE. Induction of surfactant protein in fetal lung: effects of cAMP and dexamethasone on SAP-35 RNA and synthesis. J Biol Chem 1987;262:5256–5261.

183. Whitsett JA, Weaver TE, Lieberman MA, Clark JC, Daugherty C. Differential effects of epidermal growth factor and transforming growth factor-beta on synthesis of Mr = 35,000 surfactant-associated protein in fetal lung. J Biol Chem 1987;262:7908–7913.

184. Odom MJ, Snyder JM, Boggaram V, Mendelson CR. Glucocorticoid regulation of the major surfactant associated protein (SP-A) and its messenger ribonucleic acid and of morphological development of human fetal lung in vitro. Endocrinology 1988;123:1712–1720.

185. Boggaram V, Smith ME, Mendelson CR. Regulation of expression of the gene encoding the major surfactant protein (SP-A) in human fetal lung in vitro: disparate effects of glucocorticoids on transcription and on mRNA stability. J Biol Chem 1989;264:11,421–11,427.

186. Boggaram V, Smith ME, Mendelson CR. Posttranscriptional regulation of surfactant protein-A messenger RNA in human fetal lung in vitro by glucocorticoids. Mol Endocrinol 1991;5:414–423.

187. Ballard PL, Gonzales LW, Williams MC, Roberts JM, Jacobs MM. Differentiation of type II cells during explant culture of human fetal lung is accelerated by endogenous prostanoids and adenosine 3′,5′-monophosphate. Endocrinology 1991;128:2916–2924.

188. Acarregui MJ, Snyder JM, Mitchell MD, Mendelson CR. Prostaglandins regulate surfactant protein A (SP-A) gene expression in human fetal lung in vitro. Endocrinology 1990;127:1105–1113.

189. Vanderbilt JN. Analysis of the human SP-A II gene promoter in a cell culture model. Am Rev Respir Dis 1993;147:A250.

190. O'Reilly MA, Gazdar AF, Morris RE, Whitsett JA. Differential effects of glucocorticoid on expression of surfactant proteins in a human lung adenocarcinoma cell line. Biochim Biophys Acta 1988;970:194–204.

191. Nichols KV, Floros J, Dynia DW, Veletza SV, Wilson CM, Gross I. Regulation of surfactant protein A mRNA by hormones and butyrate in cultured fetal rat lung. Am J Physiol 1990;259:L488–L495.

192. Kinnard W, Papst P, Grover F, Fisher JH. Alveolar epithelial cell function in adult lung explants. Am Rev Respir Dis 1993;147:A158.

193. McCormick SM, Mendelson CR. Human SP-A1 and SP-A2 genes are differentially regulated during development and by cAMP and glucocorticoids. Am J Physiol 1994;266:L367–L374.

194. Kumar AR, Snyder JM. Differential regulation of SP-A1 and SP-A2 genes by cAMP, glucocorticoids, and insulin. Am J Physiol 1998;274:L177–L185.

195. Scavo LM, Ertsey R, Gao BQ. Human surfactant proteins A1 and A2 are differentially regulated during development and by soluble factors. Am J Physiol 1998;275:L653–L669.

196. Li J, Gao E, Seidner SR, Mendelson CR. Differential regulation of baboon SP-A1 and SP-A2 genes: structural and functional analysis of 5′-flanking DNA. Am J Physiol 1998;275:L1078–L1088.

197. Phelps DS, Floros J. Dexamethasone in vivo raises surfactant protein B mRNA in alveolar and bronchiolar epithelium. Am J Physiol 1991;260:L146–L152.

198. Seidner S, Ikegami M, Castro R, Cox W, Correll D, Purtell J. Surfactant protein A clearance in normal adult baboons. Am Rev Respir Dis 1993;147:A143.

199. Quirk SJ, Gannell JE, Funder JW. Adrenocorticoid-dependent alpha-lactalbumin synthesis in rat mammary gland explants: antagonist studies. Clin Exp Pharmacol Physiol 1986;13:233–239.

200. Fujimoto M, Berkovitz GD, Brown TR, Migeon CJ. Time-dependent biphasic response of aromatase to dexamethasone in cultured human skin fibroblasts. J Clin Endocrinol Metab 1986;63:468–474.

201. Okret S, Poellinger L, Dong Y, Gustafsson JA. Down-regulation of glucocorticoid receptor mRNA by glucocorticoid hormones and recognition by the receptor of a specific binding sequence within a receptor cDNA clone. Proc Natl Acad Sci USA 1986;83:5899–5903.

202. Gelehrter TD, Sznycer-Laszuk R, Zeheb R, Cwikel BJ. Dexamethasone inhibition of tissue-type plasminogen activator (tPA) activity: paradoxical induction of both tPA antigen and plasminogen activator inhibitor. Mol Endocrinol 1987;1:97–101.

203. Smith CI, Rosenberg E, Reisher SR, Li F, Kefalides P, Fisher AB, Feinstein SI. Sequence of rat surfactant protein A gene and functional mapping of its upstream region. Am J Physiol 1995;269:L603–L612.

204. Chen Q, Boggaram V, Mendelson CR. Rabbit lung surfactant protein A gene: identification of a lung-specific DNase I hypersensitive site. Am J Physiol 1992;262:L662–L671.

205. Kouretas D, Karinch AM, Rishi A, Melchers K, Floros J. Conservation analysis of rat and human SP-A gene identifies 5′ flanking sequences of rat SP-A that bind rat lung nuclear proteins. Exp Lung Res 1993;19:485–503.

206. Alcorn JL, Gao E, Chen Q, Smith ME, Gerard RD, Mendelson CR. Genomic elements involved in transcriptional regulation of the rabbit surfactant protein-A gene. Mol Endocrinol 1993;7:1072–1085.

207. Young SL, Fram EK, Spain CL, Larson EW. Development of type II pneumocytes in rat lung. Am J Physiol 1991;260:L113–L122.

208. Weaver TE, Sarin VK, Sawtell N, Hull WM, Whitsett JA. Identification of surfactant proteolipid SP-B in human surfactant and fetal lung. J Appl Physiol 1988;65:982–987.

209. Bohinski RJ, Huffman JA, Whitsett JA, Lattier DL. Cis-active elements controlling lung cell-specific expression of human pulmonary surfactant protein B gene. J Biol Chem 1993;268:11,160–11,166.

210. Pilot-Matias TJ, Kister S, Fox JL, Kropp K, Glasser SW, Whitsett JA. Structure and organization of the gene encoding human pulmonary surfactant proteolipid SP-B. DNA 1989;8:75–86.

211. Lefstin JA, Yamamoto KR. Allosteric effects of DNA on transcriptional regulators. Nature 1998;392:885–888.

212. Boruk M, Savory JG, Hache RJ. AF-2–dependent potentiation of CCAAT enhancer binding protein beta-mediated transcriptional activation by glucocorticoid receptor. Mol Endocrinol 1998;12:1749–1763.

213. Glasser SW, Korfhagen TR, Bruno MD, Dey C, Whitsett JA. Structure and expression of the pulmonary surfactant protein SP-C gene in the mouse. J Biol Chem 1990;265:21,986–21,991.

214. Glasser SW, Korfhagen TR, Wert SE, Bruno MD, McWilliams KM, Vorbroker DK, Whitsett JA. Genetic element from human surfactant protein SP-C gene confers bronchiolar-alveolar cell specificity in transgenic mice. Am J Physiol 1991;261:L349–L356.

215. Rust K, Bingle L, Mariencheck W, Persson A, Crouch EC. Characterization of the human surfactant protein D promoter: transcriptional regulation of SP-D gene expression by glucocorticoids. Am J Respir Cell Mol Biol 1996;14:121–130.

# 2

# Fetal Responses to Glucocorticoids

*Alan H. Jobe, MD, PhD*
*and Machiko Ikegami, MD, PhD*

## ANTENATAL GLUCOCORTICOIDS FROM A CLINICAL PERSPECTIVE

This chapter focuses primarily on the 30 years of often conflicting responses of intact fetuses to glucocorticoid exposure following Liggins' observation in 1969 that antenatal glucocorticoids induced early lung maturation in preterm sheep *(1)*. Although the emphasis is on the surfactant system, other effects of glucocorticoid treatments on the fetal lung need to be discussed to dissociate them from effects on the surfactant system. The use of antenatal glucocorticoids is now routine for fetuses at risk of preterm delivery *(2)*. A clinical perspective on the efficacy of antenatal glucocorticoids in humans is useful to focus the interpretation of the experimental data on the important clinical questions.

Following the initial randomized controlled clinical trial of antenatal betamethasone to decrease the incidence of respiratory distress syndrome (RDS) published in 1972 *(3)*, 14 other randomized and controlled trials were included in a metaanalysis in 1995 *(2)*. Antenatal glucocorticoids decrease the incidence of RDS and death by about 50%. The benefits seem to occur at very early gestational ages, but there are limited clinical data on this point. There may be benefit for glucocorticoid treatment to delivery intervals of less than 24 h, although the 0-to 24-h interval has not been examined as to the minimal interval for effects on the incidence of RDS. There are minimal data suggesting that the beneficial effects of antenatal glucocorticoids may be lost if the treatment to delivery interval extends beyond 7 to 10 d *(4)*. Although repetitive courses of antenatal glucocorticoids are frequently used, there are no randomized and controlled trials evaluating the safety or efficacy of this approach.

From: *Contemporary Endocrinology: Endocrinology of the Lung: Development and Surfactant Synthesis*
Edited by: C. R. Mendelson © Humana Press Inc., Totowa, NJ

Liggins *(1)* proposed that the beneficial effect of antenatal glucocorticoids to decrease RDS resulted from early induction of surfactant synthesis, because the contemporary research at the time showed a close link between RDS and surfactant deficiency *(5)*. Although not supported by a number of reports *(6)*, the concepts that RDS is the result primarily of surfactant deficiency and that the primary effect of antenatal glucocorticoids is induction of surfactant synthesis continue to be generally accepted. A goal of this chapter is to develop the thesis that glucocorticoid effects on the fetus and the fetal lung are much more complex.

Although antenatal glucocorticoid treatments are a major therapeutic benefit for the fetus at risk of preterm delivery, the clinical data also provide indications of the complexities of fetal responses *(2)*. From the evolutionary perspective, the responses of the fetal lung to elevated glucocorticoids are a survival strategy to a stress signal that may protect the fetus if preterm delivery occurs. However, fetal growth restriction, premature rupture of membranes and preeclampsia can severely stress the fetus without causing early lung maturation *(7–9)*. Antenatal glucocorticoids also are not uniformly effective because optimal treatment will decrease the incidence of RDS by about 50% *(2)*. Repetitive courses of antenatal glucocorticoids may not further decrease the incidence of RDS *(10)*. Why are some fetuses apparently resistant to glucocorticoid stimulation of lung maturation? The fetal lung at 12–20 wk gestation is in glandular and then in canalicular developmental stages without terminal air spaces or a mature airway epithelium. Following explant into organ culture, the human fetal lung will develop a mature epithelium with typical type II cells, intracellular lamellar bodies, and surfactant proteins within a few days *(11,12)*. Although this process can be hastened with glucocorticoids, the rapid terminal differentiation of the lung occurs without glucocorticoids at an early point in gestation when maturation of the surfactant system does not normally occur. Is something promoting fetal lung growth and interfering with glucocorticoid responsiveness in vivo? These are clinically derived questions for which there are no answers.

## GLUCOCORTICOID EFFECTS ON THE FETAL LUNG

### *Rodents and Rabbits*

Following Liggins' observations of better aeration of the lungs of lambs that delivered prematurely after 2 to 4 d of fetal abdominal infusions of cortisol *(1)*, Kotas and Avery *(13)* demonstrated in 1971 that a combined fetal intramuscular (IM) and intraperitoneal injection of 9-fluoroprednisolone (equivalent to 75–100 mg/kg cortisol) increased lung gas volumes and deflation stability of preterm rabbit lungs. Kikkawa et al. *(14)* gave intraperitoneal and amniotic cortisol (dose estimate of about 60 mg/kg) to fetal rabbits and described early maturation of the pulmonary epithelium with anatomic evidence of surfactant production. Neither study reported fetal growth restriction after fetal glucocorticoid treatments. Kotas and colleagues *(15)* found that about 120 mg/kg cortisol given by fetal injection decreased lung cell number but did not decrease birth weight in rabbits. These early studies of direct fetal therapy are of interest because fetal growth effects of glucocorticoids were not found, despite very high doses of glucocorticoids.

Multiple investigators have consistently noted fetal growth restriction and lung maturation after maternal glucocorticoids in rodents and rabbits *(16)*. In an early and thorough study, Kauffman *(17)* reported in 1977 that low-dose maternal dexamethasone caused increased airspace volume density and no growth restriction in fetal mice. At higher doses, dexamethasone caused growth restriction and increases in lamellar bodies in type II cells. The increased airspace volume density was detected within 14 h of fetal dexamethasone exposure, while the effects on type II cells required 24 h. This anatomic study was important because it separated the more rapid changes in airspace volume from the delayed appearance of indicators of surfactant induction. The airspace components of maturation also were separated from glucocorticoid induced fetal growth restriction in mice at low doses. We and others subsequently found that in fetal rabbits the major effects of maternal glucocorticoids were increased lung gas volumes that correlated with improved compliances and decreased plasma to alveolar albumin leaks after preterm delivery and ventilation (18,19). However, the fetal rabbits had no increase in alveolar or lung surfactant phospholipid pools at gestational ages from 27 d to term at 31 d (20). Low-dose maternal glucocorticoids caused fetal growth restriction without improved postnatal lung function (21). Enhanced lung maturation could not be demonstrated in preterm rabbits without concomitant growth restriction (22). By contrast, Snyder et al. (23) found that maternal betamethasone caused not only an increase in airspace volume but an increase in type II cell number, phospholipid synthesis, and SP-A but with no effects on lamellar body volume density. Interpretation of these and other studies of antenatal glucocorticoid effects on the preterm fetal lung in rodents and rabbits are complicated by the fetal growth effects of maternal glucocorticoids (perhaps not with fetal treatments), the short gestation and rapid fetal growth in these species.

## *Monkeys*

Because of presumed comparability of lung maturation in baboons, monkeys, and humans, the effects of maternal glucocorticoids on fetal lung development were explored. Johnson and his colleagues (6,24,25) reported the effects of timing of maternal glucocorticoids on the fetal monkey lung. Daily antenatal maternal treatments with about 0.3 mg/kg betamethasone for 3 d before preterm delivery increased maximal lung gas volumes almost twofold (6,25). Lung phosphatidylcholine expressed per lung weight increased significantly by about 20%, but surface tensions of lung extracts or deflation stability on pressure–volume curves did not demonstrate enhanced surfactant function. The same dose of betamethasone given for 13 d caused fetal growth restriction and increased lung volumes measured with gas or saline but not physiologic indications of increases in surfactant (6). Subsequent measurements using the 13-d treatment course begun at 120 d gestation again demonstrated fetal growth restriction at preterm delivery at 133 d and at term delivery at 160 d gestation. The lung gas volumes of the glucocorticoid exposed fetuses were higher than controls at 133 d gestation but lower than controls at term (6). The explanation for this result was that the glucocorticoids had an acute effect on the lung to decrease the lung interstitium and to increase airspace but subsequently alveolar number and lung surface area were decreased. The physiologic changes that resulted in induced maturation were interpreted to be primarily changes in lung connective tissue and not the surfactant system (24). Bunton and Plopper (26) extended these initial observations on the effects of glucocorticoids on alveolarization in monkeys. They demonstrated that a high dose of triamcinolone acetonide given for 3 consecutive days in the midpseudoglandular (63–65 d gestation) or midcanalicular (110–112 d gestation) phases of lung development resulted in lungs that appeared more mature because less interstitial tissue was present. However, the alveoli were less numerous and larger, resulting in an "emphysematous" lung. These experiments with monkeys demonstrated large and persistent effects on lung structure, resulting from high-dose and/or prolonged fetal exposures to maternal betamethasone, even at early gestational ages. By contrast in a study focused on the surfactant system, Kessler et al. *(27)* treated pregnant monkeys with 0.2 mg/kg daily dexamethasone for 3 d before delivery and ventilation of the preterm monkeys. The antenatal glucocorticoid exposed animals had less severe respiratory distress syndrome and multiple indications of increased surfactant in the lung tissue and alveolar lavages. A recent report from Edwards et al. *(28)* did not demonstrate improved postnatal lung function of preterm monkeys after antenatal glucocorticoid treatments or increased surfactant. We found no effects of fetal or maternal treatments on postnatal lung function or on postnatal surfactant metabolism of premature baboons *(29,30)*. However, the high levels of maternal cortisol that resulted from handling the animals crossed into the fetal circulation, which may have masked any effects of the antenatal treatments. These experiments in primates demonstrated that antenatal glucocorticoids even at early gestational ages had profound effects on lung anatomy. However, consistent maturational effects of antenatal glucocorticoids on the surfactant system have not been reported in primates.

## *Sheep*

Following Liggins' initial report of improved lung aeration in lambs that delivered prematurely after an intraabdominal infusion of cortisol *(1)*, Taeusch and coworkers *(31)* used a long acting preparation of methylprednisolone (about 20 mg/kg) given intramuscularly to the surgically exposed fetus and reported preterm delivery within 85 h but no increase in fetal lung volumes or surface tensions. The explanation for no fetal lung response was not evident. Subsequently Mescher et al. *(32)* measured the amount of surfactant in tracheal fluid from 120 d gestation to term (term is 150 d) and found that surfactant increased before the normal large increase in endogenous cortisol before term. This result suggested that endogenous glucocorticoids were not responsible for the normal increases in surfactant before delivery. Hypophysectomy in sheep did delay lung maturation, an effect that was reversed by ACTH or cortisol *(33)*, demonstrating that some cortisol was required for lung maturation. Platzker et al. *(34)* found that intraperitoneal dexamethasone (about 0.2 mg/kg fetal weight) increased the amount of surfactant in tracheal fluid about 13-fold from before 120 d gestation to 134 d gestation, demonstrating that glucocorticoids could increase surfactant at quite early gestational ages.

More recent reports make a consistent interpretation of the lung maturational effects of glucocorticoids difficult. Schellenberg et al. *(35)* evaluated lung maturation after fetal cortisol, epinephrine, $T_3$, and epidermal growth factor infusions separately and in combination for 84 h. The only single agent to increase lung gas volume was cortisol (1 mg/kg · h infusion), although there were no increases in lung tissue or alveolar phospholipids after delivery at 127 d gestation. A subsequent report from the same group found no effect of fetal cortisol infusions on lung gas volumes or surfactant phospholipids *(36)*. By contrast, Warbarton et al. *(37)* found that 48 h cortisol infusions (0.45 mg/kg · h) followed by delivery at about 132 d gestation resulted in large effects — lung gas volume and lung tissue saturated phosphatidylcholine almost doubled, and alveolar saturated phosphatidylcholine increased threefold. Ikegami et al. *(38)* reported yet another pattern of lung responses in catheterized fetal sheep infused with 0.75 mg/kg · h cortisol for 60 h before preterm delivery at 128 d gestation. Lung and alveolar-saturated phosphatidylcholine and alveolar SP-A did not increase, but lung compliance increased almost twofold, lung gas volumes measured by static pressure–volume curves doubled, and the vascular to alveolar leak of albumin decreased. This series of reports demonstrated that both lung volume increases and surfactant effects could be found after cortisol infusions, but the responses were not consistent across reports.

This lack of consistency of reponses to glucocorticoids has been explained by type of glucocorticoid, duration, and dose of treatment, and gestational age at treatment. While these and other factors may contribute to the varied responses, the responsiveness of the fetus as a result of its prior history may be the major variable. Most of the research in fetal sheep has utilized surgically placed catheters, and the maternal anesthesia and surgery may alter fetal responsiveness to either endogenous or exogenous hormones. Tabor et al. *(39)* found that an interval from catheterization to cortisol infusion of 4 d before preterm delivery 60 h later at 128 d resulted in improved compliance, but no significant increase in lung tissue or alveolar saturated phosphatidylcholine or alveolar SP-A (Fig. 1). By contrast, an interval of 11 d from catheterization to the initiation of the cortisol infusion resulted in control animals that had compliance values equivalent to the cortisol-treated animals after the 4-d catheterization to treatment interval. The cortisol further augmented compliance, almost doubled alveolar and total lung-saturated phosphatidylcholine, and increased SP-A levels in alveolar wash. Although the mechanisms responsible for altered fetal responses are not known, this study demonstrated that fetal lung responses to the same glucocorticoid treatment varied strikingly.

## *Unstressed Fetal Sheep*

Interpretation of glucocorticoid effects on the fetal lungs is complicated by global fetal growth restriction in rodents and rabbits, by stress of handling and maternal to fetal cortisol transfer in primates, and by the stress of catheter placement in sheep to variable degrees in the different experiments. The responses may represent glucocorticoid effects that are augmented variably by the response state of the fetus. To avoid these problems and to evaluate the pure response of the unstressed fetus to glucocorticoids, Jobe et al. *(40)* gave fetal sheep glucocorticoid injections using an ultrasound-guided intramuscular injection technique that did not alter fetal catecholamine or cortisol levels *(41)*. Sheep were used because the placenta is impermeable to the cortisol, and as farm animals they tolerate handling without undue stress. Betamethasone (0.5 mg/kg) given by intramuscular injection to fetuses as a mixture of the acetate and sodium-phosphate salts caused consistent improvements in postnatal lung function after preterm delivery. The preterm lambs had improved lung compliances, improved gas exchange, a doubling of lung gas volume measured using static pressure–volume curves, and decreased protein losses from the vascular space into the lungs *(40,42)*. These effects on lung physiology after preterm delivery occurred after a 15-h fetal treatment to delivery interval but not within 8 h of fetal treatment *(43)*. The alveolar-saturated phosphatidylcholine pool size was very low at 121–128 d gestation (<1 μmol/kg vs about 100 μmol/kg at term), and no increases were detected for glucocorticoid treatment to delivery intervals less than 7 d *(44)* . By combining measurements from several protocols to permit comparisons of more than 20 glucocorticoid treated and 20 control fetuses for a betamethasone treatment to delivery interval of 48 h, alveolar-saturated phosphatidylcholine increased significantly from 0.9 μmol/kg to 1.8 μmol/kg without a change in saturated phosphatidylcholine in lung tissue *(45)*. This small increase may result from the more efficient lung lavage that was possible because the glucocorticoid exposed lungs were more compliant and had larger gas volumes. Saturated

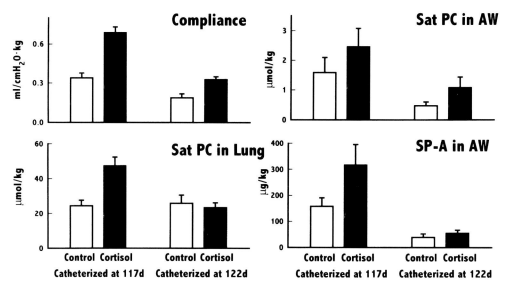

Fig. 1. Effect of time of catheterization on subsequent responses of the fetal lung to 60 h cortisol infusion (0.75 mg/kg · h). Preterm lambs were catheterized at 117 d or 122 d gestation and subsequently randomized to cortisol (0.75 mg/kg · h) or saline infusions for 60 h before preterm delivery at 128 d gestation. The measurements of lung compliance, alveolar saturated phosphatidylcholine (Sat PC in AW) and SP-A (SP-A in AW) were higher for the controls catheterized at 117 d gestation than for the controls catheterized at 122 d gestational age. The increases in compliance, alveolar and tissue Sat PC, and SP-A also were higher in the cortisol-infused fetal sheep catheterized at 117 d gestation. The responses of the fetal lung differed based on interval from catheterization to initiation of the cortisol infusion. (Data from ref. 22.)

phosphatidylcholine in lung tissue was not increased up to 4 d after fetal betamethasone treatment (44). The surfactant proteins SP-A and SP-B do not increase in lung tissue or alveolar washes for treatment to delivery intervals of 48 h or less (46).

Antenatal glucocorticoids given directly to the fetus caused a decrease in alveolar thickness and an increase in aerated parenchyma without a change in alveolar size within 48 h of treatment (47). Type II cells sampled from lungs of lambs that had physiologic responses to betamethasone demonstrated no changes in subcellular organelle volume densities. Low values for lamellar bodies (10% for controls and 12.5% for glucocorticoid treated) and high values for glycogen (28% in controls and 25% in glucocorticoid treated) indicated immaturity of the type II cells (K. Pinkerton, A. H. Jobe, and M. Ikegami, *unpublished observations*). These anatomic results and the subtle or lack of effect of antenatal betamethasone on saturated phosphatidylcholine, SP-A and SP-B pool sizes in alveolar washes and lung tissue demonstrated no physiologically important effects of glucocorticoids on surfactant pools in this animal model.

However, fetal treatments of sheep with glucocorticoids do result in more delayed effects on the surfactant system. When the fetal glucocorticoid treatment to delivery interval was extended to 7 d, the alveolar saturated phosphatidylcholine pool increased about sixfold in one experiment and doubled in another (44,48). The total lung-saturated phosphatidylcholine pools increased by 42%, demonstrating a potent but delayed effect on surfactant phospholipids in lung tissue (49). In other experiments, repetitive maternal glucocorticoid treatments given at 7-d intervals beginning at 104 d gestation resulted in large increases in alveolar and lung tissue saturated phosphatidylcholine as well as increases in alveolar and lung tissue pools of SP-A and SP-B *(46,48)* (Fig. 2). These increases in surfactant components correlated with improved postnatal lung function after preterm delivery. The effects of maternal glucocorticoid treatments on SP-A, SP-B, and SP-C mRNA levels in this in vivo model did not parallel the changes in protein levels *(50)*. The three mRNA species for the surfactant proteins were increased 24 and 48 h after fetal glucocorticoid exposure (when protein levels were unchanged) but had decreased to control levels for a treatment to delivery interval of 7 d.

An unanticipated aspect of the fetal response to antenatal glucocorticoids in sheep was the effect of the route of fetal exposure. Moraga et al. *(51)* found that maternal betamethasone (12 mg IM) given 48 and 24 h before preterm delivery at 125 d gestation doubled lung gas volume but did not significantly increase surfactant phospholipids. This result was similar qualitatively to the effects of fetal glucocorticoid treatment *(40)*. However, when directly compared, using the same dose of 0.5 mg/kg betamethasone based on maternal weight or fetal weight, maternal betamethasone resulted in a larger maturational response of the fetal lungs characterized by better compliances, improved gas exchange, larger lung volumes, and larger increases in saturated phosphatidylcholine after multiple doses given at 7-d intervals *(52)* (Fig. 3). Single or repetitive maternal betamethasone treatments resulted in proportionate fetal growth restriction following preterm delivery at 125 days gestation and at term *(48, 53)*. By contrast, single or repetitive fetal treatments did not cause growth restriction *(52)*, even though fetal betamethasone treatments result in fetal plasma levels about threefold higher than fetal plasma betamethasone levels after maternal treatments *(54)*. In this model the acute physiological lung maturational responses and the delayed increases in surfactant occurred without fetal growth restriction, disassociating these two glucocorticoid effects on the fetal sheep.

## ALTERATIONS OF GLUCOCORTICOID FUNCTION
## IN TRANSGENIC MICE

Recent experiments designed to alter endogenous glucocorticoid responsiveness in mice provide important insights into lung maturation in vivo. Disruption of the corticosteroid-releasing hormone (CRH) gene resulted in very low plasma corticosterone levels in mice *(55)* (*see* Chapter 7). The mice survived normally but required corticosterone supplementation to reproduce. Fetuses of the mating of CRH–/– mice died after birth of respiratory failure unless supplemental corticosterone was provided to the dam. The lungs were cellular and appeared to have an arrest in thinning of the saccules. The mRNAs for SP-A and SP-B were decreased on 17.5 d, but were similar to wild-type by 18.5 d; other components of the surfactant system that were evaluated appeared to be normal (*see* Chapter 7). Corticosterone supplementation in the water of the dam prevented the delayed lung development, presumably because small amounts of glucocorticoids leaked from dam to fetus. Very low levels of fetal glucocorticoid exposure were sufficient to support normal lung maturation, based on the stressed CRH–/– mice. Therefore, glucocorticoids probably are "permissive" for normal lung maturation, but large increases in fetal glucocorticoid levels are not required. In another model, targeted disruption of the glucocorticoid receptor in mice resulted in delayed anatomic maturation of the lung after about 15.5 d gestation and death after delivery *(56)*. The expression of SP-A, SP-B, and

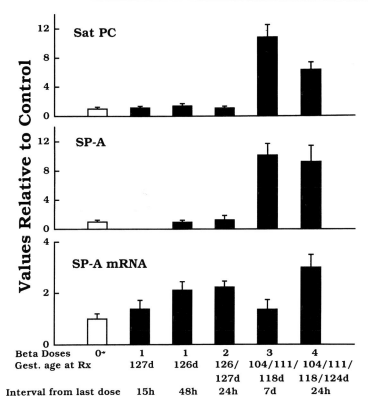

Fig. 2. Changes in saturated phosphatidylcholine (Sat PC), SP-A, and SP-A mRNA following betamethasone treatments. All values are expressed relative to values for saline injected controls. Alveolar Sat PC and SP-A did not increase for the short-term treatment to delivery intervals. Large increases in alveolar Sat PC and SP-A occurred after repetitive treatments. The mRNA for SP-A increased within 48 h of treatment but decreased to control levels even after multiple retreatments unless the last treatment was close to the time of delivery (the 4-dose beta group). (Data from refs. *46* and *51*.)

SP-C genes at birth were normal. These experiments demonstrated that the fetal lung required glucocorticoids to achieve the anatomic maturation characterized by late gestation loss of cellularity and thinning of saccules. There may be no requirement for glucocorticoid for development of the surfactant system, although this point is not clear. Glucocorticoid receptor binding to DNA was not required for normal lung maturation because disruption of the dimerization required for receptor binding to glucocorticoid response elements did not interfere with normal lung development *(57)*.

## A UNIFIED VIEW OF GLUCOCORTICOID EFFECTS ON LUNG MATURATION

In trying to integrate the multiple and often inconsistent observations about fetal lung responses in animals and in clinical practice, we will utilize a Venn diagram that separates glucocorticoid responses into three components — normal lung development, stresses on the pregnancy and the pharmacologic effects of antenatal glucocorticoids (Fig. 4). Normal lung development requires endogenous glucocorticoids at low levels to achieve anatomic maturation *(33,55)*, but the normal increase in endogenous glucocorticoids just before

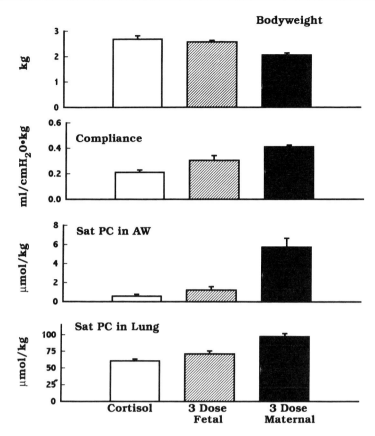

Fig. 3. Effect of fetal or maternal repetitive glucocorticoid treatments on fetal weight, compliance, and saturated phosphatidylcholine (Sat PC) in alveolar washes (AW) and the total lungs of lambs delivered prematurely at 125 d gestation. The dosing schedule was 0.5 mg betamethasone/kg maternal or fetal weight at 104, 111, and 118 d gestation. The fetal doses had less effect on compliance and Sat PC than did the maternal doses. The maternal doses decreased fetal weight. (Data from ref. 53.)

birth are not required for either anatomic maturation or maturation of the surfactant system (32). Although the information is incomplete, glucocorticoids may not be required for normal maturation of the surfactant system. Infants without adrenal function can have normal lung maturation. Transgenic mice with abnormalities in glucocorticoid function demonstrate that the major effects of endogenous fetal glucocorticoids is to permit structural maturation of the lung.

We think the fetal sheep model is the best model to date in which to evaluate glucocorticoid responses on unstressed fetuses. Maternal or fetal routes of exposure of the fetus to betamethasone cause large improvements in postnatal lung function that result from the rapid maturation of alveolar architecture (47,52). High-dose or more prolonged treatments in monkeys and rats can result in permanent alterations in alveolar development that can result in decreased alveolar numbers (6,26,58). In mice, rabbits, sheep, and monkeys the initial effects of antenatal glucocorticoid treatments are on lung anatomy and those effects can occur early in gestation and persist to term.

The fetal lung seems to respond to glucocorticoids primarily with anatomic maturation characterized by a thinning of the interstitium. Collagen may decrease, although

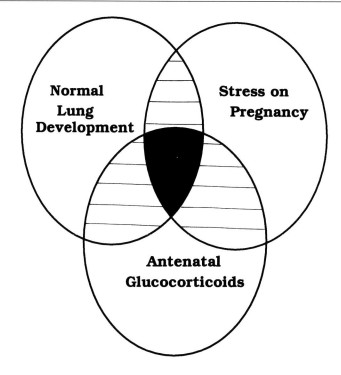

Fig. 4. Venn diagram of factors that can influence fetal lung maturation.

hyaluronan content does not change *(24,59)*. The mechanisms by which glucocorticoids can "accelerate" anatomic maturation are not known but they probably result from glucocorticoid regulation of transcription factors, because disruption of binding of the glucocorticoid receptor to glucocorticoid response elements does not alter anatomic maturation *(57)*. The characteristics of glucocorticoid induced early lung maturation are similar to the normal process of lung maturation in that the primary effect is on anatomic maturation. Increases in surfactant phospholipid pools and the amounts of the surfactant proteins are detectable after about 7 d in fetal sheep and may or may not occur in primates, depending on the experiment *(6,27,46)*. Surfactant proteins and their mRNAs have not been evaluated in primates, but the rapid induction of mRNA levels in sheep followed by a decrease to baseline parallels the reversible increases in SP-A mRNA induced by glucocorticoids in human fetal lung explants *(11,50)*. The more potent maturational responses after maternal than after fetal glucocorticoid treatments in sheep are consistent with the lung maturational response resulting from signals from the mother (placenta). The extreme interpretation of these results is consistent with glucocorticoids not being directly responsible for inducing early maturation of the preterm lung.

Stresses on a pregnancy can modulate both normal lung maturation and glucocorticoid induced early maturation. Large increases in surfactant phospholipids and proteins can occur quickly after glucocorticoid exposure of a stressed fetus *(39)*. In clinical practice, the lecithin : sphingomyelin ratio in amniotic fluid can increase rapidly with fetal stress, perhaps because of elevated glucocorticoid levels *(60)*. Infants with respiratory distress syndrome no doubt often have a combination of lung structural immaturity and surfactant deficiency, and the relative importance of each is not easily evaluated clinically. However, very preterm infants can have quite mature lungs, demonstrating that anatomic maturation and induction of surfactant can occur by 24–25 wk gestation in the human fetus with sufficient fetal stress and/or glucocorticoid exposure. Fetal stress sufficient to cause growth restriction may occur without consistent effects on lung maturation *(9)*. Fetal stress is a nonspecific designation that probably includes multiple mechanisms that contribute to fetal compromise. In both humans and sheep multiple courses of antenatal glucocorticoids (even when associated with growth restriction) can result in a preterm newborn with lung immaturity *(10)*. This result suggests that some fetuses are unresponsive to antenatal glucocorticoids. Explants of human fetal lung at midgestation will "mature" anatomically and mature type II cells will appear within a few days *(11)*. Perhaps maturation is suppressed by a factor(s) that make that lung unresponsive to exogenous glucocorticoids. Many of the inconsistencies in the effects of glucocorticoids on fetal lungs in the literature probably are explained by modulating effects of maternal and/or fetal stress on the glucocorticoid responses of the fetal lung.

Evaluations of fetal lung responses in vivo inevitably provide few answers and raise many questions. However, these integrated responses are important because of their clinical relevance and because they direct investigators toward exploring the mechanisms that are central to the regulation of maturation. A major effort needs to be directed toward understanding how glucocorticoids (or secondary signals perhaps from the placenta) alter lung anatomic development.

## REFERENCES

1. Liggins GC. Premature delivery of fetal lambs infused with glucocorticoids. J Endocrinol 1969;45:515–523.
2. Crowley P. Antenatal corticosteroid therapy: A meta–analysis of the randomized trials — 1972–1994. Am J Obstet Gynecol 1995;173:322–335.
3. Liggins GC, Howie RN. A controlled trial of antepartium glucocorticoid treatment for prevention of RDS in premature infants. Pediatrics 1972;50:515–525.
4. Howie RN, Liggins GC. The New Zealand study of antepartum glucocorticoid treatment. Farrell PM, ed. Lung development. New York: Academic Press, 1982:255–265.
5. Brumley GW, Hodson WA, Avery ME. Lung phospholipids and surface tension correlations in infants with and without hyaline membrane disease and in adults. Pediatr 1967;40:13–19.
6. Johnson JWC, Mitzner W, Beck JC, London WT, Sly DL, Lee PA, Khouzami VA, Cavalieri RL. Long–term effects of betamethasone on fetal development. Am J Obstet Gynecol 1981;141:1053–1061.
7. Hallak M, Bottoms SF. Accelerated pulmonary maturation from preterm premature rupture of membranes: A myth. Am J Obstet Gynecol 1993;169:1045–1049.
8. Friedman SA, Schiff E, Kao L, Sibai BM. Neonatal outcome after preterm delivery for preeclampsia. Am J Obstet Gynecol 1995;172:1785–1792.
9. Tyson JE, Kennedy K, Broyles S, Rosenfeld CR. The small for gestational age infant: Accelerated or delayed pulmonary maturation? increased or decreased survival? Pediatrics 1995;95:534–538.
10. French NP, Hagan R, Evans SF, Newnham, JP. Repeated antenatal glucocorticoid size at birth and subsequent development. Am J Obstet Gynecol 1999;180:114–121.
11. Liley HG, White RT, Benson BJ, Ballard PL. Glucocorticoids both stimulate and inhibit production of pulmonary surfactant protein A in fetal human lung. Proc Natl Acad Sci USA 1988;85:9096–9100.
12. Gonzales LW, Ballard PL, Ertsey R, Williams MC. Glucocorticoids and thyroid hormones stimulate biochemical and morphological differentiation of human fetal lung in organ culture. J Clin Endocrinol Metab 1986;62:678–691.
13. Kotas RV, Avery ME. Accelerated appearance of pulmonary surfactant in the fetal rabbit. J Appl Physiol 1971;30:358–361.
14. Kikkawa Y, Kaibara M, Motoyama EK, Orzalesi MM, Cook CD. Morphologic development of fetal rabbit lung and its acceleration with cortisol. Am J Pathol 1971;64:423–442.
15. Kotas RV, Mims LC, Hart LK. Reversible inhibition of lung cell number after glucocorticoid injection into fetal rabbits to enhance surfactant appearance. Pediatrics 1974;53:358–361.

16. Frank L, Roberts RJ. Effects of low–dose prenatal corticosteroid administration on the premature rat. Biol Neonate 1979;36:1–9.
17. Kauffman SL. Acceleration of canalicular development in lungs of fetal mice exposed transplacentally to dexamethasone. Lab Invest 1977;36:395–401.
18. Gladstone IM, Mercurio MR, Devenny SG, Jacobs HC. Antenatal steroids, postnatal surfactant, and pulmonary function in premature rabbits. J Appl Physiol 1989;67:1377–1382.
19. Ikegami M, Berry D, Elkady T, Pettenazzo A, Seidner S, Jobe A. Corticosteroids and surfactant change lung function and protein leaks in the lungs of ventilated premature rabbits. J Clin Invest 1987;79:1371–1378.
20. Ikegami M, Jobe AH, Seidner S, Yamada T. Gestational effects of corticosteroids and surfactant in ventilated rabbits. Pediatr Res 1989;25:32–37.
21. Sun B, Jobe A, Rider E, Ikegami M. Single dose versus two doses of betamethasone for lung maturation in preterm rabbits. Pediatr Res 1993;33:256–260.
22. Tabor BL, Rider ED, Ikegami M, Jobe AH, Lewis JF. Dose effects of antenatal corticosteroids for induction of lung maturation in preterm rabbits. Am J Obstet Gynecol 1991;164:675–681.
23. Snyder JM, Rodgers HF, Obrien JA, Mahli N, Magliato SA, Durham PL. Glucocorticoid effects on rabbit fetal lung maturation in vivo – an ultrastructural morphometric study. Anat Rec 1992;232:133–140.
24. Beck JC, Mitzner W, Johnson JWC, Hutchins GM, Foidart J, London WT, Palmer, AE, Scott, R. Betamethasone and the Rhesus fetus: Effect on lung morphometry and connective tissue. Pediatr Res 1981;15:235–240.
25. Johnson JWC, Mitzner W, London WT, Palmer AE, Scott R, Kearney, K. Glucocorticoids and the rhesus fetal lung. Am J Obstet Gynecol 1978;130:905–916.
26. Bunton TE, Plopper CG. Triamcinolone–induced structural alterations in the development of thelung of the fetal rhesus macaque. Am J Obstet Gynecol 1984;148:203–215.
27. Kessler DL, Truog WE, Murphy JH, Palmer S, Standaert TA, Woodrum DE, Hodson WA. Experimental hyaline membrane disease in the premature monkey. Am Rev Respir Dis 1982;126:62–69.
28. Edwards LA, Read LC, Nishio SJ, Weir AJ, Hull W, Barry S, Styne D, Whitsett JA, Tarantal AF, George–Nascimento C, Plopper CG. Comparison of the distinct effects of epiderman growth factor and betamethasone on the morphogenesis of the gas exchange region and differentiation of alveolar type II cells in lungs of fetal Rhesus monkeys. J Pharmacol Exp Ther 1995;274:1025–1032.
29. Seidner SR, Jobe AH, Ikegami M. Surfactant metabolism during BPD development in preterm baboons. Am J Respir Crit Care Med 1997;155:A236.
30. Ervin MG, Seidner SR, Leland MM, Ikegami M, Jobe AH. Direct fetal glucocorticoid treatment alters postnatal adaptation in premature newborn baboons. Am J Physiol 1998;274:R1169–R1176.
31. Taeusch HW, Avery JE, Sugg J. Premature delivery without accelerated lung development in fetal lambs treated with long–acting methylprednisolone. Biol Neonate 1972;20:85–92.
32. Mescher EJ, Platzker ACG, Ballard PL, Kitterman JA, Clements JA, Tooley WH. Ontogeny of tracheal fluid, pulmonary surfactant, and plasma corticoids in the fetal lamb. J Appl Physiol 1975;39:1017–1021.
33. Crone RK, Davies P, Liggins GC, Reid L. The effects of hypophysectomy, thyroidectomy, and postoperative infusion of corticol or adrenocorticotrophin on the structure of the ovine fetal lung. J Dev Physiol 1983;5:281–288.
34. Platzker ACG, Kitterman JA, Mescher EJ, Clements JA, Tooley WH. Surfactant in the lung and tracheal fluid of the fetal lamb and acceleration of its appearance by dexamethasone. Pediatrics 1975;56:554–561.
35. Schellenberg JC, Liggins GC, Manzai M, Kitterman JA, Lee CCH. Synergistic hormonal effects on lung maturation in fetal sheep. J Appl Physiol 1988;65:94–100.
36. Liggins GC, Schellenberg JC, Manzai M, Kitterman JA, Lee CCH. Synergism of cortisol and thyrotropin–releasing hormone in lung maturation in fetal sheep. J Appl Physiol 1988;65:1880–1884.
37. Warburton D, Parton L, Buckley S, Cosico L, Enns G, Saluna T. Combined effects of corticosteroid, thyroid hormones, and β–receptor binding in fetal lamb lung. Pediatr Res 1988;24:166–170.
38. Ikegami M, Polk D, Tabor B, Lewis J, Yamada T, Jobe A. Corticosteroid and thyrotropin–releasing hormone effects on preterm sheep lung function. J Appl Physiol 1991;70:2268–2278.
39. Tabor BL, Lewis JF, Ikegami M, Polk D, Jobe AH. Corticosteroids and fetal intervention interact to alter lung maturation in preterm lambs. Pediatr Res 1994;35:479–483.
40. Jobe AH, Polk D, Ikegami M, Newnham J, Sly P, Kohen R, Kelly R. Lung responses to ultrasound–guided fetal treatments with corticosteroids in preterm lambs. J Appl Physiol 1993;75:2099–2105.
41. Newnham JP, Polk DH, Kelly RW, Padbury JF, Evans SF, Ikegami M, Jobe AH. Catecholamine response to ultrasonographically guided percutaneous blood sampling in fetal sheep. Am J Obstet Gynecol 1994;171:460–465.

42. Rebello CM, Ikegami M, Polk DH, Jobe AH. Postnatal lung responses and surfactant function after fetal or maternal corticosteroid treatment. J Appl Physiol 1996;80:1674–1680.

43. Ikegami M, Polk D, Jobe A. Minimum interval from fetal betamethasone treatment to postnatal lung responses in preterm lambs. Am J Obstet Gynecol 1996;174:1408–1413.

44. Ikegami M, Polk DH, Jobe AH, Newnham J, Sly P, Kohan R, Kelly R. Effect of interval from fetal corticosteroid treatment to delivery on postnatal lung function of preterm lambs. J Appl Physiol 1996;80:591–597.

45. Willet K, Jobe AH, Ikegami M, Polk D, Newnham J, Kohan R, Gurrin L, Sly PD. Postnatal lung function after prenatal steroid treatment in sheep: Effect of gender. Pediatr Res 1997;42:885–892.

46. Ballard PL, Ning Y, Polk D, Ikegami M, Jobe A. Glucocorticoid regulation of surfactant components in immature lambs. Am J Physiol 1997;273:L1048–L1057.

47. Pinkerton KE, Willet KE, Peake J, Sly PD, Jobe AH, Ikegami M. Prenatal glucocorticoid and T4 effects on lung morphology in preterm lambs. Am J Respir Crit Care Med 1997;156:624–630.

48. Ikegami M, Jobe AH, Newnham J, Polk DH, Willet KE, Sly P. Repetitive prenatal glucocorticoids improve lung function and decrease growth in preterm lambs. Am J Respir Crit Care Med 1997;156:178–184.

49. Polk DH, Ikegami M, Jobe AH, Sly P, Kohan R, Newnham R. Preterm lung function after retreatment with antenatal betamethasone in preterm lambs. Am J Obstet Gynecol 1997;176:308–315.

50. Tan RC, Gonzales J, Strayer MS, Ballard PL, Ikegami M, Jobe AH, Possmayer F. Developmental and glucocorticoid regulation of surfactant protein mRNAs in fetal sheep. Pediatr Res 1998;43:55A.

51. Moraga FA, Riquelme RA, Lopez AA, Moya FR, Llanos AJ. Maternal administration of glucocorticoid and thyrotropin–releasing hormone enhances fetal lung maturation in undisturbed preterm lambs. Am J Obstet Gynecol 1994;171:729–734.

52. Jobe AH, Newnham J, Willet K, Sly P, Ikegami M. Fetal versus maternal and gestational age effects of repetitive antenatal glucocorticoids. Pediatrics 1998;102:1116–1125.

53. Jobe AH, Wada N, Berry LM, Ikegami M, Ervin MG. Single and repetitive maternal glucocorticoid exposures reduce fetal growth in sheep. Am J Obstet Gynecol 1998;178:880–885.

54. Berry LM, Polk DH, Ikegami M, Jobe AH, Padbury JF, Ervin MG. Preterm newborn lamb renal and cardiovascular responses after fetal or maternal antenatal betamethasone. Am J Physiol 1997;272:R1972–R1979.

55. Muglia L, Jacobson L, Dikkes P, Majzoub JA. Corticotropin–releasing hormone deficiency reveals major fetal but not adult glucocorticoid need. Nature 1995;373:427–432.

56. Cole TJ, Blendy JA, Monaghan AP, Krieglstein K, Schmid W, Aguzzi A, Fantuzzi G, Hummler E, Unsicker K, Schutz G. Targeted disruption of the glucocorticoid receptor gene blocks adrenergic chromaffin cell development and severely retards lung maturation. Gene Dev 1995;9:1608–1621.

57. Reichardt HM, Kaestner KH, Tuckermann J, Kretz O, Wessely O, Bock R, Gass P, Schmid W, Herrlich P, Angel P, Schütz, G. DNA binding of the glucocorticoid receptor is not essential for survival. Cell 1998;93:531–541.

58. Massaro GD, Massaro D. Formation of pulmonary alveoli and gas–exchange surface area: quantitation and regulation. Annu Rev Physiol 1996;58:73–92.

59. Ikegami M, Wada K, Emerson GA, Rebello CM, Hernandez RE, Jobe AH. Effects of ventilation style on surfactant metabolism and treatment response in preterm lambs. Am J Respir Crit Care Med 1998;157:638–644.

60. Gluck L, Kulovich M, Borer RC, Brenner PH, Anderson GG, Spellacy WN. Diagnosis of the respiratory distress syndrome by amniocentesis. Am J Ob Gyn 1971;109:440–445.

# 3

# Cyclic Adenosine Monophosphate and Glucocorticoid Regulation of Surfactant Protein-A Gene Expression

*Carole R. Mendelson, PhD, Laura F. Michael, PhD, Pampee P. Young, MD, PhD, Jinxing Li, MD, PhD, and Joseph L. Alcorn, PhD,*

### CONTENTS

## INTRODUCTION

Pulmonary surfactant is a developmentally and hormonally regulated phospholipid-rich lipoprotein that is synthesized exclusively by type II cells of the lung alveoli where surfactant is stored as lamellated inclusions termed lamellar bodies. The lamellar bodies are secreted into the lumens of the lung alveoli where they unwind and are transformed into the quadratic lattice structure of tubular myelin. This, in turn, gives rise to a monolayer surface film of surfactant lipids and proteins, which act to reduce surface tension, increase compliance, and prevent alveolar collapse. Prematurely born infants who manifest inadequate surfactant synthesis are at risk of developing respiratory distress syndrome, the leading cause of neonatal morbidity and mortality in developed countries. Surfactant is primarily comprised of phosphatidylcholine (PC). The principal glycerophospholipid is a disaturated form of PC, dipalmitoylphosphatidylcholine (DPPC), which has remarkable surface-active properties (Reviewed in ref. *1*).

Lung surfactant contains four associated proteins: surfactant protein (SP)-A, SP-B, SP-C and SP-D. SP-B and SP-C, are extremely hydrophobic proteins of 79 and 35 amino acids, respectively, that are derived from higher molecular weight precursors by proteolytic processing *(2,3)*. These hydrophobic proteins serve a critical role in adsorption and spreading of the surfactant surface film at the alveolar air–liquid interface *(1)*. Infants born with congenital SP-B deficiency *(4)* and mice with a targeted deletion of the SP-B gene *(5)*

From: *Contemporary Endocrinology: Endocrinology of the Lung: Development and Surfactant Synthesis*
Edited by: C. R. Mendelson © Humana Press Inc., Totowa, NJ

succumb to respiratory distress syndrome because of inadequate surfactant function. In both SP-B-deficient humans and mice, there is incomplete processing of SP-C *(6)*, suggesting a possible role of SP-B in SP-C transport and processing. SP-A and SP-D are members of the collectin subgroup of the C-type lectin family of proteins *(7)* and are comprised of N-terminal collagen-like and C-terminal lectin-like domains. In gene-targeting studies in mice, it was found that SP-D$^{-/-}$ mice develop marked accumulation of surfactant lipids and proteins within the lung alveoli and in alveolar macrophages, suggesting a major role of SP-D in reuptake and metabolism of secreted surfactant *(8,9)*. On the other hand, the lungs of SP-A$^{-/-}$ mice lack tubular myelin and clear *Pseudomonas aeruginosa* and group B streptococci less efficiently than wild-type mice, suggesting a role of SP-A in immune defense within the alveolus *(10,11)*.

Expression of the gene encoding SP-A is essentially lung-specific *(12)*, occuring primarily in alveolar type II cells and to a lesser extent in bronchioalveolar epithelial (Clara) cells of the proximal and distal airways *(13–15)*. In second-trimester human fetal lung, SP-A mRNA and protein also have been detected in nonmucus tracheal and bronchial glands and in isolated cells of conducting airway epithelium *(16)*.

SP-A expression in fetal lung is developmentally and hormonally regulated; SP-A gene transcription is initiated in fetal lung after approx 70% of gestation is completed and reaches maximal levels just before birth *(17)*. The developmental induction of SP-A gene expression in fetal lung is more closely associated with the increase in surfactant glycerophospholipid synthesis and appearance of identifiable type II cells than is the temporal regulation of the genes encoding SP-B, SP-C, and SP-D. SP-A gene expression in fetal lung appears to be regulated by a number of different hormones and factors; retinoids, insulin, growth factors and cytokines, glucocorticoids, and agents that increase formation of cAMP have been reported to serve a role (reviewed in ref. *18*). In this chapter, we focus on the effects of cAMP and glucocorticoids on the regulation of SP-A gene expression. Although, cAMP acts to increase SP-A expression at the level of gene transcription, glucocorticoid actions are far more complex, may be indirect, and appear to involve transcriptional and posttranscriptional mechanisms. We first consider the structure of the SP-A gene(s) and studies of the regulation of SP-A gene expression by glucocorticoids and by hormones and factors that increase intracellular cAMP. We then review recent studies to characterize the response elements that mediate basal and cAMP induction of SP-A gene transcription in type II cells, as well as the transcription factors that bind to these elements and our current understanding of the mechanisms involved in their regulation.

## SURFACTANT PROTEIN-A GENE STRUCTURE

SP-A is encoded by two highly similar genes (SP-A1 and SP-A2) in humans (h) *(19,20)* and baboons (b) *(21)* and by a single-copy gene in mice *(22)*, rats *(23)*, and rabbits *(12,24)*. As is the case for the rabbit SP-A gene *(24)*, SP-A mRNA transcripts encoded by hSP-A1 gene are comprised of sequences contained within 5 exons. By contrast, mRNA transcripts of the hSP-A2 gene are encoded by sequences present in 6 exons *(20)*. By comparison of 5'-flanking and intronic sequences of the bSP-A genes with those of the human, we found one to be more similar to hSP-A1 (bSP-A1) and the other to be more similar to hSP-A2 (bSP-A2). The mRNA transcripts encoded by bSP-A1 are encoded by either 5 or 6 exons, whereas those of the bSP-A2 gene are encoded by 5 exons *(21)*. In the case of all species studied to date, the SP-A proteins are encoded by sequences contained within four exons; either one or two exons encode the 5'-untranslated region.

# EFFECTS OF CYCLIC ADENOSINE MONOPHOSPHATE AND GLUCOCORTICOIDS ON MORPHOLOGIC DEVELOPMENT OF FETAL LUNG AND ON SURFACTANT PROTEIN-A GENE EXPRESSION

The majority of studies of the effects of cAMP and glucocorticoids on morphologic development and on SP-A expression in fetal lung have been carried out using explants of fetal lung maintained in organ culture. Organ culture provides a convenient model system for study of developmental and hormonal regulation of SP-A gene expression in fetal lung; the preservation of tissue architecture and appropriate cellular interactions appear to be essential for the initiation and maintenance of type II pneumonocyte differentiation *(25,26)*. Lung explants from midgestation human abortuses *(27,28)* and 19-or 21-d gestational age fetal rabbits *(29)* differentiate spontaneously when placed in organ culture in serum-free, defined medium. Before culture, the tissue is comprised of small ducts surrounded by abundant connective tissue; the ductular epithelial cells are columnar, filled with cytoplasmic glycogen, and contain no lamellar bodies. Within 2–4 d of organ culture, the ducts enlarge, the amount of connective tissue is decreased, and the epithelium differentiates into recognizable type II cells containing lamellar bodies *(27)*. These changes in morphology are associated with an induction of the levels of SP-A mRNA and protein, which are undetectable in the fetal lung before culture *(30,31)*. In association with these changes in morphology, there is an increase in synthesis of surfactant glycerophospholipids, as well as a marked increase in the specific activity of phosphatidate phosphohydrolase *(27,29)*, a key regulatory enzyme in glycerophospholipid synthesis.

## *Hormonal Regulation of Morphologic Development of Fetal Lung in Culture*
### Effects of Agents That Increase cAMP on Morphologic Development

Treatment of lung explants with dibutyryl cAMP (Bt$_2$cAMP) causes an enlargement of the prealveolar ducts and accelerates the rate of type II cell differentiation as compared to tissues cultured in control medium *(32)*. These effects of cAMP on morphologic development are apparent only at early time points of culture. After longer periods of incubation, volume densities of type II cells and of the lumens of prealveolar ducts of control explants are increased to levels comparable to those of cAMP-treated tissues *(32)*. The spontaneous differentiation of midgestation fetal lung cultured in control medium may be caused by endogenously produced prostaglandins and other factors that increase cAMP formation.

Human fetal lung in organ culture produces large amounts of prostaglandin E$_2$ (PGE$_2$) *(33)*. Indomethacin treatment of human fetal lung explants causes a marked reduction in PGE$_2$ production, cAMP formation and accumulation of SP-A protein and mRNA *(33)*. Indomethacin also reduces alveolar lumen and lamellar body volume density in the cultured fetal lung explants. The inhibitory effects of indomethacin are prevented by simultaneous incubation with Bt$_2$cAMP or PGE$_2$. These findings suggest that endogenous cAMP formation, induced by increased PGE$_2$ synthesis, causes the spontaneous enlargement of prealveolar ducts and increased SP-A expression by human fetal lung in culture *(33)*. The role of prostaglandins, such as PGE$_2$, in developmental induction of type II cell differentiation and SP-A gene expression in human fetal lung in vivo has not been determined.

In other studies, we also observed that spontaneous differentiation and cAMP induction of SP-A gene expression in the cultured lung tissue is dependent upon the oxygen tension of the environment; at environmental oxygen tensions of ≤5% the effects of

Bt$_2$cAMP on morphology and on SP-A gene expression were abolished *(34)*. Oxygen also plays a permissive role in cAMP regulation of SP-A expression (see below).

The actions of cAMP to increase transcription of a variety of genes are mediated by the activation and binding of the basic-leucine zipper (bZIP) transcription factor, cAMP-response element binding protein (CREB) to a cAMP-response element (CRE). In recent studies, mice homozygous for a targeted deletion of the gene encoding CREB were found to die within 15 min of birth from severe atelectasis *(35)*. The lungs of these animals contained normal levels of the surfactant proteins, SP-A, SP-B, and SP-C; however, SP-D levels in the lungs of CREB$^{-/-}$ mice were only 20% of those of the wild-type mice. Since mice homozygous for targeted deletion of the SP-D gene are viable *(8,9)*, it is unlikely that this decrease in SP-D expression in the CREB$^{-/-}$ contributed to their perinatal mortality.

## EFFECTS OF GLUCOCORTICOIDS ON MORPHOLOGIC DEVELOPMENT

A role for glucocorticoids in lung development was originally suggested by the finding by Liggins *(36)* that cortisol treatment of fetal lambs accelerated fetal lung maturation. Since that initial report, numerous studies have suggested that glucocorticoids enhance lung development and type II cell differentiation. Betamethasone treatment of pregnant rabbits on days 25 and 26 of gestation was found to increase the volume density of presumptive airspace and the proportion of type II cells in the prealveolar epithelium of the fetal lungs on day 27 of gestation *(37)*. The betamethasone treatment also caused a decrease in the volume density of intracellular glycogen and an increase in the volume density of mitochondria in the fetal lung type II cells *(37)*.

The importance of glucocorticoids in lung development was further indicated by findings that corticotropin-releasing hormone (CRH) knockout mice develop cyanosis and die within 24 h of birth *(38)* (*See* Chapter 7). The lungs of the CRH$^{-/-}$ mice manifested an increase in mesenchymal and epithelial cellularity due primarily to increased cell proliferation *(38)*. The finding that mice homozygous for targeted deletion of the glucocorticoid receptor (GR$^{-/-}$) die within several hours of birth as a result of respiratory failure caused by atelectatic underdeveloped lungs *(39)* emphasizes the importance of the GR in lung development. It was suggested that the lack of GR impaired development of the terminal bronchioles and alveoli beyond embryonic day (E)15.5. Of note, however, was the finding of comparable numbers of alveolar type II cells and apparently normal levels of mRNA encoding SP-A, SP-B, and SP-C in lung tissues of newborn GR$^{-/-}$ mice, as compared to heterozygous or wild-type animals *(39)*. The recent report that mice homozygous for a point mutation in the GR that prevents its dimerization and DNA-binding are viable, despite lack of inducibility of a number of GR-regulated genes, suggests that the actions of glucocorticoids to enhance lung development occur through DNA-binding independent mechanisms *(40)*.

We have observed that glucocorticoids have profound effects on morphologic development of midgestation human fetal lung in culture. Dexamethasone has dose-dependent biphasic effects on volume density of alveolar lumen and of type II cells *(41)*. At a concentration of $10^{-10}M$, dexamethasone (Dex) increased both alveolar lumen size and type II cell volume density. By contrast, after incubation with Dex at $10^{-7}M$, both type II cell and alveolar lumen volume densities were significantly decreased as compared to explants incubated in control medium. These biphasic effects of Dex on morphology of the human fetal lung tissue mirror effects on the levels of SP-A mRNA and protein (*see* the Subsection : "Effects of Glucocorticoids on SP-A Gene Expression in Fetal Lung").

## *Effect of cAMP and Glucocorticoids on SP-A Gene Expression*

EFFECTS OF CAMP ON SP-A GENE EXPRESSION IN FETAL LUNG

Cyclic AMP increases expression of the SP-A gene in rabbit, baboon, and human fetal lung tissue in culture. By contrast, the rat *(42,43)* and mouse (J. L. Alcorn and C. R. Mendelson, *unpublished data*) SP-A genes are unresponsive to cAMP. Since we have found that cAMP has a pronounced effect to stimulate promoter activity of the human, rabbit and baboon SP-A genes in transfected rat type II cells in primary culture, *(43–45)*, it is likely that differences in cAMP responsiveness are due to species-specific differences in *cis*-acting regulatory elements, rather than in *trans*-acting factors. In studies using midgestation human fetal lung explants, it was found that the hSP-A2 gene is far more responsive to the inductive effects of cAMP analogs than is the gene encoding hSP-A1 *(46,47)*, whereas both bSP-A1 and bSP-A2 genes appear to be equivalently induced by cAMP treatment *(48)*. Because the sequences of the bSP-A1 and bSP-A2 genes are more similar to each other than those of hSP-A1 and hSP-A2 *(21)*, it is likely that during evolution, divergence of the hSP-A1 gene resulted in a decrease in its responsiveness to cAMP.

The hormones and factors that act by endocrine, paracrine or autocrine mechanisms to increase cAMP formation by type II cells in fetal lung during development have not been defined. β-Adrenergic receptors have been identified in fetal lung tissues *(49)*, and the concentration of β-adrenergic receptors, as well as responsiveness of adenylyl cyclase to catecholamines, have been found to increase in fetal rabbit lung tissue with advancing gestational age *(50)*. The findings that norepinephrine levels in human fetal plasma increase during late gestation and that administration of β-adrenergic agonists as tocolytic agents to women in preterm labor results in a decreased incidence of RDS in their prematurely born infants is further suggestive of a role of the adrenergic system in fetal lung maturation and surfactant synthesis. Our findings that the β-adrenergic agonist, terbutaline, caused a dose-dependent stimulation of SP-A expression in midgestation human fetal lung explants suggests that catecholamines, acting through β-adrenergic receptors, may play a role in the regulation of type II cell differentiation and SP-A gene expression.

Vasoactive intestinal peptide (VIP) is a 28 amino acid neuropeptide produced by nerve endings in the lung *(51)*. In studies using midgestation human fetal lung in culture, we observed that VIP caused a dose-dependent increase in cAMP formation and in SP-A mRNA levels (V. Boggaram and C. R. Mendelson, *unpublished observations*). These findings suggest that VIP may play a paracrine role in the regulation of SP-A gene expression by type II cells through cAMP-mediated mechanisms.

As noted above, studies from our laboratory indicate that human fetal lung in organ culture produces large quantities of prostaglandin $E_2$ (PGE$_2$) and prostacyclin (PGI$_2$) *(33)*. Treatment of the human fetal lung explants with indomethacin markedly reduced cAMP formation by the cultured fetal lung tissue and blocked the spontaneous induction of SP-A gene expression *(33)*. The findings that treatment of the cultured fetal lung tissue with PGE$_2$ increased cAMP formation, and that PGE$_2$ or Bt$_2$cAMP had the capacity to overcome the inhibitory effect of indomethacin on SP-A gene expression, are suggestive that endogenous prostaglandins acting through cAMP may serve a role in the spontaneous differentiation of midgestation human fetal lung in culture *(33)*.

EFFECTS OF GLUCOCORTICOIDS ON SP-A GENE EXPRESSION IN FETAL LUNG

Consistent with their effects on morphologic development of human fetal lung in culture, glucocorticoids have dose-dependent, biphasic effects on SP-A gene expression that are due to differential effects on SP-A gene transcription and on SP-A mRNA stability. In studies using midgestation human fetal lung explants, we observed that Dex caused a dose-dependent induction of SP-A gene transcription and acted synergistically with $Bt_2cAMP$ (52,53); however, Dex caused a dose-dependent decrease in the levels of SP-A mRNA and protein and antagonized the stimulatory effect of $Bt_2cAMP$ on SP-A mRNA and protein levels (41). This apparent inhibitory effect of glucocorticoids is due to a dominant action to decrease SP-A mRNA stability (52,53). The inhibitory effects of Dex on SP-A mRNA stability were found to be dose-dependent, completely reversible and blocked by the glucocorticoid receptor antagonist RU486 (53). In human fetal lung explants cultured in the presence of $Bt_2cAMP$, we found that Dex had a marked effect to reduce the levels of hSP-A2 mRNA, whereas the levels of hSP-A1 mRNA were largely unaffected by glucocorticoid treatment (46). By contrast, Kumar and Snyder (47) reported that in human fetal lung explants cultured in the presence of Dex alone, there was an equivalent reduction in the levels hSP-A1 and hSP-A2 mRNA transcripts.

Similar to findings using midgestation human fetal lung, in lung explants from 90, 125, and 140-d gestational age fetal baboons (term = 184 d), Dex also caused a dose-dependent inhibition of SP-A mRNA levels and antagonized the stimulatory effect of $Bt_2cAMP$ (54). By contrast, SP-A mRNA, which was found to be present at relatively high levels in lung tissues of 160-and 174-d fetal baboons before culture, was essentially unaffected by incubation with $Bt_2cAMP$ or Dex (54). These findings suggest that with increased lung maturation and the developmental induction of SP-A gene expression, there is a decrease in responsiveness of the fetal lung to the stimulatory effects of cAMP and the inhibitory effects of glucocorticoids on SP-A gene expression.

In fetal rabbit lung, glucocorticoids have both inhibitory and stimulatory effects on SP-A gene transcription that appear to be related to the state of differentiation of the fetal lung tissue. Treatment of lung explants from 21-d fetal rabbits with cortisol or Dex ($10^{-7}M$) caused an acute (6–24 h) inhibition of SP-A gene transcription and reduced the magnitude of the stimulatory effect of $Bt_2cAMP$ (55). However, after 48–72 h of incubation, a stimulatory effect of glucocorticoid was observed and there was found to be an additive effect with $Bt_2cAMP$ on SP-A gene transcription (55). We suggest that these differentiation-related changes in glucocorticoid responsiveness may be related to changes in chromatin structure accompanying cellular differentiation that could render glucocorticoid-responsive enhancer (GRE) elements accessible to trans-acting factors (e.g., the glucocorticoid receptor). Maternal administration of synthetic glucocorticoids also has been reported to increase SP-A gene expression in lung tissues of fetal rabbits (56) and rats (57). In rats, Dex appears to have the greatest effect to stimulate SP-A gene expression during the glandular phase of lung development (57).

Despite the well-documented actions of glucocorticoids on SP-A gene expression in cultured lung tissues and in animals, the physiologic role of endogenous glucocorticoids in the regulation of SP-A gene expression in fetal lung is unclear in regard to findings in mice homozygous for targeted disruption of the glucocorticoid receptor (GR) gene (39). As discussed above, $GR^{-/-}$ mice die shortly after birth as a result of respiratory distress (39). However, the lungs of newborn $GR^{-/-}$ mice contained comparable numbers of alveolar type II cells and apparently normal levels of mRNA encoding SP-A, SP-B, and SP-C, as compared to heterozygous or wild-type animals (39). It was suggested that the respiratory failure of the $GR^{-/-}$ neonates was not due to inadequate development of the surfactant system, but rather to decreased expression of the glucocorticoid-responsive amiloride-sensitive epithelial Na$^+$ channel (ENaC), which normally is induced in alveolar epithelium after E17 in mouse and is essential for lung liquid clearance *(58)*. Since study of the lungs of the GR$^{-/-}$ mice did not include analysis of surfactant synthesis or composition, it remains possible that perinatal mortality of these animals may have been due, in part, to inadequate surfactant glycerophospholipid synthesis and/or secretion.

## MOLECULAR MECHANISMS IN THE REGULATION OF SURFACTANT PROTEIN-A GENE EXPRESSION

As discussed above, cAMP appears to regulate SP-A expression primarily through effects on gene transcription; whereas, glucocorticoids exert effects both at transcriptional and posttranscriptional levels. To identify the genetic elements that mediate transcriptional effects of cAMP and glucocorticoids on SP-A gene expression in fetal lung, we have used transfected type II cells and transgenic mice. Upon identification of critical *cis*-acting elements, the proteins that bind to these sequences have been characterized by a number of techniques, including electrophoretic mobility shift assays (EMSA), antibody supershift EMSA, ultraviolet (UV) crosslinking and expression cloning.

### *Identification of Critical cis-Acting Elements Using Transfected Type II Cells*

In consideration of the fact that the SP-A gene is expressed in a lung-specific manner and selectively in type II cells, we reasoned that reporter gene transfection studies to characterize response elements involved in the regulation of SP-A gene expression should be carried out using type II cells that have maintained phenotypic properties, particularly with regard to SP-A gene expression. Since there are no established lung cell lines that have retained the majority of type II cell characteristics, we devised a method for primary monolayer culture of type II cells isolated from rat, rabbit, mouse, and human fetal lung *(59)*. The lung cells contain osmiophilic lamellar inclusions with the ultrastructural characteristics of lamellar bodies and continue to express the SP-A gene at elevated levels for up to 3 wk of culture *(59)*. To functionally define the *cis*-acting elements required for cAMP and glucocorticoid regulation of SP-A promoter activity, fusion genes were constructed comprised of various amounts of 5'-flanking DNA from the rabbit, human, and baboon SP-A genes linked to the human growth hormone (hGH) structural gene, as reporter. Since the type II cells are resistant to conventional methods of DNA transfection, the fusion gene constructs were incorporated into a replication-defective human adenovirus vector (Ad5) and introduced into the type II cells by infection *(43)*. This results in highly efficient and reproducible transfection of fusion gene constructs. SP-A promoter activity is analyzed by radioimmunoassay of hGH protein secreted into the culture medium over each 24-h period for 5 d.

#### CHARACTERIZATION OF RESPONSE ELEMENTS REQUIRED FOR BASAL, cAMP, AND GLUCOCORTICOID REGULATION OF EXPRESSION

To begin to functionally define the genomic regions that regulate SP-A promoter activity, fusion genes were constructed comprising of -1766, -991, -378, and -47 bp of DNA flanking the 5'-end of the rabbit SP-A gene, the transcription initiation site, and 20 bp of exon I linked to the hGH structural gene, as reporter. These were incorporated into the genome of the replication-defective human adenovirus and introduced into rat type II cells by infection. In type II cells transfected with SP-A$_{-1766}$:hGH and SP-A$_{-991}$:hGH fusion genes, hGH production was induced approx 40- and 20-fold, respectively, by Bt$_2$cAMP (1m$M$) (Fig. 1). When type II cells were transfected with the SP-A$_{-378}$:hGH fusion gene, basal levels of expression were reduced by >50%, as compared to SP-A$_{-991}$:hGH; however, Bt$_2$cAMP caused an 11-fold increase in hGH production. In type II cells transfected with the SP-A$_{-47}$:hGH fusion gene, basal levels of hGH production were essentially undetectable and no stimulatory effect of Bt$_2$cAMP was apparent *(43)*. We observed that Dex (10$^{-7}M$), which had little effect when added alone, caused a 65% inhibition of cAMP-induced expression of SP-A$_{-1766}$:hGH, SP-A$_{-991}$:hGH and SP-A$_{-378}$:hGH fusion genes (Fig. 1). This inhibitory effect of Dex was unanticipated, because as discussed previously, we have found that Dex increases transcription of the endogenous SP-A gene in rabbit lung explants, and has an additive stimulatory effect with Bt$_2$cAMP *(55)*. In the cell transfection studies, we observed that the inhibitory effect of Dex on cAMP induction of SP-A$_{-1766}$:hGH expression was dose-dependent; half-maximal inhibition was observed at a Dex concentration of $8 \times 10^{-10}M$, similar to the $K_d$ for binding of Dex to the GR (Fig. 2A). The finding that this inhibitory action of Dex was blocked by the GR antagonist RU486 (Fig. 2B) *(43)* suggests an action of the GR to antagonize the cAMP induction of SP-A:hGH expression in transfected type II cells.

The mechanism(s) whereby glucocorticoids exert this inhibitory effect on cAMP induction of SP-A promoter activity has not been determined. Based on sequence analysis of the rabbit SP-A gene and surrounding genomic regions, we have been unable to find a palindromic glucocorticoid response element (GRE, AGAACAnnnTGTTCT) *(60)* within 3.0 kb of 5'-flanking DNA, or within the structural gene; however, we found two sequences with homology to GRE half-sites at -150 and -190 bp and two other GRE half-sites within the first intron. It is evident from the above-mentioned studies that the GRE half-sites at -150 and -190 bp do not function as stimulatory GREs. To determine whether one or both of the GRE-like sequences within the first intron could serve as a functional GRE, an SP-A:hGH fusion gene containing 991 bp of SP-A 5'-flanking DNA, the first exon, intron and part of the second exon of the rabbit SP-A gene linked to hGH (SP-A$_{-991+670}$:hGH) was constructed and transfected into rat type II cells. Again, we found that Dex caused a marked inhibition of cAMP induced SP-A$_{-991+670}$:hGH expression *(43)*. These findings suggest that the stimulatory effect of glucocorticoids on expression of the endogenous SP-A gene may be mediated by sequences that lie far upstream, within the SP-A structural gene downstream of the first exon, or within the 3'-flanking sequence. In the absence of a functional GRE within the fusion gene constructs, we postulate that the GR may either interact with a transcription factor(s) that mediates cAMP stimulation and inhibit its function, or else, compete for coactivators essential for cAMP induction of SP-A promoter activity. As a consequence of the perceived complexity of glucocorticoid regulation of SP-A gene expression, we subsequently have focused our studies on defining the mechanisms whereby cAMP regulates SP-A gene expression in type II cells.

The pronounced stimulatory effect of cAMP on expression of the SP-A$_{-1766}$:hGH fusion gene was apparent both in rat and human type II pneumonocytes in primary culture. In two lung adenocarcinoma cell lines of presumed type II cell origin, NCI-H358 and A549, which do not express SP-A, there were relatively high levels of basal expression; however, little or no stimulatory effect of cAMP was apparent. By contrast,

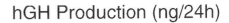

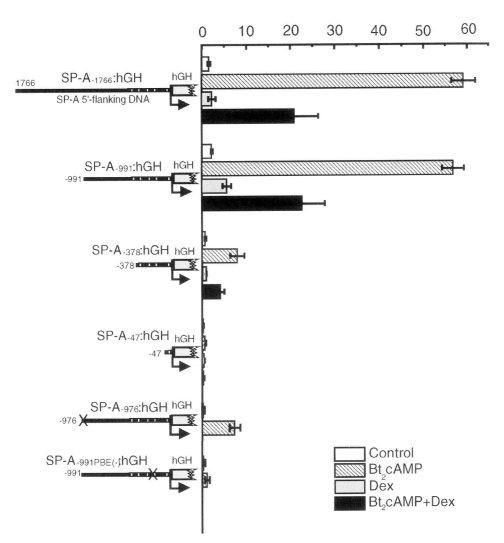

Fig. 1. Expression of rabbit SP-A:hGH fusion genes in rat type II cells cultured in the absence or presence of Bt$_2$cAMP and Dex, added alone and in combination. Rat type II cells were infected with recombinant adenoviruses containing SP-A:hGH fusion genes comprised of 1766, 991, 378 or 47 bp of 5'-flanking sequence from the rabbit SP-A gene linked to the human growth hormone (hGH) structural gene, as reporter. After infection, the cells were incubated in serum-free medium in the absence (Control) or presence of Bt$_2$cAMP (1m$M$), Dex (10$^{-7}M$), or Bt$_2$cAMP+Dex. Expression of an SP-A$_{-976}$:hGH fusion gene, which lacks the distal binding element (DBE) and an SP-A-991(PBE-):hGH fusion gene, containing a mutation in the proximal binding element PBE, also were analyzed in type II cells cultured in the absence or presence of Bt$_2$cAMP. Culture media were harvested and replaced daily. Shown are the levels of hGH that accumulated in the medium over a 24-h period between days 4 and 5 of culture. Values are the mean ± SEM of data from three independent experiments each conducted in triplicate. (Modified from ref. **43**, with permission.)

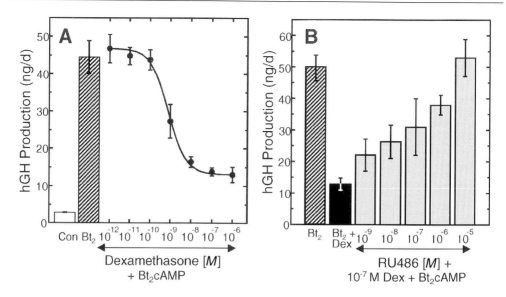

Fig. 2. The effects of Dex and RU486 on expression of SP-A$_{-1766}$:hGH fusion genes in type II cells. **(A)** Rat type II cells transfected with SP-A$_{-1766}$:hGH fusion genes were incubated in the absence (Con) or presence of Bt$_2$cAMP (Bt), in the absence or presence of Dex ($10^{-12}$ to $10^{-6}M$). **(B)** Rat type II cells were transfected with SP-A$_{-1766}$:hGH in the presence of Bt$_2$cAMP, or in the presence of Bt$_2$cAMP+Dex in the absence or presence of the glucocorticoid receptor antagonist, RU486, at concentrations from $10^{-9}$ to $10^{-5}M$. Shown are the levels of hGH secreted into the culture medium between days 4 and 5 of culture. Values are the mean± SEM of data from two independent experiments performed in triplicate. (From ref. *43*, with permission.)

in primary cultures of cAMP-responsive ovarian granulosa and thecal cells and in the cAMP-responsive adrenal cell line Y1, basal expression was barely detectable and no stimulatory effect of cAMP was apparent *(43)*. This suggests that cAMP regulation of SP-A gene expression requires the interaction of type II cell-specific transcription factors with tissue-specific enhancers. These cell-specific transcription factors may be reduced in the lung adenocarcinoma cell lines, and absent in the ovarian and adrenal Y1 cells. Alternatively, the H358 and A549 cells may be deficient in some component of the cAMP response pathway.

**E-Boxes That Bind the Basic-Helix-Loop-Helix Zipper Factor Upstream Stimulatory Factor Are Essential for Basal and cAMP Induction of SP-A Promoter Activity in Type II Cells.** By use of electrophoretic mobility shift assays (EMSA), rabbit lung nuclear proteins were found to bind to several elements within the 5'-flanking region of the rabbit SP-A gene; two of these, termed distal binding element (DBE, -986 to -977 bp) and proximal binding element (PBE, -87 to -70 bp), had related core E-box-like sequences (DBE: <u>CACGTG</u>; PBE: <u>CTCGTG</u>) *(61)*. To assess the functional role of the DBE and PBE in the regulation of SP-A promoter activity, SP-A:hGH fusion genes containing deletions or mutations in these regions were introduced into rat type II cells in primary culture. The levels of basal and cAMP-induced expression of SP-A$_{-976}$:hGH fusion genes, which lack sequences containing the DBE, were reduced markedly to levels that were comparable to those observed with SP-A$_{-378}$:hGH fusion genes (Fig. 1). The finding that expression of SP-A$_{-976}$:hGH was stimulated approx 15-fold by Bt$_2$cAMP treatment (as compared to a 22-fold stimulation of SP-A$_{-991}$:hGH), suggests that the DBE serves a more important role as a general enhancer than as a specific enhancer of cAMP regulated expression. To evaluate the functional importance of the PBE, type II cells were transfected with SP-A$_{-991}$:hGH fusion genes containing a mutation of the PBE sequence. Basal expression of SP-A$_{-991PBE(-)}$:hGH was reduced to levels comparable to those of cells transfected with SP-A$_{-47}$:hGH fusion genes, and essentially no stimulatory effect of Bt$_2$cAMP was observed (Fig. 1) *(61)*. It is apparent that the PBE serves a more critical role in basal and cAMP regulation of SP-A promoter activity than does the DBE. Whether this is due to its proximity to the promoter, or its interaction with other transcription factors bound to adjacent response elements, remains to be determined.

To characterize transcription factors that bind to these E-Box motifs, the PBE was used to screen a rabbit fetal lung cDNA expression library; a cDNA insert was isolated that is highly similar in sequence to human upstream stimulatory factor1 (hUSF1), a bHLH-ZIP transcription factor *(62)*. By use of reverse transcriptase PCR, two isoforms of rabbit USF1 (rUSF1a and 1b) mRNAs were identified in fetal rabbit lung and other tissues. The levels of rUSF1 mRNAs reach a peak in fetal rabbit lung at 23-d gestation, in concert with the time of initiation of SP-A gene transcription *(62)*. Binding complexes of nuclear proteins obtained from fetal rabbit lung tissue and isolated type II cells with the DBE and PBE were supershifted by addition of anti-rUSF1 IgG. USF1-binding activity was highly enriched in type II cells as compared with lung fibroblasts. Overexpression of rUSF1s in A549 adenocarcinoma cells positively regulated SP-A promoter activity of cotransfected reporter gene constructs *(62)*. These findings suggest that rUSF1, which binds to DBE and PBE, may serve a key role in the regulation of SP-A gene expression in pulmonary type II cells.

**A CRE-like Sequence That Likely Binds a Member of the Nuclear Receptor Superfamily Is Critical for Basal and cAMP Induction of SP-A Promoter Activity.** The results of deletion mapping studies indicate the 5'-flanking region between –47 and –378 bp is essential for cAMP induction of SP-A promoter activity in transfected type II cells *(43)*. By sequence comparison of this region with the binding site consensus sequences of known transcription factors, a *cis*-acting element was identified at -261 bp with sequence similarity to a cAMP-response element (CRE), and was termed CRE$_{SP-A}$ (TGACCTCA). CRE$_{SP-A}$ differs by one nucleotide from the palindromic consensus CRE (CRE$_{pal}$, TGACGTCA), which is known to bind the cAMP-response element-binding protein (CREB) as a homodimer *(63)*. CREB, which belongs to the basic-leucine zipper (bZIP) superfamily of transcription factors, activates transcription of target genes subsequent to PKA catalyzed phosphorylation at serine 133 *(64)*. CRE$_{pal}$ also interacts with several related, cAMP-responsive members of the bZIP superfamily, namely activating transcription factor-1 (ATF-1) and cAMP-response element modulator (CREM) *(64)*.

To determine the functional role of CRE$_{SP-A}$ in cAMP regulation of SP-A promoter activity, CRE$_{SP-A}$ was mutated either to the CRE$_{pal}$ sequence (TGACGTCA), or to a sequence known to weakly support cAMP induction of gene expression (TGACGACA; CRE[-]) *(65)* in the context of SP-A:hGH fusion genes containing 991 bp of 5'-flanking DNA and 20 bp of exon I from the rabbit SP-A gene *(44)*. In type II cells transfected with SP-A$_{-991}$:hGH fusion genes containing the wild-type CRE (CRE$_{SP-A}$), Bt$_2$cAMP caused a 22-fold increase in reporter gene expression as compared to transfected type II cells maintained in control medium (Fig. 3). By contrast, in cells transfected with the fusion gene containing the CRE(–) sequence, there was a pronounced decrease in basal and cAMP-regulated expression. Surprisingly, in cells transfected with the fusion gene containing CRE$_{pal}$, basal and cAMP-induced hGH production also were markedly reduced as compared to the wild-type

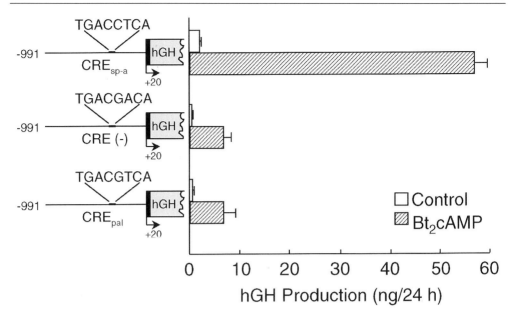

Fig. 3. Effects of mutations in $CRE_{SP-A}$ on expression of SP-A$_{-991}$:hGH fusion genes in type II cells. Rat type II cells infected with recombinant adenoviruses expressing SP-A$_{-991}$:hGH fusion genes containing the wild-type CRE (TGACCTCA), CRE-(TGACGACA), or $CRE_{pal}$ (TGACGTCA) were incubated in the absence or presence of Bt$_2$cAMP for 5 days. Shown are the levels of hGH secreted into the medium over a 24-h period between days 4 and 5 of incubation. Values are the mean ± SEM of data from three independent experiments, each conducted in triplicate. (From ref. *44*, with permission.)

construct (Fig. 3) *(44)*. Together, these findings indicate that cAMP stimulation of SP-A gene transcription is mediated, in part, through this CRE-like sequence and that *trans*-acting factors other than CREB homodimers interact with this element.

This is supported by the finding that bacterially expressed CREB, which binds to $CRE_{pal}$ does not bind to $CRE_{SP-A}$, and antibodies to CREB, CREM and ATF-1 fail to supershift the complex of type II cell nuclear proteins bound to $CRE_{SP-A}$, although they do supershift type II cell nuclear proteins bound to $CRE_{pal}$ *(44)*. Moreover, in competition EMSA using radiolabeled $CRE_{SP-A}$ and fetal rabbit lung nuclear proteins, a purified basic leucine zipper (bLZ) polypeptide failed to compete for binding. By contrast, the bLZ polypeptide competed effectively with $CRE_{pal}$ for lung nuclear protein binding. This finding suggests that leucine zipper transcription factors do not bind $CRE_{SP-A}$. Additionally, expression of a $CRE_{SP-A}$ containing HIS3 fusion gene in yeast was unaffected either by CREB or bLZ polypeptides fused to the GAL4 activation domain. By contrast, HIS3 expression was markedly induced both by CREB and bLZ fusion proteins in a yeast strain in which the HIS3 gene was under control of $CRE_{pal}$ *(44)*. By competition EMSA using radiolabeled $CRE_{SP-A}$ as probe and mutagenized nonradiolabeled $CRE_{SP-A}$ oligonucleotides as competitors, the critical protein-binding nucleotides in $CRE_{SP-A}$ were found to constitute a hexameric element, TGACCT, which corresponds to a half-site for binding members of the nuclear receptor superfamily *(44)*. Since the TGACCT motif is present in the SP-A gene as a single site, we propose that a unique orphan member of the nuclear receptor superfamily may bind to this element as a monomer.

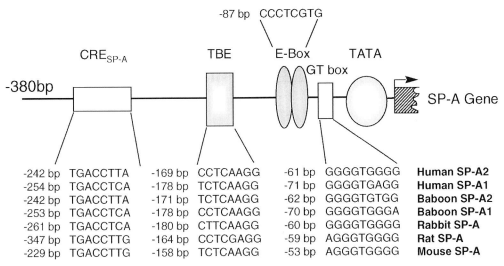

Fig. 4. The SP-A structural gene and 5'-flanking region contains response elements conserved among various species. Sequences and positions of the CRE$_{SP-A}$, TTF-1-binding element (TBE), E-box and GT-box elements relative to the start sites of transcription of the SP-A genes of various species are shown. The position of the TATA box and the start of transcription (denoted by the arrow) are indicated. (Modified from ref. 66, with permission.)

The CRE-like sequence is highly conserved in position and sequence among the SP-A genes of all species that have been thus far characterized (Fig. 4). In cell transfection studies using hSP-A2:hGH fusion gene constructs containing from 47 to 1500 bp of 5'-flanking sequence from the human (h) SP-A2 gene, we found that fusion genes containing 296 bp of hSP-A2 5'-flanking sequence mediated relatively high levels of basal and cAMP-induced expression in primary cultures of lung type II cells (Fig. 5), but not in lung adenocarcinoma cell lines or in other cell types (45). Mutagenesis of CRE$_{SP-A}$ at –242 bp caused a marked reduction in basal and loss of cAMP-induced expression (Fig. 5) (45), suggesting that this element also serves an important role in basal and in cAMP-induced expression of the human SP-A gene. As discussed above, the rat and mouse SP-A genes are not responsive to cAMP. Although the CRE$_{SP-A}$ sequences of the rat and mouse genes are highly conserved, in the case of the rat SP-A gene, the CRE-like sequence is localized approx 100 bp upstream of its localization site in the SP-A genes of humans, baboons, rabbits and mice (Fig. 4). Whether this difference in CRE$_{SP-A}$ localization contributes to the lack of cAMP responsiveness of the rat SP-A gene is not known. However, it should be noted, that cAMP induction of SP-A promoter activity is mediated by cooperative interactions of transcription factors bound to at least four enhancer elements. Therefore, alterations in any one of these, as well as in others yet to be characterized, could be responsible for the lack of cAMP induction of the rat and mouse SP-A genes.

**A GT-Box, Which Binds the Transcription Factor Sp1, Is Crucial for Basal and cAMP Induction of SP-A Promoter Activity.** A GT-box, which also is highly conserved among the SP-A genes of rats, mice, rabbits, baboons, and humans (Fig. 4), is localized approx 40 bp upstream of the TATA box. In the hSP-A2 gene, the GT-box at –61 bp contains the core sequence GGGGTGGGG (GT$_{SP-A}$) (Fig. 4). To examine its role in regulation of hSP-A2 promoter activity, GT$_{SP-A}$ was mutated in the context of the SP-A2$_{-296}$:hGH fusion gene and transfected into type II cells (66). Mutagenesis of GT$_{SP-}$

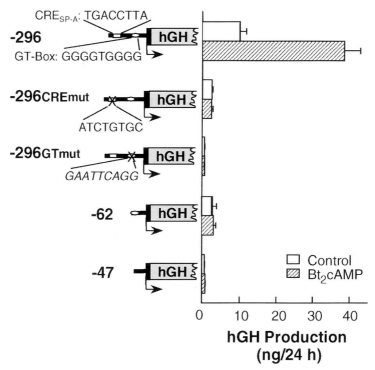

Fig. 5. CRE$_{SP-A}$ and the GT-box of the hSP-A2 gene are essential for cAMP induction of SP-A promoter activity in type II cells. Human type II cells in primary culture were infected with recombinant adenoviruses containing human (h)SP-A2:hGH fusion genes that comprise the 296, 62, and 47 bp of 5'-flanking sequence from the human SP-A2 gene, or with hSP-A2$_{-296}$:hGH containing mutations in CRE$_{SP-A}$ (-296CREmut) or GT$_{SP-A}$ (-296GTmut) and incubated for 5 d in the absence (Control) or presence of Bt$_2$cAMP. Shown are the levels of hGH that accumulated in the medium over a 24-h period between days 4 and 5 of culture. Values are the means ± SEM of data from two independent experiments, each conducted in triplicate. (From ref. 66, with permission.)

$_A$ within the -296 bp fusion gene dramatically reduced basal (by >90%) and abolished cAMP-induced expression (Fig. 5). Expression of SP-A2$_{-296GTmut}$:hGH was similar to that of the minimal promoter construct, SP-A2$_{-47}$:hGH, which lacks the GT$_{SP-A}$ sequence and includes only the TATA motif. Basal expression of the SP-A2$_{-62}$:hGH construct, which just includes GT$_{SP-A}$, was >3-fold higher than the –47 bp minimal promoter construct (Fig. 5). These findings indicate that GT$_{SP-A}$ also is essential for elevated levels of basal and cAMP induction of SP-A2 promoter activity.

By EMSA, it was observed that nuclear proteins isolated from primary cultures of type II cells bound the GT box as five specific complexes. By contrast, nuclear proteins isolated from lung fibroblasts displayed notably reduced binding activity *(66)*. Competition and supershift EMSA indicated that the ubiquitously expressed transcription factor Sp1, a GC box binding protein of approx 100 kDa, is a component of the complex of proteins that bind the GT box of SP-A2 *(66)*. The finding that only two of the five GT box-binding complexes were supershifted by incubation with Sp1 antibody suggests that a factor(s) in type II cell nuclear extracts that is distinct from Sp1 also interacts with the GT box. By UV crosslinking and SDS/PAGE/EMSA analysis, we have identified a approx 55-kDa GT-box binding factor in type II cell nuclear proteins that preferentially binds the GT box of SP-A2 over the consensus Sp1 GC box sequence. This 55-kDa factor was able to bind the GT box independently of Sp1 *(66)*. Sp1 is a ubiquitously expressed member of the Krüppel family of zinc finger-containing transcription factors. Several novel proteins belonging to the Krüppel family have recently been identified, which manifest significantly higher binding activity toward the GT/CA box than does Sp1 *(67)*. We suggest that the 55 kDa factor that interacts with the GT box of SP-A2 may be a new member of this protein family.

**Elements That Bind Thyroid Transcription Factor-1 (TTF-1) Are Essential for cAMP Induction of SP-A Promoter Activity in Type II Cells; Binding and Transcriptional Activation of TTF-1 Are Increased by cAMP-Dependent Protein Kinase.** TTF-1 is a homeodomain transcription factor expressed selectively in developing thyroid, diencephalon, and lung epithelium from the earliest stages of organogenesis *(68)*. Mice homozygous for a targeted deletion of the TTF-1 gene lacked thyroid, anterior pituitary, and lung parenchyma *(69)*, suggesting an important role in morphogenesis of these organs. TTF-1 also appears to play an important role in expression of the genes encoding SP-A *(70,71)*, SP-B *(72,73)*, SP-C *(74)* and Clara cell secretory protein (CCSP) *(75,76)*. By mutagenesis, it was found that the TTF-1 sites in the mouse SP-A gene 5'-flanking sequence were required for basal expression of the SP-A promoter in transfected mouse lung epithelial cells *(70)*. We have identified three TTF-1-binding elements (TBE) within 255 bp of 5'-flanking region of the baboon SP-A2 gene (Fig. 6A) *(48)*. One of these elements (TBE1) at −172 bp is highly conserved with regard to position and sequence among all of the SP-A genes thus far characterized (Fig. 4). In type II cell transfection experiments, we observed that mutagenesis of TBE1 had a more pronounced effect to reduce basal and cAMP-induced expression than mutagenesis of either TBE2 or TBE3 (Fig. 6B) *(71)*.

In studies to define the mechanism(s) whereby TTF-1 mediates cAMP induction of SP-A gene expression in type II cells, we observed that TTF-1 DNA binding activity of type II cell nuclear extracts was increased by cAMP treatment. By contrast, nuclear protein binding activities for $CRE_{SP-A}$ and the GT-box were unaffected by cAMP (Fig. 7) *(71)*. These findings indicate that cAMP specifically increases TTF-1 binding activity in type II cells. Our findings that the levels of immunoreactive TTF-1 in nuclear extracts, as well as the rate of incorporation of [$^{35}$S]methionine into immunoisolated TTF-1 were unaffected by cAMP treatment of type II cells *(71)*, suggest that cAMP induction of TTF-1 binding activity is not mediated by changes in its nuclear localization or expression. In association with its effect to stimulate TTF-1 DNA binding activity, we observed that cAMP treatment markedly increased the rate of [$^{32}$P]phosphate incorporation into immunoisolated TTF-1 *(71)*. The finding that phosphatase treatment effectively abolished the cAMP induction of TTF-1 DNA binding activity indicates that cAMP-induced TTF-1 phosphorylation mediates the increase in binding activity for TBEs within the bSP-A2 5'-flanking sequence *(71)*. A PKA phosphorylation site near the N-terminus (Thr$^9$) of TTF-1 was identified and found to be essential for PKA activation of the SP-B promoter in H441 cells *(76)*.

To analyze effects of PKA on TTF-1 transcriptional activity, A549 cells, a lung adenocarcinoma cell line which lacks TTF-1, were cotransfected with a bSP-A2$_{-255}$:hGH fusion gene (which contains 3 TBEs), and with expression vectors for TTF-1, and for PKA catalytic (PKA-cat) subunits α and β (Fig. 8A). Cotransfection of TTF-1 caused an induction of bSP-A2 promoter activity. The response to TTF-1 was increased further by cotransfection of PKA catalytic subunits. The finding that PKA-cat had no effect to increase bSP-A2 promoter activity in the absence of cotransfected TTF-1 and that mutation of the major TTF-1 binding site abolished PKA induction of TTF-1 transcrip-

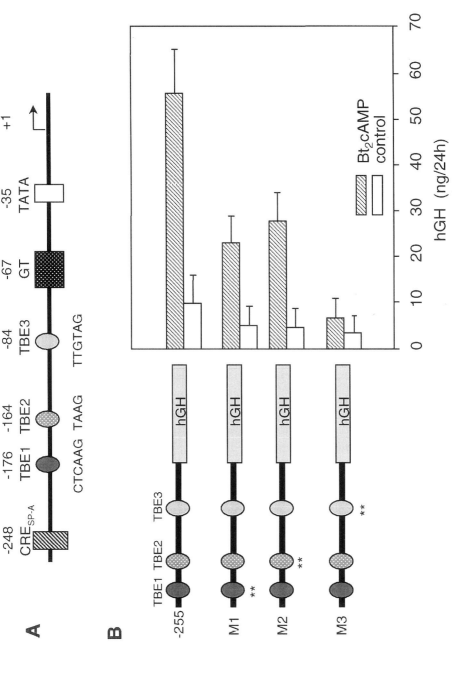

Fig. 6. TTF-1 binding elements (TBE) mediate basal and cAMP induction bSP-A2 promoter activity in type II cells. (**A**) Schematic diagram of the baboon (b) SP-A2 gene 5'-flanking region (−255 to 40 bp) showing the locations and core sequences of three TTF-1 binding elements (TBE) and of CRE$_{SP-A}$ and the GT-box. (**B**) Expression of bSP-A2$_{-255}$:hGH fusion genes with and without mutations in TBE1, TBE2, and TBE3 (M1, M2, M3, respectively) in rat fetal lung type II cells maintained in the absence or presence of Bt$_2$cAMP. After infection, the cells were incubated for up to 5 d in serum-free medium in the absence or presence of Bt$_2$cAMP. Shown are the concentrations of hGH that accumulated in the medium between days 4 and 5 of culture. Values are means ± SEM of data from two independent experiments, each conducted in triplicate. (From ref. *48*, with permission.)

74

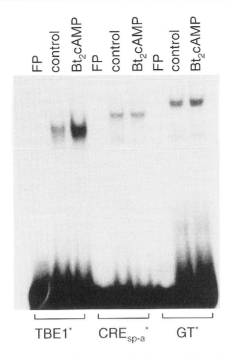

Fig. 7. cAMP treatment of type II cells increases binding activity of nuclear proteins for the TBE1, but not for $CRE_{SP-A}$, or the GT-box. Nuclear proteins from human fetal type II cells cultured for 5 d in control or $Bt_2cAMP$ (1m$M$)-containing medium were incubated with $^{32}$P-labeled TBE1, $CRE_{sp-a}$ and GT-box-containing oligonucleotides and analyzed by EMSA. FP; free probe. (From ref. 71, with permission.)

tional activity (71) suggests that the effect of PKA to induce bSP-A2 gene expression is mediated, in part, through TTF-1. We also have observed that the TTF-1 induction of bSP-A2$_{-255}$:hGH fusion gene expression in the absence of co-transfected PKA-cat was prevented by cotransfection of a dominant negative form of PKA RI$\alpha$ (71). This suggests that the inductive effect of TTF-1 on bSP-A2 promoter activity in A549 cells is dependent on phosphorylation by endogenous PKA. To further substantiate the role of TTF-1 in PKA induction of SP-A promoter activity, A549 cells transfected with a reporter gene containing three tandem TBEs fused upstream of the bSP-A2 gene TATA box and transcription initiation site (TBE$_3$SP-A2:hGH) were cotransfected with PKA-cat and TTF-1 expression vectors (Fig. 8B). The finding that PKA-cat enhanced transactivation of TBE$_3$SP-A:hGH by cotransfected TTF-1 indicates that the effect of PKA to increase SP-A promoter activity is mediated specifically by TTF-1 binding to TBEs. These findings, together with those that indicate that cAMP specifically increases TTF-1 binding activity in type II cells, suggest that TTF-1 is the cAMP-responsive transcription factor in lung type II cells.

## CONCLUSIONS

The results of our cell transfection studies indicate that conserved response elements within 400 bp upstream of the rabbit, human and baboon SP-A genes mediate elevated basal and cAMP-induced expression in lung type II cells. These response elements include a CRE-like sequence, which may bind a member of the nuclear receptor superfamily ($CRE_{SP-A}$), several TTF-1 binding sites, an E-box, that binds the transcription factor

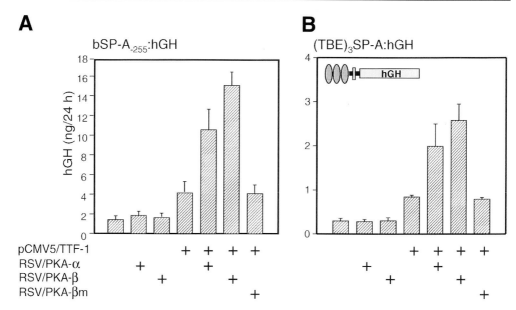

Fig. 8. PKA increases TTF-1 transcriptional activity in transfected A549 cells. A549 cells were cotransfected with either with bSP-A2$_{-255}$:hGH (**A**) or with a (TBE)$_3$SP-A2:hGH fusion gene comprised of three tandem copies of TBE1 fused to a basal bSP-A2 promoter linked to hGH, as reporter (**B**) in the absence or presence of a TTF-1 expression vector (pCMV5/TTF-1) or pCMV5 empty vector, and either with expression vectors for PKA catalytic subunit-α (RSV/PKA-cat-α), PKA catalytic subunit β (RSV/PKA-cat-β), a mutated form of PKA catalytic subunit β (RSV/ PKA-cat-βm), or the corresponding empty vector pRSV, plus internal control, RSV-βgal. The levels of hGH secreted into the medium are shown over a 24-h period, 48 h after transfection. Data are the means ± SEM from two independent experiments, each conducted in triplicate, normalized to β-galactosidase activity. (From ref. *71*, with permission.)

USF1, and a GT-box which binds Sp1 along with other proteins that may be tissue-selective members of the Krüppel family of transcription factors (Fig. 4). Each one of these elements appears to be essential for cAMP induction of the SP-A promoter, suggesting a cooperative interaction of the proteins that bind to these elements. cAMP-induced expression of the SP-A gene is associated with a PKA-catalyzed increase in TTF-1 phosphorylation, resulting in increased TTF-1 DNA binding and transcriptional activity. Thus, it appears that the PKA-mediated increase in TTF-1 phosphorylation and DNA binding activity may constitute the primary mechanism for cAMP induction of SP-A gene expression. We suggest that the increase in TTF-1 phosphorylation and DNA-binding activity may facilitate its interactions with transcription factors bound to the other cis-acting elements found to be essential for cAMP induction of SP-A promoter activity, as well as with coactivators and components of the basal transcription machinery (Fig. 9). In recent studies using transgenic mice, we have found that SP-A:hGH fusion genes comprised of as little as 378 bp of 5'-flanking sequence from the rabbit SP-A gene are expressed in a lung-selective manner, specifically in type II and bronchioalveolar epithelial cells *(77)*. The rabbit SP-A$_{-378}$:hGH transgenes are developmentally regulated in lung tissues of transgenic fetal mice in concert with the endogenous mouse SP-A gene. These findings, together with those of type II cell transfection studies suggest that the unique complement of transcription factors within this approx 400 bp region serves to

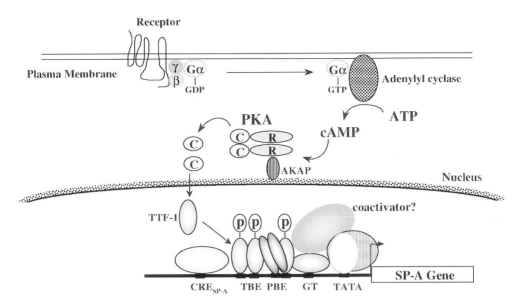

Fig. 9. Proposed mechanism for cAMP induction of SP-A gene expression in type II cells. Binding of regulatory hormone to its receptor results in activation of adenylyl cyclase, increased cAMP formation and activation of PKA tethered to the nuclear membrane by a specific A-kinase anchor protein (AKAP). Entry of activated PKA catalytic subunit (C) into the nucleus results in increased phosphorylation of TTF-1 and its enhanced binding to TBEs. This, in turn, results in the interaction of TTF-1 with transcription factors bound to CRE$_{SP-A}$, E-box and GT-box sequences. Certain of these factors have been found to be developmentally regulated in fetal lung (e.g., USF1 bound to PBE) and selectively expressed in type II cells (USF1 and GT-box-binding proteins [which include Sp1]). Cooperative interaction of these transcription factors with each other and putative coactivators leads to induction of SP-A promoter activity and increased *SP-A* gene transcription.

activate expression of the SP-A gene in a lung cell-specific, cAMP-regulated and developmentally timed manner. In future studies, we will identify the transcription factors that interact with each of the response elements found to be essential for basal and cAMP induction of SP-A promoter activity. We also will define the mechanisms by which they interact in a type II cell-specific and developmentally timed manner to mediate spatial and temporal regulation of SP-A gene expression in fetal lung.

## ACKNOWLEDGMENTS

This research was supported by NIH Grants R37 HL50022 and U01 HL52647.

## REFERENCES

1. Veldhuizen R, Nag K, Orgeig S, Possmayer F. The role of lipids in pulmonary surfactant. Biochim. Biophys Acta 1998;1408:90–108.
2. Hawgood S, Derrick M, Poulain, F. Structure and properties of surfactant protein B. Biochim Biophys Acta 1998;1408:150–160.
3. Weaver TE. Synthesis, processing and secretion of surfactant proteins B and C. Biochim Biophys Acta 1998;1408:173–179.
4. Nogee LM, deMello DM, Dehner LP, Colten HR. Deficiency of surfactant protein B in congential alveolar proteinosis. N Engl J Med 1993;328:406–410.

5. Clark JC, Wert SE, Bachurski CJ, Stahlman MT, Stripp BR, Weaver TE, Whitsett JA. Targeted disruption of the surfactant protein B gene disrupts surfactant homeostasis causing respiratory failure in newborn mice. Proc Natl Acad Sci USA 1995;92:7794–7798,

6. Vorbroker DK, Profitt SA, Nogee LM, Whitsett JA. Aberrant processing of surfactant protein C (SP-C) in hereditary SP–B deficiency. Am J Physiol 1995;268:L647–L656.

7. McCormack FX. Structure, processing and properties of surfactant protein A. Biochim Biophys Acta 1998;1408:109–131.

8. Botas C, Poulain F, Akiyama J, Brown C, Allen L, Goerke J, Clements J, Carlson E, Gillespie AM, Epstein C, Hawgood S. Altered surfactant homeostasis and alveolar type II cell morphology in mice lacking surfactant protein D. Proc Natl Acad Sci USA 1998;95:11,869–11,874.

9. Korfhagen TR, Sheftelyevich V, Burhans MS, Bruno MD, Ross GF, Wert SE, Stahlman MT, Jobe AH, Ikegami M, Whitsett JA, Fisher JH. Surfactant protein–D regulates surfactant phospholipid homeostasis in vivo. J Biol Chem 1998;273:28,438–28,443.

10. Korfhagen TR, Bruno MD, Ross GF, Huelsman KM, Ikegami M, Jobe AH, Wert SE, Stripp BR, Morris RE, Glasser SW, Bachurski CJ, Iwamoto HS, Whitsett JA. Altered surfactant function and structure in SP–A gene targeted mice. Proc Natl Acad Sci USA 1996;93:9594–9599.

11. Ikegami M, Korfhagen TR, Whitsett JA, Bruno MD, Wert SE, Wada K, Jobe AH. Characteristics of surfactant from SP–A–deficient mice. Am J Physiol 1998;275:L247–L254.

12. Boggaram V, Qing K, Mendelson, CR. Rabbit pulmonary surfactant apoprotein: Elucidation of primary sequence and hormonal and developmental regulation, J Biol Chem 1988;263:2939–2947.

13. Phelps DS, Floros J. Localization of surfactant protein synthesis in human lung by *in situ* hybridization. Am Rev Respir Dis 1988;137:939–942.

14. Auten RL, Watkins RH, Shapiro DL, Horowitz S. Surfactant apoprotein A (SP–A) is synthesized in airway cells. Am J Respir Cell Mol Biol 1990;3:491–496.

15. Wohlford–Lenane CL, Snyder JM. Localization of the surfactant–associated proteins SP–A and SP–B mRNA in fetal rabbit lung by *in situ* hybridization. Am J Respir Cell Mol Biol 1992;7:335–343.

16. Khoor A, Gray ME, Hull WM, Whitsett JA, Stallman, MT. Developmental expression of SP–A and SP–A mRNA in the proximal and distal respiratory epithelium in the human fetus and newborn. J Histochem Cytochem 1993;41:1311–1319.

17. Mendelson CR, Boggaram V. Hormonal control of the surfactant system in fetal lung. Annu Rev Physiol 1991;53:415–440.

18. Mendelson CR, Gao E, Li J, Young PP, Michael LF, Alcorn JL. Regulation of expression of surfactant protein–A. Biochim Biophys Acta 1998;1408:132–149.

19. Katyal SL, Singh G, Locker J. Characterization of a second human pulmonary surfactant associated protein SP–A gene. Am J Respir Cell Mol Biol 1992;6:446–452.

20. McCormick SM, Boggaram V, Mendelson CR. Characterization of mRNA transcripts and exon–intron organization of the human surfactant protein (SP)–A1 and SP–A2 genes. Am J Physiol 1994;266:L354–L366.

21. Gao E, Wang Y, McCormick SM, Li J, Seidner SR, Mendelson CR. Characterization of two baboon surfactant protein A genes. Am J Physiol 1996;271:L617–L630.

22. Korfhagen TR, Bruno MD, Glasser SW, Ciraolo PJ, Whitsett JA, Lattier DL, Wikenheiser KA, Clark JC. Murine pulmonary surfactant SP–A gene: cloning, sequence, and transcriptional activity. Am J Physiol 1992;263:L546–L554.

23. Fisher JH, Emrie PA, Shannon J, Sano K, Hattler B, Mason RJ. Rat pulmonary surfactant protein A is expressed as two differently sized mRNA species which arise from differential polyadenylation of one transcript. Biochim Biophys Acta 1988;950:338–345.

24. Chen Q, Boggaram V, Mendelson CR. Rabbit surfactant protein A (SP–A) gene: Identification of a lung-specific DNaseI hypersensitive site in the 5'–flanking region. Am J Physiol 1992;262:L662–L671.

25. Sorokin S. A study of development in organ cultures of mammalian lungs. Dev Biol 1961;3:60–83.

26. Masters JRW. Epithelial–mesenchymal interaction during lung development: The effect of mesenchymal mass. Dev Biol 1976;51:98–108.

27. Snyder JM, Johnston JM, Mendelson CR. Differentiation of type II cells of human fetal lung in vitro. Cell Tissue Res 1981;220:17–25.

28. Mendelson CR, Johnston JM, MacDonald PC, Snyder JM. Multihormonal regulation of surfactant synthesis by human fetal lung in vitro. J Clin Endocrinol Metab 1981;53:307–317.

29. Snyder JM, Mendelson CR, Johnston JM. The effect of cortisol on rabbit fetal lung maturation in vitro. Dev Biol 1981;85:129–140.

30. Mendelson CR, Chen C, Boggaram V, Zacharias C, Snyder JM. Regulation of the synthesis of the major surfactant apoprotein in fetal rabbit lung tissue. J Biol Chem 1986;261:9938–9943.

31. Snyder JM, Mendelson CR. Insulin inhibits the accumulation of the major lung surfactant apoprotein in human fetal lung explants maintained in vitro, Endocrinology 1987;120:1250–1257.

32. Odom MJ, Snyder JM, Mendelson CR. Cyclic AMP analogues and β–adrenergic agonists stimulate the synthesis of the major surfactant apoprotein in human fetal lung in vitro. Endocrinology 1987;121:1155–1163.

33. Acarregui MJ, Snyder JM, Mitchell MD, Mendelson CR. Prostaglandins regulate surfactant protein A (SP–A) gene expression in the human fetal lung in vitro. Endocrinology 1990;127:1105–1113.

34. Acarregui MJ, Snyder JM, Mendelson CR. Oxygen modulates the differentiation of human fetal lung in vitro and its responsiveness to cyclic AMP. Am J Physiol 1993;264:L465–L474.

35. Rudolph D, Tafuri A, Gass P, Hämmerling GJ, Arnold B, Schütz G. Impaired fetal T cell development and perinatal lethality in mice lacking the cAMP response element binding protein. Proc Natl Acad Sci USA 1998;95:4481–4486.

36. Liggins GC. Premature delivery of foetal lambs infused with glucocorticoids. J Endocrinol 1969;45:515–523.

37. Snyder JM, Rodgers HF, O'Brien JA, Mahli N, Magliato SA, Durham PL. Glucocorticoid effects on rabbit fetal lung maturation in vivo: an ultrastructural morphometric study. Anat Rec 1992;232:133–140.

38. Muglia LJ, Bae DS, Brown TT, Vogt SK, Alvarez JG, Sunday ME, Majzoub JA. Proliferation and differentiation defects during lung development in corticotropin–releasing hormone–deficient mice. Am J Respir Cell Mol Biol 1999;20:181–188.

39. Cole TJ, Blendy JA, Monaghan P, Kriegelstein K, Schmid W, Aguzzi A, Fantuzzi G, Hummler E, Unsicker K, Schütz G. Targeted disruption of the glucocorticoid receptor gene blocks adrenergic chromaffin cell development and severely retards lung maturation. Genes Dev 1995;9:1608–1621.

40. Reichardt HM, Kaestner KH, Tuchermann J, Kretz O, Wessely O, Bock R, Gass P, Schmid W, Herrlich P, Angel P, Schütz G. DNA binding of the glucocorticoid receptor is not essential for survival. Cell 1998;93:531–541.

41. Odom MJ, Snyder JM, Boggaram V, Mendelson CR.Glucocorticoid regulation of the major surfactant–associated protein (SP–A) and its mRNA and of morphologic development of human fetal lung in vitro. Endocrinology 1988;123:1712–1720.

42. Nichols KV, Floros J, Dynia DW. Regulation of surfactant protein A mRNA by hormones and butyrate in cultured fetal rat lung. Am J Physiol 1990;259:L488–L495.

43. Alcorn JL, Gao E, Chen Q, Smith ME, Gerard RD, Mendelson CR. Genomic elements involved in transcriptional regulation of the rabbit surfactant protein–A (SP–A) gene. Mol Endocrinol 1993;7:1072–1085.

44. Michael LF, Alcorn JL, Gao E, Mendelson CR. Characterization of the cAMP response element of the rabbit surfactant protein–A gene: Evidence for transactivators distinct from CREB/ATF family members. Mol Endocrinol 1996;10:159–170.

45. Young PP, Mendelson CR. A CRE–like element plays an essential role in cAMP regulation of the human surfactant protein–A2 (SP–A2) gene. Am J Physiol 1996;271:L287–L299.

46. McCormick SM, Mendelson CR. The human SP–A1 and SP–A2 genes are differentially regulated during development and by cAMP and glucocorticoids. Am J Physiol 1994;266:L367–L374.

47. Kumar AR, Snyder JM. Differential regulation of SP–A1 and SP–A2 genes by cAMP, glucocorticoids and insulin. Amer J Physiol 1998;274:L177–L185.

48. Li J, Gao E, Seidner SR, Mendelson CR. Differential regulation of the baboon SP–A1 and SP–A2 genes and structural and functional analysis of their 5'–flanking regions. Am J Physiol 1998;275:L1078–L1088.

49. Roberts JM, Jacobs MM, Cheng JB, Barnes PJ, O'Brien AT, Ballard PL. Fetal pulmonary β–adrenergic receptors: Characterization in human and in vitro modulation by glucocorticoids. Pediatr Pulmonol 1985;1:S69–S76.

50. Barrett CT, Sevanian A, Kaplan SA. Adenylate cyclase activity in immature rabbit lung. Pediat Res 1974;8:244–247.

51. Said SI, Mutt V. Polypeptide with broad biological activity: isolation from small intestine. Science 1970;169:1217–1218.

52. Boggaram V, Smith ME, Mendelson CR. Regulation of expression of the gene encoding the major surfactant protein (SP–A) in human fetal lung in vitro. J Biol Chem 1989;264:11,421–11,427.

53. Boggaram V, Smith ME, Mendelson CR. Posttranscriptional regulation of surfactant protein A (SP–A) mRNA in human fetal lung in vitro by glucocorticoids. Mol Endocrinol 1991;5:414–423.

54. Seidner SR, Smith ME, Mendelson CR. Developmental and hormonal regulation of SP–A gene expression in baboon fetal lung. Am J Physiol 1996;271:L609–L616.

55. Boggaram V, Mendelson CR. Transcriptional regulation of the gene encoding the major surfactant–associated protein (SP–A) in rabbit fetal lung. J Biol Chem 1988;263:19,060–19,065.

56. Connelly IH, Hammond GL, Harding PGR, Possmayer F. Levels of surfactant–associated protein messenger ribonucleic acids in rabbit lung during perinatal development and after hormonal treatment. Endocrinology 1991;129:2583–2591.

57. Schellhase DE, Shannon JM. Effects of maternal dexamethasone on expression of SP–A, SP–B, and SP–C in the fetal rat. Am J Respir Cell Mol Biol 1991;4:304–312.

58. Hummler E, Barker P, Gatzy J. Early death due to defective neonatal lung liquid clearance in ENaC-deficient mice. Nat Genet 1996;12:325–328.

59. Alcorn JL, Smith ME, Smith J, Margraf L, Mendelson CR. Primary cell culture of human type II pneumonocytes: maintenance of a differentiated phenotype and transfection with recombinant adenoviruses. Am J Respir Cell Mol Biol 1997;17:672–682.

60. Glass CK. Differential regulation of target genes by nuclear receptor monomers, dimers and heterodimers. Endocrine Rev 1994;15:391–407.

61. Gao E, Alcorn JL, Mendelson CR. Identification of enhancers in the 5'–flanking region of the rabbit surfactant protein–A gene and characterization of their binding proteins. J Biol Chem 1993;268:19,697–19,709.

62. Gao, E, Wang Y, Alcorn JL, Mendelson CR. The basic helix–loop–helix–zipper transcription factor USF1 regulates expression of the surfactant protein–A gene. J Biol Chem 1997;272:23,398–23,406.

63. Brindle PK, Montminy MR. The CREB family of transcription activators. Curr Opin Genet Dev 1992;2:199–204.

64. Meyer TE, Habener JF. Cyclic adenosine 3',5'–monophosphate response element binding protein (CREB) and related transcription–activating deoxyribonucleic acid–binding proteins. Endo Rev 1993;14:269–290.

65. Bokar JA, Roesler WJ, Vandenbark GR, Kaetzel DM, Hanson RW, Nilson JH. Characterization of the cyclic AMP responsive elements from the genes for the α–subunit of glycoprotein hormones and phosphoenolpyruvate carboxykinase (GTP). J Biol Chem 1988;263:19,740–19,747.

66. Young PP, Mendelson CR. A GT box element is essential for basal and cyclic adenosine 3',5'–monophosphate regulation of the human surfactant protein A2 gene in alveolar type II cells: evidence for the binding of lung nuclear proteins distinct from Sp1. Mol Endocrinol 1997;11:1082–1093.

67. Miller I, Bieker JJ. A novel, erythroid cell–specific murine transcription factor that binds to the CACCC element and is related to the krüppel family of nuclear proteins. Mol Cell Biol 1993;13:2776–2786.

68. Lazzaro D, Price M, De Felice M, Di Lauro R. The transcription factor TTF–1 is expressed at the onset of thyroid and lung morphogenesis and in restricted regions of foetal brain. Development 1991;113:1093–1104.

69. Kimura S, Hara Y, Pineau T, Fernandez–Salguero P, Fox CH, Ward JM, Gonzalez FJ. The T/ebp null mouse: thyroid–specific, enhancer–binding protein is essential for organogenesis of the thyroid, lung, ventral forebrain, and pituitary. Genes Dev 1996;10:60–69.

70. Bruno MD, Bohinski RJ, Huelsman KM, Whitsett JA, Korfhagen TR. Lung cell–specific expression of the murine surfactant protein A (SP–A) gene is mediated by interactions between the SP–A promoter and thyroid transcription factor–1. J Biol Chem 1995;270:6531–6536.

71. Li J, Gao E, Mendelson CR. Cyclic AMP–responsive expression of the surfactant protein–A gene is mediated by increased DNA–binding and transcriptional activity of thyroid transcription factor–1. J Biol Chem 1998;273:4592–4600.

72. Bohinski RJ, Di Lauro R, Whitsett JA. The lung–specific surfactant protein B gene promoter is a target for thyroid transcription factor 1 and hepatocyte nuclear factor 3, indicating common factors for organ–specific gene expression along the foregut axis. Mol Cell Biol 1994;14:5671–5681.

73. Margana RK, Boggaram V. Functional analysis of surfactant protein B (SP–B) promoter. Sp1, Sp3, TTF–1, and HNF–3α transcription factors are necessary for lung cell–specific activation of SP–B transcription. J Biol Chem 1997;272:3083–3090.

74. Kelly SE, Bachurski CJ, Burhans MS, Glasser SW. Transcription of the lung–specific surfactant protein C gene is mediated by thyroid transcription factor 1. J Biol Chem 1996;271:6881–6888.

75. Ray MK, Chen CY, Schwartz RJ, DeMayo FJ. Transcriptional regulation of a mouse Clara cell–specific protein (mCC10) gene by the NKx transcription factor family members thyroid transcription factor 1 and cardiac muscle–specific homeobox protein (CSX). Mol Cell Biol 1996;16:2056–2064.

76. Yan C, Whitsett JA. Protein kinase A activation of the surfactant protein B gene is mediated by phosphorylation of thyroid transcription factor 1. J Biol Chem 1997;272:17,327–17,332.

77. Alcorn JL, Hammer RE, Graves KR, Smith ME, Maika SD, Michael LF, Gao E, Wang Y, Mendelson CR. Analysis of genomic regions involved in regulation of the rabbit surfactant protein A gene in transgenic mice. Am J Physiol 1999;277:L349–L361.

# 4 Hormonal Regulation of Surfactant Protein-B and Surfactant Protein-C Gene Expression in Fetal Lung

*Vijayakumar Boggaram, PhD*

## INTRODUCTION

Pulmonary surfactant, a complex of lipids and proteins *(1)*, is synthesized and secreted by the type II epithelial cells of the pulmonary alveolus. Surfactant is best recognized for its ability to maintain the integrity of the lung through reduction of surface tension at the alveolar air–liquid interphase *(2)*. Surfactant also plays important roles in pulmonary defense against certain bacteria and viruses by promoting their phagocytosis by alveolar macrophages *(3)*. Deficient synthesis of surfactant as found in premature infants causes the development of newborn respiratory distress syndrome (RDS) *(4)* the leading cause of neonatal morbidity and mortality in developed countries. Surfactant levels are also significantly reduced in adult respiratory distress syndrome (ARDS) *(5)* and in acute pulmonary infections *(6)*.

Surfactant is comprised of approximately 90% lipids and 10% proteins. Four distinct lung-specific and surfactant-associated proteins have been purified and characterized *(7,8)*. These proteins, termed surfactant protein (SP)-A, SP-B, SP-C, and SP-D, have been shown to play important roles in influencing the physicochemical properties, function and metabolism of surfactant. SP-A (28,000–36,000 Dalton) and SP-D (43,000 Dalton) are hydrophilic proteins that belong to the C-type mammalian lectin superfam-

From: *Contemporary Endocrinology: Endocrinology of the Lung: Development and Surfactant Synthesis*
Edited by: C. R. Mendelson © Humana Press Inc., Totowa, NJ

ily. SP-A and SP-D contain collagenous and lectin or carbohydrate recognition domains and are referred to as collectins. SP-A and SP-D appear to play important roles in host defense within the lung through their ability to stimulate phagocytosis of bacteria and viruses by alveolar macrophages *(3)*. SP-B and SP-C are hydrophobic proteins that coisolate with surfactant phospholipids during organic solvent extraction. SP-B (9000 Dalton) and SP-C (5000 Dalton) are processed from larger precursor molecules via proteolytic processing at amino and carboxy termini. SP-B and SP-C enhance the spreading and adsorption of phospholipids to an air–liquid interphase and promote reduction of surface tension *(9)*. In particular, SP-B is believed to stabilize the phopholipid monolayer formed on the alveolar surface *(10)*. Studies have also indicated that SP-B is involved in the formation of tubular myelin that serves as an intermediate in the transformation of the lamellar body into monolayer lipid film formed on the alveolar surface *(11,12)*. The critical role of SP-B in the maintenance of surfactant activity and normal lung function is highlighted by its absence in congenital alveolar proteinosis, a fatal respiratory disease, in newborns *(13)*. The molecular defect underlying the absence of SP-B in congenital alveolar proteinosis is the result of a frame shift mutation in SP-B coding region *(14)*. Targeted disruption of the SP-B gene causes respiratory failure in newborn mice, further supporting the importance of SP-B in lung function *(15)*. Inactivation of SP-B gene also leads to the disruption of surfactant metabolism, in particular it significantly reduces the levels of fully processed SP-C peptide *(15)*.

In this chapter I review the effects of hormones on SP-B and SP-C gene expression and the mechanisms underlying the hormonal effects. The effects of hormones on the surfactant system have been reviewed extensively *(16–18)*.

## HORMONAL REGULATION OF THE SURFACTANT SYSTEM

A number of hormones, growth factors, cytokines and other agents influence fetal lung development and differentiation and in turn affect surfactant synthesis. Among hormones, glucocorticoids, and agents that act through increasing intracellular cAMP levels have profound stimulatory effects on fetal lung maturation and surfactant synthesis. Glucocorticoid, thyroid, and β-adrenergic receptors are present in the lung and glucocorticoid and thyroid hormone levels increase during development concomitant with an increase in surfactant synthesis. These data suggest that there may be a causal relationship between increasing glucocorticoid and thyroid hormone levels and surfactant synthesis. The key discovery by Liggins *(19)* that administration of glucocorticoids to fetal lambs accelerated lung maturation, and subsequent studies by a number of investigators have demonstrated that glucocorticoids serve as important regulators of fetal lung maturation and surfactant synthesis (reviewed in ref. *20*). Clinical studies have demonstrated that antenatal administration of glucocorticoids reduce the incidence of neonatal RDS and morbidity and mortality associated with neonatal RDS *(21)*. The stimulatory effects of glucocorticoids on surfactant synthesis have been suggested to be mediated by a glucocorticoid inducible lung fibroblast-derived factor, fibroblast pneumonocyte factor *(22)*. While glucocorticoids and cAMP have stimulatory effects on fetal lung maturation and surfactant synthesis, insulin *(23,24)* and androgens *(25,26)* may have inhibitory effects on surfactant synthesis and maturation of type II cells. Infants of diabetic mothers are at an increased risk of acquiring RDS *(27)* as a consequence of delayed lung maturation. The effects of hormones, cytokines, and other agents on SP-B and SP-C gene expression are summarized in Table 1 and are discussed below.

Table 1
Multifactorial Regulation of SP-B and SP-C Gene Expression in Fetal Lung
In Vitro and In Lung Cell Lines

|       | Dex | cAMP | T3 | Insulin | Retinoids | TNF-α | TGF-β |
|-------|-----|------|-----|---------|-----------|-------|-------|
| SP-B  | ↑   | ↑    | ↓   | ↓       | ↑         | ↓     | ND    |
| SP-C  | ↑   | ↑    | ND  | ↓       | ↑         | ↓     | ↓     |

↑, induction; ↓, inhibition; ND, not determined

# EFFECTS OF GLUCOCORTICOIDS
# ON SP-B AND SP-C GENE EXPRESSION

## Effects of Glucocorticoids on SP-B and SP-C mRNA Levels In Vivo

Several studies have investigated the effects of glucocorticoids on the expression of SP-B and SP-C mRNAs in vivo. Typically, in these studies, the effects of maternal administration of glucocorticoids on the fetal expression levels of SP-B and SP-C mRNAs were determined. Administration of dexamethasone (1 mg/kg) to pregnant rats for 1, 3, or 5 d resulted in an increased expression of SP-B (28,29) and SP-C mRNAs (28) in day 17 and day 19 fetal lung and in day 16 postnatal lung compared to fetal or postnatal lung from saline–treated rats. Maximum increases in the expression levels of SP-B mRNA were found in gestational age 18-d and 19-d animals compared to other gestational age animals as well as postnatal animals (29). It was also found that there were no significant gender-related differences in dexamethasone stimulation of SP-B mRNA expression (29). Tissue in situ hybridization showed that dexamethasone treatment increased SP-B mRNA content to a similar degree in both alveolar and bronchiolar epithelial cells (29). Administration of dexamethasone to adult rats cause increased SP-B and SP-C mRNA expression with the effects on SP-B mRNA levels much greater than the effects on SP-C mRNA levels (30). Adrenalectomy did not significantly alter SP-B and SP-C mRNA levels, suggesting that glucocorticoids may not play a major role in maintaining the steady-state levels of surfactant protein mRNAs (30).

Maternal administration of glucocorticoids or 17β-estradiol increase SP-B mRNA but not SP-C mRNA expression in day-26 and day-27 fetal rabbits (31,32). In fact, 17β-estradiol caused inhibition of SP-C mRNA expression in fetal rabbits (31). In contrast to the findings that maternal administration of dexamethasone increased the content of SP-B mRNA in bronchiolar epithelial cells in the fetal rat (29) SP-B and SP-C mRNA expression was not detected in the bronchiolar epithelial cells of fetal rabbits from control or dexamethasone-treated animals (32).

Investigation of the effects of dose and duration of maternal glucocorticoid treatment on lung maturation in preterm lambs (33) showed that in lambs subjected to long-term glucocorticoid exposure, SP-B levels significantly increased in tissue and lavage fluid with increases in SP-B content in lavage fluid much greater than that in the tissue. In animals treated with glucocorticoids for 48 h, SP-B content was increased only in the lung tissues.

## Effects of Glucocorticoids on SP-B and SP-C mRNA Levels In Vitro

The fetal lung explant culture system has been widely used to investigate the effects of hormones and other agents on surfactant synthesis and type II cell differentiation.

Lung tissues from midgestational age fetuses when maintained in vitro differentiate spontaneously and develop the capacity to synthesize surfactant proteins and lipids. The influence of added hormones and other agents on the spontaneously induced surfactant protein gene expression can be determined to assess the regulatory effects of the agents on surfactant protein gene expression.

Glucocorticoids act in a dose-dependent manner to increase SP-B and SP-C mRNA and protein levels in midgestational age human fetal lung tissues in vitro *(34,35)*. After 48 h of incubation in the presence of 10n$M$ dexamethasone, SP-B mRNA accumulation increased 4-fold, wheareas SP-C mRNA accumulation increased 30-fold compared to control tissues *(35)*. Dexamethasone induction of SP-B and SP-C mRNAs was associated with similar increases in the content of SP-B and SP-C proteins *(35,36)*. Exposure of 12-to 16-wk gestational age human fetal lung explants to dexamethasone markedly increased the rate of synthesis of proSP-C protein (15-fold compared to control) *(37)*. Posttranslational processing of proSP-C into mature SP-C was detected only in dexamethasone-treated explants *(37)*. These data indicate that glucocorticoids may also play important roles in the processing of SP-C. Glucocorticoids act rapidly to increase the content of SP-B and SP-C mRNAs. In fetal lung tissues incubated with 100n$M$ dexamethasone, SP-B mRNA content increased to maximum levels (3.5-fold compared to control) after 12 h of incubation, while SP-C mRNA content increased to maximum levels (30-fold compared to control) after 24 h of incubation *(38)*.

Glucocorticoids also increase SP-B and SP-C gene expression in human lung cell lines that have characteristics of bronchiolar (Clara) or alveolar (type II) epithelial cells. In NCI-H441 cells (a human lung adenocarcinoma cell line that expresses SP-A and SP-B and has characteristics of Clara cells) dexamethasone (10n$M$) significantly increased the expression of SP-B mRNA and protein *(39)*. In NCI-H820 cells (a human lung adenocarcinoma cell line that expresses SP-A, SP-B, and SP-C and has characteristics of type II epithelial cells) dexamethasone increased the expression of SP-B and SP-C mRNAs and the content of SP-B and SP-C precursor proteins in a dose-dependent manner *(40)*. Processing of SP-B and SP-C precursor proteins into mature forms was not detected in NCI-H820 cell line *(40)*.

As in the case of human fetal lung tissues, glucocorticoids act in a dose-dependent manner to increase SP-B and SP-C mRNA expression in fetal rat and rabbit lung tissues in vitro. Incubation of 18-d gestational age fetal rat lung tissues with 100n$M$ dexamethasone for 48 h increased SP-B *(41)* and SP-C *(42)* mRNA expression by 22-fold and 3-fold. Consistent with findings of the in vivo effects of glucocorticoids *(29)*, *in situ* hybridization analysis showed that dexamethasone treatment of fetal rat lung explants increased SP-B mRNA content in alveolar type II epithelial cells and in certain cells of the bronchiolar epithelium *(41)*. Incubation of 21-, 26-, or 30-d gestational age fetal rabbit lung explants with 100 nm dexamethasone for 48 or 72 h increased SP-B mRNA levels 4- to 6-fold *(43,44)*. In similar studies with 21-d gestational age fetal rabbit lung explants, dexamethasone increased SP-C mRNA content 4- and 2-fold after 24 and 48 or 72 h of incubation *(45)*. Rabbit SP-C gene is alternatively spliced to produce two mRNAs that differ by an insertion of a sequence of 31 nucleotides in the 3' untranslated regions *(45)*. Dexamethasone treatment increased the content of SP-C mRNA containing the insertion by a similar magnitude compared to the content of total SP-C mRNA, indicating that the alternatively spliced SP-C mRNAs are increased in a coordinate manner by dexamethasone *(45)*.

## EFFECT OF CAMP ON SP-B AND SP-C GENE EXPRESSION

In contrast to the marked stimulatory effects of glucocorticoids on SP-B and SP-C gene expression, cAMP analogs have modest stimulatory effects on SP-B and SP-C mRNA levels in fetal human, rat, and rabbit lung tissues in vitro. Treatment of 16- to 20-wk gestational age fetal human lung tissues in vitro for 48 h with cAMP analogs, dibutyryl cAMP or 8-bromo-cAMP, or adenylate cyclase activators, forskolin or terbutaline, increased SP-B mRNA content by 2- to 3- fold without any effect on SP-C mRNA content *(34,35)*. Although 8-bromo-cAMP increased SP-B mRNA content, it did not have any stimulatory effect on SP-B protein content *(34)*. cAMP analogs and forskolin increase SP-B mRNA expression in fetal rat *(41)* and rabbit *(44)* lung tissues similar to their effects in human fetal lung tissues. In contrast to their lack of stimulatory effects on SP-C expression in human fetal lung tissues, cAMP analogs and forskolin increase SP-C mRNA levels in fetal rat *(42)* and rabbit *(45)* tissues. In 18-d gestational age fetal rat lung explants, dibutyryl cAMP increased SP-C mRNA levels to a significantly higher level (8-fold relative to control) than 8-bromo-cAMP (2-fold relative to control) *(42)*. The action of dibutyryl cAMP to increase SP-C mRNA levels to a higher level than 8-bromo-cAMP appeared not to be due to butyric acid, a metabolite of dibutyryl cAMP. When lung explants were exposed to a combination of dexamethasone and dibutyryl cAMP or 8-bromo-cAMP, the increase in SP-C mRNA accumulation was less than the additive effects of the two agents *(42)*. This was especially true in lung explants treated with a combination of dexamethasone and dibutyryl cAMP, where SP-C mRNA accumulation was less than that caused by dibutyryl cAMP alone *(42)*.

## MECHANISMS OF GLUCOCORTICOID AND CAMP REGULATION OF SP-B AND SP-C GENE EXPRESSION

Protein synthesis inhibitors, such as cycloheximide and puromycin, block dexamethasone induction of SP-B mRNA in NCI-H441 cells indicating that continued protein synthesis is essential for SP-B mRNA induction *(46)*. Although inhibition of protein synthesis blocked dexamethasone induction of SP-B mRNA in NCI-H441 cells it had no effect on dexamethasone induction of SP-B mRNA content in human fetal lung explants *(38)*. The apparent discrepancy of the effects of cycloheximide on dexamethasone induction of SP-B mRNA may reflect differences in dexamethasone regulation of SP-B gene expression in Clara cells vs type II epithelial cells as NCI-H441 cells are thought to be of Clara cell origin and fetal lung explants after culture are enriched in type II cells and contain very few Clara cells. Although cycloheximide had no effect on dexamethasone induction of SP-B mRNA in human fetal lung explants, it blocked dexamethasone induction of SP-C transcription and mRNA content *(47)*. Treatment with cycloheximide as briefly as 1 h blocked dexamethasone induction of SP-C mRNA indicating the importance of continued protein synthesis and a labile protein factor(s) for dexamethasone induction of SP-C mRNA *(47)*.

Analyses of gene transcription rates by nuclear run-on assays and steady-state accumulation of mRNA levels have been used to assess the relative roles of transcriptional and posttranscriptional mechanisms in the regulation of gene expression. Glucocorticoid treatment of NCI-H441 cells increases SP-B mRNA accumulation by a far greater degree (60- to 150-fold) than SP-B gene transcription (2- to 4-fold) *(46)*. The discrepancy of the glucocorticoid effects on SP-B transcription and SP-B mRNA accumulation indicates that posttranscriptional mechanisms may contribute toward glucocorticoid induction of SP-B mRNA. The important role of posttranscriptional mechanisms in the glucocorticoid induction of SP-B mRNA is supported by the finding that glucocorticoids increase the half-life of SP-B mRNA in human fetal lung tissues in vitro by 2- to 3-fold compared to control tissues (control = 7.5 h; dexamethasone-treated = 18.8 h) *(38)*. As in the case of NCI-H441 cells and human fetal lung tissues in vitro, glucocorticoids increase SP-B mRNA levels disproportionately compared to SP-B transcription rate in fetal rabbit lung tissues in vitro indicating that mechanisms other than transcription may play important roles in the glucocorticoid induction of SP-B mRNA *(44)*. Determination of the stability of SP-B mRNA in control and glucocorticoid treated lung explants showed that glucocorticoids increased the half-life of SP-B mRNA by greater than 2-fold (control = 9.0 h; dexamethasone-treated = 25 h) *(44)*.

Although glucocorticoids act at transcriptional and posttranscriptional (mRNA stability) levels to increase SP-B mRNA levels in NCI-H441 cells and human fetal lung tissues in vitro, they act primarily at the transcriptional level to increase SP-C mRNA levels in human fetal lung tissues in vitro *(38,47)*. Glucocorticoids did not have any effect on the stability of SP-C mRNA *(38)*. In contrast to human fetal lung explants, glucocorticoids increase SP-C mRNA accumulation in fetal rabbit lung explants primarily through increasing the stability of SP-C mRNA *(48)*. In lung explants treated with glucocorticoids for 24 h, SP-C mRNA half-life increased by nearly 3-fold (control = 11.2 h; dexamethasone-treated = 30 h) and SP-C transcription remained unchanged *(48)*. The differences in the actions of glucocorticoids to alter SP-C gene expression in human versus rabbit fetal lung tissues may be related to the nature of the species and the gestational age of the lung.

While glucocorticoids increase SP-B mRNA accumulation by increasing SP-B gene transcription and SP-B mRNA stability, cAMP appears to act primarily at the transcriptional level to increase SP-B mRNA accumulation *(44)*. In fetal rabbit lung explants incubated with dibutyryl cAMP for 48 or 72 h, SP-B transcription and SP-B mRNA levels increase by similar magnitude indicating that increase in SP-B mRNA accumulation is primarily due to an increase in SP-B gene transcription *(44)*. Determination of the stability of SP-B mRNA in control and dibutyryl cAMP-treated lung explants showed no alteration in the half-life of SP-B mRNA (control = 9 h; cAMP-treated = 11 h) *(44)* further indicating that mRNA stability does not play a role in cAMP-dependent increase of SP-B mRNA accumulation. While glucocorticoids increase SP-C gene expression by increasing gene transcription, as in the case of human fetal lung explants, or by increasing mRNA stability, as in the case of rabbit fetal lung explants, cAMP appears to act primarily at the transcriptional level to increase SP-C mRNA accumulation in fetal rabbit lung explants. In explants incubated with dibutyryl cAMP for 48 or 72 h, increases in SP-C mRNA accumulation were associated with similar or higher levels of SP-C transcription *(48)*.

Gene regulatory elements and interacting transcription factors that mediate glucocorticoid and cAMP regulation of SP-B and SP-C gene expression, and the mechanisms underlying transcriptional regulation by glucocorticoids and cAMP are yet to be determined.

## EFFECTS OF OTHER HORMONES, CYTOKINES, AND GROWTH FACTORS

Hormones other than glucocorticoids and cAMP have no significant stimulatory effects on SP-B and SP-C gene expression. Maternal administration of 17β-estradiol to pregnant rabbits on day 26 of gestation increased SP-B mRNA levels in fetal lungs by 2-fold while SP-C mRNA levels remained unchanged *(31)*. Although 17β-estradiol increased fetal lung SP-B mRNA levels, it did not have any effect on the expression of

SP-B and SP-C mRNAs in human fetal lung in vitro *(35)*. Likewise, dihydrotestosterone and 17 α-hydroxyprogesterone did not alter SP-B and SP-C mRNA expression in human fetal lung in vitro *(35)*. Although thyroid hormone ($T_3$) reduced basal as well as dexamethasone-induced expression of SP-B mRNA in fetal rat lung in vitro *(41)* it did not have any effect on SP-C expression *(42)*.

Infants born to diabetic mothers have increased incidence of RDS compared to infants of similar gestational age born to nondiabetic mothers *(27)* (*see* Chapter 10 for further discussion). Infants of diabetic mothers have higher incidence of RDS despite that the lecithin/sphingomyelin ratio of amniotic fluid is normal, indicating lung maturity. Thus impairment of factors other than surfactant phospholipids may contribute to higher incidence of RDS in infants of diabetic mothers. In a pregnant rat model of streptozotocin-induced diabetes, the expression of SP-B and SP-C in developing fetal lung was reduced *(49)* indicating that deficiency of SP-B and SP-C may lead to increased incidence of RDS in infants of diabetic mothers. In human fetal lung in vitro, insulin at a concentration of 2500 ng/mL reduced basal level of SP-B mRNA *(50)* as well as dexamethasone induced SP-B and SP-C mRNA levels *(51)*. The inhibitory effects of insulin on SP-B gene expression in fetal lung must be at least partly due to a direct action on the lung epithelial cell since insulin inhibited SP-B mRNA levels in NCI-H441 cells *(52)*(*see* Chapter 10). The inhibitory effects of insulin on SP-B gene expression in NCI-H441 cells were mediated at the transcriptional level *(52)*. Since the fetus of the diabetic mother is frequently found to be hyperinsulinemic, decreased expression of SP-B may be one of the factors that lead to delayed lung maturation and higher incidence of RDS in infants of diabetic mothers.

The pro-inflammatory cytokine tumor necrosis factor-α (TNF-α) and transforming growth factor-β (TGF-β) have inhibitory effects on SP-B and SP-C gene expression. TGF-β, at a concentration of 5 ng/mL, decreased the abundance of SP-C mRNA, as determined by in situ hybridization, in isolated type II epithelial cells in primary culture *(53)*. Release of TNF-α induced by intratracheal administration of TNF-α or intraperitoneal administration of anti-CD3 antibody to mice decreases SP-B and SP-C mRNA levels in mice *(54)*. Treatment of NCI-H441 cells with 25 ng/mL of TNF-α decreased SP-B mRNA levels by 80% compared to control cells *(55)*. The inhibitory effects of TNF-α appeared to be due to decreased SP-B mRNA stability and not due to decreased SP-B gene transcription *(54,56)*. TNF-α (25 ng/mL) inhibited SP-C mRNA levels in murine lung epithelial cell lines, MLE-12 and MLE-15, in a time dependent manner *(57)*. After 24 h of incubation, SP-C mRNA level was reduced by 80%. Nuclear run-on assays using isolated nuclei showed that the inhibitory effects of TNF-α on SP-C mRNA expression are mediated at the transcriptional level *(57)*.

Retinoids have important effects on the morphogenesis and differentiation of a variety of target organs, including lung (*see* Chapter 9 for further discussion). Retinoids alter SP-B and SP-C gene expression in human *(58)* and rat *(59)* fetal lung in vitro and in lung cell lines *(60,61)*. While all-*trans* and 9-*cis*-retinoic acid increased SP-B mRNA accumulation in a dose-dependent manner they did not have any stimulatory effect on SP-C mRNA expression *(58)*. At a concentration of 3 µ*M*, all-*trans* retinoic acid inhibited SP-C mRNA *(58)*. Although retinoic acid did not increase SP-C mRNA expression in human fetal lung in vitro, it increased SP-C mRNA levels in fetal rat lung in vitro *(59)* and in MLE-12 cells *(61)*. The mechanism by which retinoic acid increases SP-B gene expression is unclear. While one study found that retinoic acid increased SP-B gene expression in NCI-H441cells by increasing SP-B mRNA stability rather than SP-B gene transcription *(62)*, another study found that it increased SP-B promoter activity in NCI-H441 and MLE-15 cells *(63)*.

# SUMMARY

SP-B and SP-C, the hydrophobic proteins of surfactant, are essential for the maintenance of biophysical properties and physiologic function of surfactant. Physiological agents that control fetal lung maturation also regulate the levels of surfactant proteins and lipids. Among hormones, glucocorticoids and cAMP have stimulatory effects on SP-B and SP-C gene expression, whereas insulin appears to have inhibitory effects. Apart from hormones, cytokines, growth factors and other agents also influence SP-B and SP-C gene expression. Among these TNF-α and TGF-β have significant inhibitory effects and retinoic acid has stimulatory effects on SP-B and SP-C gene expression. Whereas glucocorticoids act at transcriptional and mRNA stability levels to increase SP-B and SP-C mRNA levels, cAMP acts solely at the transcriptional level to increase SP-B and SP-C mRNA levels. *Cis*-acting DNA regulatory elements and interacting protein factors that mediate transcriptional and posttranscriptional (mRNA stabilization) effects of glucocorticoids and cAMP on SP-B and SP-C gene expression and molecular mechanisms underlying their actions remain to be determined.

# ACKNOWLEDGMENTS

My research is supported by National Institutes of Health Grant HL 48048.

# REFERENCES

1.  Clements JA, King RJ. Composition of surface-active material. In: Crystal RG, ed. The biochemical basis of pulmonary function. New York: Marcel Dekker, 1976:363–387.
2.  Goerke J, Clements JA. Alveolar surface tension and lung surfactant. In: Macklem PT, Mead J, eds. Handbook of physiology: the respiratory system. Washington, DC: American Physiological Society, 1986:47–261.
3.  Van Iwaarden JF, Van Golde LMG. (1995) Pulmonary surfactant and lung defense. In: Robertson B, Taeusch WH, eds. Surfactant therapy for lung disease. New York: Dekker, 1995:75–92.
4.  Avery ME, Mead J. Surface properties in relation to atelectasis and hyaline membrane disease. Am J Dis Child 1959;97:517–523.
5.  Lewis JF, Jobe AH. Surfactant and the adult respiratory distress syndrome. Am Rev Respir Dis 1993;147: 218–233.
6.  Gunther A, Siebert C, Schmidt R, Ziegler S, Grimminger F, Yabut M, Temmesfeld B, Walmrath D, Morr H, Seeger W. Surfactant alterations in severe pneumonia, acute respiratory distress syndrome, and cardiogenic edema. Am J Respir Crit Care Med 1996;153:176–184.
7.  Possmayer F. A proposed nomenclature for pulmonary surfactant-associated proteins. Am Rev Respir Dis 1988;138:990–998.
8.  Kuroki Y, Voelker DR. Pulmonary surfactant proteins. J Biol Chem 1994;269:25,943–25,946.
9.  Possmayer F. The role of surfactant-associated proteins. Am Rev Respir Dis 1990;142:749–752.
10. Cochrane CG, Revak SD. Pulmonary surfactant protein B (SP–B): structure–function relationships. Science 1991;254:566–568.
11. Suzuki Y, Jujita Y, Kogishi K. Reconstitution of tubular myelin from synthetic lipids and proteins associated with pig pulmonary surfactant. Am Rev Respir Dis 1989;140:75–81.
12. Williams MC, Hawgood S, Hamilton RL. Changes in lipid structure produced by surfactant proteins SP-A, SP-B and SP-C. Am J Respir Cell Mol Biol 1991;5:41–50.
13. Nogee LM, DeMello DP, Dehner LP, Colten HR. Brief report: Deficiency of pulmonary surfactant protein B in congenital alveolar proteinosis. N Engl J Med 1993;328:406–410.
14. Nogee LM, Garnier G, Dietz HC, Singer L, Murphy AM, deMello DE, Colten HR. A mutation in the surfactant protein B gene responsible for fatal neonatal respiratory disease in multiple kindreds. J Clin Invest 1994;93:1860–1863.
15. Clark JC, Wert SE, Bachurski CJ, Stahlman MT, Stripp BR, Weaver TE, Whitsett JA. Targeted disruption of the surfactant protein B gene disrupts surfactant homeostasis, causing respiratory failure in newborn micc. Proc Natl Acad Sci USA 1995;92:7794–7798.
16.  Ballard PL. Hormonal regulation of pulmonary surfactant. Endocr Rev 1989;10(2):165–181.

17. Mendelson CR, Boggaram V. Hormonal control of the surfactant system in fetal lung. Annu Rev Physiol 1991;53:415–440.

18. Weaver TE, Whitsett JA. Function and regulation of expression of pulmonary surfactant-associated proteins. Biochem J 1991;273:249–264.

19. Liggins GC. Premature delivery of fetal lambs infused with glucocorticoids. J Endocrinol 1969;45:515–523.

20. Ballard PL.Hormones and lung maturation. In: Monographs on Endocrinology. Baxter JD, Rousseau GG (eds.) New York: Springer Verlag 1986;28:24–341.Monogr Endocrinol 1986;28:24–341.

21. Crowley P, Chalmers I, Keirse MJNC. The effects of corticosteroid administration before preterm delivery: an overview of the evidence from controlled trials. Br J Obstet Gynecol 1990;97:11–25.

22. Smith BT, Post M. Fibroblast–pneumonocyte factor. Am J Physiol Lung Cell Mol Physiol 1989;257: L174–178.

23. Bourbon JR, Farrell PM. Fetal lung development in the diabetic pregnancy. Pediatr Res 1985;19: 253–267.

24. Pignol B, Bourbon J, Ktorza A, Marin L, Rieutort M, Tordet C. Lung maturation in the hyperinsulinemic rat fetus. Pediatr Res 1987;21: 436–421.

25. Nielsen HC, Zinman HC, Torday JS. Dihydrotestosterone inhibits fetal rabbit pulmonary surfactant production. J Clin Invest 1982;69:611–614.

26. Torday JS. Androgens delay human fetal lung maturation in vitro. Endocrinology 1990;126: 3240–3244.

27. Robert MF, Neff RK, Hubbell JP, Taeusch HW, Avery ME. (Association between maternal diabetes mellitus and the respiratory distress syndrome in the newborn. N Engl J Med 1996;294:357–360.

28. Schellhase DE, Shannon JM. Effects of maternal dexamethasone on expression of SP-A, SP-B, and SP-C in the fetal rat lung. Am J Respir Cell Mol Biol 1991;4:304–312.

29. Phelps DS, Floros J. Dexamethasone in vivo raises surfactant protein B mRNA in alveolar and bronchiolar epithelium. Am J Physiol Lung Cell Mol Physiol 1991;260:L146–L152.

30. Fisher JH, McCormack F, Park SS, Stelzner T, Shannon JM, Hofmann T.In vivo regulation of surfactant proteins by glucocorticoids. Am J Respir Cell Mol Biol 1991;5:63–70.

31. Connelly IH, Hammond GL, Harding PGR, Possmayer F. Levels of surfactant-associated protein messenger ribonucleic acids in rabbit lung during perinatal development and after hormonal treatment. Endocrinology 1991;129:2583–2591.

32. Durham PL, Nanthakumar EJ, Snyder JM. Developmental regulation of surfactant-associated proteins in rabbit fetal lung in vivo. Exp Lung Res 1992;18:775–793.

33. Ballard PL, Ning Y, Polk D, Ikegami M, Jobe A. Glucocorticoid regulation of surfactant components in immature lambs. Am J Physiol Lung Cell Mol Physiol 1997;273:L1048–L1057.

34. Whitsett JA, Weaver TE, Clark JC, Sawtell N, Glasser SW, Korfhagen TR, Hull WM. Glucocorticoid enhances surfactant proteolipid Phe and pVal synthesis and RNA in fetal lung. J Biol Chem 1987;262:15,618–15,623.

35. Liley HG, White RT, Warr RG, Benson BJ, Hawgood S, Ballard PL. Regulation of messenger RNAs for the hydrophobic surfactant proteins in human lung. J Clin Invest 1989;83:1191–1197.

36. Beers MF, Shuman H, Liley HG, Floros J, Gonzales LW, Yue N, Ballard PL. Surfactant protein B in human fetal lung: Developmental and glucocorticoid regulation. Pediatr Res 1995;38:668–675.

37. Solarin KO, Ballard PL, Guttentag SH, Lomax CA, Beers MF. Expression and glucocorticoid regulation of surfactant protein C in human fetal lung. Pediatr Res 1997;42:356–364.

38. Venkatesh VC, Iannuzzi DM, Ertsey R, Ballard PL. Differential glucocorticoid regulation of the pulmonary hydrophobic surfactant proteins SP–B and SP–C. Am J Respir Cell Mol Biol 1993;8: 222–228.

39. O'Reilly MA, Gazdar AF, Morris RE, Whitsett JA. Differential effects of glucocorticoid on expression of surfactant proteins in a human adenocarcinoma cell line. Biochim Biophys Acta 1988;970:194–204.

40. O'Reilly MA, Gazdar AF, Clark JC, Pilot-Matias TJ, Wert SE, Hull WM, Whitsett JA. Glucocorticoids regulate surfactant protein synthesis in a pulmonary adenocarcinoma cell line. Am J Physiol Lung Cell Mol Physiol 1989;257:L385–L392.

41. Floros J, Gross I, Nichols KV, Veletza SV, Dynia D, Lu H, Wilson CM, Peterec SM. Hormonal effects on the surfactant protein B (SP-B) mRNA in cultured fetal rat lung. Am J Respir Cell Mol Biol 1991;4:449–454.

42. Veletza SV, Nichols KV, Gross I, Lu H, Dynia DW, Floros J. Surfactant protein C: hormonal control of SP–C mRNA levels in vitro. Am J Physiol Lung Cell Mol Physiol 1992;262:L684–687.

43. Xu J, Possmayer F. Exposure of fetal lung to glucocorticoids in vitro does not enhance transcription of the gene encoding pulmonary surfactant-associated protein B (SP-B). Biochim Biophys Acta 1993;1169:146–155.

44. Margana RK, Boggaram V. Transcription and mRNA stability regulate developmental and hormonal expression of rabbit surfactant protein B gene. Am J Physiol Lung Cell Mol Physiol 1995; 268: L481–L490.

45. Boggaram V, Margana RK. Rabbit surfacatant protein C: cDNA cloning and regulation of alternatively spliced surfactant protein C mRNAs. Am J Physiol Lung Cell Mol Physiol 1992;263:L634–644.

46. O'Reilly MA, Clark JC, Whitsett JA. Glucocorticoid enhances pulmonary surfactant protein B gene transcription. Am J Physiol Lung Cell Mol Physiol 1991;260:L37–L43.

47. Ballard PL, Ertsey R, Gonzales LW, Gonzales J. Transcriptional regulation of human pulmonary surfactant proteins SP-B and SP-C by glucocorticoids. Am J Respir Cell Mol Biol 1996;14:599–607.

48. Boggaram V, Margana RK. Developmental and hormonal regulation of surfactant protein C (SP-C) gene expression in fetal lung: role of transcription and mRNA stability. J Biol Chem 1994;269: 27,767–27,772.

49. Guttentag SH, Phelps DS, Warshaw JB, Floros JS. Delayed hydrophobic surfactant protein (SP-B, SP-C) expression in fetuses of streptozotocin–treated rats. Am J Respir Cell Mol Biol 1992;7:190–197.

50. Dekowski SA, Snyder JM. Insulin regulation of messenger ribonucleic acid for the surfactant–associated proteins in human fetal lung in vitro. Endocrinology 1992;131:669–676.

51. Dekowski SA, Snyder J. The combined effects of insulin and cortisol on surfactant protein mRNA levels. Pediatr Res 1995;38:513–521.

52. Miakotina OL, Dekowski SA, Snyder JM. Insulin inhibits surfactant protein A and B gene expression in the H441 cell line. Biochim Biophys Acta 1998;1442:60–70.

53. Maniscalco WM, Sinkin RA, Watkins RH, Campbell MH. Transforming growth factor-β1 modulates type II cell fibronectin and surfactant protein C expression. Am J Physiol Lung Cell Mol Physiol 1994;267:L569–L577.

54. Whitsett JA, Clark JC, Wispe JR, Pryhuber GS. Effects of TNF-α and phorbol ester on human surfactant protein and MnSOD gene transcription in vitro. Am J Physiol Lung Cell Mol Physiol 1992;262:L688–L693.

55. Pryhuber GS, Bachurski C, Hirsch R, Bacon A, Whitsett JA. Tumor necrosis factor–α decreases surfactant protein B mRNA in murine lung. Am J Physiol Lung Cell Mol Physiol 1996;270: L714–L721.

56. Pryhuber GS, Church SL, Kroft T, Panchal A, Whitsett JA. 3'-untranslated region of SP-B mRNA mediates inhibitory effects of TPA and TNF-α on SP-B expression. Am J Physiol Lung Cell Mol Physiol 1994;267:L16–L24.

57. Bachurski CJ, Pryhuber GS, Glasser SW, Kelly SE, Whitsett JA. Tumor necrosis factor–α inhibits surfactant protein C gene transcription. J Biol Chem 1996;270:19,402–19,407.

58. Metzler MD, Snyder JM. Retinoic acid differentially regulates expression of surfactant–associated proteins in human fetal lung. Endocrinology 1993;133:1990–1998.

59. Bogue CW, Jacobs HC, Dynia DW, Wilson CM, Gross I. Retinoic acid increases surfactant protein mRNA in fetal rat lung in culture. Am J Physiol Lung Cell Mol Physiol 1996;271:L862–L868.

60. George TN, Snyder JM. Regulation of surfactant protein gene expression by retinoic acid metabolites. Pediatr Res 1997;41:692–701.

61. Grummer MA, Zachman RD. Retinoic acid and dexamethasone affect RAR–beta and surfactant protein C mRNA in the MLE lung cell line. Am J Physiol Lung Cell Mol Physiol 1998;274:L1–L7.

62. George TN, Miakotina OL, Goss KL, Snyder JM. Mechanism of all trans–retinoic acid and glucocorticoid regulation of surfactant protein mRNA. Am J Physiol Lung Cell Mol Physiol 1998;274: L560–L566.

63. Yan C, Ghaffari M, Whitsett JA, Zeng X, Sever Z, Lin S. Retinoic acid–receptor activation of SP-B gene transcription in respiratory epithelial cells. Am J Physiol Lung Cell Mol Physiol 1998;275: L239–L246.

# 5

# Glucocorticoid Regulation of Fatty Acid Synthase in Fetal Lung

*Seamus A. Rooney, PhD, ScD*

CONTENTS

## INTRODUCTION

The goal of this chapter is to review current information on the regulation of fatty acid biosynthesis and its role in surfactant production in the fetus.

Development of the surfactant system is a crucial event during the later stages of fetal lung maturation. Surfactant reduces surface tension at the air–liquid interface in the alveolar lumen and is critical for the normal ventilatory function of the lung. There is a surge in surfactant production in fetal lung toward the end of gestation in preparation for extrauterine life. A deficiency in surfactant leads to serious illness; birth before the surfactant system is sufficiently mature can lead to the respiratory distress syndrome (RDS), a major cause of illness in premature babies *(1,2)*. Glucocorticoids and other hormones can accelerate fetal lung maturation and stimulate surfactant synthesis *(3–7)*. Clinically, glucocorticoids are extensively administered to pregnant women at risk of premature delivery in order to prevent RDS *(1)*.

Surfactant is a complex material. It consists largely of lipids, which make up about 90% of surfactant by weight, and it contains four unique proteins *(8)*. Phosphatidylcholine is by far the most abundant lipid in surfactant and accounts for almost 70% of its total mass *(9)*. More than half the phosphatidylcholine in surfactant is disaturated *(10)*, principally the dipalmitoyl species, and it is dipalmitoylphosphatidylcholine that is largely responsible for the surface tension reducing property of surfactant *(11)*.

From: *Contemporary Endocrinology: Endocrinology of the Lung: Development and Surfactant Synthesis*
Edited by: C. R. Mendelson © Humana Press Inc., Totowa, NJ

Fatty acids are integral components of glycerophosphatides and consequently key substrates in the synthesis of surfactant lipids. It well established that fetal and adult lungs have the ability to synthesize fatty acids *de novo (12)*. However, fatty acids can also be supplied via the blood and the relative importance *de novo* synthesis vs extrapulmonary supply in the provision of fatty acids for surfactant synthesis has not been unequivocally established *(12,13)*. There is little blood supply to the lungs during fetal life so it is likely that *de novo* synthesis is of quantitative importance at that stage of development. As discussed subsequently, there is a developmental increase in fatty acid biosynthesis concomitant with that of phosphatidylcholine consistent with a role for fatty acid biosynthesis in overall surfactant production. However, the most compelling evidence for the importance of fatty acids in surfactant biosynthesis in fetal lung is the finding that inhibition of fatty acid biosynthesis results in abolition of the glucocorticoid-induced increase in the activity of the rate-limiting enzyme in the phosphatidylcholine biosynthetic pathway.

## FATTY ACID BIOSYNTHETIC PATHWAY

The pathway of *de novo* fatty acid biosynthesis is illustrated in Fig. 1. Fatty acid biosynthesis take place in the cytosol of the cell. Precursors such as glucose and glycogen are metabolized via the glycolytic pathway and Krebs cycle to citrate *(14)*. Mitochondrial citrate is transported across the mitochondrial membrane and into the cytosol by the tricarboxylate anion carrier where it is metabolized to acetyl-CoA by ATP-citrate lyase (EC 4.1.3.8). Acetyl-CoA is then converted to malonyl-CoA in a reaction catalyzed by acetyl-CoA carboxylase (EC 6.4.1.2). Long-chain fatty acid biosynthesis is finally completed by fatty acid synthase (FAS) in a series of seven distinct enzymatic reactions, four of which are repeated for the addition of each 2-carbon unit to the growing fatty acid chain *(15,16)*. In prokaryotes and plants the seven reactions are carried out by separate loosely associated proteins, but in animals and yeast they are carried out by single multifunctional proteins *(15,16)*. Animal FAS (EC 2.3.1.85) is a homodimer ($M_r$ approximately 570,000) of two identical subunits *(15,16)*. Palmitic acid is the usual product of *de novo* fatty acid biosynthesis in mammals.

As acetyl-CoA is a precursor for biosynthesis of cholesterol in addition to fatty acids, acetyl-CoA carboxylase is considered the first committed step in fatty acid biosynthesis *(16)*. Fatty acid biosynthesis can be regulated by both acetyl-CoA carboxylase and FAS. Acetyl-CoA carboxylase has a role in both short-term and long-term regulation *(14,16)*. Short-term regulation is mediated by phosphorylation/dephosphorylation and allosteric factors, whereas long-term regulation is mediated by gene expression *(14,16)*. By contrast, FAS regulation of fatty acid biosynthesis appears to be entirely long term and mediated by altered gene expression *(14,17)*. Until recently there was no convincing evidence that FAS is regulated by posttranslational modification or by allosteric factors. Recently, however, mammalian FAS was reported to be regulated by phosphorylation in human tumor cell lines *(18)*. Confirmation and the general applicability of that finding is needed to establish whether FAS can also be subject to short-term regulation in other mammalian systems.

## FATTY ACID BIOSYNTHESIS IN DEVELOPING FETAL LUNG

There is a developmental increase in *de novo* fatty acid biosynthesis toward the end of gestation in fetal lung *(19,20)*. In those studies *de novo* synthesis was assessed by measuring the rate of $^3H_2O$ incorporation into fatty acids, a method that avoids problems

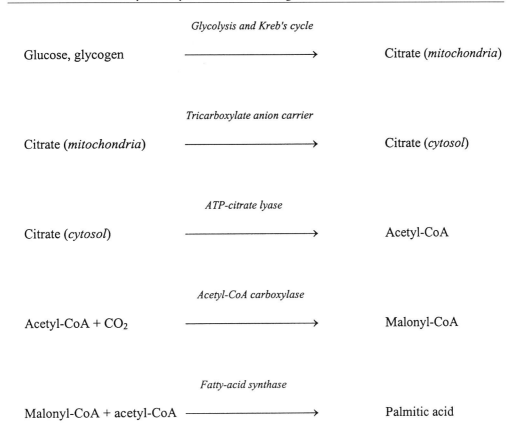

Fig. 1. Biochemical pathway of *de novo* fatty acid biosynthesis.

with the pool size of substrates and intermediate metabolites *(21)*. In the rat the increase in fatty acid biosynthesis correlates with the developmental increase in phosphatidylcholine synthesis and surfactant phospholipid content in fetal lung *(20)*.

The increase in *de novo* synthesis in fetal rat lung is accompanied by a corresponding developmental increase in FAS activity *(22,23)*. The increase in FAS activity is due to increased gene expression as shown by the fact that there is a similar developmental increase in the level of FAS mRNA *(24,25)*. There is also a developmental increase in FAS activity and FAS content in fetal rabbit lung *(26)*. In contrast to FAS, there are either no changes or minor and inconsistent increases in the activities and mRNA levels of ATP-citrate lyase and acetyl-CoA carboxylase during fetal rat *(19,22–25)* and rabbit *(27)* lung development. These data suggest that the developmental increase in *de novo* fatty acid biosynthesis is mediated by the increase in FAS gene expression. There is currently no information on whether developmental regulation of the FAS gene is at the transcriptional or posttranscriptional level.

Glycogen may be an important source of substrate for fatty acid synthesis in fetal lung. There is an inverse temporal relationship between glycogen content and the biosynthesis of fatty acids and phosphatidylcholine in developing fetal lung. As fatty acid and phosphatidylcholine biosynthesis increase glycogen content decreases *(20,28)*. The decrease in glycogen has been noted morphologically in type II cells *(29)*, the cellular source of surfactant within the lung *(8)*, and has also been shown in type II cells isolated from fetal rats *(30)*. The inverse relationship between glycogen content and phosphatidylcholine synthesis had led to speculation that glycogen provides substrate for surfactant synthesis *(28,29,31)*. However, it is equally likely that glycogen provides substrate for fatty acid biosynthesis *(12)*. A direct relationship between glycogen and either fatty acid or phosphatidylcholine biosynthesis is difficult to prove, as glycogen cannot be specifically radiolabeled with a substrate that is not also incorporated into other cellular components.

## EFFECTS OF HORMONES ON FATTY ACID BIOSYNTHESIS IN DEVELOPING FETAL LUNG

### *Glucocorticoids*

Lung maturation and surfactant production in the fetus can be accelerated by a number of hormones *(3–6)*. Glucocorticoids, the first hormones reported to stimulate fetal lung surfactant production *(32,33)*, have been the most extensively investigated with respect to their effects on fetal lung maturation *(3–8)* and remain the only hormone used clinically to prevent RDS in premature human infants *(1,2)*. Glucocorticoids accelerate surfactant phospholipid biosynthesis, glycogen depletion and fatty acid biosynthesis in the late gestation fetal lung *(6)*.

Glucocorticoids stimulate the rate of *de novo* fatty acid biosynthesis in fetal rat *(20)*, rabbit *(34)* and human *(35)* lung. As in the case of normal fetal lung development, the increase in *de novo* fatty acid biosynthesis in response to glucocorticoids appears to be entirely due to increased FAS activity. Glucocorticoids increase FAS activity in fetal rat *(22,36)* and human *(35)* lung, but they do not increase the activities of ATP-citrate lyase *(25)* or acetyl-CoA carboxylase *(22)*. In contrast to the rat, rabbit, and human, it was recently reported that betamethasone does not increase FAS activity in fetal lamb lung *(37)*. Whether that is due to a species difference or a function of the gestational age examined is not clear at present.

The glucocorticoid induced increase in fatty acid biosynthesis and FAS activity is a direct effect on the fetal lung. The effect of the hormone has been observed in cultured fetal lung explants *(25,34,35)* as well as in the lungs of fetuses exposed to glucocorticoid by maternal in vivo injection *(20,22)*. There is convincing evidence that the stimulatory effect of the hormone is mediated by the glucocorticoid receptor. The glucocorticoid $EC_{50}$s for stimulation of fatty acid biosynthesis and FAS activity are similar to or less than the $K_d$ for nuclear receptor binding. The dexamethasone $EC_{50}$ for stimulation of the rate of $^3H_2O$ incorporation into fatty acids in fetal lung is 0.5n$M$ in the rabbit *(34)* and 1.5n$M$ in the human *(35)*. Similar $EC_{50}$ values for stimulation of FAS activity in fetal rat *(36)* and human *(38)* lung were reported. Such $EC_{50}$s are less than the $K_d$s (5–10n$M$) reported for dexamethasone binding to the nuclear glucocorticoid receptor *(39,40)*. Furthermore, the potency order of steroids in stimulating fatty acid biosynthesis and FAS activity is consistent with involvement of the glucocorticoid receptor *(35,36)*.

It is clear that the glucocorticoid induced increase in FAS activity is due to increased gene expression. In fetal rat lung, dexamethasone increases the amount of FAS as measured by immunotitration *(36)* and Western blotting *(41)*. Glucocorticoids also increase FAS mRNA levels in cultured explants of fetal rat *(25,42)* and human *(38)* lung. As in the case of enzyme activities, glucocorticoids do not increase ATP-citrate lyase or acetyl-CoA carboxylase mRNA levels *(25,42)*.

The glucocorticoid induced increase in the level of FAS mRNA appears to be largely due to increased transcription. There is a biphasic increase in FAS mRNA content in response to dexamethasone in fetal rat lung; an early increase that is maximal (almost threefold) 5 h after addition of the hormone followed by a later increase of similar magnitude that reaches a plateau after 28 h *(25)*. The early increase is antagonized by actinomycin D suggesting that it is due to increased transcription. However, the later increase cannot be attributed to increased transcription as it is not antagonized by actinomycin D. Nuclear run on assays confirmed that glucocorticoids do indeed increase transcription of the FAS gene in fetal rat lung *(41)*. The increase in the rate of transcription is maximal 1 h after addition of the hormone and is still apparent for at least 48 h. However, glucocorticoids also increase FAS mRNA stability *(43)*. The apparent half-life of FAS mRNA in fetal rat lung is approx 4 h and it is increased up to 84% by dexamethasone *(43)*. Therefore glucocorticoids increase expression of the FAS gene in developing fetal lung by two mechanisms; an increase in the rate of gene transcription and an increase in the stability of the mRNA transcripts.

Although there is some variation between experiments in the extent of the increases, the hormone induces an approximately 2-fold increase in FAS activity *(25,36,41)* and mass *(41)* in the fetal rat, a 2-to 3.5-fold increase in mRNA content *(25,41–43)*, a 3-to 4-fold increase in rate of transcription *(41)* and a less than 2-fold increase in mRNA stability *(43)*. Therefore, it is likely that the major glucocorticoid effect on FAS gene expression in fetal lung is an increase in its rate of transcription.

## *Thyroid Hormone*

Thyroid hormone is another hormone that accelerates fetal lung maturation and stimulates surfactant phospholipid synthesis in the late gestation fetal lung *(5,6)*. The stimulatory effects of glucocorticoid and thyroid hormones on parameters of fetal lung phosphatidylcholine synthesis are synergistic *(2)*. Thyroid hormone, however, does not stimulate fatty acid biosynthesis in fetal lung. Injection of pregnant rats with triiodothyronine ($T_3$) results in a delay in the normal developmental increase in fatty acid biosynthesis in the lungs of their fetuses *(20)*. When $T_3$ and dexamethasone are injected together the thyroid hormone antagonizes the stimulatory effect of the glucocorticoid on *de novo* fatty acid biosynthesis *(20)*. $T_3$ also antagonizes the stimulatory effect of dexamethasone on FAS activity both in vivo *(22)* and in cultured lung explants *(36)*. Although the inhibitory effect of $T_3$ on fatty acid synthesis in vivo was observed at the same dose that stimulates phosphatidylcholine synthesis, its effect in cultured lung requires a relativity high concentration. The $T_3$ $IC_{50}$ in fetal rat lung explants is 25n$M$ *(36)*, considerably greater than the reported $K_d$ for thyroid hormone receptor binding *(40)*. The physiologic relevance of the inhibitory effect of thyroid hormone is therefore questionable. In human fetal lung explants, $T_3$ has no effect on *de novo* fatty acid biosynthesis, FAS activity or FAS mRNA level and does not antagonize the stimulatory effects of glucocorticoid on those parameters *(35,38)*. In the adult, thyroid hormone levels have no effect on lung FAS mRNA content in the rat *(44)*.

## *Cyclic Adenosine Monophosphate*

Cyclic adenosine monophosphate (cAMP) was reported to increase FAS mRNA levels in human fetal lung explants and its effect was strongly synergistic with that of dexamethasone *(38)*. In fetal rat lung explants, on the other hand, cAMP and agents that increase endogenous cAMP levels had a small stimulatory effect on FAS activity but no effect on its mRNA content *(41)*. The was no synergism between the effects of cAMP and dexamethasone in the rat system. The reason for the discrepancy between the rat and human systems is not presently clear nor is the physiologic importance of cAMP regulation of FAS gene expression. Although cAMP has been reported to stimulate phosphatidylcholine synthesis in developing fetal lung *(5)* it is known to inhibit expression of the FAS gene in liver and fat cells *(14,17)*.

### *Retinoic Acid*

Retinoic acid is an agent that has profound effects on development of many organs *(45)* including the lung *(46–48)* and that also influences surfactant phospholipid synthesis *(49)* and surfactant protein gene expression *(50–52)*. Retinoic acid antagonizes the stimulatory effect of glucocorticoid on FAS gene expression in fetal rat lung explants *(41)*. Retinoic acid antagonizes the stimulatory effects of dexamethasone on FAS activity, content, mRNA level and rate of transcription. Retinoic acid alone has no effect on any of the parameters. The physiologic relevance of the effect of retinoic acid is not clear. Its antagonism of the glucocorticoid effects occurs in a relatively narrow concentration range. Inhibition ranges from approx 25% at $5 \times 10^{-6}M$ to 100% at $5 \times 10^{-4}M$ retinoic acid *(41)*. Although in some studies in other systems, effects of retinoic acid have been noted at concentrations as low as $10^{-8}M$ *(45)*, many of its effects on the fetal lung have been noted at $10^{-6}$ to $10^{-5}M$ *(48–52)*. Furthermore, the concentration of retinol, the parent compound of retinoic acid, is approx $0.8 \times 10^{-5}M$ in fetal rat lung on day 19 of gestation *(53)*, the age at which the antagonism between retinoic acid and dexamethasone on FAS gene expression was observed *(41)*.

## FUNCTION OF FATTY ACID BIOSYNTHESIS IN GLUCOCORTICOID-INDUCED SURFACTANT PHOSPHOLIPID PRODUCTION IN FETAL LUNG

Increased expression of the FAS gene appears to be a major factor in glucocorticoid induction of surfactant phospholipid synthesis in the late gestation fetal lung. There is evidence that the glucocorticoid induced increase in choline-phosphate cytidylyltransferase (CYT; EC 2.7.7.15) activity is mediated by the increase in FAS expression. The reaction catalyzed by CYT, formation of CDPcholine from choline phosphate and CTP, is the second of three reactions in the incorporation of choline into phosphatidylcholine. It is a major rate-regulatory enzyme in phosphatidylcholine biosynthesis; altered CYT activity invariably accompanies altered phosphatidylcholine biosynthesis *(5,6,54–56)*.

The developmental increase in phosphatidylcholine biosynthesis in fetal lung is accompanied by increased CYT activity *(5,6)*. Glucocorticoids, which stimulate surfactant phospholipid production and phosphatidylcholine biosynthesis in developing fetal lung *(5,6)*, also increase CYT activity in fetal rat *(39,57,58)*, rabbit *(59,60)*, mouse *(61)*, and human *(62)* lung. Increases in the activities of other enzymes of phosphatidylcholine biosynthesis in response to glucocorticoids have also been reported, but such effects are not consistent among species or from one laboratory to another *(5,6)*. On the other hand, the increase in CYT activity is a consistent finding. CYT remains the only lipogenic enzyme activity, apart from that of FAS, that is consistently increased by glucocorticoids in fetal lung. Hence it is likely that CYT and FAS have pivotal roles in the glucocorticoid induction of surfactant phospholipid biosynthesis.

The mechanism by which glucocorticoids increase CYT activity in fetal lung has been extensively investigated. As in the case of FAS, the glucocorticoid induced increase in CYT activity is a direct effect on the fetal lung mediated by the glucocorticoid receptor. The stimulatory effect of glucocorticoids on CYT activity has been noted in cultured fetal lung explants *(39,62,63)* as well as in animals treated with the hormone in vivo *(57–61)*. The $EC_{50}$ and $K_d$ values for dexamethasone stimulation of CYT activity and binding to the receptor in nuclear fractions are identical (6.6n$M$ and 6.8n$M$, respectively) in fetal rat lung and the potency order of steroids in binding to the receptor and in stimulating CYT are the same *(39)*. The time course of the glucocorticoid stimulation of CYT activity is consistent with that of new protein synthesis as the increase does not become detectable until about 20 h after addition of dexamethasone to cultured fetal rat lung explants and cells *(64,65)*. The stimulatory effect of glucocorticoid on CYT activity is antagonized by actinomycin D *(39)* and cycloheximide *(65)*, inhibitors of transcription and protein synthesis, respectively.

The foregoing data are consistent with the stimulatory effect of CYT being due to increased mRNA and protein synthesis. However, there is compelling evidence that expression of the CYT gene is not increased by glucocorticoids in fetal lung and that the stimulatory effect of the hormone is due to activation of existing enzyme rather than synthesis of new CYT. Glucocorticoids do not increase the amount of fetal lung CYT protein *(58,66)* or mRNA levels *(42,67,68)*. CYT activity can be increased severalfold by inclusion of phosphatidylglycerol and other lipids in the assay mixture *(69–71)* and when fetal lung CYT is assayed in the presence of sufficient lipid to achieve maximum activation in vitro the stimulatory effect of glucocorticoids is markedly diminished *(39,58,64,66,72)*. As the exogenous lipids would be expected to activate newly synthesized CYT to the same extent as existing enzyme, those data strongly suggest that it is the catalytic activity rather than the amount of CYT that is increased by glucocorticoids.

CYT activity in fetal lung cytosol is markedly decreased by extraction of lipids with solvents that do not cause protein denaturation *(58,71)*. Lipid extraction under such conditions completely abolishes the stimulatory effect of glucocorticoids on the fetal rat enzyme *(58)*. CYT activity and the stimulatory effect of the hormone is fully restored on readdition of the appropriate lipid extract *(58)*. Such data establish that the stimulatory effect of the hormone is mediated by a lipid factor or factors.

Inhibitors of fatty acid biosynthesis were used to address the question of whether the increase in FAS expression is responsible for the glucocorticoid-induced increase in CYT activity *(64)*. *De novo* fatty acid biosynthesis can be inhibited early in the biosynthetic pathway by agaric and hydroxycitric acids. Agaric acid inhibits citrate transfer from mitochondria to cytosol and possibly acetyl-CoA carboxylase *(73)*, whereas hydroxycitrate inhibits ATP-citrate lyase *(74)*. Incubation of fetal rat lung explants with agaric acid or hydroxycitrate inhibited the rate of acetate or glucose incorporation into fatty acids but had no effect on FAS activity *(64)*. The inhibitors completely abolished the stimulatory effect of dexamethasone on CYT activity while only slightly diminishing the increase in FAS activity. When CYT was assayed in the presence of phosphatidylglycerol the activities in the control and dexamethasone-treated explants were both maximally increased and there was no reduction in activity on addition of the inhibitors. Thus the inhibitors did not impair the ability of the enzyme to be maximally stimulated and therefore did not directly inhibit CYT activity. Those data showed that the glucocorticoid induced increase in CYT activity is dependent on fatty acid synthesis.

The foregoing data suggest a mechanism by which glucocorticoids stimulate phosphatidylcholine synthesis in developing fetal lung. The hormone increases expression of the FAS gene. The increase in FAS content results in increased FAS activity and consequently increased fatty acid biosynthesis. The fatty acids, either as free acids or following their incorporation into lipids, activate CYT. Increased CYT activity then results in increased phosphatidylcholine biosynthesis. Whether induction of the FAS gene completely accounts for the developmental and glucocorticoid-induced increases in phosphatidylcholine synthesis in fetal lung remains to be investigated. However, it is of interest that in fetal type II cells another inhibitor of fatty acid biosynthesis, 5-tetradecyloxy-2-furoic acid, decreased the biosynthesis of both fatty acids and disaturated phosphatidylcholine to the same extent *(75)*.

Although there is good evidence that increased expression of the FAS gene is required for activation of CYT the identity of the activator has not been established. In addition to phospholipids *(69–71)*, free fatty acids *(76)* are also known to activate CYT activity in vitro and betamethasone elevates fatty acid levels in fetal rat lung *(58)*. The findings that linoleic acid was the fatty acid that was increased to the greatest extent and that it was the most effective fatty acid in activating CYT in vitro led to the suggestion that glucocorticoid stimulation of fetal lung CYT activity is mediated by linoleic acid *(77)*. However, linoleic acid is an essential fatty acid that is not synthesized by mammals and that must be provided in the diet. Therefore, it is difficult to reconcile the notions that glucocorticoid activation of CYT is mediated by both increased fatty acid biosynthesis and by linoleic acid. In summary, although there is compelling evidence that the stimulatory effect of glucocorticoids on CYT activity is mediated by endogenous lipid(s), the precise nature of the activator(s) remains to be established. Nevertheless, it appears that FAS induction is a crucial factor in glucocorticoid induction of surfactant phospholipid synthesis in developing fetal lung.

## REGULATION OF FATTY ACID SYNTHASE GENE EXPRESSION BY HORMONES AND OTHER FACTORS

Animal FAS is encoded by a single gene that is 18 kb in the rat *(15,78)*, about 19 kb in the human *(79)* and 50 kb in the goose *(80)*. The FAS gene has been localized to chromosome 17q in the human *(81,82)* and to syntenic distal chromosome 11 in the mouse *(81)*. The rat FAS gene contains 43 exons from which two equally abundant mRNAs, a consequence of two different polyadenylation signals, are transcribed *(15,78,83,84)*. Two mRNAs are also transcribed in goose *(80,85)* and chicken *(86)* but there is only one transcript in a number of other species *(79,81,87,88)*.

The FAS gene is widely expressed but is most pronounced in lung, liver and adipose tissue *(17,79,81)*. In a number of tissues, expression of the FAS gene is regulated by developmental *(89,90)* and nutritional *(14,89–93)* factors as well as by several hormones *(87,88,90,93–101)*. Insulin *(94–96)*, insulinlike growth factor *(96)* and thyroid hormone *(90,94,97)* increase expression of the FAS gene in liver and fat cells, whereas glucagon *(97,98)*, growth hormone *(88,99)* and cAMP *(87,97,98)* decrease it. Progesterone *(100)* and androgens *(101)* increase FAS expression in breast and prostate cancer cells, respectively. Indeed increased FAS expression is associated with cancer in a number of organs *(102–104)*. Most increases in expression of the FAS gene are due to increased transcription *(14)*, although increased mRNA stability has also been reported *(90,92,94,100)*.

The molecular mechanisms by which hormones and other factors regulate transcription of the FAS gene have begun to be investigated *(17)*. *cis*-Acting elements responsible for the regulatory effects of insulin *(105–108)*, cAMP *(109,110)* and nutrients *(111–114)* have been identified. Most such sequences are located in the promoter region. For instance, an insulin responsive region has been identified at 68–52 bp upstream of the transcription start site [–68/–52 bp] *(105,115)* and a cAMP-responsive region at –99/–92 bp *(109)*. However, more distal regulatory regions have also been identified both upstream and downstream of the transcription start site. Thus, an insulin-responsive region was identified at –516/–498 bp *(108)* and a glucose responsive region at +290/+316 bp *(112)*. Negative regulatory regions were reported at –319/–301, +405/+768 and +924/+1083 bp in the rat gene *(116,117)*. Several transcription factors have been shown to bind to the above and other regions of the FAS gene *(108–110,115,118–120)*.

Glucocorticoids are generally considered to stimulate lipogenesis *(14,121)*, an effect that is reasonably well characterized in liver, although less established in other organs *(14)*. However, apart from the fetal lung, there are few reports of glucocorticoid regulation of FAS gene expression in other tissues. Dexamethasone increases chloramphenicol acetyltransferase (CAT) expression in several tissues of transgenic mice containing the 2.1 kb 5' flanking promoter region of the FAS gene (–2100/+67 bp) fused with the CAT reporter gene *(122)*. The greatest increase is in white adipose tissue followed by liver and the increase is also apparent in the lung as well as brown fat, heart, spleen, and muscle *(122)*. Dexamethasone was also reported to increase FAS mRNA levels in primary cultures of rat hepatocytes *(123)*. Glucocorticoids interact with other hormones, particularly insulin and thyroid hormone, in regulating FAS gene expression *(14)*. Such effects appear to be species and/or organ specific. Thus, the thyroid hormone induced increase in FAS mRNA content is enhanced by corticosterone in chick hepatocytes *(124)* but antagonized by dexamethasone in rat hepatocytes *(123)*. Similarly, the stimulatory effect of insulin is enhanced by glucocorticoids in hepatocytes *(123)* but antagonized in adipose tissue *(98)*. There is little information on the DNA sequences responsible for glucocorticoid regulation of the FAS gene. Inspection of the FAS gene and its 5'-flanking region revealed a number of potential glucocorticoid regulatory regions. In particular, half of the glucocorticoid response element (GRE) consensus sequence is located at –422 bp in the rat gene *(78)*, and there are also tentative GREs in the first intron *(78,125)*. Putative GREs have also been noted in the human *(126)* and goose *(80)* FAS genes. To identify functional GREs or other glucocorticoid responsive regions, we transiently transfected human lung adenocarcinoma (A549) cells with chimeric constructs consisting of serial deletions of the –1592/–67 bp region of the rat FAS gene ligated to the firefly luciferase reporter gene *(127)*. Dexamethasone increased luciferase gene expression in response to all constructs as much as twofold. The full effect of the hormone was retained in response to the –33/+56 bp fragment suggesting that 89 bp region has an important role in glucocorticoid stimulation of FAS gene expression. That the glucocorticoid responsive region lies in the –1657/+65 bp fragment is in agreement with the finding that dexamethasone increases CAT expression in transgenic mice containing the –2100/+67 bp FAS fragment fused to the CAT reporter gene *(122)*. The –33/+56 bp fragment glucocorticoid responsive DNA fragment does not contain a classical GRE suggesting that the effect of the hormone may be indirect. Further studies are required to identify the precise DNA sequence responsible for the glucocorticoid effect as well as *trans*-acting factors that bind to it.

## ACKNOWLEDGMENT

Research in my laboratory was supported by a grant (HL-43320) from the National Heart, Lung and Blood Institute.

## REFERENCES

1. Gross I, Ballard PL. Hormonal therapy for prevention of respiratory distress syndrome. In: Polin RA, Fox WW, eds. Fetal and neonatal physiology. Philadelphia: Saunders, 1998:1314–1321.
2. Kresch MJ, Gross I. The biochemistry of fetal lung development. Clin Perinatol 1987;14:481–507.
3. Ballard PL Hormonal regulation of pulmonary surfactant. Endocr Rev 1989;10:165–181.
4. Mendelson CR, Boggaram V. Hormonal control of the surfactant system in fetal lung. Annu Rev Physiol 1991;53:415–440.
5. Rooney SA. The surfactant system and lung phospholipid biochemistry. Am Rev Respir Dis 1985;131:439–460.
6. Rooney SA. Regulation of surfactant–associated phospholipid synthesis and secretion. In: Polin RA, Fox WW, eds. Fetal and neonatal physiology. Philadelphia: Saunders, 1998:1283–1299.
7. Rooney SA. Regulation of surfactant phospholipid biosynthesis. In: Rooney SA, ed. Lung surfactant: cellular and molecular processing. Austin, TX: Landes, 1998: 29–45.
8. Rooney SA, Young SL, Mendelson CR. Molecular and cellular processing of lung surfactant. FASEB J 1994;8:957–967.
9. Possmayer F. Physicochemical aspects of pulmonary surfactant. In Polin R, Fox W, eds. Fetal and neonatal physiology. Philadelphia: Saunders, 1998:1259–1275.
10. Rooney SA. Phospholipid composition, biosynthesis, and secretion. In: Parent RA, ed. Comparative biology of the normal lung. Boca Raton, FL: CRC Press1992:511–544.
11. Keough KMW. Surfactant composition and extracellular transformations. In: Rooney SA, ed. Lung surfactant: cellular and molecular processing. Austin, TX: Landes, 1998:1–27.
12. Rooney SA. Fatty acid biosynthesis in developing fetal lung. Am J Physiol 1989;257:L195–L201.
13. Batenburg JJ. Surfactant phospholipids: synthesis and storage. Am J Physiol 1992;262:L367–L385.
14. Hillgartner FB, Salati LM, Goodridge AG. Physiological and molecular mechanisms involved in nutritional regulation of fatty acid synthesis. Physiol Rev 1995;75:47–76.
15. Smith S. The animal fatty acid synthase: one gene, one polypeptide, seven enzymes. FASEB J 1994;8:1248–1259.
16. Wakil SJ, Stoops JK, Joshi VC., Fatty acid synthesis and its regulation. Annu Rev Biochem 1983;52:537–579.
17. Semenkovich CF. Regulation of fatty acid synthase (FAS). Prog Lipid Res 1997;36:43–53.
18. Hennigar RA, PochetM, Hunt DA, Lukacher AE, Venema VJ, Seal E, Marrero MB. Characterization of fatty acid synthase in cell lines derived from experimental mammary tumors. Biochim Biophys Acta 1998;1392:85–100.
19. Maniscalco WM, Finkelstein JN, Parkhurst AB. De novo fatty acid synthesis in developing rat lung. Biochim Biophys Acta 1982;711:49–58.
20. Rooney SA, Gobran LI, Chu AJ. Thyroid hormone opposes some glucocorticoid effects on glycogen content and lipid synthesis in developing fetal rat lung. Pediatr Res 1986;20:545–550.
21. Jungas RL. Fatty acid synthesis in adipose tissue incubated in tritiated water. Biochemistry 1968;7:3708–3717.
22. Pope TS, Rooney SA. Effects of glucocorticoid and thyroid hormones on regulatory enzymes of fatty acid synthesis and glycogen metabolism in developing fetal rat lung. Biochim Biophys Acta 1987;918:141–148.
23. Batenburg JJ, den Breejen JN, Geelen MJH, Bijleveld C, van Golde LMG. Phosphatidylcholine synthesis in type II cells and regulation of the fatty acid supply. Prog Respir Res 1990;25:96–103.
24. Batenburg JJ, Whitsett JA. Levels of mRNAs coding for lipogenic enzymes in rat lung upon fasting and refeeding and during perinatal development. Biochim Biophys Acta 1990;1006:329–334.
25. Xu ZX, Stenzel W, Sasic SM, Smart DA, Rooney SA. Glucocorticoid regulation of fatty acid synthase gene expression in fetal rat lung. Am J Physiol 1993;265:L140–L147.
26. Das DK. Fatty acid synthesis in fetal lung. Biochem Biophys Res Commun 1980;92:867–875.
27. Gross I, Warshaw JB. Enzyme activities related to fatty acid synthesis in developing mammalian lung. Pediatr Res 1974;8:193–199.
28. Maniscalco WM, Wilson CM, Gross I, Gobran L, Rooney SA, Warshaw JB. Development of glycogen and phospholipid metabolism in fetal and newborn rat lung. Biochim Biophys Acta 1978;530:333–346.

29. Kikkawa Y, Kaibara M, Motoyama EK, Orzalesi MM, Cook CD. Morphologic development of fetal rabbit lung and its acceleration with cortisol. Am J Pathol 1971;64:423–442.

30. Carlson KS, Davies P, Smith BT, Post M. Temporal linkage of glycogen and saturated phosphatidyl-choline in fetal lung type II cells. Pediatr Res 1987;22:79–82.

31. Farrell PM, Bourbon JR. Fetal lung surfactant lipid synthesis from glycogen during organ culture. Biochim Biophys Acta 1986;878:159–167.

32. Liggins GC. Premature delivery of foetal lambs infused with glucocorticoids. Endocrinology 1969;45:515–523.

33. Liggins GC, Howie RN. A controlled trial of antepartum glucocorticoid treatment for prevention of the respiratory distress syndrome in premature infants. Pediatrics 1972;50:515–525.

34. Maniscalco WM, Finkelstein JN, Parkhurst AB Dexamethasone increases de novo fatty acid synthesis in fetal rabbit lung explants. Pediatr Res 1985;19:1272–1277.

35. Gonzales LW, Ertsey R, Ballard PL, Froh D, Goerke J, Gonzales J. Glucocorticoid stimulation of fatty acid synthesis in explants of human fetal lung. Biochim Biophys Acta 1990;1042:1–12.

36. Pope TS, Smart DA, Rooney SA. Hormonal effects on fatty–acid synthase in cultured fetal rat lung; induction by dexamethasone and inhibition of activity by triiodothyronine. Biochim Biophys Acta 1988;959:169–177.

37. Jobe AH, Ikegami M, Padbury J, Polk DH, Korirnilli A, Gonzales LW, Ballard PL. Combined effects of fetal beta agonist stimulation and glucocorticoids on lung function of preterm lambs. Biol Neonate 1997;72:305–313.

38. Gonzales LW, Ballard PL, Gonzales J. Glucocorticoid and cAMP increase fatty acid synthetase mRNA content in human fetal lung explants. Biochim Biophys Acta 1994;1215:49–58.

39. Rooney SA, Dynia DW, Smart DA, Chu AJ, Ingleson LD, Wilson CM, Gross I. Glucocorticoid stimu-lation of choline–phosphate cytidylyltransferase activity in fetal rat lung: receptor–response relation-ships. Biochim Biophys Acta 1986;888:208–216.

40. Ballard PL. Hormones and lung maturation. Berlin: Springer–Verlag, 1986.

41. Xu ZX, Viviano CJ, Rooney SA. Glucocorticoid stimulation of fatty–acid synthase gene transcription in fetal rat lung: antagonism by retinoic acid. Am J Physiol 1995;268:L683–L690.

42. Fraslon C, Batenburg JJ. Pre–translational regulation of lipid synthesizing enzymes and surfactant proteins in fetal rat lung in explant culture. FEBS Letts 1993;325:285–290.

43. Xu ZX, Rooney SA. Glucocorticoids increase fatty–acid synthase mRNA stability in fetal rat lung. Am J Physiol 1997;272:L860–L864.

44. Blennemann B, Leahy P, Kim TS, Freake HC. Tissue–specific regulation of lipogenic mRNAs by thyroid hormone. Mol Cell Endocrinol 1995;110:1–8.

45. Gudas L. Retinoids and vertebrate development. J Biol Chem 1994;269:15,399–15,402.

46. Chytil F. Retinoids in lung development. FASEB J 1996;10:986–992.

47. Schuger L, Varani J, Mitra R, Gilbride K. Retinoic acid stimulates mouse lung development by a mechanism involving epithelial–mesenchymal interaction and regulation of epidermal growth factor receptors. Develop Biol 1993;159:462–473.

48. Cardoso WV, Mitsialis SA, Brody JS, Williams MC. Retinoic acid alters the expression of pattern–related genes in the developing lung. Develop Dyn 1996;207:47–59.

49. Fraslon C, Bourbon JR. Retinoids control surfactant phospholipid biosynthesis in fetal rat lung. Am J Physiol 1994;266:L705–L712.

50. Metzler MD, Snyder JM. Retinoic acid differentially regulates expression of surfactant–associated proteins in human fetal lung. Endocrinology 1993;133:1990–1998.

51. Bogue CW, Jacobs HC, Dynia DW, Wilson CM, Gross I. Retinoic acid increases surfactant protein mRNA in fetal rat lung in culture. Am J Physiol 1996;271:L862–L868.

52. George TN, Snyder JM. Regulation of surfactant protein gene expression by retinoic acid metabolites. Pediatr Res 1997;41:692–701.

53. Geevarghese SK, Chytil F. Depletion of retinyl esters in the lungs coincides with lung prenatal mor-phological maturation. Biochem Biophys Res Commun 1994;200:529–535.

54. Tijburg LBM, Geelen MJH, van Golde LMG. Regulation of the biosynthesis of triacylglycerol, phos-phatidylcholine and phosphatidylethanolamine in the liver. Biochim Biophys Acta 1989;1004:1–19.

55. Kent C. Regulation of phosphatidylcholine biosynthesis. Prog Lipid Res 1990;29:87–105.

56. Kent C. Eukaryotic phospholipid biosynthesis. Annu Rev Biochem 1995;64:315–343.

57. Post M. Maternal administration of dexamethasone stimulates choline–phosphate cytidylyltransferase in fetal type II cells. Biochem J 1987;241:291–296.

58. Mallampalli RK, Walter ME, Peterson MW, Hunninghake GW. Betamethasone activation of CTP:cholinephosphate cytidylyltransferase in vivo is lipid dependent. Am J Respir Cell Mol Biol 1994;10:48–57.

59. Rooney SA, Gobran LI, Marino PA, Maniscalco WM, Gross I. Effects of betamethasone on phospholipid content, composition and biosynthesis in fetal rabbit lung. Biochim Biophys Acta 1979;572:64–76.

60. Freese WB, Hallman M. The effect of betamethasone and fetal sex on the synthesis and maturation of lung surfactant phospholipids in rabbits. Biochim Biophys Acta 1983;750:47–59.

61. Brehier A, Rooney SA. Phosphatidylcholine synthesis and glycogen depletion in fetal mouse lung. Exp Lung Res 1981;2:883–890.

62. Sharma AK, Gonzales LW, Ballard PL. Hormonal regulation of cholinephosphate cytidylyltransferase in human fetal lung. Biochim Biophys Acta 1993;1170:237–244.

63. Khosla SS, Brehier A, Eisenfeld AJ, Ingleson LD, Parks PA, Rooney SA. Influence of sex hormones on lung maturation in the fetal rabbit. Biochim Biophys Acta 1983;750:112–126.

64. Xu ZX, Smart DA, Rooney SA. Glucocorticoid induction of fatty–acid synthase mediates the stimulatory effect of the hormone on choline–phosphate cytidylyltransferase activity in fetal rat lung. Biochim Biophys Acta 1990;1044:70–76.

65. Viscardi RM, Weinhold PA, Beals TM, Simon, RH. Cholinephosphate cytidylyltransferase in fetal rat lung cells: activity and subcellular distribution in response to dexamethasone, triiodothyronine, and fibroblast–conditioned medium. Exp Lung Res 1989;15:223–237.

66. Rooney SA, Smart DA, Weinhold PA, Feldman DA. Dexamethasone increases the activity but not the amount of choline–phosphate cytidylyltransferase in fetal rat lung. Biochim Biophys Acta 1990;1044:385–389.

67. Hogan M, Kuliszewski M, Lee W, Post M. Regulation of phosphatidylcholine synthesis in maturing type II cells: increased mRNA stability of CTP:phosphocholine cytidylyltransferase. Biochem J 1996;314:799–803.

68. Batenburg JJ, Elfring RH. Pre–translational regulation by glucocorticoid of fatty acid and phosphatidylcholine synthesis in type II cells from fetal rat lung. FEBS Letts 1992;307:164–168.

69. Feldman DA, Kovac CR, Dranginis PL, Weinhold PA. The role of phosphatidylglycerol in the activation of CTP:phosphocholine cytidylyltransferase from rat lung J Biol Chem 1978;253:4980–4986.

70. Feldman DA, Rounsifer ME, Weinhold PA. The stimulation and binding of CTP:phosphorylcholine cytidylyltransferase by phosphatidylcholine–oleic acid vesicles. Biochim Biophys Acta 1985; 429:429–437.

71. Chu AJ, Rooney SA. Stimulation of cholinephosphate cytidylyltransferase activity by estrogen in fetal rabbit lung is mediated by phospholipids. Biochim Biophys Acta 1985;834:346–356.

72. Gross I, Dynia DW, Wilson CM, Ingleson LD, Gewolb IH, Rooney SA. Glucocorticoid–thyroid hormone interactions in fetal rat lung Pediatr Res 1984;18:191–196.

73. Freedland RA, Newton RS. Agaric acid. Methods Enzymol 1981;72:497–506.

74. Lowenstein JM, Brunengraber H. Hydroxycitrate. Methods Enzymol 1981;72:486–497.

75. Maniscalco WM, Finkelstein JN, Parkhurst AB. Effects of exogenous fatty acids and inhibition of de novo fatty acid synthesis on disaturated phosphatidylcholine production by fetal lung cells and adult type II cells. Exp Lung Res 1989;15:473–489.

76. Feldman DA, Brubaker PG, Weinhold PA. Activation of CTP:phosphocholine cytidylyltransferase in rat lung by fatty acids. Biochim Biophys Acta1981; 665:53–59.

77. Mallampalli RK, Salome RG, Li CH, VanRollins M, Hunninghake GW. Betamethasone activation of CTP:cholinephosphate cytidylyltransferase is mediated by fatty acids. J Cell Physiol 1995;162: 410–421.

78. Beck KF, Schreglmann R, Stathopulos I, Klein H, Hoch J, Schweizer M. The fatty acid synthase (FAS) gene and its promoter in Rattus norvegicus. DNA Sequence – J DNA Seq Mapp 1992;2:359–386.

79. Jayakumar A, Tai MII, Huang WY, Al–Feel W, Hsu M, Abu Elheiga L, Chirala SS, Wakil SJ. Human fatty acid synthase: properties and molecular cloning. Proc Natl Acad Sci USA 1995;92:8695–8699.

80. Kameda K, Goodridge AG. Isolation and partial characterization of the gene for goose fatty acid synthase. J Biol Chem 1991;266:419–426.

81. Semenkovich CF, Coleman T, Fiedorek FT. Human fatty acid synthase mRNA: tissue distribution, genetic mapping, and kinetics of decay after glucose deprivation. J Lipid Res 1995;36:1507–1521.

82. Jayakumar A, Chirala SS, Chinault AG, Baldini A, Abu–Elheiga L, Wakil SJ. Isolation and chromosomal mapping of genomic clones encoding the human fatty acid synthase gene. Genomics 1994;23:420–424.

83. Amy CM, Witkowski A, Naggert J, Williams B, Randhawa Z, Smith S. Molecular cloning and sequencing of cDNAs encoding the entire rat fatty acid synthase. Proc Natl Acad Sci USA 1989;86:3114–3118.

84. Amy CM, Williams–Ahlf B, Naggert J, Smith S. Intron–exon organization of the gene for the multifunctional animal fatty acid synthase. Proc Natl Acad Sci USA 1992;89:1105–1108.

85. Back DW, Goldman MJ, Fisch JE, Ochs RS, Goodridge AG. The fatty acid synthase gene in avian liver Two mRNAs are expressed and regulated in parallel by feeding, primarily at the level of transcription. J Biol Chem 1986;261:4190–4197.

86. Swierczynski J, Mitchell DA, Reinhold DS, Salati LM, Stapleton SR, Klautky SA, Struve AE, Goodridge AG. Triiodothyronine–induced accumulations of malic enzyme, fatty acid synthase, acetyl–coenzyme A carboxylase, and their mRNAs are blocked by protein kinase inhibitors: transcription is the affected step. J Biol Chem 1991;266:17,459–17,466.

87. Paulauskis JD, Sul HS. Cloning and expression of mouse fatty acid synthase and other specific mRNAs: developmental and hormonal regulation in 3T3–L1 cells. J Biol Chem 1988;263:7049–7054.

88. Mildner AM, Clarke SD. Porcine fatty acid synthase: cloning of a complementary DNA, tissue distribution of its mRNA and suppression of expression by somatotropin and dietary protein. J Nutr 1991;121:900–907.

89. Iritani N, Fukuda H, Matsumura Y. Lipogenic enzyme gene expression in rat liver during development after birth. J Biochem 1993;113:519–525.

90. Moustaid N, Sul HS. Regulation of expression of the fatty acid synthase gene in 3T3–L1 cells by differentiation and triiodothyronine. J Biol Chem 1991;266:18,550–18,554.

91. Iritani N. Nutritional and hormonal regulation of lipogenic–enzyme gene expression in rat liver. Eur J Biochem 1992;205:433–442.

92. Semenkovich CF, Coleman T, Goforth R. Physiologic concentrations of glucose regulate fatty acid synthase activity in HepG2 cells by mediating fatty acid synthase mRNA stability. J Biol Chem 1993;268:6961–6970.

93. Girard J, Perdereau D, Foufelle F, Prip–Buus C, Ferre P. Regulation of lipogenic enzyme gene expression by nutrients and hormones. FASEB J 1994;8:36–42.

94. Katsurada A, Iritani N, Fukuda H, Matsumura Y, Nishimoto N, Noguchi T, Tanaka T. Effects of nutrients and hormones on transcriptional and post–transcriptional regulation of fatty acid synthase in rat liver. Eur J Biochem 1990;190:427–433.

95. Paulauskis JD, Sul HS. Hormonal regulation of mouse fatty acid synthase gene transcription in liver. J Biol Chem 1989;264:574–577.

96. Teruel T, Valverde AM, Benito M, Lorenzo M. Insulin–like growth factor I and insulin induce adipogenic–related gene expression in fetal brown adipocyte primary cultures. Biochem J 1996;319:627–632.

97. Stapleton SR, Mitchell DA, Salati LM, Goodridge AG. Triiodothyronine stimulates transcription of fatty acid synthase gene in chick embryo hepatocytes in culture: insulin and insulin–like growth factor amplify that effect. J Biol Chem 1990;265:18,442–18,446.

98. Foufelle F, Gouhot B, Perdereau D, Girard J, Ferre P. Regulation of lipogenic enzyme and phosphoenolpyruvate carboxykinase gene expression in cultured white adipose tissue: glucose and insulin effects are antagonized by cAMP. Eur J Biochem 1994;223:893–900.

99. Donkin SS, McNall AD, Swencki BS, Peters JL, Etherton TD. The growth hormone–dependent decrease in hepatic fatty acid synthase mRNA is the result of a decrease in gene transcription. J Mol Endocrinol 1996;16:151–158.

100. Joyeux C, Rochefort H, Chalbos D. Progestin increases gene transcription and mRNA stability of fatty acid synthetase in breast cancer cells. Mol Endocrinol 1989;3:681–686.

101. Swinnen JV, Esquenet M, Goossens K, Heyns W, Verhoeven G. Androgens stimulate fatty acid synthase in the human prostate cancer cell line LNCaP. Cancer Res 1997;57:1086–1090.

102. Kuhajda FP, Jenner K, Wood FD, Hennigar RA, Jacobs LB, Dick JD, Pasternack GR Fatty acid synthesis: a potential selective target for antineoplastic therapy. Proc Natl Acad Sci USA 1994;91:6379–6383.

103. Pizer ES, Wood FD, Pasternack GR, Kuhajda FP. Fatty acid synthase (FAS): a target for cytotoxic antimetabolites in HL60 promyelocytic leukemia cells. Cancer Res 1996;56:745–751.

104. Rashid A, Pizer ES, Moga M, Milgraum LZ, Zahurak M, Pasternack GR, Kuhajda FP, Hamilton SR. Elevated expression of fatty acid synthase and fatty acid synthetic activity in colorectal neoplasia. Am J Pathol 1997;150:201–208.

105. Moustaid N, Beyer RS, Sul HS. Identification of an insulin response element in the fatty acid synthase promoter. J Biol Chem 1994;269:5629–5634.

106. Wolf SS, Hofer G, Beck KF, Roder K, Schweizer M. Insulin–responsive regions of the rat fatty acid synthase gene promoter. Biochem Biophys Res Commun 1994;203:943–950.
107. Misra S, Sakamoto K, Moustaid N, Sul HS. Localization of sequences for the basal and insulin–like growth factor–I inducible activity of the fatty acid synthase promoter in 3T3–L1 fibroblasts. Biochem J 1994;298:575–578.
108. Roder K, Wolf SS, Beck KF, Schweizer M. Cooperative binding of NF–Y and Sp1 at the DNase I–hypersensitive site, fatty acid synthase insulin–responsive element 1, located at –500 in the rat fatty acid synthase promoter. J Biol Chem 1997;272:21,616–21,624.
109. Rangan VS, Oskouian B, Smith S. Identification of an inverted CCAAT box motif in the fatty–acid synthase gene as an essential element for mediation of transcriptional regulation by cAMP. J Biol Chem 1996;271:2307–2312.
110. Roder K, Wolf SS, Beck KF, Sickinger S, Schweizer M. NF–Y binds to the inverted CCAAT box, an essential element for cAMP–dependent regulation of the rat fatty acid synthase (FAS) gene. Gene 1997;184:21–26.
111. Roder K, Klein H, Kranz H, Beck KF, Schweizer M. The tripartite DNA element responsible for diet–induced rat fatty acid synthase (FAS) regulation. Gene 1994;144:189–195.
112. Foufelle F, Lepetit N, Bosc D, Delzenne N, Morin J, Raymondjean M. DNase I hypersensitivity sites and nuclear protein binding on the fatty acid synthase gene: identification of an element with properties similar to known glucose–responsive elements. Biochem J 1995;308:521–527.
113. Magana MM, Osborne TF. Two tandem binding sites for sterol regulatory element binding proteins are required for sterol regulation of fatty–acid synthase promoter. J Biol Chem 1996;271:32,689–32,694.
114. Fukuda H, Iritani N, Noguchi T. Transcriptional regulatory regions for expression of the rat fatty acid synthase. FEBS Letts 1997;406:243–248.
115. Rolland V, Le Liepvre X, Jump DB, Lavau M, Dugail I. A GC–rich region containing Sp1 and Sp1–like binding sites is a crucial regulatory motif for fatty acid synthase gene promoter activity in adipocytes: implication in the overactivity of FAS promoter in obese Zucker rats. J Biol Chem 1996;271:21,297–21,302.
116. Oskouian B, Rangan VS, Smith S. Transcriptional regulation of the rat fatty acid synthase gene: identification and functional analysis of positive and negative effectors of basal transcription. Biochem J 1996;317:257–265.
117. Oskouian B, Rangan VS, Smith S. Regulatory elements in the first intron of the rat fatty acid synthase gene. Biochem J 1997;324:113–121.
118. Wang D, Sul HS. Upstream stimulatory factors bind to insulin response sequence of the fatty acid synthase promoter USF1 is regulated. J Biol Chem 1995;270:28,716–28,722.
119. Wang D, Sul HS. Upstream stimulatory factors bind to insulin response sequence of the fatty acid synthase promoter: a correction. J Biol Chem 1996;271:7873.
120. Wang D, Sul HS. Upstream stimulatory factor binding to the E–box at –65 is required for insulin regulation of the fatty acid synthase promoter. J Biol Chem 1997;272:26,367–26,374.
121. Berdanier CD. Role of glucocorticoids in the regulation of lipogenesis. FASEB J 1989;3:2179–2183.
122. Soncini M, Yet SF, Moon Y, Chun JY, Sul HS. Hormonal and nutritional control of the fatty acid synthase promoter in transgenic mice. J Biol Chem 1995;270:30,339–30,343.
123. Fukuda H, Katsurada A, Iritani N. Nutritional and hormonal regulation of mRNA levels of lipogenic enzymes in primary cultures of rat hepatocytes. J Biochem 1992;111:25–30.
124. Roncero C, Goodridge AG. Hexanoate and octanoate inhibit transcription of the malic enzyme and fatty acid synthase genes in chick embryo hepatocytes in culture. J Biol Chem 1992;267:14,918–14,927.
125. Amy CM, Williams–Ahlf B, Naggert J, Smith S. Molecular cloning of the mammalian fatty acid synthase gene and identification of the promoter region. Biochem J 1990;271:675–679.
126. Hsu MH, Chirala SS, Wakil SJ. Human fatty–acid synthase gene: Evidence for the presence of two promoters and their functional interaction. J Biol Chem 1996;271:13,584–13,592.
127. Lu Z, Gu Y, Rooney SA. Identification of DNA sequences responsible for glucocorticoid induction of the fatty–acid synthase gene in late gestation fetal lung. Am J Respir Crit Care Med 1998;157:A147.

# 6

# The Genetics of Glucocorticoid-Regulated Embryonic Lung Morphogenesis

## A First Approximation of the Epigenetic Rules

*Tina Jaskoll, PhD and Michael Melnick, DDS, PhD*

### CONTENTS

Prenatal lung development is the result of complex interactions between epithelial and mesenchymal primordia, which require a relatively precise program of signal transduction and specific gene regulation. Elucidating the details of this program is important for understanding the etiology of pulmonary immaturity associated with respiratory distress syndrome (RDS), as well as for the development of effective preventive and treatment strategies. Lung morphogenesis has conclusively been shown to be under steroidal control (reviewed in refs. *1–30, see also* Chapters 1–5, 7). Antenatal glucocorticoid (CORT) administration accelerates both morphogenesis and maturation (surfactant synthesis) of fetal lungs, reducing the incidence of neonatal RDS. Yet, in premature human births, significant racial, gender, and familial differences in the success of this steroid therapy are well known. Given the genetic susceptibility of infants to RDS *(4,5)*, the observation of a maternal effect, the association between specific HLA haplotypes and glucocorticoid responsiveness *(6)*, and the results of mouse studies *(7–9)*, we postulated that the gene(s) at or near the major histocompatibility complex [(MHC), HLA in humans, H-2 in mice] may be related to the risk for developing RDS and the relative response to CORT treatment. The observation by Hafez and coworkers *(10)* of an association between specific HLA haplotypes and RDS supports this hypothesis.

From: *Contemporary Endocrinology: Endocrinology of the Lung: Development and Surfactant Synthesis*
Edited by: C. R. Mendelson © Humana Press Inc., Totowa, NJ

Experimentally, the most important mammalian model is the genetically defined laboratory mouse because large segments of chromosomes have been identified in mice and humans that are conserved *(11)*. These syntenic segments, which include genes for lung-relevant hormones and growth factors and their respective receptors can be used to provide important insight into the developmental genetics of human lung morphogenesis. Since the H-2 complex in mice is homologous to the HLA complex in humans, one can use H-2 congenic mouse strains to investigate the relationship of the MHC-associated genes and lung development. Significantly, these H-2 congenic strains share identical genetic backgrounds except for a 3–18c$M$ region of chromosome 17 (i.e., the congenic region) that encompasses the H-2 gene complex and defines each haplotype *(12)*. Studies in our laboratory, as well as others, have shown that differential CORT responsiveness is related to genetic variation at or near the H-2 complex *(7–9,13,14)*. Using the B10 and B10.A congenic mouse pair, we have been investigating the relationship between genes at or near the MHC, CORT responsiveness, and lung morphogenesis. Our studies indicate that haplotype-dependent growth factor-mediated heterochronic development plays a key role in different pulmonary responses to CORT.

## H-2 HAPLOTYPE AND LUNG MORPHOGENESIS

Our laboratory has demonstrated haplotype-specific rates of development (heterochrony) in B10.A (H-2$^a$, a/a) and B10 (H-2$^b$, b/b) congenic mice. B10.A mice produce smaller fetuses exhibiting delays in lung development and skeletal development compared to B10 mice at identical Theiler (1989) stages *(7,9,15,16)*. B10.A lungs are a full developmental stage behind B10 lung on embryonic days 12–17 (E12–E17) *(15,16)*. As shown in Fig. 1, B10.A lung primordium is clearly smaller and has undergone less branching than the B10 lung primordium when isolated on day 12 of gestation from embryos with external features (e.g., craniofacial development and handplate shape) that stage identically (i.e., Theiler stage 20)*(17)*. This heterochrony persists throughout *in utero* development (Fig. 2); E17 B10 lungs are significantly more mature than E17 B10.A lungs *(7,8)*. In addition, the rate of pulmonary development is subject to a maternal effect; the maturation rate of heterozygous offspring from reciprocal crosses (e.g., B10.A ♀ × B10 ♂ and B10 ♀ × B10.A ♂) is dependent upon the maternal H-2 haplotype (Fig. 2)*(7)*. Given the above, we cultured E12 B10 and B10.A lung primordia under chemically defined conditions to determine if haplotype-specific rates of lung morphogenesis persist outside the maternal environment. After 7 days in vitro, B10.A primordia are substantially smaller and exhibit less epithelial branching compared to B10 primordia (Fig. 1C,D), indicating that haplotype-specific rates of lung morphogenesis already exist in early embryonic lung and that these haplotype-specific rates are independent of a continued maternal effect.

In addition, a strong association has consistently been shown between H-2 haplotype and susceptibility to CORT-induced cleft palate and fetal loss in congenic mouse strains *(9,18)*. Different degrees of CORT-induced susceptibility are shown to be related to specific haplotypes. These results indicate that H-2 haplotype differences alone are sufficient to alter CORT-induced susceptibility to cleft palate; other genes need not be present. Based on these observations, we postulated that a significant association exists between H-2 haplotype and CORT enhancement of lung morphogenesis *(7,8)*. With CORT treatment *in utero* on day 12 of gestation, only mice with the *a* haplotype became more mature; no differences were observed between control and CORT-treated *b* mice (Fig. 2) *(7)*. Thus, congenic mice can achieve haplotype-specific developmental

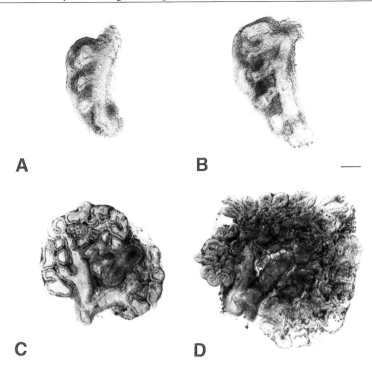

Fig. 1. Heterochronic development in H-2 congenic embryonic lungs. Panels A and B show early embryonic lung development in vivo. (**A**) E12 B10.A pulmonary left lobe. (**B**) E12 B10 pulmonary left lobe. Although the lungs were collected from embryos on day 12 of gestation and identified by external features as being at Theiler stage 20, substantial differences in the size and extent of epithelial branching are observed. The B10.A lung is markedly smaller and less branched than the B10 lung. Panels C and D show early embryonic lung development in vitro. (**C**) E12 B10.A lung primordium cultured for 7 days. (**D**) E12 B10 lung primordium cultured for 7 d. When E12 B10.A and B10 lung primordia were cultured for 7 d under chemically defined conditions as previously described *(76)*, the B10 explants are substantially larger and exhibit greater branching morphogenesis than the B10.A explants. Bar = 50 μm.

maturation, and the expression of these potentials is regulated by CORT. The results of our studies lead us to postulate that there exists on mouse chromosome 17 at or near the H-2 region a "developmental gene(s)" (DG) and a "glucocorticoid responsiveness gene(s)" (GRG) *(8)*. The GRG is not the structural gene for the glucocorticoid receptor (GR), which has previously been mapped to mouse chromosome 18 *(19)*. During development, we postulated that the GRG regulates CORT or receptor function. The GRG, through H-2 haplotype-specific CORT-GR activity, could then indirectly regulate the expression of the DG, modulate a cascade of developmental gene(s) and growth factors or increase the expression of regulatory factor(s) necessary to induce these DGs *(7,20,21)*. Thus, the combined GRG and DG influences will regulate the rate of embryonic and fetal morphogenesis. Under physiologic conditions, the GRG influences the DG to express the maximal developmental potential in the 17-d B10 fetal lung; thus exogenous steroids do not elicit further development (Fig. 3). By contrast, equivalent levels of endogenous CORT are inadequate to stimulate the DG to achieve maximal phenotypic expression in the B10.A mouse lungs; this results in an immature (pedomorphic) lung (Fig 3). During B10.A lung development, the regulatory clock was delayed by genetic,

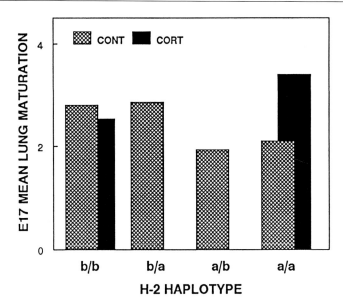

Fig. 2. H-2 haplotype-specific rates of fetal lung development. Mean E17 lung maturation (mm/mm$^2$) of control (CONT) and CORT-treated (CORT) lungs was determined by morphometric analyses (7). B10 (b/b) mouse lungs are significantly more mature than B10.A (a/a) lungs ($p < .025$). With CORT treatment, a/a lungs are significantly more mature than control a/a lungs ($p < .001$); there was no significant difference between control and treated b/b mice ($p > .05$). A significant maternal effect is seen in reciprocal crosses, B10 × B10.A (b/a) and B10.A × B10 (a/b): b/a mice are significantly more mature lungs than a/b mice ($p < .025$) and are similar to b/b mice; a/b lungs are similar to a/a lungs. [Data from ref. 8]

epigenetic, or environmental factors; changes in these factors alter the timing of the clock and change the developmental rate. Exogenous CORT treatment induces the B10.A mouse lung to develop and reach its maximal potential (Fig. 3). We have conducted a series of experiments in an attempt to identify the putative GRG and DG.

## H-2, LUNG MORPHOGENESIS, AND CORT RESPONSIVENESS

CORT-elicited responses are mediated by specific high-affinity cytoplasmic receptors (reviewed in refs. 21 and 22). In the presence of CORT, the hormone-bound receptor is activated to translocate into the nucleus where it binds to specific glucocorticoid response elements (GRE) in the regulatory regions of target genes, inducing or repressing de novo mRNA (21,22). Strain differences in CORT-GR responses can be mediated through ligand and/or GR differences between haplotypes. To determine if endogenous levels of corticosterone, the active glucocorticoid in mice, differ in B10 and B10.A lungs, we measured its level in E14 to E17 lungs by radioimmunoassay; no significant difference in endogenous CORT levels was seen between congenic strains (7). Given that (i) endogenous embryonic and fetal CORT levels are equivalent in developing B10 and B10.A lungs that exhibit different responses to CORT (7); (ii) the GR structural gene, encoded on chromosome 18 (19), is identical in both members of the congenic pair, which differ genetically only at a short segment of chromosome 17; and (iii) qualitative and quantitative differences in GR have been shown to be associated with tissue-specific CORT responsiveness (22–24), it was reasonable to postulate that H-2 associated gene(s)

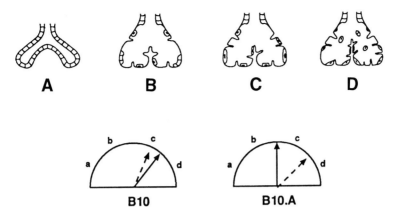

Fig. 3. A modified clock model of heterochronic lung development illustrates pulmonary development of E17 fetal lungs with or without CORT treatment *(67)*. (**A**) Stages of lung development: *a:* pseudoglandular stage; *b:* early canalicular stage; *c:* late canalicular stage; *d:* terminal sac stage. (**B**) B10 and B10.A each have different developmental potentials. No difference in lung maturation was observed between control (→) and CORT-treated (--->) B10 lungs. The B10.A control lung was less mature when compared to B10 lung; after CORT treatment; it became more mature than B10.A and B10 controls. The intervals shown on the clocks *(a–d)* represent the different lung maturation stages described in Fig. A above. [From ref. *8* with permission].

transregulate pulmonary GR expression. To address this question, we investigated possible translational and/or posttranslational modifications of the GR in B10 and B10.A mouse lungs. Since a significant maternal effect had been seen in CORT-induced lung morphogenesis (Fig. 2)*(7)*, we first evaluated GR characteristics in adult lungs. GR binding characteristics, receptor levels, and ligand-GR binding to the GRE were similar in both strains *(25)*. Our data indicated that, if gene(s) at or near the H-2 complex mediate differential *in utero* responses to CORT by modifying the GR, receptor differences should exist in the embryo/fetus. We analyzed embryonic B10 and B10.A pulmonary GR with immunochemical and biochemical methodologies. Western blot (Fig. 4) and ELISA analyses demonstrate no haplotype-specific qualitative or quantitative differences in the 96 kDa receptor. To determine if haplotype-specific variation in the GR pathway (e.g., CORT-GR complex binding to GRE DNA) is associated with differential CORT responsiveness, we evaluated GR-GRE binding by electrophoretic mobility-shift assays (EMSA); no qualitative differences in the GR-GRE complex are seen (Fig. 4). Quantitation of the EMSA data by phosphor image analysis and ANOVA demonstrated that the amount of GR activated in vitro significantly increases with development from E13 to E17 ($F = 24.148; p <.01$). Equivalent amounts of activatable GR are seen on each gestational day in both strains ($F = 0.296; p > .50$). The increase with gestational age was equivalent in B10 and B10.A congenic strains ($F = 1.482; p > .25$), indicating that the GR could be transformed and translocated into the nucleus in both strains with equal efficacy. We conclude that H-2 associated gene(s) do *not* transregulate either GR expression or function. Thus, a putative "glucocorticoid responsiveness gene" in the H-2 complex can effectively be discounted. The different responses to CORT seen between H-2 haplotypes are most probably consequent to different rates of embryonic morphogenesis (heterochrony) mediated by developmental genes which map at or near the H-2 region of mouse chromosome 17. The most likely candidate are growth factors or their receptors.

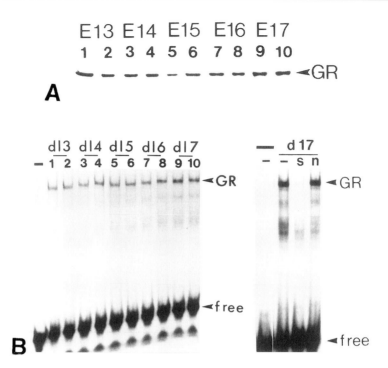

Fig. 4. Characterization of embryonic B10 and B10.A GR. (**A**) Western blot analysis of E13 to E17 B10 (odd-numbered lanes) and B10.A (even-numbered lanes) shows that the relative mobility of the GR protein is similar on all gestational days in both strains. (**B**) Functional analysis of the GR-GRE pathways. GRE binding by E13 to E17 B10 (odd-numbered lanes) and B10.A (even-numbered lanes) pulmonary GR demonstrates that the receptor is functional on all gestational days evaluated. No qualitative differences in GR-GRE interactions were observed between strains or days of gestation; quantitative differences were observed between days of gestation, but not between strains. Western blot analysis and electrophoretic mobility-shift assays were performed as previously described *(57)*. Unbound (free), GR-bound GRE, and the control BSA lane (-) are indicated. (**C**). To identify that the retarded complexes represent specific GR-GRE binding, E 17 extracts were incubated with no competitor (-) or in the presence of excess unlabeled GRE (s) or nonspecific (n) oligodeoxyribonucleotides; BSA control lane (—) is indicated. [From ref. *57* with permission].

## H-2 HAPLOTYPE-SPECIFIC EXPRESSION OF INSULIN-LIKE GROWTH FACTOR-IIR AND EMBRYONIC LUNG DEVELOPMENT

Because B10 and B10.A mice are genetically identical except for a 3–18c*M* region of chromosome 17 *(12)*, we sought promising candidate genes encoded in this region that regulate embryonic growth. The best candidate is the gene for IGF-IIR, mapped at approximately 8c*M* from the centromere and 10c*M* from the more telomeric H-2 *(20)*. IGF-IIR is a large, membrane-bound glycoprotein (approx 300 kDa) that contains distinct binding sites for two ligands, IGF-II growth factor and mannose-6-phosphate (M6P)-bearing molecules such as lysosomal enzymes and latent TGF-β *(26,27)*(*see* Chapter 11 for further discussion). This receptor does not appear to transduce mitogenic signals *(28)*; instead it sequesters IGF-II from type I IGF receptors (IGF-IR), which mediate IGF-II growth signal transduction (reviewed in refs. *29* and *30*). This sequestation of IGF-II appears to regulate the level of ligand available for use in promoting growth *(29,31)*. Significantly, the *Igf2r* locus is genomically imprinted; primarily the maternal copy is expressed in postimplantation embryos *(29,32,33)*. We first investigated the spatial distribution of IGF-II signaling molecules in B10 and B10.A embryonic lungs (Fig. 5). Although B10 embryonic lungs are developmentally 1 gestational day ahead of B10.A lungs, the *stage-specific* pattern of IGF-IIR immunolocalization is similar (data not shown). Our colocalization of IGF-II and IGF-IR in the epithelia suggests that the IGF-II/IGF-IR mitogenic signal promotes bronchiolar growth. By contrast, the localization of both IGF-II and IGF-IIR in the mesenchyme suggests that IGF-II/IGF-IIR sequestation of the ligand negatively regulates IGF-II-mediated mesenchymal growth. These observations indicate a segregation of IGF-II/IGF-IR growth promotion and IGF-II/IGF-IIR growth inhibition in embryonic lungs and suggest that IGF-II/IGF-IR promotes epithelial, and not mesenchymal, growth. To determine if quantitative differences in IGF-IIR exist between B10 and B10.A lungs, the steady-state levels of IGF-IIR transcripts were determined in E13 and E15 lungs (Fig. 6)*(16)*; we chose to analyze E13 and E15 lungs because these days encompass the critical period of mouse pulmonary branching morphogenesis. A significant increase in IGF-IIR mRNA from day 13 to day 15 is seen, regardless of strain. Further, the IGF-IIR mRNA levels in B10.A lungs are very significantly greater than that seen in B10 lungs. B10.A lungs also exhibit higher levels of IGF-IIR protein compared to B10 lungs *(16)*. These results, together with previous findings that IGF-IIR is required for embryogenesis *(34–37)*, suggest that IGF-IIR not only regulates the progressive differentiation of embryonic lungs but also the rate at which it proceeds.

Most importantly, we have demonstrated a significant haplotype-dependent variation in IGF-IIR levels during mouse embryogenesis *(16,38)*. B10.A lungs exhibit significantly greater IGF-IIR mRNA levels than in B10 lungs; the mean level for B10 on E15 is approximately that for B10.A on E13 (Fig. 6). This significant IGF-IIR variation is correlated with haplotype-specific rates of embryonic lung maturation. Clearly, developing B10.A lungs are paedomorphic ("underdeveloped") with respect to their B10 congenic partner *(7,16)*. However, it is not yet clear whether this results from a slower rate of morphogenesis or late induction of the initial bud, or both. Our IGF-IIR data would suggest that, at the very least, the rate of development is slower in B10 than in B10.A lungs in a way that is related to both cell number and IGF-IIR-regulated cell division.

A schematic model of IGF-IIR-mediated different pulmonary morphogenetic rates is shown in Fig. 7. Haplotype-specific differences in the amount of IGF-II available to transduce the mitogenic signal results in heterochronic development. Although IGF-II binds to both IGF-IR and IGF-IIR, it has approximately a sixfold higher affinity for IGF-IIR than for IGF-IR *(39)*. Higher levels of IGF-II/IGF-IIR binding in B10.A lungs decreases the amount of ligand available to bind to the growth-promoting IGF-IR, thereby delaying morphogenesis. Lower levels of IGF-IIR in B10 lungs would enable more ligand to bind IGF-IR. This would result in a morphogenetic signal of greater magnitude in B10 lungs than in B10.A lungs and acceleration of their morphogenetic rate. Differences in IGF-II/IGF-IIR levels can account for haplotype-specific differences in the rate of lung development; nevertheless, the IGF-II/IGF-IIR pathway has not been shown to be CORT-responsive. Clearly, other growth factor-directed signal transduction pathways must be involved.

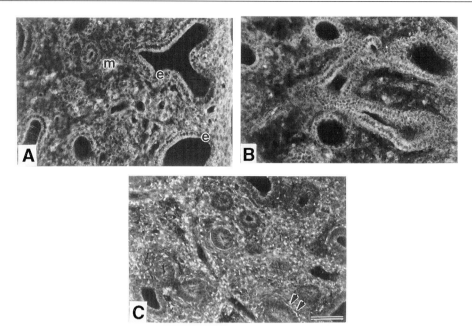

Fig. 5. Immunolocalization of IGF-II signaling molecules in embryonic (E15) lungs. **(A)** IGF-II. **(B)** IGF-IR. **(C)** IGF-IIR. IGF-II is immunodetected throughout epithelia (e) and mesenchyme (m). IGF-IR, the signal-transducing receptor, is only seen in epithelial cells. IGF-IIR is seen throughout the mesenchyme, with an increase in immunostain being seen in the aligned mesenchyme (arrowheads) adjacent to the branching epithelia and in the connective tissue surrounding blood vessels (data not shown). Bar = 50 µm.

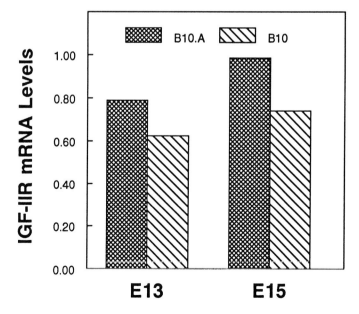

Fig. 6. Comparison of B10 and B10.A IGF-IIR transcript levels. IGF-IIR transcript levels were determined in E13 and E15 B10 and B10.A lungs by RNase protection assays *(16)*. Between E13 and E15, there is a significant (p > .05) increase in IGF-IIR mRNA levels. In addition, A significant 26–33% greater level of IGF-IIR mRNA is seen in B10.A lungs compared to B10 lungs (p < .01); IGF-IIR protein levels are also higher in B10.A lungs compared to B10 lungs (data not shown; *16*)[Data from ref. *16*].

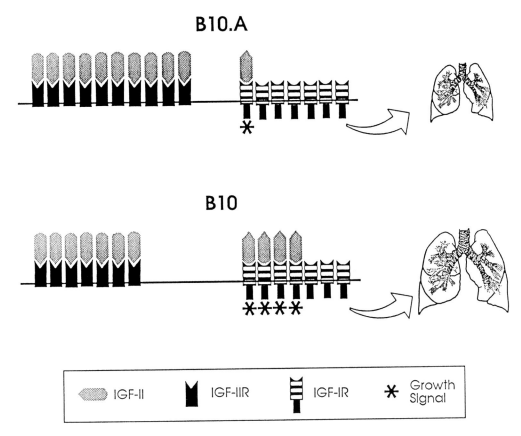

Fig. 7. Schematic of IGF-IIR's role during lung development. IGF-II binds to IGF-IR and IGF-IIR, having a higher affinity for IGF-IIR than for IGF-IR. The lower level of IGF-IIR in B10 lungs results in increased availability of IGF-II, thereby enabling more of the ligand to bind the IGF-IR in B10 lungs compared to B10.A lungs. Because only IGF-II/IGF-IR transduces a mitogenic signal (*), the result is an accelerated rate of morphogenesis in the B10 lungs compared to the B10.A lungs. [From ref. *16* with permission].

## TRANSFORMING GROWTH FACTOR BETA SIGNALING PATHWAYS DURING EMBRYONIC LUNG DEVELOPMENT

TGF-β is a member of an extensively studied family of growth factors. The TGF-β family of autocrine/paracrine growth factors participates in regulating cell proliferation and differentiation and extracellular matrix formation and degradation (reviewed in refs. *39a* and *40*). Newly synthesized TGF-β protein is noncovalently bound to the proregion dimer, the latency-associated peptide (LAP) and must be activated before binding to its receptor. TGF-β signaling is effected through a set of transmembrane Ser/Thr kinase receptors (reviewed in refs. *39a* and *40*). TGF-βs and their receptors have been shown to be present in embryonic lungs *(41–45)*. TGF-β ligand binding to the type II receptor (TGF-βRII) triggers heterodimerization with the TGF-β type I receptor (TGF-β RI), phosphorylation of TGF-β RI, and the propagation of the TGF-β signal to downstream substrates, including Smad2 or Smad3. Upon phosphorylation, Smad2 or Smad3 binds to Smad4 to form a heteromer complex, which then translocates into the nucleus to mediate the transcription of TGF-β - responsive genes.

Numerous investigations have indicated that TGF-β is an important morphoregulator of embryonic and fetal lung development (*see* Chapter 13 for further discussion). Beginning with the observation of different and possibly overlapping cell-specific distribution of TGF-β isoforms (β1,β2, and β3) in embryonic mouse lungs, researchers have speculated that different TGF-β isoforms differentially affect lung morphogenesis *(41,42,44,46)*. TGF-β2 (and TGF-β1) is immunolocalized in branching epithelia and, to a lesser extent, throughout the mesenchyme whereas TGF-β3 is only immunodetected in the aligned mesenchyme adjacent to branching epithelia (Fig. 8). TGF-βRII, the signal transducing receptor, is immunolocalized throughout both the epithelia and mesenchyme (Fig. 8); thus all three TGF-β isoforms can locally bind TGF-βRII to transduce the TGF-β signal. Several mechanistic studies have shown that TGF-β inhibits branching morphogenesis and lung maturation *(45, 47–51a)*. *First*, exogenous TGF-β supplementation in vitro has been shown to inhibit epithelial branching, lung maturation, and SP-A and SP-C expression *(45,47–49, 52–54)*. *Second*, organ-specific overexpression of TGF-β1 in transgenic mice bearing a chimeric SP-C promotor-directed TGF-β1 expression construct results in hypoplastic lungs *(51)*. *Third*, the inhibition of endogenous TGF-βRII or downstream effectors (i.e., Smad2, Smad3, or Smad4) expression prevents TGF-β-mediated inhibition of epithelial cell proliferation and branching morphogenesis *(45,50)*. When exogenous TGF-β is added to the culture medium, no pulmonary response is elicited. Taken together, these results indicate that TGF-β inhibits lung morphogenesis and that this inhibition must be overcome in order for lung maturation to occur.

TGF-β has been shown to negatively regulate epithelial and mesenchymal cell growth in vivo and in vitro. A better understanding of endogenous levels of TGF-β would help in understanding the role of TGF-β in regulating in vivo lung morphogenesis and histodifferentiation. Thus we characterized the steady-state levels of TGF-β1, TGF-β2, and TGF-β3 in E13 to E17 mouse lungs. Between E13 and E17, TGF-β2 transcript levels decrease approximately 40% and TGF-β3 transcript levels decrease approximately 25% (Fig. 9); no marked change in TGF-β1 mRNA level is seen (data not shown). This decrease in TGF-β2 and TGF-β3 levels is concomitant with the reported reduction in pulmonary TGF-β receptor number and activity in fetal lungs with gestational age *(55)*. Based on the above, we conclude that the substantial decrease in TGF-β2, TGF-β3, and TGF-βRII levels reduces TGF-β-mediated cell cycle arrest, resulting in cell proliferation and lung maturation.

Recently, our laboratory has demonstrated that CORT treatment in vivo significantly modulates TGF-β2 and/or TGF-β3 expression in embryonic mouse salivary glands and palates *(38,56)*. To determine if exogenous CORT treatment *in utero* also regulates embryonic pulmonary TGF-β expression, pregnant mice were injected on day 12 of gestation and lungs were collected on E15, 3 d postinjection. CORT-exposed lungs exhibit a significant 16% decrease in TGF-β3 mRNA level, whereas we find no significant change in TGF-β1and TGF-β2 mRNA levels (Fig. 7)*(57)*. This precocious downregulation of TGF-β3 expression on E15 is correlated with a marked decrease in TGF-β signal transduction, including a decrease in immunodetectable effector proteins (Smad2/3) in branching epithelia, as well as a substantial increase in cell proliferation and SP-A expression (Fig. 10). Our data indicate that CORT enhancement of branching morphogenesis and SP-A expression is, in part, mediated through the downregulation of the TGF-β3 signal transduction pathway.

However, it is very perplexing that only the precocious downregulation of TGF-β3 is a prerequisite for pulmonary histodifferentiation, since both TGF-β2 and TGF-β3

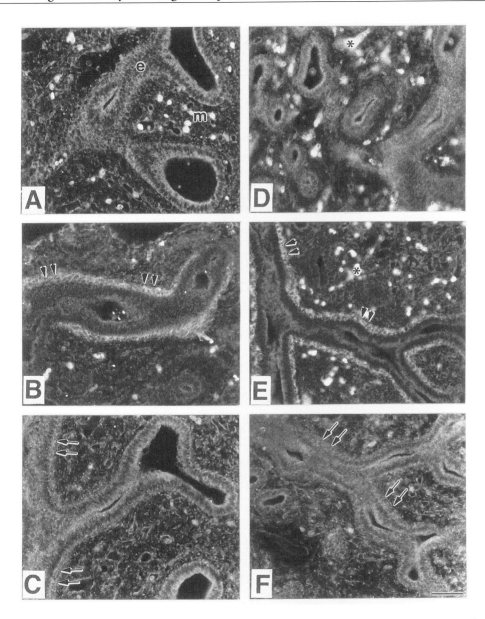

Fig. 8. Spatial distribution of TGF-β2, TGF-β3 and TGF-βRII during embryonic lung development. (**A, B, C**). E13. (**D, E, F**). E15. Panels A and D: TGF-β2 protein is primarily immunodetected throughout the epithelia (e) and to a lesser extent, in the mesenchyme (m) (Panels A and D); a similar spatial distribution is seen for TGF-β1 protein (data not shown). Panels B and E: TGF-β3 protein is immunolocalized in the aligned mesenchymal cells adjacent to the epithelia (arrowheads) and is absent from the epithelia. Panels C and F: TGF-βRII is immunolocalized throughout the both the epithelia and mesenchyme; by E15 (Panel F), a high level of TGF-βRII immunostain is detected in the aligned adepithelial mesenchyme (arrows). Note that TGF-β is also immunolocalized in blood vessels (*). Bar = 50 µm.

transcript levels normally decrease with gestational age (Figs. 9). One likely explanation is the *unique* spatial distribution of the TGF-β3 protein. TGF-β3, but not TGF-β1 or

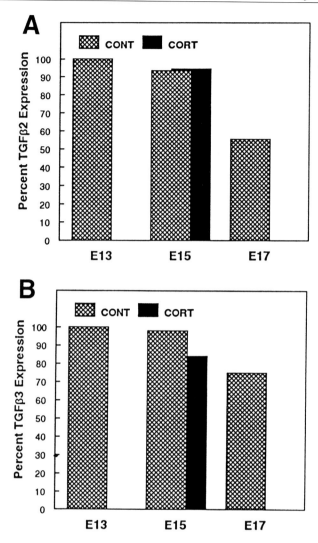

Fig. 9. Quantitative analysis of TGF-β2 and TGF-β3 transcript levels in control (CONT) and CORT-treated (CORT) lungs. During progressive development from E13 to E17, there was a 40% decrease in TGF-β2 and a 25% decrease in TGF-β3 mRNA levels; no substantial difference was seen for TGF-β1 (data not shown). CORT-treated E15 lungs exhibited almost no change in TGF-β1 and TGF-β2 mRNA expression and a significant 16% decrease in TGF-β3 mRNA expression compared with controls (*p* < .01). Northern blot and RNase protection assays were conducted and the blots were analyzed by Phosphorimager as previously described *(16,57)*. The data are presented as percent E13 transcript level.

TGF-β2, protein is immunolocalized in the aligned adepithelial mesenchyme (Figs. 8 and 11). Lung morphogenesis has conclusively been shown to be regulated by epithelial–mesencymal interactions and these adepithelial cells have been shown to be important for these cell–cell interactions *(58–60)*. The alignment of these mesenchymal cells adjacent to the epithelia, with the associated basal lamina discontinuities and transient direct-epithelial–mesenchymal cell–cell contacts *(58,59,61,62)* is believed to induce epithelial cytodifferentiation and surfactant synthesis *(58,62)*. Our immunolocalization data suggests that adepithelial mesenchymal TGF-β3 level is pivotal for pulmonary cell

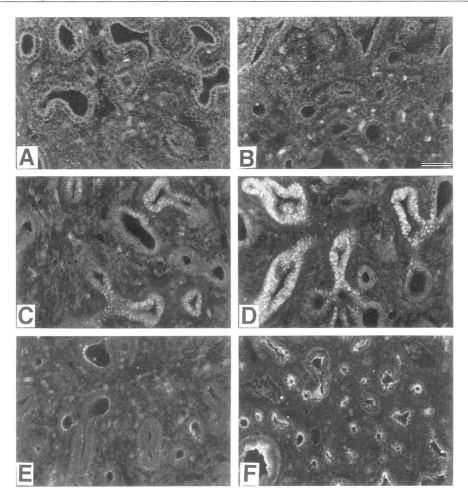

Fig. 10. Embryonic pulmonary responses to *in utero* CORT treatment. *(A,C,E)*. E15 control lung. *(B,D,F)*. CORT-treated E15 lung. Panels A and B: The spatial distribution of TGF-β effector proteins, Smad2/3. During development, TGF-β binding to its receptors induces Smad2/3 expression, formation of the Smad2/3–Smad4 heteromer and translocation into the nucleus to mediate the TGF-β signal. With CORT treatment (Panel **B**), there is a decrease in immunodetectable Smad2/3 compared to control lungs (Panel **A**). Panels C and D: Cell proliferation studies. CORT-treated lungs (Panel **D**) exhibit a marked increase in immunodetectable Cdk4 (cell proliferation) in epithelial cells compared to control lungs (Panel **C**). Panels E and F: SP-A expression. A marked increase in immunodectable SP-A is seen in CORT-treated lungs (Panel **F**) compared to controls (Panel **E**). Bar = 50 μm.

proliferation, maturation, and surfactant synthesis (Fig. 12). The CORT-induced preco-cious downregulation of adepithelial TGF-β3 on E15 negatively regulates the antimitogenic effect of TGF-β3's and inhibition of surfactant synthesis. We conclude that the highly localized expression and signaling of TGF-β3 at the epithelial–mesen-chymal interface is essential for lung maturation. A similar association between pulmo-nary cell proliferation and TGF-β3 reduction is seen in AEC2 pulmonary cells during recovery from hypoxia *(63)*. The level of active TGF-β3 peptide is significantly decreased during hypoxia and recovery in AEC2 pulmonary cells, with the greatest reduction in active peptide being seen during the proliferative phase of recovery *(63)*.

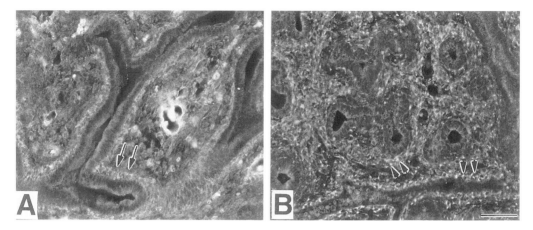

Fig. 11. Colocalization of TGF-β3 and IGF-IIR in E15 pulmonary mesenchyme. (**A**) TGF-β3 is immunodetected in the aligned adepithelial mesenchyme (arrows). (**B**) IGF-IIR is distributed throughout the mesenchyme; the immunolocalization of IGF-IIR in the aligned adepthelial mesenchymal cells is shown (arrow heads). Bar = 50 µm.

The aligned adepithelia are also important for CORT-enhanced lung development. Since the capability of the GR to transactivate a GRE on target genes is dependent on direct cell–cell contacts *(64)*, the observations of GR immunolocalization in these cells in fetal mouse lungs *(57)* and the increase in the number of epithelial–mesenchymal cell–cell contacts with *in utero* CORT treatment of fetal rabbits lungs *(60)* provide supporting evidence that CORT's influence on epithelial histodifferentiation is mediated through these adepithelial cells. Thus it appears that the CORT-induced downregulation of TGF-β3 is permissive of pulmonary branching morphogenesis (Fig. 12). The identification of a putative GRE in the promotor region of the SP-A *(65)*, as well as the observations that TGF-βs inhibit surfactant synthesis *(11,48,53,54,66)*, suggest that CORT might directly upregulate SP-A expression. Thus, the decrease in TGF-β3 expression is merely permissive for surfactant expression (Fig. 12). The ontogenic sequence would be CORT downregulation of TGF-β3, followed by growth factor-enhanced branching morphogenesis (Fig. 12, *pathway 1*), followed by CORT-enhanced histodifferentiation and SP-A synthesis (Fig. 12, *pathway 2*). The word permissive in this general model is shorthand for the as yet undetermined series of steps between CORT downregulation of TGF-β3 and the resulting phenotypes. Further studies are needed to delineate the molecular details of TGF-β3 regulation of surfactant expression.

Our designation that TGF-β3 is an important morphoregulator of embryonic lung development is supported by other reports *(66,67)*. *First,* immature lungs are seen in TGF-β3 null mice *(67)*. *Second,* exogenous TGF-β3 appears to inhibit CORT induction of surfactant expression *(66)*. The fact that TGF-β3 appears to be the most potent inhibitor of epithelial cell proliferation because of the differing ability of the TGF-β isoforms to bind to TGF-βRII and initiate signal transduction *(68)* helps to explain why the small, but significant, CORT-induced downregulation of TGF-β3 expression negatively regulates the $G_1$ arrest of the cell cycle. The endogenous levels of TGF-β1 and TGF-β2 proteins do not appear to be as important as the level of TGF-β3 protein.

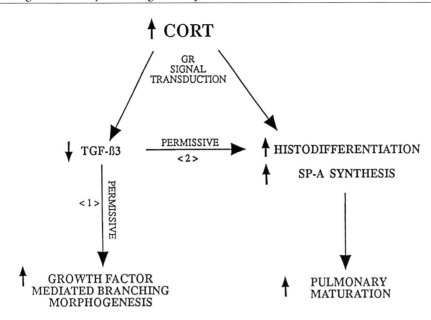

Fig. 12. Sequence of events consequent to administration of CORT to E12 mouse embryos *in utero*. CORT-induced down-regulation of TGF-β3 expression is followed by enhanced epithelial branching *(pathway 1)*; these developmental events are then followed by CORT- stimulated pulmonary histodifferentiation and SP-A expression *(pathway 2)*. [From ref. *57* with permission].

## RELATIONSHIP BETWEEN HAPLOTYPE-SPECIFIC INSULIN-LIKE GROWTH FACTOR-IIR LEVELS, TRANSFORMING GROWTH FACTOR BETA, AND LUNG MORPHOGENESIS

The association among H-2 haplotype, CORT-modulation of TGF-β expression, and lung morphogenesis requires further clarification. The relationship between TGF-β3 activation and IGF-IIR seems to us to be a key one. Strain differences in growth rate are associated with IGF-IIR expression *(16,38)* and cellular activation of latent TGF-β appears to require LAP binding to the mannose-6-phosphate (M6P) binding site of the IGF-IIR (Fig. 13) *(69,70)*. It was, therefore, reasonable to hypothesize that greater availability of the IGF-IIR receptor in B10.A embryos would result in a higher level of *activated* TGF-β. That is precisely what was seen in E14 palates; more IGF-IIR in B10.A palates, more active TGF-β protein and smaller palatal shelves *(38)*. The colocalization of TGF-β3 and IGF-IIR in embryonic p              ulmonary adepithelial mesenchyme (Fig. 11) suggests that IGF-IIR may play a similar role in pulmonary TGF-β3 protein activation. Since TGF-β inhibits the $G_1$-S transition of the cell cycle, one would expect an inverse relationship between activated TGF-β and cell proliferation.

During development, there exists a delicate balance between growth-promoting and growth-inhibiting factors. The complementary relationship between IGF-II and TGF-β signaling molecules is shown in Fig. 13. The IGF-II system promotes cell proliferation and growth by binding to the IGF-1R. Growth inhibition can be achieved in two ways: the decrease of the positive growth regulator (IGF-II/IGF-IIR) and the increase of the negative growth regulator (TGF-β3/IGF-IIR). (i) IGF-II/IGF-IIR binding sequesters the IGF-II ligand and negatively regulates the level of ligand available for the growth-

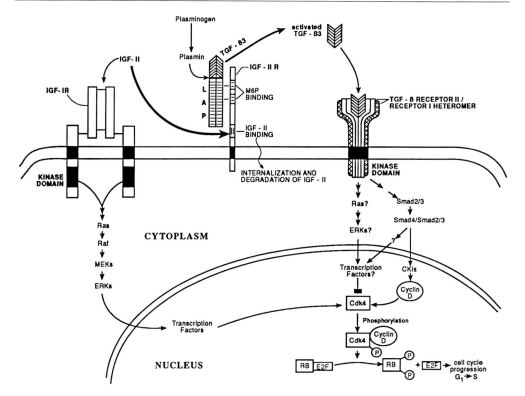

Fig. 13. This dynamic epigenetic model shows the complementary relationship between IGF-IIR and TGF-β. IGF-II promotes cell proliferation and growth by binding to IGF-IR. Two growth inhibitory pathways are shown: IGF-II/IGF-IIR and TGF-β3/IGF-IIR. First, IGF-II/IGF-IIR binding sequesters the IGF-II ligand and negatively regulates the level of ligand available for the growth promoting IGF-IR. Second, TGF-β protein is activated through TGF-β/IGF-IIR binding. TGF-β inhibition of the G$_1$-S cell cycle transition may be mediated through specific transcription factors, Smad2/3–Smad4 translocation into the nucleus, and/or the induction of cyclin-dependent kinase inhibitors (CKIs) MEK, mitogen-activated protein kinase kinase; ERK, mitogen-activated protein kinase; RB, retinoblastoma protein; E2F, a family of transcription factors.

promoting IGF-IR. Since IGF-II binds to the IGF-IIR with a significantly greater affinity than to the IGF-IR, less IGF-II will be available to bind IGF-IR and transduce the mitogenic signal (*see* Fig. 7). (ii) TGF-β protein is activated through TGF-β/IGF-IIR binding. Newly synthesized TGF-β protein is a large inactive molecule consisting of a mature TGF-β molecule noncovalently bound to the latency-associated peptide (LAP); latent TGF-β cellular activation appears to require TGF-β/LAP binding to the M6P binding site of IGF-IIR *(70)*. Once activated, TGF-β binding to its receptors induces the downregulation of Cdk4, and perhaps other G$_1$ factors, like cyclin E and/or Cdk2 expression, and the arrest of the G$_1$-S transition of the cell cycle (reviewed in refs. *32, 40,* and *71*). The antimitogenic effect of TGF-β is mediated through Smad2/3–Smad4 heteromer translocation from the cytoplasm into the nucleus. IGF-II and TGF-β competitively bind to the IGF-IIR, since the binding of either ligand (IGF-II or TGF-β) induces steric hindrance or conformational changes that prevent the other from binding *(68)*.

Based on this epigenetic model, we can outline the "putative" mechanism for H-2 haplotype-specific heterochronic lung development. Slower developing B10.A embryos have higher levels of IGF-IIR that serves to sequester IGF-II from the growth-promoting IGF-IR or to bind latent TGF-β3. Reduced levels of IGF-II/IGF-IR signal transduction and higher levels of TGF-β3/IGF-IIR growth inhibition in the late $G_1$ phase of the cell cycle would account for the slower growth and development of B10.A lungs relative to its B10 congenic partner. By contrast, B10 lung morphogenesis proceeds at a faster rate due to an increased level of IGF-II/IGF-IR growth-promoting signal and a decreased level of TGF-β3-mediated growth inhibition. CORT treatment induces precocious downregulation of TGF-β3 expression; this reduction of TGF-β3/IGF-IIR activated protein markedly reduces the mesenchymally derived inhibition of epithelial cell proliferation and histodifferentiation. Thus, we see increased cell proliferation and histodifferentiation. On the other hand, since B10 lungs are developmentally more advanced than B10.A lungs, CORT has no effect on lung morphogenesis because the CORT-induced downregulation of TGF-β3 coincides with the normal reduction of TGF-β3. A further reduction by CORT is not required for epithelial histodifferentiation and surfactant synthesis. Based on our data, we conclude that heterochronic rates of lung development is key for haplotype-specific responses to CORT.

In summary, we have reviewed the data demonstrating a relationship between H-2 haplotype, lung morphogenesis, and CORT responsiveness. Our studies indicate that H-2 haplotype-specific levels of IGF-IIR regulate the rate of lung morphogenesis by decreasing IGF-II/IGF-IR growth promotion and increasing activated TGF-β3/IGF-IIR growth inhibition. The haplotype-specific differences in IGF-IIR levels in embryonic lungs emphasizes the importance of the MHC haplotype in developing lungs. HLA in humans is the homolog of H-2 mice; the HLA complex and *IGF2R* gene are both mapped to chromosome 6. Since *IGF2R* is polymorphic in humans *(72)*, and RDS is associated with HLA haplotype differences *(10)*, this may have important implications for the treatment of RDS in premature infants. Finally, given that pulmonary morphogenesis, mouse or human, is characterized by an ordered and precise schedule of cellular spatiotemporal events *(62,73–75)*, a better understanding of the gestational endocrinology regulating these morphogenetic events is critical for elucidating the pathogenesis of RDS and developing effective treatment strategies. Our data indicates that CORT enhancement of lung morphogenesis and surfactant production is likely mediated through the precocious decrease in TGF-β3 signal transduction. Finally, the observation that CORT induces lung maturation in TGF-β3-null mice to a lesser degree than that seen in wild-type mice provides additional evidence that TGF-β3 is involved in CORT modulation of lung development *(77)*.

Clearly other signal transduction pathways influence embryonic lung morphogenesis. We have limited our focus to the IGF-II and TGF-β signaling pathways to discuss their complementary relationship as it relates to haplotype-specific pulmonary responses to CORT. Further studies are needed to determine if other pathways (e.g., TNF-α, EGF) also play important roles in haplotype-specific lung morphogenesis and CORT responsiveness.

## REFERENCES

1. Ballard PL. Hormonal regulation of pulmonary surfactant. Endocr Rev 1989;10:165–181.
2. Rooney SA, Young SL, Mendelson CR. Molecular and cellular processing of lung surfactant. FASEB J 1994;8:957–967.
3. Weaver TE, Whitsett JA. Function and regulation of expression of pulmonary surfactant-associated proteins. Biochem J 1991;273:249–264.

3a. Muglia LJ, Bar DS, Brown TT, Vogt SK, Alvarez JG, Sunday ME, Majzoub JA. Proliferation and differentiation defects during lung development in corticotropin-releasing hormone-deficient mice. Am J Resp Cell Mol Biol 1999;20:181–188.

4. Graven SN, Misheimer HR. Respiratory distress syndrome and the high risk mother. Am J Dis Child 1965;109:489–494.

5. Lankenau HM. A genetic and statistical study of the respiratory distress syndrome. Eur J Pediatr 1976;123:167–177.

6. Becker B, Shin DH, Palmberg PF, Waltman SR. HLA antigens and corticosteroid response. Science 1976;194:1427–1428.

7. Hu CC, Jaskoll TF, Minkin C, Melnick M. Mouse major histocompatibility complex (H-2) and fetal lung development: implications for human pulmonary maturation. Am J Med Genet 1990;35:126–131.

8. Jaskoll T, Hu CC, Melnick M. Mouse major histocompatibility complex and lung development: haplotype variation, H-2 immunolocalization, and progressive maturation. Am J Med Genet 1991;39:422–436.

9. Melnick M, Jaskoll T, Slavkin HC. Corticosteroid-induced cleft palate in mice and H-2 haplotype: maternal and embryonic effects. Immunogenetics 1981;13:443–450.

10. Hafez M, el Salleb F, Khashabe M, Risk MS, el Morsey Z, Bassinoy MR, el K'enawy F, Zaqhloul W. Evidence of HLA-linked susceptiblity gene(s) in respiratory distress syndrome. Dis Markers 1989;7:201–208.

11. Winter RM. The importance and methods of using animal models to study human disease. Growth Gen Horm 1993;9:6–8.

12. Vincek V, Sertie J, Zaleska-Rutczynska Z, Figuero F, Klein J. Characterization of H-2 congenic strains using DNA markers. Immunogenetics 1990;31:45–51.

13. Bonner JJ, Slavkin HC. Cleft palate susceptibility linked to histocompatibility-2 (H-2) in the mouse. Immunogenetics 1975;2:213–218.

14. Goldman AS. Biochemical mechanism of glucocorticoid- and phenytoin-induced cleft palate. In: Zimmerman EF, ed. Current topics in developmental biology, New York: Academic Press,1984:217–239.

15. Good L, Jaskoll T, Melnick M, Minkin C. The major histocompatibility complex and murine fetal development. J Dent Res 1991;70:579.

16. Melnick M, Chen H, Rich KA, Jaskoll T. Developmental expression of insulin-like growth factor II receptor in congenic mouse embryonic lungs: correlation between IGF-IIR mRNA and protein levels and heterochronic lung development. Mol Reprod Dev 1996;44:159–170.

17. Theiler K. The house mouse. Berlin: Springer-Verlag, 1989.

18. Melnick M, Jaskoll T, Slavkin HC. The association of H-2 haplotype with implantation, survival, and growth of murine embryos. Immunogenetics 1981;14:303–308.

19. Francke U, Gehring U. Chromosome assignment of a murine glucocorticoid receptor gene (GRl-1) using intraspecies somatic cell hybrids. Cell 1980;22:657–664.

20. Lyon MF, Kirby MC. Mouse chromosome atlas. In: Lyon MF, Raston S, Brown SDM. eds. Genetic variants and strains of the laboratory mouse. Oxford, UK: Oxford University Press, 1996:881–924.

21. Yamamoto KR. Steroid regulated transcription of specific genes and gene networks. Annu Rev Genet 1985;19:209–252.

22. Meisfeld R. The structure and function of steroid receptor proteins. Crit Rev Biochem Mol Biol 1989;24:101–117.

23. Kalimi M, Hubbard J, Gupta S. Modulation of glucocorticoid receptor from development to aging. Ann NY Acad Sci 1988;521:149–154.

24. Kalinyak JE, Griffin CA, Hamilton RW, Bradshaw JG, Perlman AJ, Hoffman AR. Developmental and hormonal regulation of glucocorticoid receptor messenger RNA in the rat. J Clin Invest 1989;84:1843–1848.

25. Jaskoll T, Luttge WG, Sakai DD, Nichols NR, Melnick M. H-2 gene complex and corticosteroid responsiveness: evidence that the corticosteroid hormone signal transduction pathway in the adult mouse lung is not associated with halplotype-specific responses to corticosteroids. Steroids 1993;58:400–406.

26. Jones JI, Clemmons DR. Insulin like growth factors and their binding proteins: biological actions Endocr Rev 1995;16:3–34.

27. Vignon F, Rochefort H. Interactions of pro-cathepsin D and IGF-II on the mannose-6-phosphate/IGF-II receptor. Breast Cancer Res Treat 1992;22:47–57.

28. Moats–Staats BM, Price WA, Xu L, Jarvis HW, Stiles AD. Regulation of the insulin-like growth factor system during normal rat lung development. Am J Res Cell Mol Biol 1995;12:56–64.

29. Barlow DP. Gametic imprinting in mammals. Science 1995;270:1610–1613.

30. Haig D, Graham C. Genomic imprinting and the strange case of the insulin-like growth factor II receptor. Cell 1991;64:1045–1046.

31. Ellis MJC, Leav BA, Yang Z, Rasmussen EJ, Pearce A, Zwiebel JA, Lippman ME, Cullen KJ. Affinity for the insulin-like growth factor II (IGF-II) receptor inhibits autocrine IGF-II activity in MCF-7 breast cancer cells. Mol Endocrinol 1996;10:286–297.

32. Hu JF, Oruganti H, Vu TH, Hoffman AR. Tissue-specific imprinting of the mouse insulin-like-growth-factor-II receptor gene correlates with differential allele-specific DNA methylation. Mol Endocrinology 1998;12:220–232.

33. Lerchner W, Barlow DP. Paternal repression of the imprinted mouse Igf2r locus occurs during implantation and is stable in all tissues of the postimplantation mouse embryo. Mech Dev 1997;61:141–149.

34. Baker J, Liu JP, Robertson EJ, Efstratiadis A. Role of insulin–like growth factors in embryonic and postnatal growth. Cell 1993;75:73–82.

35. Filson AJ, Louvi A, Efstratiadis A, Robertson EJ. Rescue of the T-associated maternal effect in mice carrying null mutations in Igf-2 and Igf2r, two reciprocally imprinted genes. Development 1993;118:731–736.

36. Lau MMH, Stewart CEH, Liu Z, Bhatt H, Rotwein P, Stewart CL. Loss of the imprinted IGF2/cation-independent mannose 6-phosphate receptor results in fetal overgrowth and perinatal lethality. Genes Dev 1994;8:2953–2963.

37. Wang Z-Q, Fung MR, Barlow DP, Wagner EF. Regulation of embryonic growth and lysosomal targeting by the imprinted Igf2/Mpr gene. Nature 1994;372:464–467.

38. Melnick M, Chen HM, Buckley S, Warburton D. Insulin-like-growth-factor-II receptor, transforming-growth-factor-beta, and CDK4 expression and the developmental epigenetics of mouse palate morphogenesis and dysmorphogenesis. Dev Dyn 1998;211:11–25.

39. Rechler MM, Nissley SP. Insulin-like growth factors. In: Peptide growth factors and their receptors. New York: Springer Verlag, 1991:263–367.

39a Hu PP-C, Datto MB, Wang X-F. Molecular mechanisms of transforming growth factor-β signaling. Endocr Rev 1998;19:349–363.

40. Kretzschmar M, Massague J. SMADs: mediators and regulators of TGF-beta signaling. Curr Opin Genet Dev 1998;8:103–111.

41. Heine UI, Munoz E, Flanders KC, Roberts AB, Sporn MB. Colocalization of TGF-β 1 and collagen I and II, fibrinectin and glycosaminoglycans during lung branching morphogenesis. Development 1990;109:29–36.

42. Pelton RW, Dickinson ME, Moses HL, Hogan BL. In situ hybridization analysis of TGF-β3 RNA expression during mouse development: comparative studies with TGF-β1 and TGF-β2. Development 1990;110:609–620.

43. Pelton RW, Moses HL. The Beta-type transforming growth factor: Mediators of cell regulation in the lung. Am Rev Respir Dis 1990;142:S31–S35.

44. Pelton RW, Saxena B, Jones M, Moses HL, Gold LI. Immunohistochemical localization of TGFβ1, TGFβ2, and TGFβ3 in the mouse embryo: Expression patterns suggest multiple roles during embryonic development. J Cell Biol 1991;115:1091–1105.

45. Zhao J, Bu D, Lee M, Slavkin HC, Hall FL, Warburton D. Abrogation of transforming growth factor-β type II receptor stimulates embryonic mouse lung branching morphogenesis in culture. Dev Biol 1996;180:242–257.

46. Millan FA, Denhez F, Kondaiah P, Akhurst RJ. Embryonic gene expression patterns of TGFβ1, β2 and β3 sugggest different developmental functions in vivo. Development 1991;111:131–144.

47. Chinoy MR, Zgleszewski SE, Cilley RE, Blewett CJ. Krummel TM, Reisher SR, Feinstein SI. Influence of epidermal growth-factor and transforming-growth-factor beta–1 on patterns of fetal mouse lung branching morphogenesis in organ–culture. Pediatr Pulmonol 1998;25:244–256.

48. Torday JS, Kourembanas S. Fetal rat lung fibroblasts produce a TGFb homolog that blocks alveolar type II cell maturation. Dev Biol 1990;139:35–41.

49. Whitsett JA, Budden A, Hull WM, Clark JC, O'Reilly MA. Transforming growth factor-β inhibits surfactant protein A expression in vitro. Biochim Biophys Acta 1992;1123:257–262.

50. Zhao J, Lee M, Smith S, Warburton D. expression positively regulates murine embryonic lung branching morphogenesis in culture. Dev Biol 1998;194:182–195.

51. Zhou L, Dey CR, Wert SE, Whitsett JA. Arrested lung morphogenesis in transgenic mice bearing an SP-C-TGF-β1 chimeric gene. Dev Biol. 1996;175:227–238.

51a. Beers MF, Solarin KO, Guttentag SH, Rosenbloom J, Kormilli A, Gonzales LW, Ballard PL. TGF-β1 inhibits surfactant component expression and epithelial cell maturation in cultured human feta lung. Am J Physiol 1998;275:L950–L960.

52. Serra R, Pelton RW, Moses HL. TGFβ1 inhibits branching morphogenesis and N-myc expression in lung bud organ cultures. Development 1994;120:2153–2161.
53. Torday JS. Cellular timing of fetal lung development. Semin Perinatol 1992;16:130–139.
54. Whitsett JA, Weaver TE, Lieberman MA, Clark JC, Daugherty C. Differential effects of epidermal growth factor and transforming growth factor-β in synthesis of $M_r$ = 35,000 surfactant–associated protein in fetal lung. J Biol Chem 1987;262:7908–7913.
55. Pereira S, Dammann CEL, McCants D, Nielsen HC. Tranforming-growth-factor-beta 1 binding and receptor kinetics in fetal mouse lung fibroblasts. Proc Soc Exp Biol Med. 1998;218:51–61.
56. Jaskoll T, Choy HA, Melnick M. Glucocorticoids, TGF-β, and embryonic mouse salivary gland morphogenesis. J Craniofacial Genet Dev Biol 1994;14:217–230.
57. Jaskoll T, Choy HA, Melnick M. The Glucocorticoid–glucocortidoid receptor signal transduction pathway, transforming growth factor-b, and embryonic mouse lung development in vivo. Pediatr Res 1996;39:749–759.
58. Adamson IYR, King GM. Epithelial–interstitial cell interactions in fetal rat lung development accelerated by steroids. Lab Invest 1986;50:456–460.
59. Grant MM, Cutts NR, Brody JS. Alterations in lung basement membrane during fetal growth and type-2 cell development. Dev Biol 1983;97:173–183.
60. Snyder JM, Rodgers H, O'Brien J, Mahli N, Magliato S, Durham P. The effects of glucocorticoids on rabbit fetal lung maturation in vivo: an ultrastructural morphometric study. Anat Rec 1992;232:133–140.
61. Bluemink JG, Van Maurik P, Lawsen KA. Intimate cell contacts at the epithelial/mesenchymal interface in embryonic mouse lung. J Ultrstruct Res 1976;56:257–270.
62. Jaskoll TF, Slavkin HC. Ultrastructural and immunofluorescence studies of basal–lamina alterations during mouse-lung morphogenesis. Differentiation 1984;28:36–48.
63. Buckley S, Bui KC, Hussain M, Warburton D. Dynamics of TGF-β3 peptide activity during rat alveolar epithelial–cell proliferative recovery from acute hyperoxia. Am J Physiol-Lung Cell Mol Physiol 1996;15:L54–L60.
64. Reisfeld S, Vardimon L. Cell to cell contacts control the transcription activity of the glucocorticoid receptor. Mol Endocrinol 1994;94:1224–1233.
65. Lacaze-Masmonteil T, Fraslon C, Bourbon J, Raymondjean M, Kahn A. Characterization of the rat pulmonary surfactant protein A promoter. Eur J Biochem 1992;206:613–623.
66. Wang XC, Jin QL, Xu J, Shen WT, Wang JX, Post M. TGF-beta 3 inhibits the increased gene expressions of pulmonary surfactant proteins induced by dexamethasone in fetal-rat lung in-vitro. Chinese Med J 1997;110:590–593.
67. Kaartinen V, Voncken JW, Schuler C, Warburton D, Bu D, Heisterkamp N, Groffen J. Abnormal lung development and cleft palate in moce lacking TGF-β3 indicates defects of epithelial–mesenchymal interactions. Nat Genetics 1995;11:415–421.
68. Cheifetz S, Hernandez H, Laiho M, ten Dijke P, Iwata KK, Massagues J. Distinct tranforming growth factor-β (TGFβ) receptor subsets as determinants of cellular responsiveness to three TGF-β isoforms. J Biol Chem 1990;265:20,533–20,538.
69. Dennis PA, Rifkin DB. Cellular activation of latent transforming growth factor β requires binding to the cation–independent mannose 6-phosphate/insulin-like growth factor type II receptor. Proc Natl Acad Sci USA 1991;88:580–584.
70. Gleizes P-E, Munger JS, Nunes I, Harpel JG, Mazzieri R, Noguera I, Rifkin DB. TGF-β latency: biological significance and mechanisms of activation. Stem Cells 1997;15:190–197.
71. Piek E, Heldin C-H, Dijke PT. Specificity, diversity, and regulation in TGF-β superfamily signaling. Faseb J 1999;13:2105–2124.
72. Xu Y, Goodyear CC, Deal C, Polychronakis C. Functional polymorphism in the parental imprinting of the human IGF2R gene. Biochem Biophys Res Commun 1993;197:747–754.
73. Farell PM. Morphologic aspects of lung maturation. In: Farrell, PM, ed. Lung development: biological and clinical perspectives. New York: Academic Press, 1992:13–26.
74. Jaskoll TF, Phelps D, Taeusch HW, Smith BT, Slavkin HC. Localization of pulmonary surfactant protein during mouse lung development. Dev Biol 1984;106:256–261.
75. Stiles AD, D'Ercole AJ. The insulin-like growth factors and the lung. Am J Respir Cell Mol Biol 1990;3:93–100.
76. Jaskoll TF, Don-Wheeler G, Johnson R, Slavkin HC. Embryonic mouse lung morphogenesis and type II cytodifferentiation in serumless, chemically defined medium using prolonged in vitro culture. Cell Differ 1988;24:105–118.
77. Shi W, Heisterkamp N. Groffen J, Zhao J, Warburton D, Kaartinen V. TG-β3-null mutation does not abrogate fetal lung maturation in vivo by glucocorticoids. Am J Physiol 1999;277:L1205–L1213.

# 7

# Corticotropin-Releasing Hormone and the Lung

*Maria Venihaki, PHD, Louis J. Muglia, MD, PHD, and Joseph A. Majzoub, MD*

## CONTENTS

INTRODUCTION
COMPONENTS OF THE HYPOTHALAMIC–PITUITARY–ADRENAL AXIS
CORTICOTROPIN-RELEASING HORMONE EXPRESSION DURING
    EMBRYONIC LIFE
CORTICOTROPIN-RELEASING HORMONE KNOCKOUT MICE
EFFECTS OF GLUCOCORTICOID
    ON LUNG DEVELOPMENT AND MATURATION
SUMMARY

## INTRODUCTION

Thirty years ago, Liggins *(1)* made the observation that treatment of pregnant sheep with glucocorticoid caused the preterm delivery of lambs at 124 d instead of the usual 145 d of gestation. Even more remarkably, the lambs survived despite their prematurity, a puzzling finding, given that lambs delivered at the same gestational age by cesarean section died soon after birth with respiratory insufficiency. Avery *(2)* suggested that the administered glucocorticoid had accelerated the lung development of the treated fetal lambs and was responsible for their postnatal survival due to an increase in surfactant content in the lung, which she proved in subsequent studies in sheep and rabbits. Since that time, how glucocorticoid affects fetal lung development has been the subject of much study *(3,4)*. At the clinical level, pregnant women with threatened preterm labor are now routinely given prenatal glucocorticoid treatment to accelerate lung maturation and diminish or prevent neonatal respiratory distress syndrome *(5)*. There is now heightened interest in the impact of glucocorticoids on lung development, as increasing numbers of pematurely born infants are being treated postnatally with high doses of potent glucocorticoid in an attempt to decrease the severity of chronic lung diseases of the newborn *(6)*.

In this chapter, we review the influence of the hypothalamic–pituitary–adrenal (HPA) axis upon lung development during fetal life. We will highlight contributions that have come from the analysis of mouse models employing targeted inactivation of genes encoding corticotropin-releasing hormone (CRH) and other components of the HPA axis.

6ng

From: *Contemporary Endocrinology: Endocrinology of the Lung: Development and Surfactant Synthesis*
Edited by: C. R. Mendelson © Humana Press Inc., Totowa, NJ

# COMPONENTS
## OF THE HYPOTHALAMIC–PITUITARY–ADRENAL AXIS

CRH is a 41-amino acid neuropeptide isolated from ovine hypothalamic extracts and characterized by Vale and his colleagues in 1981 *(7)*. The primary amino acid structure of CRH is highly conserved among species, with the human peptide identical to that in rats and mice and different only by seven amino acids from ovine *(8)*.

CRH is the major regulator of the HPA axis during postnatal life. It is synthesized in the parvocellular neurons of the paraventricular nucleus of the hypothalamus (PVH), released into the hypophysial portal blood system, and carried to the anterior pituitary gland. At this site, CRH stimulates the synthesis of proopiomelanocortin (POMC) mRNA and peptide, (the precursor of ACTH), and the release of ACTH from pituitary corticotrophs *(9,10)*. Secreted ACTH in turn acts on the adrenal gland via specific receptors to stimulate the secretion into the bloodstream of glucocorticoid, either corticosterone in rodents or cortisol in humans. A CRH-related molecule, urocortin, has also been recently described *(11)*. It is 45% identical to CRH and 63% identical to fish urotensin, which may be involved in salt regulation in fish *(12)*. Urocortin is found principally in the Edinger–Westphal nucleus of the rodent brain. Its functions are unknown.

CRH exerts its actions in the pituitary through receptors located on corticotrophs. Two specific CRH receptors, termed CRHR1 and CRHR2, have been identified *(13)*. CRHR1 is expressed in anterior pituitary corticotrophs and several brain regions. Its expression is regulated by psycholgical and physiologic stressors as well as by CRH *(14–16)*. CRHR2 is expressed in peripheral tissues, including the heart, skeletal muscle, gastrointestinal tract, and epididymis, as well as in some brain regions *(17,18)*. CRHR2 is also expressed in lung, albeit at low levels *(18,19)*.

ACTH, acting on steroidogenic cells of the adrenal cortex via the specific melanocortin receptor type 2 *(20)*, stimulates the synthesis and secretion of glucocorticoid. In postnatal life, a major function of glucocorticoid is the maintenance of blood glucose levels during fasting by stimulating gluconeogenesis and glycogenolysis *(21)*. In addition, glucocorticoid may protect against excessive immune system responses to inflammation, as well as maintain vascular responsiveness to vasoconstrictors *(22)*. Glucocorticoid in turn exerts a negative feedback effect on hypothalamic CRH and pituitary ACTH synthesis and secretion *(23–25)*. In light of these important functions of glucocorticoid, it is not surprising that adrenal insufficiency (Addison's disease) is lethal. However, mice with targeted inactivation of the CRH gene, which have very low basal and stressor-stimulated glucocorticoid levels, have normal longevity and are able to respond to most stressors as well as do normal mice *(26)*. This suggests that the low levels of glucocorticoid present in these mice are sufficient to maintain life, or that something other than glucocorticoid deficiency per se causes death in normal animals with adrenal insufficiency.

# CORTICOTROPIN-RELEASING HORMONE
## EXPRESSION DURING EMBRYONIC LIFE

### *Placental CRH*

The hypothalamus is the main source of CRH. However, CRH mRNA and peptide have been found in many extrahypothalamic sites as well as in a plethora of peripheral tissues *(27–31,49)*. In humans and other primates, the placenta is a major source of CRH

*(27,32–34)* but CRH is not present in the placentae of nonprimate mammals *(35).* In human placenta, CRH is made primarily by syncytiotrophoblasts and intermediate tro- phoblasts, but not cytotrophoblasts *(36).*

Placental CRH is under developmental regulation, with its mRNA expression increas- ing markedly during the last 6–8 wk of gestation *(37).* CRH made in the placenta is secreted into both the maternal and fetal circulations, with levels rising from approx 50 to 5000 pg/mL in the mother during gestation *(38).* The regulation of placental CRH has been studied in vitro, where it has been shown that glucocorticoid exerts a stimulatory effect on CRH gene expression, in contrast to its inhibitory effect on hypothalamic CRH *(39).* In contrast to the effect of glucocorticoid, progesterone has been found to inhibit the synthesis and release of CRH from the placenta *(40).*

The role of placental CRH is not well understood. Although its secretion into the mother may stimulate maternal HPA axis and thus contribute to the observed hypercortisolemia *(41,42),* a CRH-binding protein present in human plasma may limit its action in the mother *(43).* In the fetus, placental CRH may activate the fetal HPA axis *(40).* The concentration of CRH in fetal plasma is similar to that in hypophysial portal blood *(33),* consistent with a role in the stimulation of fetal pituitary ACTH secretion. In humans pituitary ACTH expression starts as early as 8 wk of gestation *(44)* and human fetal pituitary cells can respond to CRH in vitro at the earliest time tested (14 wk of gestation) *(45).* The human fetal HPA axis is active as early as 10 wk of gestation, as is clear in fetuses with congenital adrenal hyperplasia who are virilized by that time *(46).* Placental CRH and fetal cortisol may stimulate each other in a positive feedback loop *(38,39),* consistent with the observed exponential rise in both hormones during gestation *(47).* Thus stimulated, the rising fetal cortisol promotes the maturation of many fetal organs, including the lung.

## *Hypothalamic and Lung CRH*

The HPA axis is one of the first endocrine systems to develop during fetal life. Despite the potentially important role of placental CRH in promoting maturation in the human fetus, nonprimate mammals do not express CRH in their placentae *(35).* How- ever, CRH is highly expressed in the fetal mouse lung *(48).* Lung CRH expression starts on embryonic d 12.5 (e12.5), preceding the expression of hypothalamic CRH by 1 d, which suggests that lung-derived CRH may have a role to stimulate the pituitary– adrenal axis. Lung CRH mRNA is undetectable in 1-d-old mice using *in situ* hybrid- ization mRNA analysis *(48),* but is detectable in adult murine lung using reverse transcription PCR *(49).* The onset of expression of POMC mRNA and peptides in the murine pituitary starts as early as e12.5 *(50–52).* The onset of POMC expression becomes apparent at a stage when brain development is far from complete. Thus, the activation of POMC expression is probably independent of the formation of hypotha- lamic and extrahypothalamic brain structures, which suggests that CRH from other sources may enter the hypophysial portal circulation to stimulate the release of ACTH and adrenal corticosterone synthesis and secretion during early fetal life. CRH has recently been found to promote angiogenesis, being chemotactic for endothelial cells in vitro, as well as causing angiogenesis and tumor growth in vivo *(53).* This raises the intriguing possibility that fetal lung CRH, whose expression coincides with the peak timing of pulmonaryvasculogenesis *(54),* may function to augment pulmonary angio- genesis during fetal development.

## CORTICOTROPIN-RELEASING HORMONE KNOCKOUT MICE

### *Production of CRH Knockout Mice*

CRH knockout (KO) mice were produced by targeted gene inactivation. The targeting construct was generated from the *Eco*RI-*Sal*I 5 kb mouse CRH 5' flanking region extending from –5000 to –50 nucleotides and the 0.85 kb *Eco*RI-*Dra*I 3' CRH flanking region beginning within the 3' untranslated region. Homologous recombination resulted in replacement of the entire preproCRH coding region with the neomycin resistance gene. Of 127 clones 2 proved to have undergone gene targeting. The clones were injected into 3.5-d C57Bl/6 postcoital blastocysts to generate chimeras capable of transmitting the mutant allele to their offspring *(49)*. Chimeras transmitted the changed embryonic-stem-cell genome to their offspring, yielding mice heterozygous for CRH deficiency. Heterozygotes were then bred to each other to create mice homozygous for CRH deficiency *(26)*. CRH deficiency was confirmed by RNA and protein analyses of homozygous mutant and wild-type animals. Reverse-transcription polymerase chain reaction (RT-PCR) analysis of whole-brain RNA from these mice at e18.5 was done using CRH-specific primers. The products, expected for the wild-type CRH gene (1267 bp) and messenger RNA (585 bp), were seen in normal mice, whereas in homozygous mice neither product was observed.

### *Survival of CRH Knockout Mice*

CRH KO mice born from a heterozygous mother (CRH±) have normal longevity and are fertile, despite their low basal glucocorticoid levels. They are equal in size to their wild type (WT) littermates and appear healthy without glucocorticoid replacement. Matings between homozygous CRH KO mice result in fetuses delivered at term with a normal appearance, but which all die on the first day of life, with respiratory insufficiency and abnormal lung architecture (Fig. 1). Since there was no mortality in CRH-deficient neonates from heterozygote matings, the altered *in utero* environment of the homozygote mother must contribute to the neonatal demise *(26)*. Fetal glucocorticoid deficiency in the setting of concomitant maternal glucocorticoid deficiency was the suspected cause of abnormal pulmonary development in CRH KO fetuses carried by CRH KO mothers. It was reasoned that lung development in CRH KO fetuses carried by heterozygote mothers would be rescued by transplacental passage of glucocorticoid from mother to fetus, thus explaining the different outcomes of neonates produced by the two maternal genotypes. Indeed, CRH KO fetuses carried by heterozygous mothers have normal corticosterone levels, whereas those carried by CRH KO mothers have corticosterone levels approx 30% of normal during the last third of gestation *(55)*.

To further investigate maternal as well as fetal corticosterone deficiency as the basis for neonatal demise, corticosterone (30 μg/mL) was administered in the drinking water to pregnant CRH KO mice beginning at 12 d of gestation and extending through postpartum day 14. CRH KO offspring from these treated pregnancies were again viable without further postnatal glucocorticoid supplementation. Histologic examination of treated CRH KO neonates revealed normal lung architecture (Fig. 1). Thus, prenatal glucocorticoid treatment, or transfer of glucocorticoid from a glucocorticoid-sufficient mother, can reverse the pulmonary abnormality of CRH KO fetuses despite

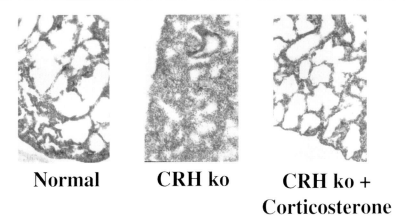

**Normal          CRH ko          CRH ko +
                                  Corticosterone**

Fig. 1. Lung dysplasia in CRH-deficient offspring of homozygous CRH-deficient matings is rescued by in utero corticosterone replacement. (Left) Wild-type lung on day of life 1 demonstrates thin alveolar septae and prominent air space expansion. Lungs were fixed in 4% paraformaldehyde, cut into 20-μ sections, and hematoxylin-eosin stained. The area shown is from the lateral region of the left lower lobe, as are the following sections from knockout mice. (Middle) Lung histology on day of life 1 from offspring of homozygous CRH knockout matings reveals dense, hypercellular lungs, thick alveolar septae, and a paucity of air spaces. (Right) In utero treatment of offspring of homozygous matings with corticosterone (30 μg/mL) in the maternal drinking water results in normalization of lung architecture and neonatal viability. (Reproduced with permission from ref. 26).

the presence of fetal CRH deficiency. Transfer of glucocorticoid from mother to fetus is probably also important in other disorders. For example, children with in the DAX-1 gene mutations (56) and mice with SF-1 gene mutations (57) are born lacking any adrenocortical tissue. Despite this, their pulmonary development is normal. Likewise, anencephalic infants and those with defects in adrenocortical steroidogenesis such as 21-hydroxylase deficiency have never been reported to be born with defective pulmonary development. This suggests that despite severe or even complete fetal glucocorticoid insufficiency, fetal maturation can be sustained by the transfer of maternal glucocorticoid to the fetus. This calls into question the degree to which placental 11-beta-hydroxysteroid dehydrogenase type 2 inactivates cortisol as it passes from mother to fetus (58).

Several other murine gene knockout models address the role of CRH and glucocorticoid in lung development. Mice with targeted inactivation of the CRHR1 gene have a neonatal phenotype indistinguishable from that of the CRH KO mouse, dying of respiratory failure on the first day of life unless treated prenatally with glucocorticoid (59). Also consistent with findings in the CRH KO mouse, targeted deletion of the glucocorticoid receptor gene results in neonatal death of respiratory insufficiency, with lung pathology similar to that found in the CRH KO newborn (60). As expected, prenatal glucocorticoid therapy is unable to rescue these mice. Mice with Brain-2 gene deletion lack hypothalamic CRH (61). Despite this, they are born with apparently normal lungs, but die several days later of an unclear cause, possibly related to concomitant vasopressin deficiency. This suggests that hypothalamic CRH is not absolutely required for activation of adrenocortical secretion during fetal life.

# EFFECTS OF GLUCOCORTICOID
# ON LUNG DEVELOPMENT AND MATURATION

## Lung Cell Proliferation and Differentiation

Since the early 1970s, it has been known that glucocorticoid can accelerate pulmonary epithelial cell differentiation *(2,62)*. Steroid-injected rabbit fetuses had lower lung weights, less protein and lung water, accelerated differentiation and a lower mitotic index compared to their non-injected littermates *(63)*. In vivo, Crone et al. *(64)* showed that hypophysectomy of fetal ovine fetuses and replacement therapy with either ACTH or cortisol had a marked effect on the differentiation and the number of type I and type II pneumocytes. Fetal rat lungs, when treated in an early stage of gestation with dexamethasone, show a pattern of maturation normally observed in late gestational ages *(65,66)*.

The CRH KO model offers a unique opportunity to investigate the effects of glucocorticoid deficiency in a setting independent of other factors which change during gestation. Fetal CRH KO mice carried in CRH KO mothers without prenatal steroid treatment are glucocorticoid insufficient, as described previously. The histologic appearance of their lungs is normal before e17.5, with normal bronchial branching morphogenesis and distribution of mesenchymal and epithelial cells *(67)*. However, on e17.5, a failure of septal thinning and airspace formation is observed, with maintenance of a dense pseudoglandular appearance (Fig. 2). Consistent with this, lung weight and total DNA content are increased in CRH KO mice compared to WT littermates *(67)* (Table 1). Immunostaining for proliferating cell nuclear antigen (PCNA, an index of cell proliferation) and total cell number are significantly elevated in CRH KO in proximal and distal airways between e17.5 and e18.5 (Fig. 3A, 3B). Levels of apoptosis in normal and CRH-deficient fetal lung are not different *(67)*. These data are in agreement with previous studies showing that exogenously administered glucocorticoid accelerates epithelial cell maturation *(2,62)*, and indicate that the lung hypercellularity observed in CRH KO fetuses is due to excessive cell proliferation, rather than a failure of apoptosis.

In addition to differences in mesenchymal and epithelial cellularity, examination of other specific cell types revealed differences between normal and CRH KO fetal lungs. CC10, a specific marker for Clara cells, remains undetectable in KO mice on e18.5 compared to WT mice, which shows prominent CC10 immunoreactivity in bronchial airway epithelium at this time point *(67)*. PGP9.5, a pulmonary neuroendocrine cell marker, which is restricted to these cells at e18.5 in normal mice, is found not only in neuroendocrine cells but also in the majority of the epithelial cells in CRH KO at this time point, as observed earlier in gestation in WT mice. This suggests that glucocorticoid-deficient CRH KO fetuses may have a delay in their developmental program of lung maturation.

## Effect of Glucocorticoid on Pulmonary Surfactant: Lipids

Production and secretion of pulmonary surfactant is under developmental and hormonal regulation. Liggins *(1)* was the first to recognize the effect of glucocorticoid treatment on the synthesis of surfactant lipids and proteins, when he reported that dexamethasone treatment of sheep resulted in partial aeration and survival of lambs for several hours at a point of gestation when survival would not otherwise have been possible. Since then, several studies in vitro and in vivo have shown the effect of glucocorticoid on surfactant proteins and lipids *(2,68–70)*. Glucocorticoid exerts its effects via specific types of receptors. Specific binding sites for the synthetic and the natural glu-

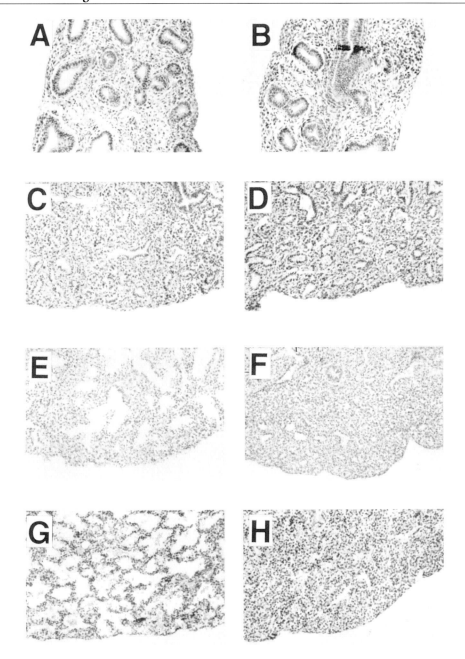

Fig. 2. Developmental analysis of lung histology in CRH KO and WT mice. Hematoxylin and eosin stained sections from 14.5, 16.5, 17.5, and 18.5 d of gestation photographed at 200× magnification are shown. (A) WT 14.5 d; (B) KO 14.5 d; (C) WT 16.5 d; (D) KO 16.5 d; (E) WT 17.5 d; (F) KO 17.5 d; (G) WT 18.5 d; (H) KO 18.5 d. (Reproduced with permission from ref. 67).

cocorticoid are present in fetal lungs of different species and the number of cytoplasmic receptors during the last days of pregnancy is increased (71). In human embryos binding was present as early as 12 wk of gestation. Dexamethasone binding capacity has also been found in fetal lungs of other species (71,72).

Table 1
Lung Weight and DNA Content at 18.5 d of Gestation in CRH-Deficient (KO)
and Wild-Type (WT) Fetuses

|  | WT | KO |  |
|---|---|---|---|
| Body weight (g) | $1.206 \pm 0.029$ | $1.172 \pm 0.026$ | $p = 0.4$ |
| Lung wet weight (mg/g body weight) | $31.3 \pm 0.9$ | $38.7 \pm 1.5$ | $p = 0.001$ |
| Lung dry weight (mg/g body weight) | $3.8 \pm 0.1$ | $5.4 \pm 0.2$ | $p < 0.0001$ |
| Wet/dry | $8.2 \pm 0.1$ | $7.1 \pm 0.1$ | $p < 0.0001$ |
| Total lung DNA (g/g body weight) | $289 \pm 14$ | $405 \pm 12$ | $p = 0.0001$ |

(Reproduced with permission from ref. 67)

Phosphatidylcholine (PC) is the most abundant component of surfactant, making up over two thirds of the molecule by weight in all mammalian species (73). Most PC in mammalian surfactant is present in the disaturated form as dipalmitoylphosphatidylcholine (DPPC) comprising about 45% of lung lipid, and responsible for most of the surface-active properties of surfactant. The content of DPPC and PC increases in amniotic fluid during the third trimester of human pregnancy. These lipids are used as markers for fetal lung maturity (74,75), and to monitor the response to prenatal glucocorticoid therapy (76).

A variety of enzymes that catalyze the biosynthesis of surfactant lipids are responsive to glucocorticoid. Cholinephosphate cytidyltransferase (CYT) catalyzes the conversion of choline–phosphate to cytidine–diphosphate–choline and is rate-limiting in the choline incorporation pathway. The activity of CYT is stimulated in vivo by dexamethasone in rats and other species and is developmentally regulated during gestation (68,69,77–79).

The activity of fatty acid synthase is similarly stimulated by in vivo treatment with dexamethasone, and also increases before birth (68,80,81).

Several in vitro and in vivo studies have been used to characterize the effect of glucocorticoid on surfactant phospholipids synthesis. It has been shown that glucocorticoid accelerates the appearance of lamellar bodies, increases the rate of choline incorporation into PC, the tissue content of DPPC and PC, and saturation of PC, reflecting synthesis and remodeling of PC to the disaturated species (70,82,83). In all cases, their effect on lung lipids is dose-dependent, receptor-mediated, and similar among different species.

Studies in CRH KO mice have provided information regarding the role of glucocorticoid on phospholipid biosynthesis. Fatty acid synthase mRNA is low in CRH KO mice on e17.5 but it goes back to normal levels by e18.5 (Fig. 4A). Amniotic fluid concentrations of DPPC on e18.5 (Fig. 4B) and the time of appearance of lamellar bodies in type II pneumocytes are normal in CRH KO fetuses, suggesting that glucocorticoid deficiency has no marked effect on surfactant phospholipids (67).

### Effect of Glucocorticoid on Pulmonary Surfactant: Proteins

Surfactant proteins comprise 5–10% of the total mass of pulmonary surfactant. Of the four proteins characterized thus far, surfactant protein A (SPA) and SPD are hydrophilic and may play a major role in host defense, while SPB and SPC are the major regulators of surface tension (84). SPA, the most abundant of the surfactant proteins, is a water-

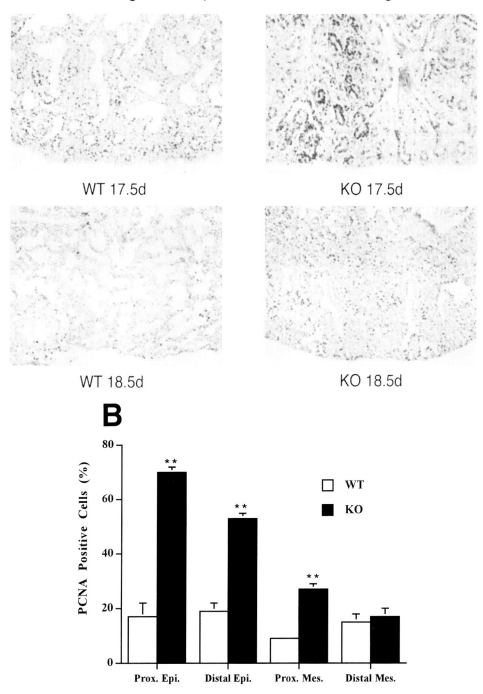

**A** Lung Development: PCNA Staining

WT 17.5d      KO 17.5d

WT 18.5d      KO 18.5d

**B**

Fig. 3. Analysis of proliferating cell nuclear antigen (PCNA) in CRH KO and WT mice at 17.5 and 18.5 d of gestation. (**A**) Immunohistochemical analysis. PCNA-positive cells are visualized by peroxidase staining resulting in formation of a brown nuclear precipitate. Sections are counterstained with methyl green for demonstration of architecture and photographed at 200× magnification. (**B**) Mophometric analysis of pulmonary development at 18.5 d of gestation. Prevalence of PCNA immunoreactivity in epithelial (Epi.) and mesenchymal (Mes.) cells in proximal and distal airways. **$p < 0.001$. (Reproduced with permission from ref. *67*).

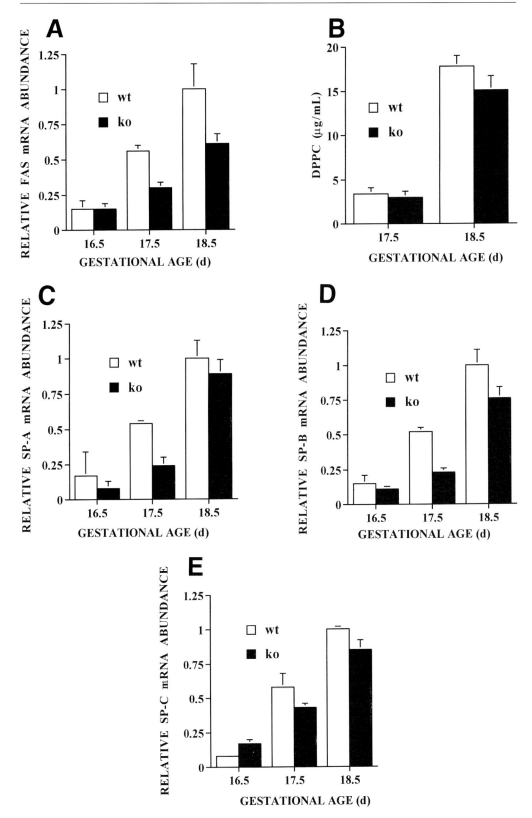

soluble glycoprotein. The SPA gene has been cloned and characterized in a variety of mammalian species *(85–87)*. SPA is developmentally regulated in human fetal lung tissue, being almost undetectable before the third trimester, after which it increases exponentially until delivery *(88–90)*. The effects of glucocorticoid on SPA mRNA and peptide content are contradictory. In vivo and in vitro, low doses of natural or synthetic glucocorticoid cause a marked stimulatory effect on SPA mRNA and protein expression in different species *(88,90–92)*. In other in vitro studies it has been reported that dexamethasone causes a marked inhibitory effect of accumulation of SPA protein *(93)* or had a biphasic dose- and time-dependent effect on the accumulation of SPA mRNA and immunoreactivity *(94,95)*. The inhibitory effect is receptor-mediated since it is blocked by specific glucocorticoid antagonists, and may involve decreased gene transcription and/or transiently reduced mRNA stability *(96,97)* *(see also* Chapters 1 and 3 for discussion).

SPD, the last surfactant protein to appear during gestation, is also under developmental regulation, with the levels of mRNA increasing before birth and diminishing during neonatal life before attaining adult levels *(98)*. Glucocorticoid stimulates SPD mRNA accumulation in vitro as well as in vivo in humans and rodents *(99–101)*.

SPB and SPC are small, hydrophobic proteins. They both enhance lipid spreading and the formation of a monolayer film. The genes for both SPB and SPC have been found and characterized in different species *(102)*. Both proteins are under developmental and glucocorticoid regulation. They are detected in human fetal lung as early as 13 wk of gestation, with levels increasing to approximately 50% (SPB) and 15% (SPC) of adult values by 24 wk of gestation *(70)*. Dexamethasone and cortisol increase levels of both mRNAs in vitro *(103–105)* as well as in vivo in fetal and adult lung *(106–108)*. SPB and SPC mRNAs are differentially regulated, with glucocorticoid enhancing both the rate of transcription and the stability of SPB mRNA, while affecting only the transcription rate of SPC *(109)* *(see also* Chapters 1 and 4 for discussion).

The expression of surfactant proteins is altered in CRH KO fetal mice, but it is to a lesser extent than expected given the known regulation of these proteins by glucocorticoid and the reduction in CRH KO fetuses of corticosterone levels to approximately 30% of normal during from e16.5 to birth *(55)*. Although levels of SPA and SPB mRNA are reduced by approximately 50% in CRH KO mice on e17.5, they return to normal by e18.5. SPC mRNA levels are normal in CRH KO fetuses at both time points (Fig. 4C–E). Together with the finding of normal DPPC lipid content of surfactant in CRH KO fetuses, these data suggest that the surfactant system is not the major pulmonary target of glucocorticoid during fetal development. Rather, glucocorticoid more broadly affects pulmonary epithelial and mesenchymal maturation, leading to alterations in cell proliferation and Clara cell differentiation, with surprisingly mild effects on the induction of surfactant protein and lipid synthesis *(67)*.

---

Fig. 4. *(opposite page)* Quantitation of parameters of type II pneumocyte maturation in WT and CRH KO mice. Northern blot analysis at 16.5–18.5 d gestation for **(C)** SP-A mRNA; **(D)** SP-B mRNA; **(E)** SP-C mRNA; and **(A)** fatty acid synthase (FAS) mRNA. Average hybridization intensity as fraction of the d 18.5 average for the indicated probe, with standard error of the mean, is shown (*$p < 0.01$). **(B)** Amniotic fluid concentration of dipalmitoyl phosphatidylcholine (DPPC) during late gestation in KO and WT mice determined by high-performance thin layer chromatography. (Reproduced with permission from ref. *67*).

## SUMMARY

During the past three decades, the importance of glucocorticoid for normal lung development has become more apparent. Initially thought principally to regulate the expression of lung surfactant, glucocorticoid has more recently been recognized to more broadly orchestrate pulmonary development, with surfactant expression being but one aspect of this. The CRH knockout model has revealed the importance of maternal glucocorticoid for lung development in the glucocorticoid-deficient fetus. Furthermore, this model, in which glucocorticoid deficiency is separable from other developmental processes, should prove valuable for ongoing evaluation of the mechanisms of glucocorticoid action and investigation of the program of cell differentiation in the lung.

## REFERENCES

1. Liggins GC. Premature delivery of foetal lambs infused with glucocorticoids. J Endocrinol 1969;45:515–523.
2. Kotas RV, Avery ME. Accelerated appearance of pulmonary surfactant in the fetal rabbit. J Appl Physiol 1971;30:358–361.
3. Ballard PL. Glucocorticoid regulation of lung maturation. Mead Johnson Symp Perinat Dev Med 1987;22–27.
4. Mendelson CR, Boggaram V. Hormonal control of the surfactant system in fetal lung. Annu Rev Physiol 1991;53:415–440.
5. Consensus development conference on the effect of corticosteroids for fetal maturation and perinatal outcome. Publication 95–3784. National Institutes of Health, Bethesda, MD, 1994.
6. Bancalari E. Corticosteroids and neonatal chronic lung disease. Eur J Pediatr 1998;157:S31–S37.
7. Vale W, Spiess J, Rivier C, Rivier J. Characterization of a 41-residue ovine hypothalamic peptide that stimulates secretion of corticotropin and beta-endorphin. Science 1981;213:1394–1397.
8. Rivier J, Spiess J, Vale W. Characterization of rat hypothalamic corticotropin-releasing factor. Proc Natl Acad Sci USA 1983;80:4851–4855.
9. Rivier C, Rivier J, Vale W. Inhibition of adrenocorticotropic hormone secretion in the rat by immunoneutralization of corticotropin-releasing factor. Science 1982;218:377–379.
10. Bruhn TO, Sutton RE, Rivier CL, Vale WW. Corticotropin-releasing factor regulates proopiomelanocortin messenger ribonucleic acid levels in vivo. Neuroendocrinology 1984;39:170–175.
11. Vaughan J, Donaldson C, Bittencourt J, Perrin MH, Lewis K, Sutton S, Chan R, Turnbull AV, Lovejoy D, Rivier C. Urocortin, a mammalian neuropeptide related to fish urotensin I and to corticotropin-releasing factor. Nature 1995;378:287–292.
12. Lederis K, Fryer J, Rivier J, MacCannell KL, Kobayashi Y, Woo N, Wong KL. Neurohormones from fish tails. II: actions of urotensin I in mammals and fishes. Recent Prog Horm Res 1985;41:553–576.
13. Dieterich KD, Lehnert H, De Souza EB. Corticotropin-releasing factor receptors: an overview. Exp Clin Endocrinol Diabetes 1997;105:65–82.
14. Mansi JA, Rivest S, Drolet G. Regulation of corticotropin-releasing factor type 1 CRF1) receptor messenger ribonucleic acid in the paraventricular nucleus of rat hypothalamus by exogenous CRF. Endocrinology 1996;137:4619–4629.
15. Rabadan-Diehl C, Kiss A, Camacho C, Aguilera G. Regulation of messenger ribonucleic acid for corticotropin releasing hormone receptor in the pituitary during stress. Endocrinology 1996;137:3808–3814.
16. Rivest S, Rivier C. The role of corticotropin-releasing factor and interleukin-1 in the regulation of neurons controlling reproductive functions. Endocr Rev 1995;16:177–199.
17. Chalmers DT, Lovenberg TW, De Souza EB. Localization of novel corticotropin-releasing factor receptor CRF2) mRNA expression to specific subcortical nuclei in rat brain: comparison with CRF1 receptor mRNA expression. J Neurosci 1995;15:6340–6350.
18. Lovenberg, TW, Chalmers DT, Liu C, De Souza, EB. CRF2 alpha and CRF2 beta receptor mRNAs are differentially distributed between the rat central nervous system and peripheral tissues. Endocrinology 1995;136:4139–4142.

19. Stenzel P, Kesterson R, Yeung W, Cone RD, Rittenberg MB, Stenzel-Poore, MP. Identification of a novel murine receptor for corticotropin-releasing hormone expressed in the heart. Mol Endocrinol 1995;9:637–645.

20. Mountjoy KG, Robbins LS, Mortrud MT, Cone RD. The cloning of a family of genes that encode the melanocortin receptors. Science 1992;257:1248–51.

21. Cryer PE, Fisher, JN, Shamoon H. Hypoglycemia. Diabetes Care 1994;17:734–755.

22. Munck A, Guyre PM, Holbrook NJ. Physiological functions of glucocorticoids in stress and their relation to pharmacological actions. Endocr Rev 1984;5:25–44.

23. Keller-Wood ME, Dallman MF. Corticosteroid inhibition of ACTH secretion. Endocr Rev 1984;5:1–24.

24. Plotsky PM, Sawchenko PE. Hypophysial-portal plasma levels, median eminence content, and immunohistochemical staining of corticotropin-releasing factor, arginine vasopressin, and oxytocin after pharmacological adrenalectomy. Endocrinology 1987;120:1361–1369.

25. Young WS, Mezey E, Siegel RE. Quantitative in situ hybridization histochemistry reveals increased levels of corticotropin-releasing factor mRNA after adrenalectomy in rats. Neurosci Lett 1986;70:198–203.

26. Muglia L, Jacobson L, Dikkes P, Majzoub JA. Corticotropin-releasing hormone deficiency reveals major fetal but not adult glucocorticoid need. Nature 1995;373:427–432.

27. Sasaki A. Tempst P, Liotta AS, Margioris AN, Hood LE, Kent SB, Sato S, Shinkawa O, Yoshinaga K, Krieger DT. Isolation and characterization of a corticotropin-releasing hormone- like peptide from human placenta. J Clin Endocrinol Metab 1988;67:768–773.

28. Potter E, Behan DP, Linton EA, Lowry PJ, Sawchenko PE, Vale WW. The central distribution of a corticotropin-releasing factor CRF- binding protein predicts multiple sites and modes of interaction with CRF. Proc Natl Acad Sci USA 1992;89:4192–4196.

29. Bruhn TO, Engeland WC, Anthony EL, Gann DS, Jackson IM. Corticotropin-releasing factor in the dog adrenal medulla is secreted in response to hemorrhage. Endocrinology 1987;120:25–33.

30. Karalis K, Sano H, Redwine J, Listwak S, Wilder RL, Chrousos GP. Autocrine or paracrine inflammatory actions of corticotropin-releasing hormone in vivo. Science 1991;254:421–423.

31. Emanuel RL, Thull DL, Girard DM, Majzoub JA. Developmental expression of corticotropin releasing hormone messenger RNA and peptide in rat hypothalamus. Peptides 1989;10:1165–1169.

32. Sasaki A, Liotta AS, Luckey MM, Margioris AN, Suda T, Krieger DT. Immunoreactive corticotropin-releasing factor is present in human maternal plasma during the third trimester of pregnancy. J Clin Endocrinol Metab 1984;59:812–814.

33. Goland RS, Wardlaw SL, Blum M, Tropper PJ, Stark RI. Biologically active corticotropin-releasing hormone in maternal and fetal plasma during pregnancy. Am J Obstet Gynecol 1988;159:884–890.

34. Smith R, Chan EC, Bowman ME, Harewood WJ, Phippard AF Corticotropin-releasing hormone in baboon pregnancy. J Clin Endocrinol Metab 1993;76:1063–1068.

35. Robinson BG, Arbiser JL, Emanuel RL, Majzoub JA. Species-specific placental corticotropin releasing hormone messenger RNA and peptide expression. Mol Cell Endocrinol 1989;62:337–341.

36. Riley SC, Walton JC, Herlick JM, Challis JR. The localization and distribution of corticotropin-releasing hormone in the human placenta and fetal membranes throughout gestation. J Clin Endocrinol Metab 1991;72:1001–1007.

37. Frim DM, Emanuel RL, Robinson BG, Smas CM, Adler GK, Majzoub JA. Characterization and gestational regulation of corticotropin-releasing hormone messenger RNA in human placenta. J Clin Invest 1988;82:287–292.

38. Emanuel RL, Robinson BG, Seely EW, Graves SW, Kohane I, Saltzman D, Barbieri R, Majzoub JA. Corticotrophin releasing hormone levels in human plasma and amniotic fluid during gestation. Clin Endocrinol (Oxf) 1994;40:257–262.

39. Robinson BG, Emanuel RL, Frim DM, Majzoub JA. Glucocorticoid stimulates expression of corticotropin-releasing hormone gene in human placenta. Proc Natl Acad Sci USA 1988;85:5244–5248.

40. Karalis KP, Goodwin G, Majzoub JA. Cortisol blockade of progesterone: a possible mechanism involved in the initiation of human labor. Nat Med 1996;2:556–560.

41. Goland RS, Jozak S, Conwell I. Placental corticotropin-releasing hormone and the hypercortisolism of pregnancy. Am J Obstet Gynecol 1994;171:1287–1291.

42. Magiakou MA, Mastorakos G, Rabin D, Margioris AN, Dubbert B, Calogero AE, Tsigos C, Munson PJ, Chrousos GP. The maternal hypothalamic-pituitary-adrenal axis in the third trimester of human pregnancy. Clin Endocrinol (Oxf) 1996;44:419–428.

43. Linton EA, Behan DP, Saphier PW, Lowry PJ. Corticotropin-releasing hormone CRH)-binding protein: reduction in the adrenocorticotropin-releasing activity of placental but not hypothalamic CRH. J Clin Endocrinol Metab 1990;70:1574–1580.

44. Holm IA, Majzoub JA. Adrenocorticotropin. In: The Pituitary (Melmed S, ed), Blackwell Scientific, Cambridge, 1995, pp. 45–97.

45. Blumenfeld Z, Jaffe RB. Hypophysiotropic and neuromodulatory regulation of adrenocorticotropin in the human fetal pituitary gland. J Clin Invest 1986;78:288–294.

46. Majzoub JA, McGregor JA, Lockwood CJ, Smith R, Taggart MS, Schulkin J. A central theory of preterm and term labor: putative role for corticotropin-releasing hormone. Am J Obstet Gynecol 1999;180:S232–S241.

47. Fencl MD, Stillman RJ, Cohen J, Tulchinsky D. Direct evidence of sudden rise in fetal corticoids late in human gestation. Nature 1980;287:225, 226.

48. Keegan CE, Herman JP, Karolyi IJ, O'Shea KS, Camper SA, Seasholtz AF. Differential expression of corticotropin-releasing hormone in developing mouse embryos and adult brain. Endocrinology 1994;134:2547–2555.

49. Muglia LJ, Jenkins NA, Gilbert DJ, Copeland NG, Majzoub JA. Expression of the mouse corticotropin-releasing hormone gene in vivo and targeted inactivation in embryonic stem cells. J Clin Invest 1994;93:2066–2072.

50. Carr GA, Jacobs RA, Young IR, Schwartz J, White A, Crosby S, Thorburn GD. Development of adrenocorticotropin-(1–39) and precursor peptide secretory responses in the fetal sheep during the last third of gestation. Endocrinology 1995;136:5020–5027.

51. Japon MA, Rubinstein M, Low MJ. In situ hybridization analysis of anterior pituitary hormone gene expression during fetal mouse development. J Histochem Cytochem 1994;42:1117–1125.

52. Ma E, Milewski N, Grossmann R, Ivell R, Kato Y, Ellendorff F. Proopiomelanocortin gene expression during pig pituitary and brain development. J Neuroendocrinol 1994;6:201–209.

53. Arbiser JL, Karalis K, Viswauathan A, Koike C, Anand-Apte B, Flynn E, Zetter B, Majzoub JA. Corticotropin-releasing hormone stimulates angiogenesis and epithelial tumor growth in the skin. J Invest Dermatol 1999;113:838–842.

54. Roman J. Cell-cell and cell-matrix interactions in development of the lung vasculature. In: Lung Growth and Development (MacDonald, J, ed.) Marcel Dekker, New York, 1997, pp. 365–399.

55. Venihaki M, Majzoub JA. The ontogeny of the hypothalamic-pituitary-adrenal axis in the CRH knockout fetal mice. 80th Annual Endocrine Society meeting, 1998;#P1–414.

56. Guo W, Mason JS, Stone CGJ, Morgan SA, Madu SI, Baldini A, Lindsay EA, Biesecker LG, Copeland KC, Horlick MN. Diagnosis of X-linked adrenal hypoplasia congenita by mutation analysis of the DAX1 gene. JAMA 1995;274:324–330.

57. Luo X, Ikeda Y, Parker KL. A cell-specific nuclear receptor is essential for adrenal and gonadal development and sexual differentiation. Cell 1994;77:481–490.

58. Benediktsson R, Calder AA, Edwards CR, Seckl JR. Placental 11 beta-hydroxysteroid dehydrogenase: a key regulator of fetal glucocorticoid exposure. Clin Endocrinol (Oxf) 1997;46:161–166.

59. Smith GW, Aubry JM, Dellu F, Contarino A, Bilezikjian LM, Gold LH, Chen R, Marchuk Y, Hauser C, Bentley CA, Sawchenko PE, Koob GF, Vale W, Lee KF. Corticotropin releasing factor receptor 1-deficient mice display decreased anxiety, impaired stress response, and aberrant neuroendocrine development. Neuron 1998;20:1093–1102.

60. Cole TJ, Blendy JA, Monaghan AP, Krieglstein K, Schmid W, Aguzzi A, Fantuzzi G, Hummler E, Unsicker K, Schutz G. Targeted disruption of the glucocorticoid receptor gene blocks adrenergic chromaffin cell development and severely retards lung maturation. Genes Dev 1995;9:1608–1621.

61. Schonemann MD, Ryan AK, McEvilly RJ, O'Connell SM, Arias CA, Kalla KA, Li P, Sawchenko PE, Rosenfeld MG. Development and survival of the endocrine hypothalamus and posterior pituitary gland requires the neuronal POU domain factor Brn-2. Genes Dev 1995;9:3122–3135.

62. Kotas RV, Avery ME. The influence of sex on fetal rabbit lung maturation and on the response to glucocorticoid. Am Rev Respir Dis 1980;121:377–380.

63. Carson SH, Taeusch HWJ, Avery ME. Inhibition of lung cell division after hydrocortisone injection into fetal rabbits. J Appl Physiol 1973;34:660–663.

64. Crone RK, Davies P, Liggins GC, Reid L. The effects of hypophysectomy, thyroidectomy, and postoperative infusion of cortisol or adrenocorticotrophin on the structure of the ovine fetal lung. J Dev Physiol 1983;5:281–288.

65. Oshika E, Liu S, Ung LP, Singh G, Shinozuka H, Michalopoulos GK, Katyal SL. Glucocorticoid-induced effects on pattern formation and epithelial cell differentiation in early embryonic rat lungs. Pediatr Res 1998;43:305–314.

66. Kinnard WV, Tuder R, Papst P, Fisher JH. Regulation of alveolar type II cell differentiation and proliferation in adult rat lung explants. Am J Respir Cell Mol Biol 1994;11:416–425.

67. Muglia LJ, Bae DS, Brown TT, Vogt SK, Alvarez JG, Sunday ME, Majzoub JA. Proliferation and differentiation defects during lung development in corticotropin-releasing hormone-deficient mice. Am J Respir Cell Mol Biol 1999;20:181–188.

68. Sharma A, Gonzales LW, Ballard PL. Hormonal regulation of cholinephosphate cytidylyltransferase in human fetal lung. Biochim Biophys Acta 1993;1170:237–244.

69. Rooney SA, Dynia DW, Smart DA, Chu AJ, Ingleson LD, Wilson CM, Gross I. Glucocorticoid stimulation of choline-phosphate cytidylyltransferase activity in fetal rat lung: receptor-response relationships. Biochim Biophys Acta 1986;888:208–216.

70. Ballard PL. Hormonal regulation of pulmonary surfactant. Endocr Rev 1989;10:165–181.

71. Ballard PL, Ballard RA. Glucocorticoid receptors and the role of glucocorticoids in fetal lung development. Proc Natl Acad Sci USA 1972;69:2668–2672.

72. Ballard PL. Glucocorticoid receptors in the lung. Fed Proc 1977;36:2660–2665.

73. King RJ. Pulmonary surfactant. J Appl Physiol 1982;53:1–8.

74. Spillman T, Cotton DB. Current perspectives in assessment of fetal pulmonary surfactant status with amniotic fluid. Crit Rev Clin Lab Sci 1989;27:341–389.

75. Gluck L. Fetal maturity and amniotic fluid surfactant determinations In: Management of the High Risk Pregnancy Spellacy WN, ed.), University Park Press, Baltimore, MD, 1976, pp. 189–207.

76. Torday J, Carson L, Lawson EE. Saturated phosphatidylcholine in amniotic fluid and prediction of the respiratory–distress syndrome. N Engl J Med 1979;301:1013–1018.

77. Oldenborg V, Van Golde LM. The enzymes of phosphatidylcholine biosynthesis in the fetal mouse lung. Effects of dexamethasone. Biochim Biophys Acta 1977;489:454–465.

78. Rooney SA, Gobran LI, Marino PA, Maniscalco WM, Gross I. Effects of betamethasone on phospholipid content, composition and biosynthesis in the fetal rabbit lung. Biochim Biophys Acta 1979;572:64–76.

79. Brehier A, Rooney SA. Phosphatidylcholine synthesis and glycogen depletion in fetal mouse lung: developmental changes and the effects of dexamethasone. Exp Lung Res 1981;2:273–287.

80. Pope TS, Rooney SA. Effects of glucocorticoid and thyroid hormones on regulatory enzymes of fatty acid synthesis and glycogen metabolism in developing fetal rat lung. Biochim Biophys Acta 1987;918:141–148.

81. Gonzales LW, Ertsey R, Ballard PL, Froh D, Goerke J, Gonzales J. Glucocorticoid stimulation of fatty acid synthesis in explants of human fetal lung. Biochim Biophys Acta 1990;1042:1–12.

82. Gross I, Ballard PL, Ballard RA, Jones CT, Wilson CM. Corticosteroid stimulation of phosphatidylcholine synthesis in cultured fetal rabbit lung: evidence for de novo protein synthesis mediated by glucocorticoid receptors. Endocrinology 1983;112:829–837.

83. Mendelson CR, Snyder JM. Effect of cortisol on the synthesis of lamellar body glycerophospholipids in fetal rabbit lung tissue in vitro Biochim Biophys Acta 1985;834:85–94.

84. Creuwels LA, Van Golde LM, Haagsman HP. The pulmonary surfactant system: biochemical and clinical aspects. Lung 1997;175:1–39.

85. White RT, Damm D, Miller J, Spratt K, Schilling J, Hawgood S, Benson B, Cordell B. Isolation and characterization of the human pulmonary surfactant apoprotein gene. Nature 1985;317:361–363.

86. Korfhagen TR, Bruno MD, Glasser SW, Ciraolo PJ, Whitsett JA, Lattier DL, Wikenheiser KA, Clark JC. Murine pulmonary surfactant SP-A gene: cloning, sequence, and transcriptional activity. Am J Physiol 1992;263:L546–L554.

87. Chen Q, Boggaram V, Mendelson CR. Rabbit lung surfactant protein A gene: identification of a lung-specific DNase I hypersensitive site. Am J Physiol 1992;262:L662–L671.

88. Ballard PL, Hawgood S, Liley H, Wellenstein G, Gonzales LW, Benson B, Cordell B, White RT. Regulation of pulmonary surfactant apoprotein SP 28-36 gene in fetal human lung. Proc Natl Acad Sci USA 1986;83:9527–9531.

89. Snyder JM, Mendelson CR. Induction and characterization of the major surfactant apoprotein during rabbit fetal lung development. Biochim Biophys Acta 1987;920:226–236.

90. Mendelson CR, Chen C, Boggaram V, Zacharias C, Snyder JM. Regulation of the synthesis of the major surfactant apoprotein in fetal rabbit lung tissue. J Biol Chem 1986;261:9938–9943.

91. Liley HG, Hawgood S, Wellenstein GA, Benson B, White RT, Ballard PL. Surfactant protein of molecular weight 28,000–36,000 in cultured human fetal lung: cellular localization and effect of dexamethasone. Mol Endocrinol 1987;1:205–215.
92. Mendelson CR, Acarregui MJ, Odom MJ, Boggaram V. Developmental and hormonal regulation of surfactant protein A (SP-A) gene expression in fetal lung. J Dev Physiol 1991;15:61–69.
93. Whitsett JA, Pilot T, Clark JC, Weaver TE. Induction of surfactant protein in fetal lung. Effects of cAMP and dexamethasone on SAP-35 RNA and synthesis. J Biol Chem 1987;262:5256–5261.
94. Odom MJ, Snyder JM, Boggaram V, Mendelson CR. Glucocorticoid regulation of the major surfactant associated protein SP-A and its messenger ribonucleic acid and of morphological development of human fetal lung in vitro. Endocrinology 1988;123:1712–1720.
95. Liley HG, White RT, Benson BJ, Ballard PL. Glucocorticoids both stimulate and inhibit production of pulmonary surfactant protein A in fetal human lung. Proc Natl Acad Sci USA 1988;85:9096–9100.
96. Iannuzzi DM, Ertsey R, Ballard PL. Biphasic glucocorticoid regulation of pulmonary SP-A: characterization of inhibitory process. Am J Physiol 1993;264:L236–L244.
97. Boggaram V, Smith ME, Mendelson,CR. Posttranscriptional regulation of surfactant protein-A messenger RNA in human fetal lung in vitro by glucocorticoids. Mol Endocrinol 1991;5:414–423.
98. Crouch E, Rust K, Marienchek W, Parghi D, Chang D, Persson A. Developmental expression of pulmonary surfactant protein D (SP-D). Am J Respir Cell Mol Biol 1991;5:13–18.
99. Deterding RR, Shimizu H, Fisher JH, Shannon JM. Regulation of surfactant protein D expression by glucocorticoids in vitro and in vivo. Am J Respir Cell Mol Biol 1994;10:30–37.
100. Ogasawara Y, Kuroki Y, Tsuzuki A, Ueda S, Misaki H, Akino T. Pre- and postnatal stimulation of pulmonary surfactant protein D by in vivo dexamethasone treatment of rats. Life Sci 1992;50:1761–1767.
101. Dulkerian SJ, Gonzales LW, Ning Y, Ballard PL. Regulation of surfactant protein D in human fetal lung. Am J Respir Cell Mol Biol 1996;15:781–786.
102. Hawgood S, Shiffer K. Structures and properties of the surfactant-associated proteins. Annu Rev Physiol 1991;53:375–394.
103. Phelps DS, Floros J. Dexamethasone in vivo raises surfactant protein B mRNA in alveolar and bronchiolar epithelium. Am J Physiol 1991;260:L146–L152.
104. Whitsett JA, Weaver TE, Clark JC, Sawtell N, Glasser SW, Korfhagen TR, Hull WM. Glucocorticoid enhances surfactant proteolipid Phe and pVal synthesis and RNA in fetal lung. J Biol Chem 1987;262:15,618–15,623.
105. Floros J, Gross I, Nichols KV, Veletza SV, Dynia D, Lu HW, Wilson CM, Peterec, SM. Hormonal effects on the surfactant protein B (SP-B) mRNA in cultured fetal rat lung. Am J Respir Cell Mol Biol 1991;4:449–454.
106. Fisher JH, McCormack F, Park SS, Stelzner T, Shannon JM, Hofmann T. In vivo regulation of surfactant proteins by glucocorticoids. Am J Respir Cell Mol Biol 1991;5:63–70.
107. Schellhase DE, Shannon JM. Effects of maternal dexamethasone on expression of SP-A, SP-B, and SP-C in the fetal rat lung. Am J Respir Cell Mol Biol 1991;4:304–312.
108. Veletza SV, Nichols KV, Gross I, Lu H, Dynia, DW, Floros J. Surfactant protein C: hormonal control of SP-C mRNA levels in vitro. Am J Physiol 1992;262:L684–L687.
109. Venkatesh VC, Iannuzzi DM, Ertsey R, Ballard PL. Differential glucocorticoid regulation of the pulmonary hydrophobic surfactant proteins SP-B and SP-C. Am J Respir Cell Mol Biol 1993;8:222–228.

# 8 Sex Differences in Fetal Lung Development
## Biology, Etiology, and Evolutionary Significance

*Heber C. Nielsen and John S. Torday, PhD*

### CONTENTS

## HISTORICAL PERSPECTIVE

Interest in the relationship between sexual dimorphism and lung maturation emerged in the late 1970s for one specific reason: it had been observed among pregnant women treated antenatally with glucocorticoids for lung immaturity that the risk of respiratory distress syndrome (RDS) was halved in females, but had no effect on males [1]. Because of our mutual interest in fetal lung development, particularly its relationship to fetal endocrinology [2], we decided to determine the biologic basis for this phenomenon, thinking that if there were a sex-specific steroid effect, that this experiment of nature could be exploited as a means of discovering the underlying nature of the cellular machinery that mediates the processes of lung development. The global strategy we used was

From: *Contemporary Endocrinology:* Endocrinology of the Lung: *Development and Surfactant Synthesis*
Edited by: C. R. Mendelson © Humana Press Inc., Totowa, NJ

to exploit the spontaneous sex difference in fetal lung development that occurs across species *in utero*. This "tool" would allow us to tease out the clinically significant, albeit small, differences in the timing of fetal lung maturation. With the advantage of 20/20 hindsight, we should have realized that this phenomenon comprises the "small, incremental steps" that typify self-organizing systems with respect to both their ontogeny and their homeostatic control *(3)*. Our hope was that such extensive studies would reveal the mechanisms underlying this process to better predict and prevent neonatal lung disease.

## *A PRIORI* EVIDENCE FOR THE EXISTENCE OF A SEX DIFFERENCE IN THE DEVELOPMENT OF PULMONARY SURFACTANT

Our first step in the study of sexual dimorphism of fetal lung development was to scour the literature for prior empiric evidence of such a phenomenon, particularly with respect to pulmonary surfactant ontogeny, since this process would provide a mechanistic link between lung development *(4), s*teroid therapy *(5), an*d RDS *(6)*. At that time there was fairly extensive literature documenting the interrelationship between the structural development of the fetal lung and its direct relationship to the ontogeny of the surfactant system *(7)*. The causal nature of this structure–function relationship has subsequently been elucidated, in large part, by using steroids and other hormones to influence the timing *(8)* and extent *(9)* of surfactant ontogeny. For example, glucocorticoids *(10)*, thyroid hormone *(11)*, and retinoic acid *(12)* will all accelerate both the structural maturation of the lung and the rate of surfactant production; in contrast to this, such hormones as insulin *(13)* and testosterone *(14)* delay lung development pathophysiologically; antiglucocorticoids *(15)* do so pharmacologically. Liggins' *(16)* seminal observation of a dramatic effect of exogenous steroid treatment on lung maturation and precocious survival of fetal sheep was rapidly translated to human subjects, demonstrating an effective reduction in the risk of RDS *(17)*.

A large number of randomized controlled trials demonstrated that prenatal glucocorticoid treatment reduced the risk of RDS in premature infants, generally between 28 and 32 wk. These trials culminated in an NIH-sponsored multicenter collaborative double-blind, randomized trial that showed an overall 30% reduction in the risk of RDS after prenatal dexamethasone therapy *(1)*. One serendipitous finding in the Collaborative Trial was the observation that the statistical effect of prenatal steroids was stronger in females than in males. Others also evaluated their studies for evidence of a male–female difference in response; a stronger effect in female infants than in males was noted by some *(18–20)* but not by all *(21)*. Overall, the beneficial effect of prenatal glucocorticoid was strongly substantiated by a metaanalysis of all randomized, blinded controlled trails *(22)*, and supported by a recent NIH consensus conference and official NIH Consensus Statement *(22)*.

## DIRECT EVIDENCE FOR A SEX DIFFERENCE IN HUMAN FETAL LUNG DEVELOPMENT

The first empiric evidence of a link between fetal sex and lung maturation came from our observational study of sex-specific surfactant ontogeny in human amniotic fluid *(23)*. Gluck had previously demonstrated the principle that surfactant phospholipid kinetics in amniotic fluid could be used to predict the risk of RDS in the newborn *(24)*. We (J.T.) expanded on the precept by devising a more sensitive and specific assay to measure the major surface-active component of the surfactant complex *(24)*, saturated phosphatidylcholine (DSPC) *(25)*. Using either the L/S ratio or the DSPC assay *(25)*, we were able to show a significant sex difference in the timing of surfactant appearance in amniotic fluid, male levels lagging behind females by about 2 wk *(23)*. This male–female difference in lung maturation was significant because a difference in surfactant concentration in amniotic fluid of that magnitude between 26 and 34 wk gestation is equivalent to as much as a 20% increase in the risk of RDS at birth *(26)*. In this study we also observed that male amniotic fluid cortisol concentrations were significantly lower than females, suggesting an endocrine link to the apparent delay in male fetal lung development, though it was not apparently due to cortisol deficiency per se, since exogenous glucocorticoid administration failed to correct this deficit *(1,18–20)*. It is more likely that this difference in amniotic fluid cortisol levels is a consequence of delayed lung maturation due to decreased pulmonary fibroblast conversion of circulating cortisone to cortisol *(27)* and its subsequent secretion by the lung into the amniotic cavity *(28,29)*. Our report of a sex difference in amniotic fluid surfactant phospholipids was subsequently confirmed and expanded by Fleisher et al. *(30)* to include phosphatidylglycerol, the other surface-active phospholipid component of pulmonary surfactant *(25)*.

## EVIDENCE FOR A SPONTANEOUS SEX DIFFERENCE USING ANIMAL MODELS

### *Observational Differences in Fetal Lung Structure and Growth*

Kotas and Avery *(31)* were the first to report a sex-related difference in fetal lung structure, finding that at 27 days postconceptual age (pca) lungs from female fetal rabbits were more stable upon deflation (an indirect measure of surface activity *in situ*) than males, and had larger airspaces (indicative of accelerated alveolar acinar development). Adamson and King's *(32)* laboratory characterized sex-specific fetal rat lung development in a subsequent series of studies of cytoarchitecture and surfactant. Initially they reported finding more lamellar bodies per type II alveolar cell in female fetal rat lung (days 20 and 21 pca) and more epithelial cells in female than in male lung on days 18–20 pca. In a follow-up autoradiographic analysis Adamson and King *(33)* reported finding more rapid epithelial growth in females (days 17–20 pca), indicating that structural changes predate differences in surfactant ontogeny. On closer inspection they observed earlier interruption of the basement membrane and greater and more frequent numbers of foot processes in female lung associated with more lamellar bodies per cuboidal epithelial cell on day 20 pca *(34)*.

As a unifying mechanism for both the androgen delay of differentiation and stimulation of growth, we *(35)* showed that spontaneous fetal mouse lung growth peaks earlier in females than males (day 17 v day 18 pca). Exogenous androgen treatment stimulates tissue and cell growth in vivo, directly stimulates mitosis of both type II cells and fibroblasts in cell culture, and concomitantly blocks their differentiation. Therefore, *the controls of growth and differentiation of fetal lung appear to be reciprocally linked (8)*, which is an important clue to the central mechanism that regulates lung development.

Early, independent studies by Torday *(36)* and by Nielsen *(37)* demonstrated a spontaneous sex difference in surfactant synthesis by fetal rat and rabbit lungs, respectively. Torday and colleagues *(38)* subsequently demonstrated that the sex difference in *de novo* surfactant synthesis could be observed in cultured fetal rat lung type II cells ex vivo beginning on day 20 pca.

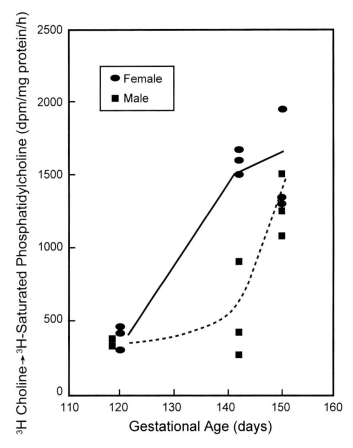

Fig. 1. Earlier rise in surfactant synthesis in female fetal sheep lung compared to male fetal sheep lung. Surfactant synthesis was measured as the incorporation of [³H-]choline into saturated phosphatidylcholine, the major surface active component of surfactant. Females appeared to reach a plateau of maximum production 1 wk before the males.

## *Observational Differences in Biochemical Fetal Lung Development*

Based on the epidemiologic evidence that males are at greater risk of developing RDS *(6,14,38,39)* and dying of HMD *(40)*, combined with direct evidence for delayed surfactant production in males *(23)*, our laboratory began a series of experiments to test the hypothesized role of androgens in sexually dimorphic fetal lung development. Our earliest studies utilized the rabbit model of fetal lung development, in which surfactant physiology had already been well characterized *(41–43)*, and in which one of us (J.T.) had already done some endocrine-related studies *(41)*. We first determined that there was a spontaneous sex difference in the onset of lung surfactant phospholipid production between days 26 and 28 pca *(44)*. In subsequent studies we showed similar spontaneous sex differences in surfactant phospholipid synthesis in fetal rat *(45)*, mouse *(46)*, sheep (Fig. 1) and human lung *(22)*. We observed a similar pattern of timing and kinetics of surfactant elaboration in all of these species (Fig. 2) as follows: (i) there appeared to be a significant difference in the timing of the surfactant phospho-lipid surge, although (ii) there was no difference in the rate of increase, and (iii) the

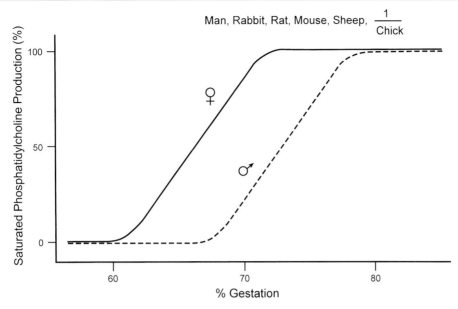

Fig. 2. Sex difference in pulmonary surfactant production across species. The diagram shows, as a percentage of gestation, the difference between females and males in the timing of increased production of saturated phosphatidylcholine. Data have been summarized from man, rabbit, mouse, sheep, and chick (in whom the increase occurs first in the male, consistent with a reversal of the homogametic and heterogametic sex; *see* the subheading "Sex Chromosomes.")

rise in surfactant production was followed by a significant plateau period, which allowed the males to "catch up" to the females in late gestation (Fig. 2). This "windowing" effect was of great help in allowing us to understand the nature of this mechanism for two reasons: First, it explained why the sex difference in the risk of RDS was transient, that is, there is no male–female difference in surfactant production at term. Second, since this "window" coincided with the time-frames for both endogenous *(47)* and exogenous glucocorticoid stimulation of fetal lung maturation *(48–50),* it suggested that *the mechanism of androgen action might be as an antiglucocorticoid.* Both Adamson and King *(32)* and Freese and Hallman *(51)* observed similar windowing of the sex difference during the period between the glandular and the saccular phases of lung development in their studies of sex-specific lung maturation. Such an androgen-as-antiglucocorticoid mechanism was also consistent with both the observed resistance of males to exogenous glucocorticoid stimulation *(52)* and our earlier observation that amniotic fluid cortisol levels are lower in males than females *(22),* since the ability of the lung to generate cortisol from circulating (biologically inactive) cortisone is developmentally dependent *(28,53,54)* and is inhibited by androgens, both endogenous *(27)* and exogenous *(52,53).* Taken together, these observations were also pivotal because they suggested that the sex difference was due to differential regulation of the triggering mechanism for fetal lung maturation *(47,52).* Armed with this cumulative knowledge, we hypothesized that *the sex difference in fetal lung maturation was due to androgen delay of surfactant production.* To test this hypothesis we treated pregnant rabbits with dihydrotestosterone (DHT), the bioactive form of testosterone in peripheral organs *(54–56).* We observed delayed surfactant production by both male and female fetuses, the males being 100-fold more sensitive than the females *(57)*. In further support of the hypothesized role of endogenous androgens in delayed male surfactant production, treatment of fetal rabbits with the antiandrogen Flutamide "neutralized" the spontaneous sex difference in surfactant production by raising the male surfactant phospholipid values up to the females, *with no effect on the females (57)*. Further documentation of the male delay was provided by examining surfactant production as a function of fetal littermate "neighbors." This experimental stratagem has been used to account for variations in anogenital distance among female littermates due to neighboring males *(58)*. This effect is due to male hormone spilling into female fetal circulation *(59)*. When the amounts of pulmonary surfactant in male and female littermates were examined on this basis *(57)*, there were no significant differences in surfactant production among the males, all male:female groupings (i.e., male with two male neighbors, male with one male neighbor, male with no male neighbor) being low compared to females. In contrast to this, among the females, those fetuses between two females were highest in surfactant content, those between two males were lowest, and those with only one male neighbor were intermediate, resulting in a significant dose-response relationship between surfactant production and the levels of androgen the fetuses were exposed to as a result of their positions *in utero (57–59)*. These data indicate that androgens in fetal circulation delay surfactant production; furthermore, these data indicate that the hormonal mechanism is one of androgen delaying, not estrogen accelerating surfactant production, since the males inhibited the females, and there was no empiric evidence for the females accelerating development of the males in the neighbor experiment.

## HORMONAL INDUCTION OF SEX DIFFERENCES IN LUNG PULMONARY SURFACTANT MATURATION

### *By Androgens*

The hypothesized role of androgens in delayed male lung maturation was based on the hormonal theory of sex differentiation *(60)*. Androgen effects on lung maturation have been examined using a variety of in vitro, in vivo, and ex vivo models. The Torday laboratory investigated the automaturational model of human fetal lung development to test the effects of both testicular androgens (i.e., testosterone) and the "weak androgens" (e.g.. dehydroepiandrosterone, androstenedione) that are of fetal adrenal origin *(61)*. DHT delayed both spontaneous maturation and dexamethasone-stimulated surfactant synthesis; dehydroepiandrosterone and androstenedione had the same inhibitory effect on *de novo* synthesis and tissue content of surfactant phospholipid.

### *Müllerian Inhibiting Substance*

Catlin et al. *(62)* have investigated the role of müllerian inhibiting substance (MIS) in the sex-specific development of the fetal lung, since both testosterone and MIS control male genital development *in utero*. Initially they reported significant inhibition of female fetal lung DSPC accumulation. This in vitro study was followed by *in utero* treatment of fetal rats *(63)* in which MIS inhibited surfactant synthesis by both female and male fetuses, indicating that both androgens and MIS may play a role in the sexual dimorphism of fetal lung development.

## MECHANISMS BY WHICH THE SEX DIFFERENCE MAY OCCUR

### *Hormones That Are Different in Male and Female Fetuses*

Surveying *(64)* the hormones in fetal circulation that might be responsible for the hormonal basis of the sex difference in fetal lung development, there were three candidates: androgens, müllerian inhibiting substance, and follicle-stimulating hormone (FSH). Evidence from this and other laboratories indicates that the spontaneous sex difference in fetal lung development is due to androgens in fetal circulation *(53)*. MIS may also play a role in this process of dimorphic fetal lung maturation *(62,63)*; whether FSH affects fetal lung maturation is not known, although we have previously tested a variety of pituitary hormones–prolactin, adrenocorticotropin, and luteinizing hormones— none of which affected surfactant phospholipid synthesis in cultured fetal rabbit lung cells *(65)*. Ballard and colleagues *(66)* tested the effect of prolactin on pulmonary surfactant production in fetal lambs and found no effect either. However, Liggins et al. *(67,68)* have demonstrated a direct effect of ACTH on lung development in the lamb model.

The classic physiologic effect of androgens on peripheral tissues is dependent on local activation of testosterone by 5α-reductase, followed by binding to the androgen receptor *(54,56)*. In our pursuit of the androgen-mediated sex difference in fetal lung maturation we began systematically evaluating these aspects of androgen metabolism in the developing lung.

### *Androgen Receptor*

Nielsen *(46)* has demonstrated the dependence of the sex difference on the androgen receptor using the mouse model of testicular feminization (Tfm), which is devoid of androgen receptors *(69,70)*. As in the rat and rabbit, there is a spontaneous sex difference in the mouse on day 17 pca *(46)*. This sex difference was not detectable in Tfm mouse fetuses, indicating the dependence of the spontaneous sex difference on the androgen receptor; androgen receptor activity has been demonstrated in human fetal lung fibroblasts *(71)*.

In our study of the role of androgens in the sex-specific regulation of surfactant production we observed that the androgen receptor antagonist Flutamide eradicated the sex difference in surfactant production by fetal rabbits, having no effect on female surfactant production *(57)*. We further demonstrated that the androgen (specifically) blocked the cortisol upregulation of fibroblast–pneumonocyte factor (FPF) mRNA transcription, but had no effect on cortisol stimulation of FPF by fetal lung fibroblasts derived from Tfm males *(46)*. As for the dependence of the sex difference on 5α-reductase, testosterone was found to be as effective in inhibiting lung maturation as DHT *(57,58,72)*. Additionally, 4-MA, a potent and specific inhibitor of 5α-reductase, failed to eliminate the spontaneous sex difference in fetal rabbit lung surfactant production *(72)*. These data indicate that lung fibroblast activation of testosterone to DHT is not necessary for androgen delay of fetal lung development. We have also found (H.C. Nielsen and J.S. Torday, unpublished results) that 5α-reductase activity is present in fetal rat lung fibroblasts derived from both males and females, but is not sexually dimorphic. These data indicate that the sex difference in fetal lung maturation is dependent on both the amount of androgen in fetal circulation *(57)* and on its binding to the androgen receptor in lung fibroblasts, consistent with our earlier finding that at high doses DHT delayed both male and female fetal lung development *(57)*. However, in contrast to other androgen-sensitive peripheral tissues, testosterone does not have to be converted to DHT to be biologically active in fetal lung.

## *Müllerian Inhibiting Substance*

As indicated above, MIS produced by the fetal testes can inhibit fetal rat lung development either by adding it to cultured fetal lungs or by administering it to the fetus *in utero*. Catlin et al. *(62,63)* subsequently demonstrated that the MIS receptor is present in fetal rat lung, further supporting a role for MIS in the regulation of fetal lung development. It should be noted, however, that unlike the modulatory effect of androgens on fetal lung surfactant, MIS had a direct inhibitory effect on surfactant production.

## *Follicle-Stimulating Hormone*

The only other hormone known to be sexually dimorphic during fetal development is follicle-stimulating hormone (FSH). Whether FSH affects fetal lung development has not been determined. However, other pituitary peptide hormones, such as luteinizing hormone, prolactin, and adrenocorticotrophin, have no direct effect on surfactant phospholipid synthesis *(65,66)*.

## *Sex Chromosomes*

The bulk of the evidence regarding the nature of the sex difference in lung development *in utero* has pointed to the effect of circulating male hormones. However, the origins of these differences must ultimately lie in their genetic control. To determine the role of the sex chromosomes in the sex-specific ontogeny of surfactant we studied the developmental patterns of surfactant production in male and female chick embryos *(73)*, since the sex karyotype is reversed in birds, that is, the homogametic sex (i.e., ZZ) is male, and because the relationship between sex phenotype and sex-specific mortality is also reversed in birds *(74–76)*. Surfactant production, in general, follows a developmental pattern *in ovo* similar to that observed for mammals *in utero*—increasing beginning on day 19 postsetting (term = 21) and plateauing just before hatching. However, in *Galus domesticus,* male surfactant production increases 1 d earlier than in females. Furthermore, when treated with glucocorticoids *in ovo*, the males are responsive earlier than the females *(73)*. Based on these observations, we have concluded that it is specifically the heterogametic sex which is at a disadvantage for timing of lung development, suggesting that there is a biologic advantage in having two complete sex chromosomes. The possible evolutionary implications for this phenomenon are addressed in the section "A Unifying Mechanism for Heterochronic Fetal Lung Development."

## MECHANISMS CONTROLLING SEX-SPECIFIC LUNG DEVELOPMENT AT THE CELL/MOLECULAR LEVEL

Our contemporary understanding of the cellular control of lung development is that it is due to the interaction between mesenchyme and epithelium *(77,78)*. Based on this precept, we have conducted studies to elucidate these cell/molecular mechanisms and how they are affected by sex steroids.

## *Fibroblast Pneumonocyte Factor*

In an initial study designed to investigate the cellular mechanisms underlying the sex difference in fetal lung maturation, the cellular origin of the sex difference was examined; it was observed in the rat that before the onset of the sex difference in type II cell surfactant synthesis there was an inherent difference in the production of fibroblast pneumonocyte factor (FPF) activity *(37)* by sex-specific fibroblasts, males producing less FPF than females *(79)*. It was also found that male fetal lung fibroblasts possessed less 11-oxidoreductase activity than females, resulting in a diminished response to exogenous cortisone (the principal glucocorticoid in fetal circulation) stimulation of FPF activity *(27)*. Based on these observations it was concluded that *the sex difference originates in the fibroblast*. Further examination of spontaneous FPF expression revealed that the number of mRNA transcripts for FPF was greater in female than in male fetal rat lung fibroblasts, but only on day 19 pca, suggesting that induction of FPF expression is also sex-specific. In companion studies we observed that glucocorticoids increased FPF production and expression by both male and female fetal rat lung fibroblasts on day 19 pca, but the sex difference persisted; in contrast to the effect of glucocorticoids on day 19 pca, there was no effect on day 17 pca and the steroid downregulated FPF expression on day 21, similar to the effects of cortisol on FPF first observed by Smith *(78)*. Androgen treatment inhibited FPF production by fetal rat lung fibroblasts only in the presence of cortisol, having no effect on the baseline activity in either sex, suggesting that the androgen interferes with the mechanism that initiates FPF production but has no effect on constitutive FPF elaboration.

The sex-specific ontogeny of FPF activity was also described in fetal mouse lung fibroblasts *(80)*. Fibroblasts from male or female day 16 pca fetal lung (term = day 18 pca) exhibited no FPF activity. Female fibroblasts, but not male fibroblasts, produced FPF activity in response to cortisol stimulation on day 17 pca. Both sexes exhibited constitutive FPF activity on day 18 pca. Additional studies in the mouse model of testicular feminization (Tfm mouse) showed that the sexual dimorphism in the timing of FPF production in fetal mouse lung fibroblasts is androgen receptor-dependent *(46)*. Studies in fetal rabbit lung organ culture indicated that the effect of androgen was to inhibit FPF production, but not the ability of the fetal lung to respond to FPF if supplied exogenously *(81)*. By contrast, TGFβ inhibited both FPF production and the ability of the lung to respond to FPF.

### *Growth Factors That Influence Lung Surfactant Production*

Growth factors are known to influence the progression of lung maturation and the onset of surfactant synthesis. Sex-specific differences in the action and/or regulation of their effects have been described for some. Epidermal growth factor (EGF), a 6-kD peptide produced in the fetal lung and elsewhere, stimulates the development of surfactant synthesis *(80,82,83)*. EGF acts on fetal lung through fibroblast-type II cell communication, promoting the expression of FPF. Exposure of fetal mouse lung fibroblasts to EGF in culture advances the gestational timing of FPF production described above, such that the specific FPF phenotype occurs 1 d earlier in development *(80)*. Similarly, the gestational development of surfactant synthesis in fetal rabbit lung organ culture was promoted by EGF in a sex-specific manner; at an earlier stage of development surfactant DSPC synthesis was promoted in female but not male fetal lung, while later in development DSPC synthesis was promoted in male fetal lung and somewhat down-regulated in female fetal lung *(84)*. Again, the effect of EGF was to advance, in a sex-specific fashion, the timing of the pattern of surfactant synthesis previously described for that model.

The female–male difference in response to EGF is due, at least in part, to differences in the development of EGFR in the fetal lung. EGFR-specific binding and receptor phosphorylation in response to EGF in fetal rabbit lung plasma membrane preparations peaked in females on day 19 pca of a 31-d gestation, but in males on day 21 pca *(85)*. Cell-specific binding studies and Western blot analyses in fetal rat lung fibroblasts show an earlier increase in the female than in the male *(86,87)*. Binding increased just before the onset of FPF production, in agreement with the earlier appearance of FPF production in the female. Conversely, binding was very low in cultured fetal lung type II cells, did not change with gestation, and showed no female–male differences. The cell-specific nature of EGFR development in fetal lung was also confirmed in mice and rats by immunocytochemistry *(86,88)*. However, these studies were not sufficiently sensitive to identify female–male differences. In all studies, the maximum specific EGF binding was similar for both sexes. Specific binding also demonstrated a decrease in very late gestation.

Signal transduction in response to EGF follows the developmental pattern of the EGFR. Diacylglycerol production in response to EGF is induced in fetal rat lung fibroblasts 1 d earlier in females than in males, at the time of increasing EGFR expression *(89)*. Consistent with the cell-specificity, there was no stimulation of diacylglycerol production by EGF in the type II cells. This developmental response in fibroblasts may be due to more than just sex differences in EGFR development, as similar results for diacylglycerol production were obtained through a non-EGFR mediated mechanism *(90)*.

Transforming growth factor beta (TGFβ) is a 9 kD protein produced in many bodily tissues, including the developing lung. As mentioned, TGFβ is a potent inhibitor of FPF production, activity, and type II cell surfactant synthesis. As receptors for TGFβ are present in fetal lung from early development onward, mechanisms to minimize the inhibitory influence of TGFβ must exist to allow the development of surfactant synthesis. Early studies by Torday and Kourembanas *(91)* had demonstrated glucocorticoid downregulation of TGFβ bioactivity in fetal rat lung fibroblast conditioned medium, and upregulation by DHT. Pereira et al. *(92)* subsequently proposed that alterations in TGFβR binding exist in late lung development. Specific binding studies performed on fetal mouse lung fibroblasts demonstrated a decrease of 50% from day 16 to day 28 pca in females and 29% in males. In addition, crosslinking studies showed that the relative preponderance of the nonsignaling type III TGFβ receptor, when compared to the signaling type I and type II receptors, increased significantly during this time. Response to TGFβ treatment also changed, with females exhibiting a more developmentally advanced response at all gestations compared to males.

Recent studies by Dammann et al. *(93)* show that chronic *in utero* DHT exposure significantly increased TGFβ receptor specific binding in both male and female fetal mouse lung fibroblasts (day 18 pca).

## *Regulatory Genes*

Significant recent progress has been made in the identification of genes that influence lung structural development. However, for only a few is information available relative to female–male differences. The homeobox protein Hoxb-5 is strongly expressed in embryonic lung fibroblasts, then in late gestation expression is seen in fewer and fewer cells, primarily fibroblasts underlying conducting airways and some overlying epithelial cells. Expression of the protein peaks on day 15 pca in female mouse lung and on day 16 pca in male mouse lung *(88)*. The function of Hoxb-5 may be related to determination of specific patterns of proximal airway branching *(94)*. Female–male differences in the peak expression may underlie subsequent structural differences in female and male lungs.

The c-*myc* oncogene is normally expressed in dividing cells and becomes down-regulated with cell differentiation. Studies show that c-*myc* expression in fetal mouse and rat lung is markedly down–regulated in late gestation just before the onset of FPF production and augmented surfactant synthesis *(95)*, consistent with evidence that androgen causes increased fetal lung growth *(35)*.

## CONTROL MECHANISMS OF FETAL LUNG DEVELOPMENT: INFLUENCE OF FACTORS THAT INDUCE SEX DIFFERENCES

### *Androgens*

In initial studies of the mechanism of androgen action on fetal lung development we had observed that DHT blocked the production of FPF by fetal lung fibroblasts, but had no effect on the type II cell response to FPF *(27)*, indicating that *the primary cellular site of androgen action is the developing fetal lung fibroblast.* These experimental results were consistent with the observation that there was a constitutive difference in the ability of male and female fetal lung fibroblasts to produce FPF in culture, but that the type II cells were able to respond to FPF independent of the sex of the donor *(27)*. To test the hypothesized effect of androgen on the fibroblast glucocorticoid-response mechanism, fetal rats were treated with DHT *in utero* and the fetal rat lung tissue was assayed for both glucocorticoid receptor and 11-oxidoreductase activities; DHT delayed the onset of both mechanisms. We then isolated the fibroblasts from the fetal lung tissue and observed the same inhibitory effects on glucocorticoid receptor and 11-oxidoreductase activities by the isolated fibroblasts ex vivo. Furthermore, DHT inhibits FPF production and expression (see above) by fetal rat lung fibroblasts, probably by down-regulating these glucocorticoid-responsive mechanisms since the DHT-treated fibroblasts were also refractory to exogenous glucocorticoid *(36,38,61)*. In support of this mechanism of androgen action, Sweezey et al. *(96)* have shown that DHT decreases the expression of the glucocorticoid receptor by fetal rat lung.

### *Transforming Growth Factor beta*

Because it had repeatedly been observed that both glucocorticoids and androgens could alter the phenotype of developing lung fibroblasts—e.g., FPF production, 11-oxidoreductase, glucocorticoid receptor—Torday and Kourembanas *(91)* performed bioassays to determine if immature fibroblasts constitutively produced inhibitory factors that might mediate the androgen effect on type II cell maturation. [There was already a precedent for the existence of such an endogenous inhibitor based on both observational *(97)* and empiric *(98)* evidence in the literature.] We observed that conditioned medium from immature fetal rat lung fibroblasts inhibited type II cell surfactant-stimulatory bioactivity from day 21 fibroblasts. This inhibitory activity was neutralized by an antibody to TGFβ; moreover, TGFβ mimicked the inhibitory effect of the endogenous factor on FPF, and day 17 pca fetal rat lung fibroblasts expressed TGFβ. Androgen treatment in vivo maintained the otherwise precipitous decline beginning on day 20 pca in the production of TGFβ-like activity by fetal rat lung fibroblasts ex vivo; conversely, glucocorticoid treatment in vivo caused a precocious decrease in the production of TGFβ activity ex vivo.

DHT affects the expression of growth factors involved in lung development. Exposure of fetal rabbits to a continuous maternal infusion of DHT beginning at the time of onset of sexual differentiation inhibited the late gestation surge in lung plasma membrane EGFR density (85). This study, however, was unable to address the cell-specific nature of EGFR expression. In recent studies, chronic infusion of DHT into pregnant mice, followed by isolation and study of the fetal lung fibroblasts ex vivo, decreased EGFR-specific binding. Further, TGFβR binding was increased, and cell proliferation in response to TGFβ treatment was increased (93).

It is important to note that just as the inhibitory effect of DHT on lung surfactant maturation arises from early developmental exposure, the effects of DHT on EGFR and TGFβR also result from exposure in early lung development. Cultured fetal rat lung fibroblasts from days 17 to 21 pca that are exposed to DHT or to TGFβ exhibit different responses than above. EGFR binding is minimally affected by DHT, and is stimulated by acute TGFβ exposure (87). These studies indicate that it is the development of EGFR expression, rather than acute regulation of expression, which is regulated by DHT in the fetal lung.

The effect of DHT on early lung development per se has not received much attention. Recent studies suggest that DHT in embryonic lung acutely increases branching morphogenesis (99,100). This stimulation is accompanied by increased cell proliferation, and by alteration of the process of programmed cell death to allow the development of new branches. It was speculated that these effects reflect the first changes which result ultimately in larger lungs in males compared to females.

Another growth factor important in the process of masculinization during development is müllerian inhibiting substance (MIS). Produced by the Sertoli cells of the fetal testis with the onset of sexual differentiation, MIS is responsible for inhibiting the development of the müllerian duct, causing it to regress. MIS also inhibits the development of fetal lung DSPC synthesis (62,63), inhibits lung branching morphogenesis and stimulates programmed cell death (101), and reduces the activity of the EGFR in fetal rat lung plasma membranes (102). MIS is a member of the large family of TGFβ-like molecules, acting through a TGFβR-type of mechanism. It is not known if the effects of MIS on lung development and surfactant production represent an alternative method of activating TGFβR signal transduction mechanisms or whether these are separate effects in addition to those activated by DHT.

## A UNIFYING MECHANISM
## FOR HETEROCHRONIC FETAL LUNG DEVELOPMENT
### Hormones and Heterochronic Lung Development

There is now ample evidence that endogenous glucocorticoids promote lung development and time the onset of lung surfactant production in a wide variety of mammals (8). There is also compelling evidence that androgens act as natural antiglucocorticoids (35,36,38,46,47,52,53,61,96) delaying the initiation of lung maturation; this difference in the timing of lung development is what the evolutionary biologists refer to as heterochrony. The concomitant effects of glucocorticoids and androgens on lung maturation lead to the paradoxical conclusion that the independent endocrine mechanisms that determine physiologic lung development and male phenotype results in increased male-specific mortality. Such male-specific mortality must exist in order to account for the striking reduction in the sex ratio (male:female) (103) during intrauterine development. There are more males than females at conception due to more frequent fertilization of ova by Y-bearing sperm *(104)*. In order to account for the reduced sex-ratio from approx 4:1 at conception *(103)* down to 1:1 at birth *(105)* mechanisms for male-specific mortality must exist. The largest decline in male embryos occurs in the first trimester *(106)* and is thought to be due to sex-linked genes *(106)*. There is a gradual decline in the sex ratio over the next 3 months, followed by a secondary peak of male losses at 7–9 mo. It is in this stage of embryonic development that more males succumb due to lung immaturity at birth *(1,14,18,19,20,23,39,40)*. Our own experimental evidence points to an androgen-mediated mechanism underlying this excess male mortality.

## Genetics and Heterochronic Lung Development

There is also extensive evidence that there is a genetic basis for sex-specific mortality during embryonic development. For example, we have observed that lung maturation *in ovo* is delayed in females, suggesting that this mechanism is not so much male vs female as it is *homogametic versus heterogametic sex* in nature. A biologic relationship between homo- and heterogametic sex and perinatal viability is supported by the observations that among mammals it is the males who are at increased risk *(14)*, whereas among birds it is the females that are at increased risk of death in the newborn period *(74–76)*. These genetically based phenotypic characteristics of sexually dimorphic fetal lung development point to an evolutionary mechanism since dioecious sex evolved from monoecious sex *(107)*. In the process of converting from a single-sex phenotype to two sexes during intrauterine development all conceptuses begin as the phenotype of the homogametic sex (XX) and the genetically determined males (XY) must be actively transformed to the phenotype of the heterogametic sex by androgens *(60)*. The converse is true in birds— all embryos begin life as the homogametic (ZZ) male phenotype and will be transformed into females if they are genetically heterogametic (ZW) *(108)*. Based on these observations, testosterone appears to be used as a proxy to dampen undesirable androgenous genetic characteristics in the population. Similarly, the absence of a second allele on the Y chromosome places male embryos at greater risk of demise if a deleterious mutation or deletion of the single gene copy on the X chromosome occurs. Quantitatively, the number of genetic stillbirths in the first trimester is much greater than the number of males that die due to the androgen effect on lung development in the third trimester. However, the "biologic investment" *(105)* is much greater by the third trimester; furthermore, the androgen will also affect fetal size *(109)*, putting the mother at increased risk of death during childbirth due to cephalopelvic disproportion; loss of the mother is the highest price that the species pays regarding contribution to the gene pool. In this context it is also well recognized that as sexually reproducing species evolve the disparity in size between the two sexes decreases—the male-specific culling mechanisms may help to explain this evolutionary phenomenon.

This hormonal strategy for evolving the second sex would be expected to have built-in safeguards against males producing excessive amounts of androgens in order to protect the species against such predictably aggressive individuals *(107)*. This may also be a biologic strategy for selecting for males with optimal genetic traits for the survival of the species. The experimental model for fusion of the genetic and endocrine mechanisms may be the B10/B10A congenic strains of mice, which are characterized by spontaneous differences in glucocorticoid-sensitive developmental mechanisms such as cleft palate *(110)* and lung maturation *(111)*. Significantly, it is the slower developing B10A males which exhibit increased androgen activity as adults, as predicted by the genetic–endocrine interactive model. Nature appears to have developed a comprehensive genetic-endocrine mechanism for evolving the second sex, while at the same time damping this process using the very same genetic–endocrine strategy.

## Evidence for an Association Between the "Steroid-Resistant/Responsive" Phenotypes and HLA Haplotypes

Observational studies have linked glucocorticoid-sensitivity with genetic variation related to the major histocompatibility complex (MHC). Ironically, these descriptive studies have now lead to "consilience" *(112)* of the phenotype and genotype, providing a unifying mechanism at the cell/molecular level for this process. In 1976 Becker et al. *(113)* first reported that *different human lymphocyte antigens (HLA, chromosome 6) of the major histocompatibility complex (MHC) are associated with differential sensitivities to corticosteroids.* Bonner and Slavkin *(114)* subsequently identified two congenic strains of mice, B10 and B10A, which exhibited differential sensitivies to induction of cleft palate by exogenous steroid treatment, providing a genetic link between the endocrine phenotype and heterochronic development of the palate in these two strains of mice *(110)*. This was a key observation because these two strains of mice only differ genetically with respect to their H-2 haplotype, representing relatively few genes that may be functionally related to postimplantation development within this locus *(115)*. Studies conducted in Slavkin's laboratory *(114)* demonstrated that in addition to palatal development, lung development was also heterochronic in these two strains of mice, and that the slower developing B10A strain was resistant to the acceleratory effect of both exogenous and endogenous glucocorticoids.

Recently, Melnick and Jaskoll have identified the gene product that mediates heterochronic development of the palate and lung in the B10/B10A congenic mouse strains; they have found that *TGFβ is differentially elaborated during development in both lung and palate,* being elaborated longer during gestation in the B10A than in the B10 strain (*see* Chapter 6 for further discussion). Since TGFβ blocks epithelial type II cell maturation *(52,91,92,98)*, the development of these cells is delayed in the B10As, resulting in delayed surfactant production. Dominance of the developing lung alveolar acinus by TGFβ results in prolonged lung growth and delayed lung differentiation *(116)*. The exploitation of TGFβ by both the endocrine and genetic mechanisms of heterochrony is an apparent example of evolutionary convergence; it is particularly striking, considering that in both cases they are terminal differentiation processes, that is, palatal closure (determined by mesenchymal differentiation) and surfactant production (determined by epithelial differentiation), which independently result in heterochrony. The use of the ubiquitous TGFβ-regulated differentiation pathway observed to "time" development in many tissues *(117)* also suggests that the steroid-resistant and nonresistant populations *(18–21)* may reflect different HLA haplotypes. Consistent with this hypothesis, there is clinical evidence *(118)* that premature infants with and without RDS differ in their HLA haplotypes; it was observed in that study that the RDS infants were comprised by two specific HLA haplotypes, $A_3$ and $B_{14}$, which are distinctly different from the haplotypes comprising the non-RDS group. The relationship between TGFβ, endocrine, and genetic mechanisms of heterochrony during fetal lung development are depicted in Fig. 3.

It was the linkage of human HLA haplotypes to glucocorticoid sensitivity that first led investigators to the B10/B10A phenotype/genotype relationship. The observation that

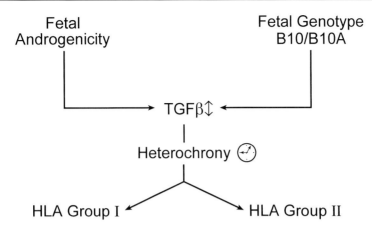

Fig. 3. Heterochronic development and maturation of specific fetal tissues may arise through differential regulation of TGFβ expression and activity between females and males. Both the fetal androgen state and the fetal genotype may contribute to the differential regulation of TGFβ. In addition, the HLA may influence the outcome of the heterochronicity of TGFβ timing of developmental events.

the timing of palate and lung development is the result of TGFβ dynamics unifies the endocrine and genetic heterochronic models mechanistically.

The identification of TGFβ as the common mechanism for both endocrine and genetic delay of lung development merges these two models into one unified mechanism. This is highly significant because it links the endocrine pathways timing lung development to HLA haplotypes associated with functionally relevant candidate genes controlling the process of lung development. This focus will ultimately lead to novel diagnostic and therapeutic tools for the prediction and prevention of neonatal lung disease.

## REFERENCES

1. Collaborative Group of Antenatal Steroid Therapy. Effect of antenatal dexamethasone administration on the prevention of respiratory distress syndrome. Am J Obstet Gynecol 1981;141:276–285.
2. Mendelson CR, Boggaram V. Hormonal control of the surfactant system in fetal lung. Annu Rev Physiol 1991;53:415–440.
3. Bak P, Paczuski M. Complexity, contingenc, and criticality. Proc Natl Acad Sci, USA 1995;92:6689–6696.
4. Brumley GW, Chernick V, Hodson WA, Normand C, Fenner A, Avery ME. Correlations of mechanical stability, morphology, pulmonary surfactant, and phospholipid content in the developing lamb lung. J Clin Invest 1967;46:863–873.
5. Ballard PL. Hormonal regulation of pulmonary surfactant. Endocr Rev 1989;10:165–181.
6. Farrell PM, Avery ME. Hyaline membrane disease: state of the art Am Rev Respir Dis 1975;111:657–688.
7. Fujiwara T, Adams FH, Sipos S, El-Salawy A. "Alveolar" and whole lung phospholipids of the developing fetal lamb lung. Am J Physiol 1968;215:375–382.
8. Torday JS, Zinman HM, Nielsen HC. Glucocorticoid regulation of DNA, protein and surfactant phospholipid in developing lung. Dev Pharm Ther 1986;9:124–131.
9. Kotas RV, Avery ME. Accelerated appearance of pulmonary surfactant in the fetal rabbit. J Appl Physiol 1971;30:358–361.
10. Kikkawa Y, Kaibara M, Motoyama EK, Orzalesi MM, Cook CD. Morphologic development of fetal rabbit lung and its acceleration with cortisol. Am J Pathol 1972;64:423–442.
11. Ballard PL. Hormones and lung maturation. Monogr Endocrinol 1986;28:1–354.
12. Chytil F. Retinoids in lung development. FASEB J 1996;10:986–992.
13. Robert MF, Neff RK, Hubbell JP, Taeusch HW, Avery ME. Association between maternal diabetes and the respiratory distress syndrome in the newborn. N Engl J Med 1976;294:357–360.

14. Naeye RL, Freeman RK, Blanc WA. Nutrition, sex, and fetal lung maturation. Pediatr Res 1974; 8:200–204.
15. Vidyasagar D, Chernick V. Effect of metopirone on the synthesis of lung surfactant in does and fetal rabbits. Biol Neonate 1975;27:1–16.
16. Liggins GC. Premature delivery of fetal lambs infused with glucocorticoids. J Endocrin 1969; 45:515–523.
17. Liggins GC, Howie RN. A controlled trial of antepartum glucocorticoid treatment for prevention of the respiratory distress syndrome in premature infants. Pediatrics 1972;50:515–525.
18. Ballard PL, Ballard RA, Granberg PJ, Sniderman S, Gluckman PD, Kaplan SL, Grumbach MM. Fetal sex and prenatal betamethasone therapy. J Pediatr. 1980;97:451–454.
19. Taeusch HW Jr, Frigolettto F, Kitzmiller J, Avery ME, Hehre A, Frann B, Lawson EE, Neff RK. Risk of respiratory distress syndrome after prenatal dexamethasone treatment. Pediatrics 1979;63:64–72.
20. Papageorgiou AN, Colle E, Farri-Kostopoulos E, Gelfand MM. Incidence of respiratory distress syndrome following antenatal betamethasone: role of sex, type of delivery, and prolonged rupture of membranes. Pediatrics 1981;67:614–617.
21. National Institutes of Health. Report of the consensus development conference on the effect of corticosteroids for fetal maturation on perinatal outcomes. NIH Publication 1994;95–3784.
22. Crowley P, Chalmers I, Keirse MJ. The effects of corticosteroid administration before preterm delivery: an overview of the evidence from controlled trials. Br J Obstet Gynecol. 1990;97:11–25.
23. Torday JS, Nielsen HC, Fencl M deM, Avery ME. Sex differences in fetal lung maturation. Am Rev Respir Dis 1981;123:205–208.
24. Torday J, Carson L, Lawson EE. Saturated phosphatidylcholine in amniotic fluid and prediction of the respiratory distress syndrome. N Engl J Med. 1979;301:1013–1018.
25. King RJ. The surfactant system of the lung. Fed Proc 1974;33:2238–2247.
26. Hunink MG, Richardson DK, Doubilet PM, Begg CB. Testing for fetal pulmonary maturity: ROC analysis involving covariate, verification bias, and combination testing. Med Decis Making 1990;10:201–211.
27. Torday JS. The sex difference in type II cell surfactant synthesis originates in the fibroblast in vitro. Exp Lung Res 1984;7:187–194.
28. Torday JS, Olson EB, First NL. Production of cortisol from cortisone by the isolated, perfused fetal rabbit lung. Steroids 1976;27:869–880.
29. Smith BT, Worthington D, Maloney A. The amniotic fluid cortisol- cortisone ratio in preterm human delivery and the risk of respiratory distress syndrome. Obstet Gynecol 1977;49:527–531.
30. Fleisher B, Kulovich MV, Hallman M, Gluck L. Lung profile: sex differences in normal pregnancy. Obstet Gynecol 1985;66:327–330.
31. Kotas RV, Avery ME. The influence of sex on fetal rabbit lung maturation and on the response to glucocorticoid. Am Rev Respir Dis 1980;121:377–380.
32. Adamson IYR, King GM. Sex-related differences in cellular composition and surfactant synthesis of developing fetal rat lungs. Am J Respir Dis 1984;129:130–134.
33. Adamson IYR, King GM Sex differences in development of fetal rat lung. I. Autoradiographic and biochemical studies. Lab Invest 1984;50:456–460.
34. King GM, Adamson IYR. Quantitative morphology of epithelial- mesenchymal interactions. Lab Invest 1984;50:461–468.
35. Nielsen HC, Kirk WO, Sweezey N, Torday JS. Coordination of growth and differentiation in the fetal lung. Exp Cell Res 1990;188:89–96.
36. Torday JS. Dihydrotestosterone antagonizes glucocorticoid-dependent surfactant synthesis in explant culture. Pediatr Res 1985;19:164A..
37. Nielsen HC. The development of surfactant synthesis in fetal rabbit lung organ culture exhibits a sex dimorphism. Biochim Biophys Acta 1986;883:373–379.
38. Floros J, Nielsen HC, Torday JS. Dihydrotestosterone blocks fetal lung fibroblast-pneumonocyte factor at a pretranslational level. J Biol Chem 1987;262:13592–13598.
39. Perelman RH, Palta M, Kirby R, Farrell PM. Discordance between male and female deaths due to respiratory distress syndrome. Pediatrics 1986;78:238–244.
40. Miller HC, Futrakul P. Birthweight, gestational age, and sex as determining factors in the incidence of respiratory distress syndrome of prematurely born infants. J Pediatr 1968;72:628–635.
41. Kotas RV, Fletcher BD, Torday JS, Avery ME. Evidence for independent regulators of organ maturation in fetal rabbits. Pediatrics 1971;47:57–64.

42. Carson SH, Taeusch HW Jr, Avery ME. Inhibition of lung cell division after hydrocortisone injection into fetal rabbits. J Appl Physiol 1973;34:660–663.

43. Torday JS, Nielsen HC. Surfactant phospholipid ontogeny in fetal rabbit lung lavage and amniotic fluid. Biol Neonate 1981;39:266–271.

44. Nielsen HC, Torday JS. Sex differences in fetal rabbit pulmonary surfactant production. Pediatr Res 1981;15:1245–1247.

45. Torday JS, Dow KE. Synergistic effect of triiodothyroxine and dexamethasone on male and female fetal rat lung surfactant synthesis. Dev Pharmacol Ther 1984;7:133–139.

46. Nielsen HC. Androgen receptors influence the production of pulmonary surfactant in the testicular feminization mouse fetus. J Clin Invest 1985;76:177–181.

47. Torday JS, Nielsen HC. The sex difference in fetal lung surfactant production. Exp Lung Res 1987;12: 1–19.

48. Baden M, Bauer CR, Colle E, Klein G, Tauesch HW Jr. A controlled trial of hydrocortisone therapy in infants with respiratory distress syndrome. Pediatrics 1972;50:526–534.

49. Ward RM. Pharmacologic enhancement of fetal lung maturation. Clin Perinatol 1984;21:523–542.

50. Kattner E, Metze B, Weiss E, Obladen M. Accelerated lung maturation following maternal steroid treatment in infants born before 30 weeks gestation. J Perinatal Med 1992;20:449–457.

51. Freese WB, Hallman M. The effect of betamethasone and fetal sex on the synthesis and maturation of lung surfactant phospholipids in rabbits. Biochim et Biophys Acta 1983;750:47–59.

52. Torday JS. Cellular timing of fetal lung development. Semin Perinatol 1992;16:130–138.

53. Torday JS. Dihydrotestosterone inhibits fibroblast-pneumonocyte factor- mediated synthesis of saturated phosphatidylcholine by fetal rat lung cells. Biochim Biophys Acta 1985;835:23–28.

54. Bardin CW, Catteral JF. Testosterone: a major determinant of extragenital sexual dimorphism. Science 1981;211:1285–1293.

55. Wilson JD, George FW. The hormonal control of sexual development. Science 1981;211:1278–1284.

56. Bardin CW, Bullock LP, Sherins RP, Mowskowicz I. Androgen metabolism and mechanism of action in male pseudohemaphroditism: a study of testicular feminization. Recent Prog Horm Res 1973;29:65–109.

57. Nielsen HC, Zinman HM, Torday JS. Dihydrotestosterone inhibits fetal rabbit pulmonary surfactant production. J Clin Invest 1982;69:611–616.

58. Meisel RL, Ward IL. Fetal female rats are masculinized by male littermates located caudally in the uterus. Science 1981;213:239–242.

59. vom Saal FS, Bronson FH. Sexual characteristics of adult female mice are correlated with their testosterone levels during prenatal development. Science 1980;208:597–599.

60. Jost A, Vigier B, Prepin J, Perchellet JP. Studies on sex differentiation in mammals. Recent Prog Horm Res 1973;29:1–41.

61. Torday JS. Androgens delay human fetal lung maturation in vitro. Endocrinology 1990;126:3240–3244.

62. Catlin EA, Manganaro TF, Donahoe PK. Müllerian inhibiting substance depresses accumulation in vitro of disaturated phosphatidylcholine in fetal rat lung. Am J Obstet Gynecol 1988;159:1299–1303.

63. Catlin EA, Powell SM, Manganaro TF, Hudson PL, Ragin RC, Epstein J, Donahoe PK. Sex-specific fetal lung development and müellerian inhibiting substance. Am Rev Respir Dis 1990;141:466–470.

64. Grumbach MM, Gluckman PD. The human fetal hypothalamus and pituitary gland: the maturation of neuroendocrine mechanisms controlling the secretion of fetal pituitary growth hormone, prolactin, gonadotropins, adrenocorticotropin-related peptides, and thyrotropin. In: Maternal-fetal endocrinology. Philadelphia: Saunders, 1994. Tulchinsky D, Little AB, eds.

65. Cox MA, Torday JS. Pituitary oligopetide regulation of phosphatidylcholine synthesis by fetal rabbit lung cells: lack of effect with prolactin. Am Rev Respir Dis 1981;123:181–184.

66. Ballard PL, Gluckman PD, Brehier A, Kitterman JA, Kaplan SL, Rudolph AM, Grumbach MM. Failure to detect an effect of prolactin on pulmonary surfactant and adrenal steroids in fetal sheep and rabbits. J Clin Invest 1978;62:879–883.

67. Liggins GC, Kitterman JA, Campos GA, Clements JA, Forster CS, Lee CH, Creasy RK. Pulmonary maturation in the hypophysectomized ovine fetus: differential responses to adrenocorticotropin and cortisol. J Dev Physiol 1981;3:1–14.

68. Crone RK, Davies P, Liggins GC, Reid LR. The effects of hypophysectomy, thyroidectomy, and postoperative infusion of cortisol or adrenocorticotrophin on the structure of the ovine fetal lung. J Dev Physiol 1983;5:281–288.

69. Lyon MF, Hawkes SG. X-linked gene for testicular feminization in the mouse. Nature 1970; 227:1217–1219.

70. Griffin JE, Wilson JD. Studies on the pathogenesis of the incomplete forms of androgen resistance in man. J Clin Endocrinol Metab. 1977;45:1137–1143.

71. Sultan C, Migeon BR, Rothwell SW, Maes M, Zerhouni N, Migeon CJ. Androgen receptors and metabolism in cultured human fetal fibroblasts. Pediatr Res 1980;13:67–69.

72. Nielsen HC Testosterone regulation of sex differences in fetal lung development. Proc Soc Exp Biol Med. 1992;199:446–452.

73. Nielsen HC, Torday JS. Sex differences in avian embryo pulmonary surfactant production: evidence for sex chromosome involvement. Endocrinology 1985;117:31–37.

74. Kohler VD Lebensdauer japanischer Wachteln bei Kafigeinzelhaltung kurze Mitterlung. Versuchstier 1981;2:239–241.

75. Levi WM. The pigeon. Sumter, SC: Levi Publishing, 1953.

76. Eisner, E. Actuarial data for the Bengales finch (Lonchura striata: Fam. Estrildidae) in captivity. Exp Gerontol 1967;2:187–189.

77. Taderera JV. Control of lung development in vitro. Dev Biol 1967;16:489–512.

78. Smith BT. Fibroblast-pneumonocyte factor: intercellular mediator of glucocorticoid effect on fetal lung. Neonat Intens Care 1978;11:25–32.

79. Floros J, Phelps DS, Taeusch HW. Biosynthesis and in vitro translation of the major surfactant-associated protein from human lung. J Biol Chem 1985;260:495–500.

80. Nielsen HC. Epidermal growth factor influences the developmental clock regulating maturation of the fetal lung fibroblast. Biochim Biophys Acta 1989;1012:201–206.

81. Nielsen HC, Kellogg CK, Doyle CA. Development of fibroblast-type II cell communications in fetal rabbit lung organ culture. Biochim Biophys Acta 1992;1175:95–99.

82. Gross I, Dynia DW, Rooney SA, Smart DA, Warshaw JB, Sissom JF, Hoath SB. Influence of epidermal growth factor on fetal rat lung development in vitro. Pediatr Res 1986;20:473–477.

83. Sen N, Cake MH. Enhancement of disaturated phosphatidylcholine synthesis by epidermal growth factor in cultured fetal lung cells involves a fibroblast-epithelial cell interaction. Am J Respir Cell Mol Biol 1991;5:337–343.

84. Klein J, Nielsen HC. Epidermal growth factor regulation of rabbit fetal lung maturation depends on the stage of maturation. Biochim Biophys Acta 1992;1133:121–126.

85. Klein JM, Nielsen HC. Androgen regulation of epidermal growth factor receptors during fetal rabbit lung development. J Clin Invest 1993;91:425–431.

86. Rosenblum DA, Volpe MV, Dammann CEL, Lo Y-S, Thompson JF, Nielsen HC. Expression and activity of epidermal growth factor receptor in late fetal rat lung is cell- and sex-specific. Exp Cell Res 1998;239:69–81.

87. Dammann CEL, Nielsen HC. Regulation of the epidermal growth factor receptor in fetal rat lung fibroblasts during late gestation. Endocrinology 1998;139:1671–1677.

88. Volpe MV, Martin A, Vosatka RJ, Mazzoni CL, Nielsen HC. Hoxb-5 expression in the developing mouse lung suggests a role in branching morphogenesis and epithelial cell fate. Histochem Cell Biol 1997;108:405–504.

89. Yerozolimsky GB, Zagami M, McCants D, Nielsen HC. Cell- and sex- specific development of diacylglycerol production by EGF receptor activation in fetal rat lung. [Abstract] Pediatr Res 1994;35:80A.

90. Yerozolimsky GB, Nielsen HC. $Ca^{+2}$-ionophore A-23187 induction of cell- specific diacylglycerol production during fetal rat lung development. [Abstract] Pediatr Res 1995;37:73A.

91. Torday JS, Kourembanas S. Fetal rat lung fibroblasts produce a TGFβ homolog that blocks alveolar type II cell maturation. Dev Biol 1990;139:35–41.

92. Pereira S, Dammann CEL, McCants D, Nielsen HC. Transforming growth factor beta 1 binding and receptor kinetics in fetal mouse lung fibroblasts. Proc Soc Exp Biol Med 1998;218:51–61.

93. Dammann CE, Ramadurai SM, McCants DD, Pham LD, Nielsen HC. Androgen controls transforming growth factor-β receptor and epidermal growth factor receptor regulation and surfactant protein gene expression in the developing lung. [Abstract] Pediatr Res 1999;45:55A.

94. Volpe MV, Nielsen HC. Control of proximal airway branching in developing mouse lung morphogenesis. [Abstract] Pediatr Res 1998;43:57A.

95. Kellogg CK, Nielsen HC, Cochran B. C-myc expression in fetal lung development suggests a positive regulatory role in lung growth. [Abstract] Am Rev Respir Dis 1991;143:159A.

96. Sweezey NB, Ghibu F, Gagnon S, Schotman E, Hamid Q. Glucocorticoid receptor mRNA and protein in fetal rat lung in vivo: modulation by glucocorticoid and androgen. Am J Physiol 1998;275:L103–L109.

97. Mendelson CR, Johnson JM, McDonald PL, Snyder JM. Multihormonal regulation of surfactant synthesis by human fetal lung in vitro. J Clin Endocrinol Metab 1981;53:307–317.
98. Whitsett JA, Weaver TE, Lieberman MA, Clark JC, Daugherty C. Differential effects of epidermal growth factor and transforming growth factor-b on synthesis of $M_r$-35,000 surfactant-associated protein in fetal lung. J Biol Chem 1987;262:7908–7913.
99. Levesque BM, Nielsen HC. Dihydrotestosterone stimulates branching morphogenesis in embryonic lung explants. [Abstract] Pediatr Res 1996;39:63A.
100. Levesque BM, Nielsen HC. The progression of branching morphogenesis in the embryonic lung involves apoptosis. [Abstract] Pediatr Res 1997;41:48A.
101. Catlin EA, Tonnu VC, Ebb RG, Pacheco BA, Manganaro TV, Ezzell RM, Donahoe PK, Teixeira J. Muellerian inhibiting substance inhibits branching morphogenesis and induces apoptosis in fetal rat lung. Endocrinology 1997;138:790–796.
102. Catlin EA, Uitvlugt ND, Donahoe PK, Powell DM, Hayashi M, MacLaughlin DT. Muellerian inhibiting substance blocks epidermal growth factor receptor phosphorylation in fetal rat lung membranes. Metabolism 1991;40:1178–1184.
103. McMillan MM. Differential mortality by sex in fetal and neonatal deaths. Science 1979;204:89–91.
104. Watkins AM, Chan PJ, Patton WC, Jacobson JD, King A. Sperm kinetics and morphology before and after fractionation on discontinuous Percoll gradient for sex preselection: computerized analyses. Arch Androl 1996;37:1–5.
105. Fisher RA. The genetical theory of natural selection. New York: Oxford University Press, 1930.
106. Hassold T, Chen N, Funkhouser J, Jooss T, Munuei B, Matsuura J, Matsuyama A, Wilson C, Yamane JA, Jacobs PA. A cytogenic study of 1,000 spontaneous abortions. Ann Hum Genet 1980;44:151–178.
107. Charnoff EL. The theory of sex allocation. Princeton, NJ: Princeton University Press, 1982:104.
108. Williams GC. Sex and Evolution. Princeton, NJ: Princeton University Press, 1975.
109. Cavalli-Sforza LL, Bodmer WF. The genetics of human populations. New York: Freeman, 1971.
110. Fraser FC, Fainstat TD. Production of congenital defects in the offspring of pregnant mice treated with cortisone. Pediatrics 1951;8:527–533.
111. Jaskoll T, Melnick M. Mouse fetal lung development and MHC-associated glucocorticoid receptor variation. Dev Biol 1992;44A.
112. Wilson EO. Consilience. New York: Knopf, 1998.
113. Becker B, Shin DH, Plamberg PF, Waltman SR. HLA antigens and corticosteroid response. Science 1976;194:1427–1428.
114. Bonner JJ, Slavkin HC. Cleft palate susceptibility linked to histocompatibility-2 (H-2) in the mouse. Immunogenetics 1975;2:213–218.
115. Hu CC, Jaskoll TF, Minkin C, Melnick M. Mouse major histocompatibility complex (H-2) and fetal lung development: implications for human pulmonary maturation. Am J Med Gen 1990;35:126–131.
116. Melnick M, Chen H, Buckley S, Warburton D, Jaskoll T. Insulin-like growth factor-β, and cdk4 expression and the developmental epigenetics of mouse palate morphogenesis and dysmorphogenesis. Dev Dynamics 1998;211:11–25.
117. Alevizopoulos A, Mermod N. Transforming growth factor-beta: the breaking open of a black box. Bioessays 1997;19:581–591.
118. Hafez M, El-Sallab SH, Khashaba M, Risk MS, El-Morsy Z, Bassiony MR, El- Kenawy F, Zaghloul W. Evidence of HLA-linked susceptibility gene(s) in respiratory distress syndrome. Disease Markers 1989;7:201–208.

# 9    Retinoids and Lung Development

*Richard D. Zachman,* PhD, MD
*and Mary A. Grummer,* PhD

## VITAMIN A AS A MEDIATOR IN EMBRYOGENESIS AND DIFFERENTIATION

The term vitamin A is used to describe the biologic activity of a group of compounds that includes both the naturally occurring and synthetically derived retinoids. Ingested vitamin A precursors such as β-carotene and natural retinyl esters are hydrolyzed forming retinol, which is absorbed and then transported to tissue for metabolic action or storage (Fig. 1). The major storage site is the liver, primarily as retinyl esters, but most other tissues are able to convert some retinol to retinyl esters *(1)*. There are precise control mechanisms for the formation, release, and metabolism of these stored retinyl esters. Loss of regulatory control of retinoids due to either deficiency or excess can cause a large number of pathologic abnormalities, varying with tissue and cell type. Retinol, a lipophilic alcohol, is released by the enzymatic hydrolysis of retinyl esters. Retinol is transported in blood bound to a specific retinol binding protein (RBP), which is complexed with transthyretin. This complex delivers retinol to target tissues for metabolic reactions that result in retinoid cellular functions and eventual turnover.

Pregnant mice and rats on a liberal supply of retinol transfer an adequate portion of the vitamin to the fetus. Maternal transplacental transfer of adequate retinol to the fetal rat is maintained until the mother is made very deficient by low dietary vitamin A *(2)*. The regulation of retinol transport from the maternal circulation to the fetus through the placenta is not well established in any species. Human cord blood concentrations of retinol are relatively constant over a wide range of maternal blood retinol levels, so it seems that the fetus is supplied with enough retinol unless the mother has obvious clinical signs of vitamin A deficiency *(3)*. Many synthetic teratogenic retinoids also freely reach the fetus.

From: *Contemporary Endocrinology: Endocrinology of the Lung: Development and Surfactant Synthesis*
Edited by: C. R. Mendelson © Humana Press Inc., Totowa, NJ

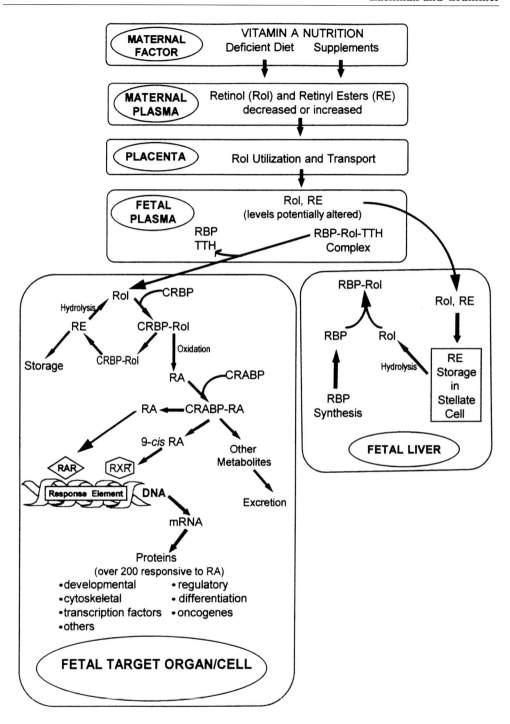

Fig. 1. General scheme of vitamin A metabolism and function. Fetal tissue accumulation of retinoids can be potentially influenced by maternal vitamin A status, length of gestation and placental passage. The uptake of retinol (Rol), its storage as retinyl ester (RE) and subsequent hydrolysis and release as retinol circulating as the retinol-binding protein–transthyretin complex (Rol-RBP-TTR) for delivery to target tissue is under tight regulation. Further metabolism of retinol is regulated by binding to cellular retinol binding protein (CRBP). An important oxidation

Specific cytosolic and nuclear binding proteins are essential for the metabolism and function of retinoids. Cellular retinol binding protein (CRBP) plays a central role in the regulation of retinol distribution and metabolism *(4)*. The apo-CRBP binds the hydrophobic retinol, possibly protecting the cell from retinol toxicity. Localization of CRBP suggests a role in specific tissue delivery of retinol through blood organ barriers *(5)*. CRBP-retinol serves as the substrate for oxidation of retinol to the aldehyde, retinal, which is then irreversibly oxidized to retinoic acid (RA). RA is bound in the cytoplasm by its own specific binding protein, cellular retinoic acid binding protein (CRABP). Spatiotemporal differences in expression during development and multiple forms have been demonstrated by *in situ* methods for both CRBP and CRABP *(4–8)*. The function of CRABP is not totally clarified, but it might serve to transport RA and, as well, might involve sequestration of RA within a cell, to alter the activity of RA in regulation of gene expression *(4)*.

RA is transferred to the nucleus, where it affects the expression of many cell genetic products *(9,10)*, mediated through its interaction with nuclear retinoic acid receptors (RAR). These protein receptors are transcription factors, members of the steroid hormone superfamily of regulatory factors, which, when bound specifically by ligands, control expression of genes affecting differentiation, growth, and homeostasis *(11)*. Three distinct types of RARs ($\alpha$, $\beta$, and $\gamma$) bind the ligand RA and then interact with specific DNA sequences, called retinoic acid response elements (RARE), on a number of RA target genes.

During development the differential patterns of expression of RAR $\alpha$, $\beta$, and $\gamma$ mRNA suggest specific role of the receptors *(12–18)*. Using transgenic mice *(13–14)*, RA responsive RAR-$\beta$ promoter activity was demonstrated in spinal cord, sensory organs, limb buds, and various endodermal and mesodermal derivations. Recently, it has been shown that there are rapid changes in RAR-$\beta$2 mRNA and protein during RA-induced fetal dysmorphogenesis *(15)*. The localization of RAR-$\gamma$ suggests its involvement in chondrogenesis and in differentiation, while RAR-$\alpha$ gene expression in mouse embryos is relatively ubiquitous *(12)*.

A single gene deletion of CRABP I or II does not seem to cause deformation problems *(18)*. Possibly other less specific fatty acid binding proteins can adequately carry out their function. Likewise, it takes double deletion of the RAR isoforms to cause lethality and malformations of various organ systems *(16,17)*. Despite the considerable amount of underlying redundancy in receptor function, it is clear the RARs are essential for the transduction of the retinoid signal during development. Further research with the null transgenic model should clarify specific effects of each RAR combination.

---

product is retinoic acid (RA) which also has its own cytosolic retinoic acid binding protein (CRABP). CRABP helps traffic RA and regulates it availability to bind to nuclear receptors (RAR) with specific response elements (RARE). Some RA is converted to 9-*cis* RA, which binds to its own family of nuclear retinoid X receptors (RXR). These interactions influence the expression of many genes that affect differentiation and growth.

BPD, bronchopulmonary dysplasia; CRBP, cellular retinol-binding protein; CRABP, cellular retinoic acid-binding protein; DEX, dexamethasone; DSPC, disaturated phosphatidylcholine; PC, phosphatidylcholine; RA, retinoic acid; RAR, retinoic acid receptor; RARE, retinoic acid response element; RBP, retinol-binding protein; RXR, retinoid X receptors; RP, retinyl palmitate; IM-RDR, Intramuscular relative dose response; SP, surfactant protein; EGF, epidermal growth factor.

A second class of nuclear retinoic acid receptors, the retinoid X receptors (RXRs), specifically bind and are activated by 9-*cis*-RA, a metabolite of RA *(19)* (Fig. 1). The RXRs also demonstrate different patterns of expression in the embryo. RXR-α is found predominately in epithelia of the digestive tract, skin, and liver of mouse embryo. Significant levels of RXR-β are detected in CNS. The RXR-γ transcript, displaying the greatest restriction pattern of the three receptors, is found primarily in the corpus striatum and pituitary, and is weakly expressed in neck, skeletal muscle, and tongue. In the chick, RXRs are expressed in nerves and neural crest cells. Mutation of the RXR/RAR-α genes results in embryonic lethality due to hypoplastic development of the ventricular chambers of the heart, a phenotype similarly seen in embryogenic vitamin A deficiency. A fundamental property of the RXRs is their interaction with other members of the steroid nuclear receptor superfamily, forming heterodimers which contribute to the diversity of the effects of retinoid signaling. These complexes also are being shown to have important roles in embryonic development and differentiation *(16,17,19,20)*.

It is clear that retinoids can potentially regulate the expression and products of many different genes in many cell types. The networks of genes eventually activated or repressed are complex because of the variety of response elements, autoregulatory loops, and positive and negative gene regulation that could vary in different cell types.

## RETINOIDS AND LUNG DEVELOPMENT

Lung differentiation, growth, and health are affected by vitamin A. It has been known for over 75 years that human neonates with vitamin A deficiency suffer from respiratory problems *(21)*. Vitamin A deficiency causes replacement of mucus-secreting epithelium by stratified squamous keratinizing epithelium in the trachea and bronchi. The differentiation of various pulmonary cells studied in culture requires retinoids *(22)*. Respiratory tract developmental defects found with various combinations of RAR-α, β, γ double mutants include agenesis of left lung, hypoplasia of right and left lung, and the lack of an esophageal–tracheal septum *(23)*. Pulmonary morbidity is frequently associated with human vitamin A deficency*(24)*. There are data and speculation that vitamin A has a role in the prevention and/or repair of lung injury in human premature newborns *(22,25–28)*. This review summarizes research evidence showing that retinoids do influence lung development.

### *Retinoid Availability and Fetal Lung Development*

An important aspect of retinoids and lung development is to determine the availability and functions of retinoids and their binding proteins during various lung development stages. These stages include branching morphogenesis, morphogenic remodeling (pseudoglandular, canalicular, and terminal saccular stages), and alveolar formation with septation *(29)*. Striking changes in retinoids occur during all developmental stages.

#### FETAL RAT MODELS

Retinyl ester stores, mostly retinyl palmitate (RP), are high in fetal rat lung from gestational days 16 to 19 (glandular to early canalicular stage of lung development), after which a marked decline occurs during development by 19–21 d (mostly saccular) *(26,30)*. This decrease of retinyl esters can be produced by cesarean birth *(31)* and programmed a day earlier by antenatal maternal dexamethasone (DEX) *(32)*. The rapid depletion in lung retinyl esters is in contrast to an increase in liver RP stores that occurs during the same time period *(25)*. This suggests that the depletion of fetal lung retinyl ester stores has an important metabolic function in lung development. Since isolated perfused neonatal rabbit lung *(33)* and adult rat type II cells *(34)* both can synthesize retinyl esters, it is likely that the endogenous fetal lung retinyl esters are synthesized in fetal lung, but this observation has not yet been made by direct experimentation. Fetal rat lung retinyl ester stores can be increased by prenatal maternal administration of a massive RP dose (15 mg per rat)*(26)*. The concentration of both RA and 9-*cis*-RA in fetal rat lung rise after day 18 gestational age and peak at postnatal day 2 and then decline to essentially undetectable levels by postnatal age of 8–12 d *(35)*.

Recent work has demonstrated that vitamin A-deficient, retinoic acid-supplemented pregnant rats cannot complete gestation *(36)*. While as little as 2 µg of retinol administered on day 10 of gestation prevents this fetal resorption, the newborn pups die within a few minutes of being born. The pups, initially healthy in appearance, begin (within seconds of birth) to gasp for air and become cyanotic, dying within several minutes from an apparent hypoxia. Histologic examination of these rat pups demonstrated delayed pulmonary development *(37)*. Branching and scalloping of ducts and saccule and subsaccule formation are decreased, similar to premature human infant with respiratory distress syndrome (RDS) *(29,37)*.

## RETINOID STATUS AND HUMAN LUNG DEVELOPMENT

The disruptive pathology of bronchopulmonary dysplasia (BPD) that occurs during the period of alveolarization in human premature infants has many pathologic features of retinoid deficiency *(38)*.These include atelectasis, loss of ciliated cells, keratinizing metaplasia, and necrotizing bronchiolitis *(22,25,26,38)*. Low liver retinyl ester stores have been documented after death in premature infants weighing <1500 g *(39)*. Many reports show that plasma retinol concentrations in premature infants <36 wk gestation are lower than those in term infants *(25,26,39,40)*. This has led to the testing of the hypothesis that premature infants who will develop BPD have lower initial plasma retinol concentrations than do those who will not develop BPD *(40–45)*. It is implied that the lower plasma retinol levels indicate less tissue retinol stores, which will then be detrimental to the developing lung, which then is in part responsible for the development of BPD.

Several clinical trials have used supplemental vitamin A and report a decrease in the incidence of BPD and its associated morbidity in premature infants *(43,46–48)*. However, these results are controversial *(49)*, and such supplements are not in common use. A meta-analysis has not helped to establish vitamin A supplementation to prevent BPD as a universal standard of care *(50)*. In most of the trials, a supplement of 5000 IU (as retinyl palmitate, RP) three times a week is given, which results frequently in a rise in serum retinol levels. However, even when infants are treated with supplemental vitamin A, 30–50% of those patients still develop BPD *(43,47,49)*. A recent multicenter study in premature infants with birthweight <1000 g showed that such supplementation decreased death or BPD at 36 wk gestation from 62% in controls to 55% in the supplemented group *(51)*. These authors have suggested that higher supplements might be needed to produce a better effect *(50,51)*.

Several factors interfere with clarification of the relation between vitamin A and BPD. First, all conclusions of previous studies were based on a single plasma retinol value, which unfortunately, does not correlate well with liver storage until it becomes very low [< 0.35 µmol/L (< 10.0 µg/dL)] *(52,53)*. In some populations, correlation is not found until even lower [< 0.17 µmol/L (< 5 µg/dL)] liver concentrations *(54)*.Despite this fact, the use of a single retinol concentration continues in the evaluation of the retinoid status of premature infants.

A hypothesis has been recently tested showing that an intramuscular relative dose response (IM-RDR) on day 1 of life more accurately predicts which premature infants will develop BPD than single measurements of retinol, RP or retinol binding protein (RBP) *(55)*. A day 1 RDR ≥ 25% (representative of low retinol stores) occurred in only 6 of 37 premature infants ≤32 wk who did not develop BPD, compared with 15 of 38 infants who developed BPD ($p < .025$). Retinol, RP, and RBP on day 1 were not different between the groups, thus not predictive of infants that will develop BPD. Other confounding variables to establishing the role of retinoids in BPD include changed criteria for the diagnosis of BPD *(56)*, and an unknown lower limit of tissue vitamin A concentration that might cause functional defects in the premature infant lung. Finally, a major factor, as will be discussed below, is the increased use of antenatal and postnatal glucocorticoids, since these cause alterations in vitamin A metabolism.

## Retinoid Binding Proteins: Levels and Gene Expression

The expression of RARs in branching fetal mouse lung at midgestation has been studied by *in situ* hybridization *(57)*. All three RAR types were expressed in 12.5-d fetal lung. RAR-α was light and rather diffuse (all cells). RAR-γ was strictly mesenchymal but widely expressed. RAR-β had a more specific pattern of expression, present linearly in the tubular epithelium and being higher in proximal epithelial tubules with little or no expression in distal tubules. With branching, the RAR-β message remained proximal in the epithelium of the intrapulmonary segmental bronchi, but lung parenchyma and alveolar ducts were not labeled. CRBP was strongly expressed in tracheal mesenchyme, tracheal, and bronchial epithelium but was only present in mesenchyme at 14.5 d. CRABP was detected between the trachea and heart but not in trachea or lung tissue. Thus, several retinoid binding proteins in the early bronchial tree are developmentally regulated and specifically localized. This suggests that retinoids do have a role in airway formation during the branching morphogenesis of lung development.

The levels of binding activity of CRBP and CRABP in fetal rat lung from day 18 gestation to birth undergo no remarkable change. After birth, there is a striking increase in the CRABP level, which peaks on postnatal day 10, and then falls to nondetectable levels again by day 21 *(58)*. CRABP mRNA and CRBP mRNA follow a similar pattern, rising to peak at postnatal day 8 and then declining *(59)*. This postnatal surge of CRABP and CRBP suggests a role in rat lung alveolarization.

RAR-specific binding studies in fetal rat lung nuclear extracts suggest a single class of receptor binding sites with high affinity ($K_d$ approx $10^{-9}M$) for RA and RAR saturation at 2–5nM RA *(60)*. RA binding by RAR at 18 d gestation is two- to threefold greater than in 20- to 21-d fetuses, newborn pup, or adult lung. Lung nuclear extract from vitamin A-deficient fetuses had higher RAR binding. These observations suggest that both gestational age and vitamin A are possible regulators of RAR binding in developing lung. However, the sequelae of this regulation are not clear.

An evaluation of RAR gene expression in whole fetal lung during gestation demonstrated that, at day 17 gestation, there were significantly higher amounts of a 2.7 kb RAR-α species than from day 19 to the newborn *(61)*. In contrast to RAR-α, fetal lung RAR-β mRNA levels from day 17 through day 22 gestation were significantly lower relative to newborn levels. The level of expression of RAR-γ mRNA at various gestations was too low to be detected by Northern blot analysis, although PCR demonstrated its presence. This transcript is very easily demonstrated postnatally and in adult rat lung *(62,63)*. These data suggest that RAR-α is related to cell type or structural changes during the transition from the glandular to canalicular stage of lung development. The surge in RAR-β mRNA just after birth implies a role in the terminal phase of the saccular period, when both type I and type II pneumocytes are clearly defined. It has not been determined whether these observations are actually cell type-specific or related to retinoic acid availability. *In situ* hybridization studies and isolated cell analyses are needed to more precisely clarify the functional significance of these RAR mRNA changes.

## *Retinoids and Fetal Lung Surfactant*

During the saccular stage of fetal lung development (rat, 20–22 d gestation; human, 24–36 wk gestation) there is histologic evidence of definite alveolar type II cells, which are responsible for surfactant synthesis *(29)*. Since the development of lung surfactant is all-important in survival after birth, factors regulating its production and turnover need to be defined. The effects of retinoids on the surfactant system has been studied in several models, although the results do not always give consistent information.

### ISOLATED TYPE II CELLS

In isolated 19 d gestation fetal rat type II cells, RA stimulates choline incorporation into phosphatidycholine (PC) *(64)* despite its effect on inhibition of type II cell proliferation *(65)*. Type II cells isolated from vitamin A-deficient adult rats incorporate less choline into PC and disaturated PC (DSPC) compared with controls *(66)*. Adding RA to these isolated adult rat cells stimulates choline incorporation into both PC and DSPC in control and deficient cells *(66)*, similar to the findings in fetal type II cells.

### EXPLANTS AND CELL CULTURES

Fetal lung explants and lung adenocarcinoma cells have been utilized to determine the effect of RA on surfactant protein (SP). In 13.5-d fetal rat lung cultured for up to 19 d, RA added to the media augments the pattern of lung development toward more growth of proximal airways. This treatment also suppresses the expression of the SP genes SP-A, SP-B and SP-C, which usually occurs in the peripheral portions of lung during alveolar development *(67)*. In 17-or 19-d fetal rat lung explants, exposure to RA results in increases in SP-A, SP-B, and SP-C mRNA, although each shows different dose-response characteristics *(68)*. At $10^{-10}M$ RA, SP-A mRNA maximally increases, but at $10^{-5}M$ RA, it decreases. By contrast, $10^{-5}M$ RA maximally stimulates SP-C and SP-B mRNA. Human fetal lung explants treated with RA for 6 d show dose-dependent decreases in SP-A protein and mRNA levels, a decrease in SP-C mRNA, and an increase in SP-B mRNA *(69)*. When H441 human lung adenocarcinoma cells are treated with RA, SP-A mRNA levels are unaffected, but SP-B mRNA levels increase in a dose-dependent manner *(70)*. Together, these results are suggestive that RA generally decreases SP-A mRNA expression, increases SP-B mRNA expression, and has a more variable effect on SP-C mRNA in the systems studied thus far. Cell source, the concentration and length of exposure time to RA, and other factors could account for the variable responses noted. One study with 19-d fetal lung explants did show that choline incorporation into PC was enhanced by RA *(71)*, similar to the findings in isolated type II cells *(64)*. RA also enhanced the effect of epidermal growth factor (EGF) on choline incorporation *(71)*.

In Vivo Fetal Rat Lung

Treating pregnant rats with one dose of RP on day 16 resulted in an increase of day 19 fetal lung total phospholipid and DSPC *(64)*. Chronic RP to the rat mother from day 16–20 gestation also increased fetal lung DSPC analyzed on day 20. By contrast, SP-A concentrations underwent no significant change after one RP dose, and were reduced in fetal lung after repetitive administration *(64)*.

To date, there are two reports that have explored the effect of maternal–fetal vitamin A deficiency on fetal lung surfactant. In one, the purpose of the experiments was to determine whether maternal–fetal vitamin A deficiency in vivo had an effect on fetal lung SP *(72)*. Weanling female rats at 21 d were fed control (C) or a vitamin A-deficient (D) diet. These females were mated, kept on their specific diet, and fetal and maternal tissues were obtained on day 20 gestation. Control mothers had liver RP concentrations of 246 ± 32 nmol/g wet weight; those in the D group had 6.1 ± 2.9 nmol/g wet weight. Control fetal liver RP was 12-fold higher and control fetal lung RP was threefold higher than in the D group. Neither fetal lung surfactant protein SP-C mRNA nor SP-A mRNA was affected by vitamin A deficiency.

Additionally, pregnant rats from both C and D groups were injected with either dexamethasone (DEX) or an equal volume of saline on days 15 through 17, and killed on day 18 *(72)*. As expected, DEX increased fetal lung SP-C mRNA twofold over the level found in the saline-injected group. This increase in SP-C mRNA also occurred in fetal lungs from the D group. Thus, fetal rat lung development, as measured by SP-C and SP-A mRNA, and the SP-C mRNA response to DEX, were not affected by vitamin A deficiency *(72)*. Although the results obtained in this rat model of vitamin A deficiency cannot be directly applied to human fetal lung development, it appears likely that mild vitamin A deficiency in humans would not affect *in utero* fetal lung SP maturation.

Using a different protocol, in which the maternal rats were deprived of vitamin A for a shorter time (delivery at 19 d gestation after maternal vitamin A deprivation from day 5 or day 12; or deprived from vitamin A for 2 or 7 d before pregnancy and again sacrificed at 19 d) fetal lung RP and PC were lower after maternal vitamin A deprivation of 14, 21, and 28 days than controls. *(71)*. RAR-β mRNA was lower in fetal lungs after 28 days of maternal deprivation, while RAR-α mRNA was higher than control. It was somewhat surprising to see that such short time periods of adult maternal rat vitamin A deprivation caused an effect on fetal lung RP, since others *(2,72)* have found it necessary to restrict vitamin A from the weanling through adulthood in order to affect fetal lung and liver RP stores.

Retinoid data in relation to lung development, discussed above, are summarized in part according to various stages of lung development in Table 1.

# RETINOID INTERACTIONS AND REGULATION OF LUNG DEVELOPMENT

## *Interaction with Glucocorticoids*

Early in the 1940s, it was noted that the stress of certain diseases and acute infections lowered the blood level and liver storage of vitamin A. There was an apparent association between susceptibility to rheumatic fever and low plasma vitamin A *(73)*. The plasma vitamin A increased with clinical improvement, but then decreased again if acute rheumatic fever recurred, with the lowest level accompanying the most severe attacks. During the next decade, further reports confirmed these observations *(74,75)*. During

Table 1
Retinoids and Lung Development

---

**Stages of lung development**

*Branching morphogenesis*
- *In situ* studies show receptor proteins localized in specific fashion
- RA favors proximal airway growth; suppresses peripheral epithelial buds

*Morphogenic remodeling stages*
- *Ligand*: Rapid decrease of fetal lung RP before delivery; RA increases from day 18 to postnatal day 2
- *Protein*: Levels of CRBP, CRABP unchanged; RAR binding highest at 18-d gestation
- *Gene expression*: Fetal lung RAR mRNA changes with gestation

*Period of alveolarization*
- CRABP levels and binding activity peak at postnatal days 7-10
- Rat lung RAR β mRNA peaks at postnatal day 3
- Lack of RA in retinol supported gestation causes neonatal rat respiratory death

**Fetal lung surfactant**
- RA slows fetal type II cell proliferation
- RA stimulates choline incorporation into surfactant phospholipid
- RA decreases expression of SP-A and SP-B in fetal lung explants, accompanying its affect on distal airway growth
- In vivo maternal vitamin A deficiency has no effect on fetal lung SP A, SP-C mRNA
- In vivo maternal vitamin A deprivation decreases fetal lung phospholipid content

**Clinical observations on retinoids and premature infant lung**
- Retinol deficiency shows lung histopathologic appearance similar to BPD
- Infants dying of BPD have low liver retinyl ester stores
- Clinical trials suggest vitamin A therapy decreases BPD morbidity

---

experiments in 1955, the color of the livers of rats treated with cortisone was less yellow than controls. Experiments showed that large doses of cortisone given to normal or adrenalectomized rats on stock or vitamin A-deficient diets resulted in a measurable loss of vitamin A from the liver and kidney, suggesting a role of glucocorticoids in the regulation of vitamin A storage, mobilization, or metabolism *(76)*. Other work confirmed that cortisone and ACTH lowered liver vitamin A stores, which was accompanied by a transient rise in serum retinol *(77)*. DEX is known to stimulate the release of plasma retinol-binding protein (RBP) from cultured rat liver cells *(78)*. Dietary vitamin A modulates the properties of both retinoic acid and glucocorticoid receptors in rat liver *(79)*. Receptors for glucocorticoids, which belong to the same steroid hormone superfamily of regulatory factors as the RARs, are present in lung and it is well known that many aspects of perinatal lung development are sensitive to glucocorticoid homones

*(80,81)*. Therefore, it seems rational to consider that an interaction between glucocorticoids and retinoids has relevance during lung development.

## ANTENATAL STEROIDS

Antenatal steroids (primarily betamethasone and DEX), used with increasing frequency in perinatal medicine to promote fetal lung maturation *(80,81)*, have profound effects on vitamin A. It was first shown that intramuscular DEX, given to pregnant rhesus monkeys 33 d before term, increased both maternal and fetal serum concentrations of RBP at delivery 3 d later *(82)*. There was a dose-dependent response. This primate study was supported by observations on 30 premature human infants whose mothers were treated with prenatal steroids, which resulted in elevated neonatal serum retinol and RBP at birth compared with a control group *(83)*. Finally, as noted above in the discussion of fetal lung retinoid stores, antenatal DEX given to pregnant rats caused the mobilization of rat fetal lung retinyl ester stores to occur a day earlier in gestation *(32)*. It is tempting to speculate that part of the mechanism of DEX stimulation of fetal lung maturation is through retinoids. However, at this time it is not clear that is the case. Indeed, it is not clear whether these effects of antenatal steroids are useful or detrimental to the newborn premature infant. Perhaps mobilizing the fetal retinoid stores would actually make it more likely for the infant to be born with less available retinoid stores for pulmonary development and extrauterine adaptation.

Antagonistic effects of DEX and RA were demonstrated recently in fetal rat lung *(84)*. Treatment of day 14 and 15 lung explants with RA ($10^{-6}M$ to $10^{-5}M$) decreased branching and caused dilatation of distal tubules and caused dilatation of proximal tubules destined to form the trachea and main bronchi. These are findings similar to those noted above *(67)*. The DEX effects on these fetal explants, such as distorted patterns of branching, reduced lung growth and inhibition of epithelial cell proliferation, were prevented by RA. RA also antagonized DEX-induced increased levels of SP-A and SP-B mRNAs, the distribution of cells expressing SP-C mRNA, and the attenuation of mesenchymal tissue, which are all factors indicating accelerated lung maturation. These authors suggested that a balance in the action of endogeneous retinoids and glucocorticoids is needed for normal lung development *(84)*. Obviously, such a balance in fetal lung could be influenced by the clinical use of antenatal steroids.

## POSTNATAL STEROIDS

DEX is now also frequently used in neonates for the treatment of neonatal BPD *(56,85)*. One could speculate that some of the lung improvement after DEX is mediated by mobilization of retinoid stores, which then facilitate lung repair required to improve BPD outcome. This hypothesis seems plausible, considering the observation that in human neonates, serum retinol increases to peak about 7 d after starting postnatal DEX treatment *(55,86)*.

Postnatal effects of exogenous DEX on rat liver and lung vitamin A content has been studied in several models. In one neonatal rat study, two groups of 1-d-old rat pups received either 1 mg/kg DEX or saline subcutaneously, at 0, 24, and 48 h and were sacrificed at 72 h *(87)*. DEX decreased liver RP between 33% and 55% and decreased lung RP by over 60%. In addition, RAR binding activity in DEX-treated lungs was also decreased. This work demonstrated for the first time an interaction between DEX and retinoids at the functional level of RA binding proteins. The postnatal effect of DEX on the expression of RAR mRNA has also been studied in neonatal rats treated with DEX at 3–7 d after birth *(88)*. Northern analyses showed that DEX specifically inhibited the expression of RAR-β mRNA. By contrast, the expression of lung RAR-α and RAR-γ were not affected by DEX *(88)*. In a somewhat related study in 3-mo-old rats, DEX treatment for 7 d depleted lung and liver retinol and RP *(89)*.

The effect of DEX and RA at the level of the alveoli in postnatal rat lung has recently been studied using serial lung sections *(90)*. Three-day-old rats were injected intraperitoneally with RA or diluent, and half of both groups were subcutaneously injected with DEX (0.25 μg/d) for 13 d. DEX treatment inhibited the number of alveoli formed and produced low body mass-specific gas-exchange surface areas (Sa). These effects were prevented by RA treatment. In rats receiving only RA treatment, the number of alveoli increased 50%, but there was no increase in Sa, suggesting the action of a regulatory mechanism to prevent unneeded Sa *(90)*. The authors hypothesize these findings support the possibility that treatment with a pharmacologic agent may provide preventive or remedial therapy for individuals with too few alveoli for adequate gas exchange *(91)*. These investigators have also shown an effect of DEX on CRABP and CRBP mRNA *(59)*.

A more basic approach in an attempt to understand the DEX-RA interaction has been recently published. A mouse lung epithelial cell line was used to explore RA and DEX effects on RAR and surfactant SP-C mRNA expression *(92)*. RA increased mRNA expression of RAR-β (5.5 times) and SP-C (two times) mRNA, with maximal effects at 24 h and at $10^{-6}M$. The RA induction was not inhibited by cycloheximide, suggesting RA affects transcription. With added actinomycin D, RA did not affect the disappearance rate of RAR-β mRNA, but SP-C mRNA degradation was slowed, indicating an effect on SP-C mRNA stability. DEX decreased RAR-β and SP-C expression to 75% and 70% of control values, respectively, with greatest effects at 48 h and at $10^{-7}M$. There was no effect of DEX on either RAR-β or SP-C mRNA disappearance in the presence of actinomycin D. However, cycloheximide prevented the effect of DEX. Despite DEX, RA increased both RAR-β and SP-C mRNA. This work suggests that RA and DEX affect RAR-β and SP-C genes by different mechanisms.

## POSSIBLE MECHANISMS OF INTERACTION BETWEEN STEROIDS AND RETINOIDS

There are several mechanisms that could be hypothesized to explain the effect of DEX on retinoids. There is the possibility that steroids have an inductive effect on enzymes of retinoid metabolism. For example, increased hydrolysis of retinyl esters in the liver would result if steroids specifically increased retinyl ester hydrolase activity. This could account for the effect of DEX reducing retinyl ester stores in lung and liver as described above *(32,87,89)*. A short-term consequence of the increased ester hydrolysis would be the transient rise in serum retinol, as described *(55,86)*, followed by a decrease in serum retinol due to the expenditures of the retinyl ester stores.

Steroid induction of enzymes associated with nonspecific oxidation of retinoids, such as the inducible cytochrome P-450 2E1 *(93)* could result in increased degradation of retinol and its tissue depletion. Steroid induction of the enzymes causing increased hydroxylation has been reported *(94)*. This could result in increased hydroxylation of the functional metabolite RA, to inactive metabolites. A resultant decrease in the ligand RA would then decrease the expression of RAR-β, as observed in DEX treatment *(88,92)*, since RAR-β is very sensitive to RA concentration *(62,63)*.

Since both RA and steroids bind to proteins belonging to a common nuclear receptor superfamily, it is possible that some of the synergistic and antagonistic effects of steroids and RA occur at this level. The DNA binding domain of RAR has a 45% homology with the glucocorticoid receptor DNA binding domain *(11,19)*. It is thus possible for mechanisms to occur in which the steroid receptor might interfere with RAR binding to DNA of target genes, which then could act at the transcriptional level to affect gene expression. As noted in the lung cell studies, cycloheximide inhibited the DEX effect on RAR-β; hence somewhere in the interaction protein synthesis is necessary. Alternative interaction mechanisms are possible and further studies are required to clarify these matters.

### *Interaction With Other Factors To Potentially Regulate Lung Development*

The possible role of retinoids in lung development in relation to two neonatal clinical lung diseases, respiratory distress syndrome with surfactant deficiency (RDS), and BPD, has been alluded to in some of the discussion above. Another potentially relevant clinical area is the respiratory problems of the very immature birth. A significant effort in time and health dollar expense is now increasingly spent on treating the human "micropreemie" — a term used frequently in clinical medicine in reference to immature/premature infants of 23–25 wk gestation, and birth weights in the range of 600–850 g *(95,96)*. These immature infants have a number of problems, but lung development and need of respiratory support is a primary concern. These infants are at the lung development stage of finishing the canalicular phase and just progressing into the saccular phase — with its associated cell differentiation of the important type I and type II cells. Clearly, if success in helping these births to intact survival is a priority, one necessary goal of basic and clinical research is to try to accelerate the emergence of the saccular stage of lung development. Retinoids, owing to their diverse and extensive interaction with transcription factors and other regulatory mechanisms, might well have a significant role in this area. Of the many RA-responsive genes, several are relevant and important to lung development and integrity *(9,10)*. A few examples will be cited here.

#### HOMEOBOX GENES

The homeobox genes are a family of related regulatory factors that are involved in specification of cell fate during development. The *Hox* genes, a subfamily of homeobox genes, are known to be responsive to RA and it has been postulated that RA influences morphogenesis by modifying *Hox* genes expression. A number of *Hox* genes are present in the developing lung, and several have been shown to decrease with advancing gestational age. Treatment of day 17 fetal rat lung explants with RA ($10^{-5}M$) causes an increase in the *Hox* A5, B5, and B6 mRNA levels, an activation that occurs within 2 h of treatment *(97)*. Through use of *in situ* hybridization, the variations in spatiotemporal localization throughout development of *Hox* A2, B6, and another patterning gene, *Sonic hedgehog*, suggest that the genes have different developmental roles. RA treatment causes upregulation of all three genes and alters their normal development changes *(98)*. It was suggested that elevated RA levels promote expression of factors involved in maintaining typical proximal lung structures of the immature lung, while preventing formation of the distal structures of the mature lung. These studies were done with a relatively high concentration of RA, so interpretation should be made with caution.

## CELL–CELL INTERACTIONS

The process of lung morphogenesis is complex and involves the coordination of collaborative activities of various cell types. Understanding this communication between cells could lead to methods to accelerate fetal lung growth. An interaction between cell types has been demonstrated in cocultures of epithelial and mesenchymal cells from 15–17 d fetal mouse lungs, where RA stimulates proliferation of both cell types *(99)*. However, when cultured separately, only the mesenchymal cells responded to RA. In organ cultures, RA caused an increase of epithelial branching activity. These results suggest that the cell proliferation and branching activity occurring in developing mouse lungs involves epithelial-mesenchymal interactions. The response to RA was accompanied by an increase in the expression of the receptor EGF. EGF, which was produced primarily in mesenchymal cultures, increased proliferation of both mesenchymal and epithelial cells and stimulated branching activity in organ cultures. It may be that the effect of RA in the developing lung is mediated through EGF receptor upregulation, with the mesenchyme producing the necessary ligand.

The pulmonary lipofibroblast, located in the alveolar interstitium, participates in alveolar development. It acts as an accessory cell to the type II cell, providing triglycerides for surfactant synthesis *(100)*. During lung development, retinoid metabolism in these cells undergoes changes in retinyl ester stores (decreasing from day 19 to postnatal day 2) accompanied by an increase in the metabolically active ligands RA and 9-*cis*-RA *(35)*. There are also significant changes in the levels of expression of retinoid cytosolic binding proteins and nuclear RARs. The results suggest that the lipofibroblast is a storage site for retinoids during later stages of lung development *(100)*. This cell also contributes to the synthesis of several extracellular matrix proteins, such as elastin and collagen, during lung development. RA has been shown to upregulate gene expression of elastin *(101)* and other essential lung matrix structural protein genes *(102)*. Laminin has a RA response element identified on the gene *(103)*.

## GROWTH FACTORS

Several growth factors are thought to be important in lung *(104)*, many of which are responsive to RA in a variety of experimental models *(9,10)*. Retinoids stimulate EGF receptor, transforming growth factor (TGF-$\beta$-1) and insulin-like growth factor (IGF-2). On the other hand, IGF-1, and TGF-$\alpha$ are downregulated by RA. Thus, the question is, could retinoid metabolism and function play a basic role in controlling lung development through its influence on these growth factors which are known to affect lung development? If alterations in these mechanisms were to modify the rate of development from the canalicular to saccular stage, the respiratory support of micropremature human infants born at 23–25 wk gestation might be helped.

## HORMONES AND NUCLEAR RESPONSE ELEMENTS

The extensive and potentially important interaction of RA with DEX was reviewed in detail above. RA also has the opportunity to interact with other homones. As noted, RA can be metabolized to 9-*cis* RA, which is the ligand for the RXRs. The RXRs form heterodimers with RARs, the vitamin D receptor, the thyroid hormone receptor and others *(19)*. This ability of RXR to dimerize with other receptors requiring hormonal ligands establishes RA metabolism and the RXR as having a central role in hormone signaling. However, the effect of most of these interactions is still unknown, and, as yet, not examined for relevance in the regulation of fetal lung. Further studies on the relationship between retinoids and these factors will undoubtedly help clarify the role of retinoids in lung development.

Table 2
Other Retinoid Interactions and Effects that have the Potential
for Regulation of Lung Development

**Interaction with glucocorticoids**
- Antenatal and postnatal steroids decrease tissue/serum storage and elevate retinol and RBP in rats, primates and humans
- Postnatal DEX decreases RAR β mRNA in rat lung
- The DEX effect on lung cell RAR β mRNA requires translation
- DEX decreases RAR β mRNA in adult rat liver
- The binding by liver glucocorticoid receptors is higher in vitamin A deficient rats than controls, restored by RA
- RA overcomes the DEX effect of suppressing rat lung septation

**Interaction with transcription factors, matrix molecules, and growth factors**
- *Homeobox genes*: RA influences Hox gene expression in many cell lines
- *Matrix molecules*: Laminin-RA response elements identified on gene
- *Response of growth factors to RA*
  - ↑ EGF
  - ↑TGF-β1
  - ↑ IGF-2
  - ↓ TGF-α
  - ↓ IGF-1

# SUMMARY

It is clear that retinoids have an enormous potential to influence lung development. The natural retinoids ultimately influence development and differentiation of lung by metabolites like RA and 9-*cis* RA acting through nuclear receptors, which themselves are major factors in embryology and organogenesis.

There are numerous lines of evidence showing that retinoids affect lung development (Tables 1 and 2). There is specific localization of the binding and receptor proteins. There are developmental and retinoid status regulation effects on cell retinoid content, cytosolic and nuclear receptor proteins and retinoid effects on other factors known to be important to lung development. Many aspects of lung development including organogenesis, cell type, surfactant component synthesis, and expression certainly do respond to retinoids. Interaction of retinoids and glucocorticoids in lung is very evident, but its meaning is not completely understood. Interaction of retinoids with other factors affecting lung development also occurs.

Presently, some roles of retinoids in lung development and repair of lung injury associated with human preterm birth and lung immaturity are being investigated in clinical studies on BPD. On the other hand, possibly only extreme maternal/fetal vitamin A deficiency will cause respiratory failure at birth. A closer evaluation of clinical material from geographic regions with a high rate of documented vitamin A deficiency might provide important information on this point. Further studies are required to clarify the actual importance and mechanisms of the role of retinoids in lung development.

# ACKNOWLEDGMENTS

This work was supported by NIH-HD 33916.

# REFERENCES

1. Blaner WS, Olson JA. Retinol and retinoic acid metabolism. In: Sporn MB, Roberts, AB, Goodman DS, eds. The retinoids. New York: Lippincott-Raven,1994:229–255.
2. Gardner EM, Ross AC Dietary vitamin A restriction produces marginal vitamin A status in young rats. J Nutr 1993; 123:1435–1443.
3. Wallingford JC, Underwood BA. Vitamin A deficiency in pregnancy lactation and the nursing child. In: Bauermfield CJ, ed. Vitamin A Deficiency and Its Control. New York: Academic Press,1986:101–151.
4. Ong DE, Newcomer ME, Chytil F. Cellular retinoid binding proteins. In: Sporn MB, Roberts AB, Goodman DS, eds. The retinoids. New York: Lippincott-Raven, 1994:283–317.
5. Maden M, Ong DE, Chytil F. Retinoid–binding protein distribution in the developing mammalian nervous system. Development 1990;109:75–80.
6. Perez–Castro AV, Toth–Rogler LE, Wei LN, Nguyen–Huu, MC. Spatial and temporal pattern of expression of the cellular retinoic acid–binding protein and the cellular retinol–binding protein during mouse embryogenesis. Proc Natl Acad Sci USA 1989;86:8813–8817.
7. Giguere V, Lyn S, Yip P, Siu CH, Amin S. Molecular cloning of a cDNA encoding a second cellular retinoic acid–binding protein. Proc Natl Acad Sci USA 1990;87:6233–6237.
8. Boylan JF, Gudas LJ. Overexpression of the cellular retinoic acid–binding protein–I CRABP–I; results in a reduction in differentiation–specific gene expression in F9 teratocarcinoma cells. J Cell Biol 1991;112:965–972.
9. Chytil F, Haq R. Vitamin A mediated gene expression. Crit Rev Eukaryot Gene Expr 1990;1:61–73.
10. Gudas IJ, Sporn MB, Roberts AB, Cellular biology and biochemisry of the retinoids. In: Sporn MB, Roberts AB, Goodman DS, eds. The retinoids. New York: Lippincott-Raven, 1994:443–520.
11. Kastner P, Chambon P, Leid M. Role of nuclear retinoic acid receptors in the regulation of gene expression. In: Blomhoff R, ed. Vitamin A in health and disease. New York: Marcel Dekker,1994:189–238.
12. Dolle P, Ruberte E, Kastner P, Petkovich M, Stoner CM, Gudas LJ, Chambon P. Differential expression of genes encoding $\alpha$, $\beta$, and $\gamma$ retinoic acid receptors and CRABP in the developing limbs of the mouse. Nature 1989;342:702–704.
13. Mendelsohn C, Larkin S, Mark M, LeMeur M, Clifford J, Zelent A, Chambon P. RAR $\beta$ isoforms: distinct transcriptional control by retinoic acid and specific spatial patterns of promoter activity during mouse embryonic development. Mech Dev 1994;45:227–241.
14. Rossant J, Zirngibl R, Cado D, Shago M, Giguere V. Expression of a retinoic acid response element–hsplacZ transgene defines specific domains of transcriptional activity during mouse embryogenesis. Genes Dev 1991;5:1333–1344.
15. Soprano DR, Gyda M, Jiang H, Harnish DC, Ugen K, Satre M, Chen L, Soprano KJ, Kochhar DM. A sustained elevation in retinoic acid receptor–b2 mRNA and protein occurs during retinoic acid–induced fetal dysmorphogenesis. Mech Dev 1994;45:243–253 .
16. Lohnes D, Mark M, Mendelsohn C, Dolle P, Dierich A, Gorry P, Gansmuller A, Chambon P. Function of the retinoic acid receptors (RARs); during development (I) Craniofacial and skeletal abnormalities in RAR double mutants. Development 1994;120:2723–2748.
17. Mendelsohn C, Lohnes D, Decimo D, Lufkin T, LeMeur M, Chambon P, Mark M. Function of the retinoic acid receptors RARs; during development II; Multiple abnormalities at various stages of organogenesis in RAR double mutants. Development 1994;120:2729–2771.
18. Lampron C, Rochette–Egly CR, Gorry P, Dolle P, Mark M, Lufkin T, LeMeur M, Chambon P. Mice deficient in cellular retinoic acid binding protein II CRABP II; or in both CRABP I and CRABP II are essentially normal. Development 1995;121:539–548 .
19. Mangelsdorf DJ, Umesono K, Evans RM. The retinoid receptors. In Sporn MB, Roberts AB, Goodman DS, eds. The retinoids. New York:Lippincott-Raven, 1994:319–350.
20. Love JM, Gudas LJ. Vitamin A differentiation and cancer. Curr Opin Cell Biol 1994;6:825–831 .
21. Bloch CE. Clinical investigations of xerophthalmia and dystrophy in infants and young child (xerophthalmia et dystroophia alipogenetica) J Hyg1921;19:283–307.

22. Chytil F. The lungs and vitamin A. Am J Physiol 1992;262:L517–L527.
23. Chambon P. The retinoid signaling pathway: molecular and genetic analyses. Cell Biology 1994; 5:115–125.
24. Fawzi WW, Chalmors TC, Herrera MG, Mosteller F. Vitamin A supplementation and child mortality: a meta analysis. JAMA 1993;269:898–903.
25. Zachman RD. Retinol vitamin A; and the neonate: special problems of the human premature infant. Am J Clin Nutr 1989;50:413–424.
26. Shenai JP. Vitamin A in lung development bronchopulmonary dysplasia. In: Blomhoff R ed. Vitamin A in health and disease. New York: Marcel Dekker,1994:323–343.
27. Zachman RD. Role of vitamin A in lung development. J Nutr 1995;125:16345–16385.
28. Chytil F. Retinoids in lung development. FASEB J 1996;10:986–992.
29. Farrell PM. Morphologic aspects of lung maturation. Biol Clin Perspect 1981;1:13–25.
30. Zachman RD, Kakkad B, Chytil F. Prenatal rat lung retinol vitamin A; and retinyl palmitate. Pediatr Res 1984;18:1297–1299.
31. Zachman RD, Valischini G. Effects of premature delivery on rat lung retinol vitamin A; and retinyl ester stores. Biol Neonate 1988;54:285–288.
32. Geevarghese SK, Chytil F. Depletion of retinyl esters in the lungs coincides with lung prenatal morophological maturation. Biochem Biophys Res Commun 1994;200:529–535.
33. Zachman RD. Retinyl ester synthesis by the isolated perfused–ventilated neonatal rabbit lung. Int J Vit Nutr Res 1994;55:371–376.
34. Zachman RD, Tsao FHC.Retinyl ester synthesis by isolated adult rabbit lung Type II cells. Int. J Vit Nutr Res 1988;58:161–165.
35. McGowan SE, Harvey CS, Jackson SK. Retinoids retinoic acid receptors and cytoplasmic retinoid binding proteins in perinatal rat lung fibroblasts. Am J Physiol 1995;269:L463–L472.
36. Wellik DM, DeLuca HF. Retinol in addition to retinoic acid is require for successful gestation in vitamin A deficient rats. Biol Reprod 1995;53:1392–1397.
37. Wellik DM, Norback DH, DeLuca HF. Retinol is specifically required during midgestation for neo-natal survival. Am J Physiol 1997;272,E25–E29.
38. Blackfan KD, Wolbach SB. Vitamin A deficiency in infants: a clinical and pathological study. J Pediatr 1933;3:679–706.
39. Shenai JP, Chytil F, Stahlman MT. Liver vitamin A reserves of very low birth weight neonates. Pediatr Res 1985;19:892–893.
40. Hustead VA, Gutcher GR, Anderson SA, Zachman RD. Relationship of vitamin A (retinol) status to lung disease in the preterm infant. J Pediatr 1984;105:610–615.
41. Mupanemunda RH, Lee DS, Fraher LJ, Koura IR, Chance GW. Postnatal change in serum retinol status in very low birthweight infants. Early Hum Dev 1994;38:45–54.
42. Shenai JP, Chytil F, Stahlman MT. Vitamin A status of neonates with bronchocpulmonary dysplasia. Pediatr Res 1985;19:185–188.
43. Shenai JP, Kennedy KA, Chytil F, Stahlman MT. Clinical trial of vitamin A supplementation in infants susceptible to bronchopulmonary dysplasia. J Pediatr 1987;111:269–277.
44. Chan V, Greenough A, Cheeseman P, Gamsu HR. Vitamin A levels at birth of high risk preterm infants. J Perinat Med 1993;21:147–151.
45. Verma RP, McCulloch KM, Worrell L, Vidyasagar D. Vitamin A deficiency and severe bronchopul-monary dysplasia in very low brithweight infants. Am J Perinatal 1996;13:389–393.
46. Papagaroufalis C, Caires M, Pantazatou E, Megreli CH, Xanthou M. A trial of vitamin A supplemen-tation of the prevention of bronchopulmonary dysplaisa (BPD) in very low-birthweight (VLBW) infants. [Abstract].Pediatr Res 1988;23:518A.
47. Shenai JP, Rush MG, Stahlman MT, Chytil F. Plasma retinol binding protein response to vitamin A administration in infants susceptible to bronchpulmonary dysplasia. J Pediatr 1990;116:607–614.
48. Robbins ST, Fletcher AB. Early vs delayed vitamin A supplementation in very low birth weight infants. J Parenter Enteral Nutr 1993;17:220–225.
49. Pearson E, Bose C, Snidow T, Ranson L, Young R, Bose G, Stiles A. Trial of vitamin A supplemen-tation in very low birth weigh infants at risk for bronchopulmonary dysplasia. J Pediatr 1992; 121:420–427.
50. Kennedy KA, Stoll BJ, Ehrenkranz RA, Oh W, Wright LL, Stevenson DK, Lemmons JA, Sowell A, Mele L, Tyson JE, Verter J, for the NICHD Neonatal Research Network. Vitamin A to prevent

bronchopulmonary dysplasis in very low birth weight infants: has the dose been too low? Early Hum Dev 1997;49:19–31.

51. Tyson JE, Ehrenkranz RA, Stoll BJ, Wright LL, Mele L, Kennedy KA, Oh W, Lemons JA, Stevenson DK, Verter J, for the NICHD Neonatal Research Network Vitamin A supplementation to increase survival without chronic lung diseases (CLD) in extremely low birth weight (ELBW) infants: a 14-center randomized trial [Abstract]. Pediatr Res 1998;43:199A.

52. Underwood BA. Vitamin A in animal and human nutrition. In: Sporn MG, Goodman DS, eds. The retinoids, Vol I. New York: Academic Press 1984:281–392.

53. Olson JA. Serum levels of vitamin A and carotenoids as reflectors of nutritional status. J Natl Cancer Inst 1984;73:1439–1444 .

54. Montreewasuant N, Olson JA. Serum and liver concentrations of vitamin A in Thai fetuses as a function of gestational age. Am J Clin Nutr 1979;32:601–606.

55. Zachman RD, Samuels DP, Brand JM, Winston JF, Pi JT. Use of the intramuscular relative dose response test to predict bronchopulmonary dysplasia in premature infants. Am J Clin Nutr 1996;63:123–129.

56. Abman SH, Groothius JR. Pathobiology and treatment of bronchopulmonary dysplasia: current issues. .Pediatr Clin North Am 1994;41:277–315.

57. Dolle E, Ruberte R, Leroy P, Morriss–Kay G, Chambon P. Retinoic acid receptors and cellular retinoid binding proteins 1 A systematic study of their differential pattern of transcription during mouse organogenesis. Development 1990;110:1133–1151.

58. Ong DE, Chytil F. Changes in levels of cellular retinol and retinoic acid binding proteins of liver and lung during prenatal development of rat. Proc Natl Acad Sci USA 1976;73:3976–3978.

59. Whitney DC, Massaro GD, Massaro D, Clerch LB. Cellular retinoid binding proteins and retinoic acid receptor $\beta$ are modulated by retinoic acid and dexamethasone in postnatal rat lung. Pediatr Res 1998;43:303A.

60. McMenamy KM, Zachman RD. Effect of gestational age and retinol (vitamin A) deficiency in fetal rat lung nuclear retinoic acid receptors. Pediatr Res 1993;33:251–255.

61. Grummer MA, Thet LA, Zachman RD. Expression of retinoic acid receptor genes in fetal and newborn rat lung. Pediatr Pulmonol 1994;17:234–238.

62. Haq RR, Pfahl M, Chytil F. Retinoic acid affects the expression of nuclear retinoic acid receptors in tissues of retinol deficient rats. Proc Natl Acad Sci USA 1991;88:8272–8276.

63. Verma AK, Shoemaker A, Simsiman R, Denning M, Zachman RD. Expression of retinoic acid nuclear receptor and tissue transglutaminase is altered in various tissues of rats fed a vitamin A deficient diet. J Nutr 1992;122:2144–2152.

64. Fraslon C, Bourbon JR. Retinoids control surfactant phospholipid biosynthesis in fetal rat lung. Am J Physiol 1994;266:L705–L712.

65. Fraslon C, Bourbon JR. Comparison of effects of epidermal and insulin–like growth factors gastric releasing peptide and retinoic acid in fetal lung cell growth and maturation in vitro. Biochem Biophys Acta 1992;1123:65–75.

66. Zachman RD, Chen M, Verma AK, Grummer M. Some effects of vitamin A deficiency on the isolated lung alveolar Type II cell. Int J Vit Nutr Res 1992;62:113–120.

67. Cardoso WV, Williams MC, Mitsialis SA, Joyce–Brady M, Riski AK, Brody JS. Retinoic acid induces changes in the pattern of airway branching and alters epithelial cell differentiation in the developing lung in vitro Am J Respir Cell Mol Biol 1995;12:464–476.

68. Bogue CW, Jacobs JC, Dynia DW, Wilson CM, Gross I. Retinoic acid increases surfactant protein mRNA in fetal rat and mouse lung in culture. Am J Physiol 1996;271:L862–L868.

69. Metzler MD, Snyder JM. Retinoic acid differentially regulates expression of surfactant–associated proteins in human fetal lung. Endocrinology 1993;133:1990–1998.

70. George TN, Snyder JM. Regulation of surfactant protein gene expression by retinoic acid metabolites. Pediatr Res 1997;41:692–701.

71. Masuyama H, Hiramatsu Y, Kudo T. Effect of retinoids on fetal lung development in the rat. Biol Neonat 1995;67:264–273.

72. Zachman RD, Grummer MA. Effect of maternal fetal vitamin A deficiency on fetal rat lung surfactant protein expression and the response to prenatal dexamethasone. Pediatr Res 1998;45:178–183.

73. Shank RE, Coburn AF, Moore LV, Hoaglund CL. The level of vitamin A and carotene in the plasma of rheumatic subjects. J Clin Invst 1944;23:289–295.

74. Jacobs AL, Leitner ZA, Moore T, Sharman IM. Vitamin A in rheumatic fever. J Clin Nutr 1954; 2:155–161.

75. Wang P, Glass HL, Goldenberg L, Stearns G, Kelly HG, Jackson RL. Serum vitamin A and carotene levels in children with rheumatic fever. Am J Dis Child 1954;87:659–672.

76. Clark I, Colburn RW. A relationship between vitamin A metabolism and cortisone. Endocrinology 1955;56:232–238.

77. McGillivray WA. Some factors influencing the release of vitamin A from the liver. Br J Nutr 1961;15:305–312.

78. Borek C, Smith JE, Soprano DR, Goodman DS. Regulation of retinoid–binding protein metabolism by glucocoticord hormones in cultured H4 IIEC₃ liver cells. Endocrinology 1981;109:386–391.

79. Audouin–Chevallier I, Higuiret P, Veronique P, Higuiret D, Garcin H. Dietary vitamin A modulates the properties of retinoic acid and glucocorticoid receptors in rat liver. J Nutr 1993;123:1195–1202.

80. Ballard PL. Glucocorticords and differentiation. Monogr Endocrinol 1986;12:493–516.

81. Venkatesh VC, Ballard PL. Glucocorticords and gene expression. Am J Respir Cell Mol Biol 1991; 4:301–303.

82. Hustead VA, Zachman RD. The effect of antenatal dexamethasone on maternal and fetal retinol–binding protein. Am J Obstet Gynecol 1986;154:203–205.

83. Georgieff MK, Chockalingan UM, Sasanow SR, Gunter EW, Murphy E, Ophoven JJ. The effect of antenatal betamethasone on cord blood concentrations of retinol–binding–protein transthyretin transferring retinol and vitamin E. J Pediatr Gastroenterol Nutr 1988;7:713–717.

84. Oshika E, Liu S, Singh G, Michalopoulos GK, Shinozuka H, Katyal SL, Antagonistiac effects of dexamethasone and retinoic acid on rat lung morphogenis. Pediatr Res 1998;43:315–324.

85. Rush MG, Hazinski TA. Current therapy of bronchopulmonary dysplasia. Clin Perinatol 1992; 19:563–590.

86. Georgieff MK, Mannel MC, Mills MM, Gunter EW, Johnson DE, Thompson TR. Effect of postnatal steroid administration on serum vitamin A concentrations in newborn infants with respiratory compromise. J Pediatr 1989;114:301–304.

87. McMenamy KR, Anderson MJ, Zachman RD. Effect of dexamethasone and oxygen exposure on neonatal rat lung retinoic acid receptor proteins. Pediatr Pulmonol 1994;18:232–238.

88. Grummer MA, Zachman RD. Postnatal rat lung retinoic acid receptor (RAR) mRNA expression and effects of dexamethasone on RAR β mRNA. Pediatr Pulmonol 1995;20:234–241.

89. Georgieff MK, Rudmer WJ, Sowell AL, Yeager PR, Blaner WS, Gunter EW, Johnson DE. The effects of glucocorticosteroids on serum liver and lung vitamin A and retinyl ester concentrations. J Pediatr Gastroenterol Nutr 1991;13:376–382.

90. Massaro GD, Massaro D. Postnatal treatment with retinoic acid increases the number of pulmonary alveoli in rats. Am J Physiol 1996;270:L305–L310.

91. Massaro GD, Massaro D. Retinoic acid treatment abrogates elastase–induced pulmonary emphysema in rats. Nat Med 1997;3:675–677.

92. Grummer MA, Zachman RD. Retinoic acid and dexamethasone affect RAR β and surfactant protein C mRNA in the MLE lung cell line. Am J Physiol 1998;274:L1–L7.

93. Lieber CS. Cytochrome P45 2E1: its physiological and pathological role Physiol Rev 1997; 77:517–544.

94. Pallet V, Audouin–Chevallier I, Higueret D, Garcin H, Higueret P. Dexamethasone decreases the expression or retinoic acid receptors (RARs) in rat liver. J Steroid Biochim Mol Biol 1996; 57:161–165.

95. Nshida H, Oishi M. Survival and disability in extremely tiny babies less than 600 g birthweight. Semin Neonat 1996;1:251–256.

96. American Academy of Pediatrics and the American College of Obstetricians and Gynecologists. Perinatal care at the threshold of viability. Pediatrics 1995;96;974–976.

97. Bogue CW. Gross I. Vasavada H. Dynia EW. Wilson CM. Jacobs HC. Identification of Hox genes in newborn lung and effects of gestational age and retinoic acid on their expression. Am J Physiol 1994;266:L448–L454.

98. Cardoso WV, Mitsialis SA, Brody JS, Williams MC. Retinoic acid alters the expression of pattern–related genes in the developing rat lung. Dev Dyn 1996;207:47–59.

99. SchugerL, Varani J, Mitra R, Gilbride K. Retinoid acid stimulates mouse lung development by a mechanism involving epithelial – mesenchymal interaction and regulation of epidermal growth factor receptors. Dev Biol 1993;159:462–473.

100. McGowan SE, Torday JS. The pulmonary lipofibroblast (lipid interstitial cell) and its contribution to alveolar development. Annu Rev Physiol 1997;59:43–62.

101. Liu C, Harvey CS, McGowan SE. Retinoic acid increases elastin in neonatal rat lung fibroblast cultures. Am J Physiol 1993;265:L430–L437.
102. Veness–Mecham KA, Mathias A. The effects of peroxia and retinol deficiency on type I collagen genes expression in lung [Abstact]. Pediatr Res 1992;31:325A .
103. Vasios GW, Gold JD, Petkovich M, Chambon P, Gudas LJ. A retinoic acid–responsive element is present in the 5' flanking region of the laminin 31 gene. Proc Natl Acad Sci USA 1989;86:9099–9103.
104. Klein JM. Fetal lung development: role of growth factors. In: Franz ID, ed. Neonatal respiratory disease, Vol. 3; Columbus OH: Ross Laboratories, 1993.

# 10
## Insulin and Lung Development

*Jeanne M. Snyder,* PhD, *Thomas N. George,* MD, *and Olga L. Miakotina,* PhD

CONTENTS

## INTRODUCTION

Infants of diabetic mothers have an elevated incidence of respiratory distress syndrome of the newborn (RDS), a disease which is caused by pulmonary surfactant deficiency associated with inadequate numbers of differentiated alveolar type II cells in the lung *(1,2)*. Pulmonary surfactant, which functions to reduce surface tension at the air–alveolar interface, is made up of glycerophospholipids (approx 80% by weight), cholesterol (approx 10%) and the surfactant-associated proteins (approx 10%) *(3)*. The fetus of the diabetic mother tends to have high serum glucose and insulin levels as a result of maternal hyperglycemia *(4)*. Robert et al. *(1)* first advanced the hypothesis that high levels of insulin might delay lung development in the fetus of the gestational diabetic woman. In this chapter, we will review the literature concerning the effects of maternal diabetes, glucose, and, in particular, insulin on fetal lung development.

## RESPIRATORY DISTRESS SYNDROME IN THE INFANT OF THE DIABETIC MOTHER

It has been estimated that 100,000 infants of diabetic mothers are born in the United States every year, a large group of infants at risk for developing RDS and other morbidities

From: *Contemporary Endocrinology: Endocrinology of the Lung: Development and Surfactant Synthesis*
Edited by: C. R. Mendelson © Humana Press Inc., Totowa, NJ

associated with a diabetic pregnancy (5). Using the White classification system, infants born to mothers with type A diabetes (gestational onset diabetes) and types B and C have been found to have a higher incidence of RDS than infants born to mothers with more severe, insulin-dependent diabetes mellitus (classes D, E, F, and R) (6). More recently, it has been shown that infants of mothers whose diabetes is well controlled have a risk for RDS that is no different than that of the general population (7,8). While universal screening of pregnant women for gestational onset diabetes is recommended, women who receive inadequate prenatal care and develop uncontrolled diabetes still exist in the population (9).

## Pathophysiology of Delayed Lung Maturation in the Diabetic Pregnancy

Two physiologic situations exist in diabetic pregnancies in which the diabetes is poorly controlled, namely, hyperinsulinemia and hyperglycemia (4). Diabetic mothers whose diabetes is poorly controlled with persistent hyperglycemia have been shown to have infants who are hyperinsulinemic at birth, with elevated proinsulin and C-peptide levels in cord blood when compared to levels in control infants (10–12). The levels of plasma insulin in infants of pregnancies complicated by diabetes have been reported to be as high as 112 µU/mL vs 11 µU/mL in control infants (13). In diabetic pregnancies with a glucose load, insulin levels in infants may rise to 200–300 µU/mL (14). Maternal blood glucose can reach levels greater than 150 mg/dL in diabetic pregnancies that are poorly controlled as compared to approx 90 mg/dL in controls (13,15). Infants of diabetic mothers have significantly higher blood glucose levels than control infants (13).

## Lecithin : Sphingomyelin Ratio

Toward the end of gestation, fetal lung type II cells differentiate and begin to secrete surfactant into the amniotic fluid (16). Lecithin (specifically dipalmitoylphosphatidylcholine, a disaturated phosphatidylcholine) is the most abundant surfactant phospholipid produced by the fetal lung and is secreted into amniotic fluid in greater amounts toward the end of gestation (16). By contrast, the concentration of another lipid, sphingomyelin, remains constant in amniotic fluid throughout gestation. Thus, the ratio of lecithin to sphingomyelin (L:S) can be used to determine fetal lung maturity, with a ratio of greater than 2:1 predictive of maturity (6,17). In early studies, several investigators observed delayed fetal lung maturation as assessed by L:S ratios in diabetic pregnancies (Table 1) (6,18,19). By contrast, in more severe classes of diabetes, D, E, F, fetal lung maturity was accelerated (Table 1) (6). It was proposed that chronic intrauterine stress experienced by fetuses of severely diabetic mothers contributed to the accelerated lung maturation observed in this group (6). There are many more studies in which no evidence of delayed lung maturation in diabetic pregnancies was observed when using the L:S ratio as a guide (Table 1) (20–34). In many of the latter studies, good metabolic control of the diabetic pregnancies was reported (Table 1) (24,28–31,33). However, several investigators have described a high incidence of false-positive L:S ratios in diabetic pregnancies, that is, infants who develop RDS at birth despite L:S ratios predictive of pulmonary maturity (Table 1) (18,20,22,23,26,27,31,35–38). Thus, the L:S ratio may not be a reliable predictor of fetal lung maturity in the diabetic pregnancy.

## Phosphatidylglycerol

When surfactant secretion begins in the fetus, at about 30–32 wk of gestation, the major anionic phospholipid present in surfactant is phosphatidylinositol (PI) (39). Then, as gestation proceeds, the level of PI falls while the level of phosphatidylglycerol (PG)

Table 1
L:S Ratio, PG Levels and Incidence of RDS in Diabetic vs
Normal Pregnancies

| Reference | L:S Ratio [a] Diabetic vs Control | PG [b] Diabetic vs Control | Presence of RDS with L:S > 2.0 [c] |
|---|---|---|---|
| 35 | NR | NR | Yes |
| 6 | Delayed in A,B,C Accelerated in D,E,F | NR | No |
| 18 | Delayed | NR | Yes |
| 19 | Delayed in A,B,C | NR | NR |
| 20 | No difference | NR | Yes |
| 36 | NR | NR | Yes |
| 21 | No difference | NR | NR |
| 22 | No difference | NR | Yes |
| 23 | No difference | Delayed | Yes (if PG -) |
| 24 | No difference | NR | No |
| 37 | Accelerated | NR | Yes |
| 25 | No difference | Delayed | NR |
| 26 | No difference | Delayed | Yes (if PG -) |
| 27 | No difference | Delayed R | Yes (if PG-) |
| 38 | NR | NR | Yes (if PG -) |
| 28 | No difference | No difference | No |
| 29 | No difference | No difference | No |
| 30 | No difference | NR | No |
| 31 | No difference | No difference | Yes (if PG -) |
| 32 | No difference | NR | No |
| 33 | No difference | No difference | NR |
| 34 | No difference | No difference | NR |

NR, not reported.
a Comparison of amniotic fluid L:S ratio in diabetic vs normal pregnancies.
b Comparison of amniotic fluid PG in diabetic vs normal pregnancies.
c Presence of RDS with an L:S ratio greater than 2.0 in diabetic pregnancies.

increases *(39)*. Cunningham and coworkers *(23)* were the first to report a deficiency of amniotic fluid PG in pregnancies in which infants subsequently developed neonatal RDS. It has been demonstrated that in pregnancies complicated by type A diabetes, there is a significant delay in the appearance of PG in amniotic fluid (Table 1) *(25)*. It is now accepted that the absence of amniotic fluid PG, even in the presence of a mature L:S ratio, is predictive of an increased risk of RDS (Table 1) *(23,26,27,31,38)*. Bleasdale and coworkers *(40)* have suggested that the inhibition of surfactant PG production in the fetal lung in the diabetic pregnancy is the result of elevated fetal myoinositol that shifts the synthesis of lamellar body anionic phospholipids from PG to PI. In well-controlled diabetic pregnancies, PG is detected at gestational ages similar to those of nondiabetic pregnancies, data suggestive that fetal lung maturity is not delayed in the presence of well-controlled maternal diabetes (28,29,33).

## Surfactant-Associated Proteins

Four surfactant-associated proteins (SP) have been identified to date (41). Surfactant protein A (SP-A) regulates both the secretion and reutilization of surfactant, and along with SP-D, appears to be involved in host defense mechanisms (41). SP-B and SP-C facilitate surfactant phospholipid adsorption and together with SP-A, play a role in the ability of surfactant to reduce surface tension (41). SP-A is not detected in human fetal lung tissue before 20 wk gestational age and is detected in amniotic fluid starting at around 30 weeks gestational age (42,43). The increase in amniotic fluid SP-A levels correlates with increases in both the L/S ratio and the concentration of PG during the end of gestation. It has been shown that in pregnancies complicated by diabetes, amniotic fluid SP-A levels are significantly decreased when compared to amniotic fluid SP-A levels in pregnancies without complications (32,38). As shown in Fig. 1, amniotic fluid SP-A content was reduced by about 60% in diabetic pregnancies when compared to levels in nondiabetic pregnancies. McMahan et al. (30) did not find decreased amounts of SP-A in amniotic fluid from diabetic pregnancies when compared to levels in nondiabetic pregnancies. In the McMahan study, however, the maternal diabetes was well controlled. These observations are suggestive that the appearance of SP-A in the surfactant secreted by the fetal lung into amniotic fluid may be delayed in the fetus of the diabetic mother.

## THE DIRECT EFFECTS OF INSULIN ON LUNG DEVELOPMENT

### In Vitro Studies

Cortisol increased choline incorporation into phosphatidylcholine (PC) in dispersed rabbit fetal lung cells (day 28 gestational age, term = 31 days) maintained in vitro (44). Cortisol stimulates fetal lung development, and glucocorticoids are used clinically to accelerate lung maturation in utero (45). Insulin significantly decreased the cortisol-induced increase in PC synthesis and had a small stimulatory effect on PC synthesis when added alone (44). Neufeld and coworkers (46) found that 100 µU/mL of insulin inhibited the synthesis of PC and disaturated PC in fetal rabbit lung slices (day 27.5 gestational age). Disaturated PC is a more specific marker for pulmonary surfactant phospholipids than PC.

Insulin (≥100 µU/mL) inhibited glucose incorporation into surfactant PC in organotypic cultures of rat fetal lung type II cells (47). Insulin had no effect on choline incorporation into total or disaturated PC in rat fetal lung explants, and further, did not antagonize the glucocorticoid-stimulated increase in choline incorporation into PC (48). In the same study, however, insulin decreased incorporation of acetate into disaturated PC and blocked the stimulatory effect of glucocorticoids on acetate incorporation into disaturated PC (48). Morphologic analysis of the rat fetal lung explants showed that insulin treatment decreased the number of type II cells and lamellar bodies (48). In another study using a rat fetal lung model, Bourbon and coworkers (49) showed that insulin (0.1 U/mL) decreased disaturated PC and phosphatidylglycerol (PG) synthesis as reflected by the incorporation of previously labeled $^{14}C$ glycogen pools. Thus, studies in the rat and rabbit species are in general consistent and suggestive that high levels of insulin decrease surfactant phospholipid synthesis in fetal lung tissue.

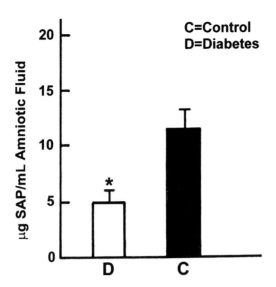

Fig. 1. Surfactant protein A (SAP) concentration in amniotic fluid samples obtained from diabetic pregnancies and in matched control pregnancies. There was a statistically significant difference ($p < .05$, Student's $t$-test) between the diabetic group and its matched control group. (Adapted from ref. *32* .)

The direct effects of insulin on surfactant phospholipid synthesis have also been examined in an in vitro model of human fetal lung development *(50,51)*. Insulin, at a concentration of 2.5 µg/mL, (0.07 U/mL) had no effect on PC synthesis in the human fetal lung explants *(50)*. On the other hand, when insulin was combined with cortisol ($10^{-7}M$) or prolactin (2.5 µg/mL), there was a significant increase in explant PC synthesis when compared to untreated controls or to explants treated with each of the hormones added alone *(50)*. In another study, the effects of insulin, cortisol, and prolactin on lamellar body PI and PG were examined in human fetal lung explants *(51)*. Insulin, added alone, had no significant effect on lamellar body PG content *(51)* (Fig. 2). By contrast, insulin in combination with cortisol or with cortisol plus prolactin significantly increased lamellar body PG content *(51)* (Fig. 2). These data are suggestive that hyperinsulinemia does not decrease surfactant PC or PG production in the human fetal lung.

## *In Vivo Studies*

Insulin infusion into pregnant rabbits (from day 26 to day 29 of gestation) decreased fetal insulin and glucose levels and appeared to accelerate fetal lung development to an even greater extent than maternal glucocorticoid treatment *(52)*. The infusion of high amounts of glucose into the pregnant rabbit resulted in hyperinsulinemia and hyperglycemia in the fetuses, as well as increased fetal body weights *(52)*. However, there was no effect of the hyperinsulinemia and hyperglycemia on the amount or composition of alveolar lavage phospholipids in the fetuses of the glucose-infused pregnant rabbits *(52)*. Levine *(53)* used litter reduction to produce a hyperinsulinemic state and macrosomia in fetal rabbits. He found that fetal insulin levels were inversely correlated with the L/S ratio, data suggestive that high fetal insulin levels depress disaturated PC levels in the developing rabbit lung in vivo.

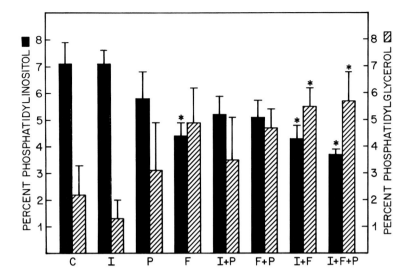

Fig. 2. The percentages of PI and PG synthesized in human fetal lung explants incubated for 7 d in control medium (C) or in medium containing insulin (I), cortisol (F), and/or prolactin (P). The percentages of PI and PG in lamellar bodies synthesized between days 6 and 7 of culture were calculated from the percentage of ($^{14}$C) glycerol incorporated into each lipid. The data are the mean ± SEM of four experiments. Significant difference between experimental values and control values ($p < .05$), as determined by analysis of variance and Newman-Keuls multiple comparison. (From ref. 51, with permission.)

The injection of insulin (0.1 to 0.2 units) into the rat fetus *in utero* resulted in decreased levels of disaturated PC in partially purified fetal lung surfactant preparations as well as decreased numbers of lamellar bodies in fetal lung type II cells (54). When the pregnant rats were infused with large amounts of glucose, both disaturated PC and PG levels were decreased in the fetal lung (54). These data are consistent with the hypothesis that hyperinsulinemia in the rat fetus decreases surfactant phospholipid production in the fetal lung.

Insulin infusion into the sheep fetus was shown to decrease serum glucose levels and decrease the flux of surface active material into tracheal fluid (55). In a subsequent study, Warburton (56) reported that hyperinsulinemia (approx 45 μU/mL), produced by glucose infusion into the fetus (serum levels approx 48 mg/dL), also decreased surface active material flux. When the control and glucose-infused sheep fetuses were treated with cortisol, there was a striking decrease in surfactant flux when compared to the non-glucose-infused controls (56). The disaturated PC and PG contents of lung washes obtained after delivery were significantly decreased in the hyperglycemic, hyperinsulinemic fetuses (56). In addition, pressure volume curves obtained after delivery showed that lung function was impaired in the glucose-infused fetuses (56).

Rooney and coworkers (57) infused insulin into fetal rhesus monkeys from 134 to 148 d of gestation (term = 165 d). The treated animals were slightly hypoglycemic and very hyperinsulinemic (approx 2400 μU/mL). No effects of insulin on choline incorporation into PC or disaturated PC in either lung lavage or lung tissue were observed. Based on these observations, the authors suggested that hyperinsulinemia may not play a role in delaying lung development in the primate. However, the authors did not perform morphologic studies of the fetal lung tissue nor did they assess lung function in the control vs insulin-treated animals. Levels of the surfactant proteins were also not measured. The results of this study are consistent with the hypothesis that in primate species, including the human, hyperinsulinemia does not affect surfactant phospholipid metabolism (except for PG levels). However, these results do not rule out the existence of inhibitory effects of insulin on other aspects of lung development.

### Alloxan-Induced Diabetes

Rabbit fetal lung development, as assessed by pressure–volume curves, is delayed by maternal alloxan-induced diabetes *(58)*. Blood glucose levels were elevated to about 260 mg/dL in the fetuses of the alloxan-treated does (glucose levels in controls = 115 mg/dL). In addition, the levels of disaturated PC in lung lavage were decreased in fetuses of the diabetic does *(58)*. Sosenko and coworkers *(59)* also observed inhibitory effects of alloxan-induced maternal diabetes on fetal lung function, but found no effects of the maternal diabetes on disatured PC levels in either lung lavage or lung tissue of the fetuses. Morphologic parameters of lung development were delayed in the fetuses of diabetic rabbits *(60)*. Cortisol injection into the diabetic pregnant rabbit reversed some of the deficits in lung function in their fetuses, however, the beneficial effects of cortisol in the diabetic pregnancies were not achieved via effects on fetal lung disaturated PC levels *(61)*. Bhavnani and coworkers *(62)* also showed that the lung phospholipid content in control fetuses and fetuses of alloxan-induced diabetic rabbits did not differ. However, pressure-volume curves revealed that the lungs of the fetuses of the diabetic rabbits did not expand as well and retained less air, evidence of functional immaturity *(62)*. These data in the diabetic rabbit model show that hyperglycemia in the rabbit fetus causes delayed lung development as determined by morphologic and functional measurements. In all of the rabbit studies however, fetal plasma insulin values were not reported and the fetuses of the alloxan-treated does were reported to be growth retarded. It is also of interest that while fetal lung function was inhibited by maternal diabetes, in most cases this was not accompanied by a decrease in surfactant phospholipids.

### Streptozotocin-Induced Diabetes

Pregnant rhesus monkeys were made diabetic by streptozotocin administration and were shown to be glucose intolerant *(63)*. The L/S ratio in the diabetic pregnancies was greater than that observed in the age-matched normal pregnancies *(63)*. In addition, PC synthesis in the fetal lung tissue was elevated when compared to controls *(63)*. These results in a primate model are in good agreement with observations in the human where normal or elevated L/S ratios are frequently observed in diabetic pregnancies. Unfortunately, no observations concerning lung function, morphologic development, PG levels or surfactant protein levels were reported in this study.

The lungs of the fetuses of streptozotocin-induced diabetic rats (day 20 gestational age, term = 22 d) are characterized by delayed morphologic maturation and decreased PC synthesis *(64)*. Insulin treatment of the mother reverses both of these effects. By contrast, in another study, Tsai and coworkers *(65)* showed that on day 19 of gestation, PC and disaturated PC synthesis were not different in fetal lungs from control animals as compared to the offspring of diabetic rats. However, cortisol treatment of the diabetic rats failed to increase PC and disaturated PC synthesis *(65)*. Mulay and McNaughton *(66)* also used a streptozotocin model of rat maternal diabetes which resulted in fetal hyperglycemia (approx 400 mg/dL) and mild hyperinsulinemia (approx 2 times control levels). In the fetuses of the diabetic mothers, evidence of delayed lung maturation included increased glycogen content of the fetal lung tissue as well as lower disaturated PC content *(66)*. In another study, which used the rat streptozotocin model, maternal diabetes decreased the incorporation of $^{14}$C-glucose into PC and PG, and this effect could be reversed by the administration of insulin to the mother *(67)*. In agreement with the findings of Mulay and McNaughton *(66)*, Eriksson and coworkers *(68)* showed in a subsequent publication that the presence of maternal diabetes decreased PC synthesis and increased the glycogen content of the fetal lung. Gewolb and coworkers *(69)* found that the fetuses of the streptozotocin-treated diabetic rats are hyperglycemic (approx 350 mg/dL) but not hyperinsulinemic. On day 21 of gestation, lung PC and disaturated PC levels, as well as morphologic parameters such as the number of type II cells and number of lamellar bodies per type II cell were reduced in the fetuses of the diabetic mothers *(69)*. In a later study, Rotenberg and Gewolb *(70)* showed that glucocorticoids and thyroid hormone could reverse the inhibitory effects of streptozotocin-induced maternal diabetes on glycogen content and on the PC and disaturated PC content of the fetal lung. Finally, in an interesting study, Bourbon and coworkers *(71)* showed that they could achieve a wide range of fetal insulin and glucose levels in streptozotocin-induced diabetic pregnant rats. In all of the animals, no matter how high or low the insulin and glucose levels were, disaturated PC levels in lung tissue and lung lavage were reduced *(71)*. By contrast, PG was absent only in fetuses of mothers with the most severe diabetes, that is, those who were hyperglycemic and hypoinsulinemic *(71)*. Together, these studies are suggestive that in the rat streptozotocin-induced diabetic model, which is characterized by fetal hyperglycemia and growth retardation, maternal diabetes delays lung development.

In summary, delayed fetal lung maturation is observed in both the rabbit and rat chemically induced models of maternal diabetes. In general, the fetuses in these animal models of diabetes are growth-retarded and hyperglycemic. Data from numerous investigators document decreases in fetal lung PC and disaturated PC synthesis as well as delays in morphologic parameters of lung development, that is, increased glycogen content of epithelial cells, decreased numbers of alveolar type II cells, and decreased numbers of lamellar bodies. These observations are consistent with the hypothesis that hyperglycemia inhibits normal lung development in these species. However, in general, the fetuses in these animal models do not reflect two characteristics observed in the human fetus of a gestational diabetic pregnancy, that is, hyperinsulinemia and macrosomia. In addition, the levels of serum glucose in these models are much greater than levels present in the infant of the diabetic mother. Thus, the results of studies in the rat and rabbit models of diabetes do not exclude the possibility that high levels of insulin delay lung development in the human fetus.

## EFFECTS OF HYPERGLYCEMIA ON FETAL LUNG DEVELOPMENT

In fetal rat lung explants maintained in vitro, Gewolb *(72)* showed that glucose causes a dose-dependent decrease in choline incorporation into PC and disaturated PC. Significant effects were observed at 50 and 100m*M* glucose (equivalent to 900–1800 mg/dL). These levels of the glucose are in great excess of glucose levels observed in diabetic women and their fetuses *(13,15)*. The maximum effect of glucose on phospholipid synthesis, observed at the 100m*M* concentration, was approximately a 30% decrease in PC and disaturated PC synthesis *(72)*. In the same study, no effect of insulin (1 U/mL) was observed on phospholipid synthesis *(72)*. Glucose only inhibited PC, PG, and PI synthesis in rat fetal lung obtained late in gestation, that is, from days 20 to 22 of gestation *(73)*. Inhibitory effects of high glucose levels were also observed on the percentage of type II cells in rat fetal lung explants and on the number of secreted lamellar bodies when using tissue obtained at days 19 and 20 of gestation but not at later time points *(74)*. Gewolb and O'Brien *(75)* showed that high glucose levels decrease baseline and secretogogue-stimulated surfactant phospholipid secretion in cultured fetal rat type II cells in monolayer culture.

## INSULIN, DIABETES, AND THE SURFACTANT-ASSOCIATED PROTEINS

It has been reported that SP-A levels are decreased in amniotic fluid obtained from diabetic pregnancies when compared to SP-A levels in normal pregnancies *(32,38)*. In an additional study, in which the glucose levels in the diabetic women were well-controlled, no difference in amniotic fluid SP-A levels was found *(30)*. These observations are suggestive that factors in the fetus of the gestational diabetic woman, that is, hyperinsulinemia and/or hyperglycemia, may inhibit SP-A production in the human fetal lung. Because insulin had no inhibitory effects on surfactant lipid synthesis in human fetal lung explants, it was hypothesized that high insulin might inhibit the induction of the surfactant-associated proteins *(42,50,51)*. In support of this hypothesis, Snyder and Mendelson *(42)* reported that insulin inhibited the accumulation of SP-A in human fetal lung explants in a dose- and time-dependent manner. Insulin, added alone at concentrations as high as 250 ng/mL (6.9 mU/mL), did not affect the rate of PC synthesis in the explants; furthermore, in combination with cortisol ($10^{-7}M$), insulin significantly increased PC synthesis *(42)*. Insulin treatment of human fetal lung explants decreased SP-A mRNA and protein levels in a similar dose- and time-dependent manner *(76)* (Figs. 3 and 4). Significant inhibitory effects of insulin on SP-A mRNA levels were observed at concentrations as low as 25 ng/mL (approx 690 µU/mL), which is close to the levels observed in the infant of the diabetic mother *(14)*. SP-B mRNA levels in human fetal lung explants were also significantly decreased by high levels of insulin, while SP-C mRNA levels were unaltered *(76)*. Insulin significantly inhibited the levels of SP-A, SP-B, and SP-C mRNA in the presence of 1n*M* cortisol *(77)*. Human SP-A is encoded by two very similar genes, SP-A1 and SP-A2 *(78)*. In a recent study, it was shown that insulin decreases the levels of both SP-A1 and SP-A2 mRNA transcripts in human fetal lung explants and in H441 cells, a human pulmonary adenocarcinoma epithelial cell line *(79)*. Miakotina and coworkers *(80)* have shown that insulin decreases SP-A and SP-B mRNA levels in H441 cells in a dose- and time-dependent manner (Fig. 5). Furthermore, they showed an inhibitory effect of insulin on SP-A and SP-B gene transcription and no effect on SP-A or SP-B mRNA stability *(80)* (Fig. 6). Together, these studies are suggestive that levels of insulin that are close to the levels observed in vivo in infants of diabetic mothers can inhibit SP-A and SP-B gene expression in human fetal lung epithelial cells.

The induction of SP-A, SP-B, and SP-C is delayed in the fetus of the streptozotocin-treated rat *(81,82)*. These results are consistent with the delays observed in other aspects of fetal lung development in this animal model. Dexamethasone treatment increased surfactant protein gene expression in control fetuses and in fetuses of streptozotocin-treated diabetic rats *(83)*. In a recent study, Moglia and Phelps *(84)* showed that insulin infusion (40 U/kg) into diabetic pregnant rats increased fetal lung SP-A mRNA levels, but failed to elevate them to control levels. Glucose levels were close to normal in the insulin-treated mothers and their fetuses, and thus factors other than glucose may be involved in the delayed lung development observed in this animal model *(84)*.

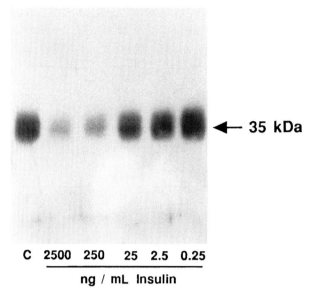

Fig. 3. Immunoblot analysis of SP-A protein content of human fetal lung explants. Human fetal lung explants were maintained for 4 d in serum-free medium that contained either no additions (C) or insulin at various concentrations. Homogenate proteins (75 µg per lane) were separated by polyacrylamide gel electrophoresis, transferred to nylon membranes, then probed using antibodies directed against human SP-A. (From ref. 76, with permission.)

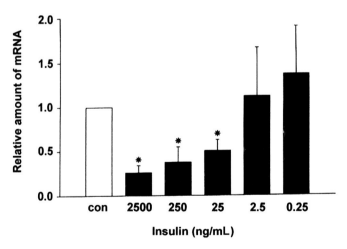

Fig. 4. The effect of insulin on SP-A mRNA levels in human fetal lung explants. Human fetal lung explants were maintained for 4 d in serum-free medium that contained either no additions (C) or insulin at various concentrations. (From ref. 76, with permission.)

## INSULIN RECEPTORS IN THE FETAL LUNG

The insulin receptor is a member of the tyrosine kinase family of growth factor receptors (85). The human insulin receptor is a heterotetrameric protein that consists of two extracellular α subunits and two transmembrane β subunits linked by disulfide bonds (85). The insulin receptor is expressed in most cell types. The human fetal lung

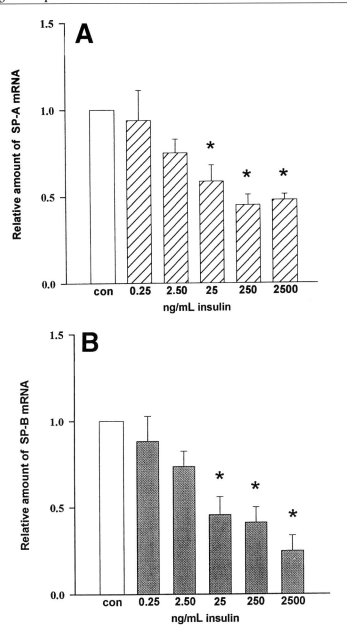

Fig. 5. The effects of insulin on SP-A and SP-B mRNA in H441 cells as determined by densito-metric analysis of Northern blots. (**A**) The effect of insulin on SP-A mRNA levels in the H441 cells. Cells were incubated for 48 h in the absence (CON) or presence of insulin at the indicated concentrations. (**B**) The effects of a 48 h exposure to insulin on SP-B mRNA levels. Cells were incubated in the absence (CON) or presence of insulin at the indicated concentrations. (Adapted from ref. *80.*)

contains large amounts of insulin-like growth factor I (IGF-I) *(86)*. The structure of the insulin-like growth factor-I receptor is closely related to that of the insulin receptor *(87)*. The insulin receptor binds IGF-I with 100-fold less affinity than insulin, while the IGF-I receptor binds insulin with 1000-fold less affinity than IGF-I *(87)*. Two major signal

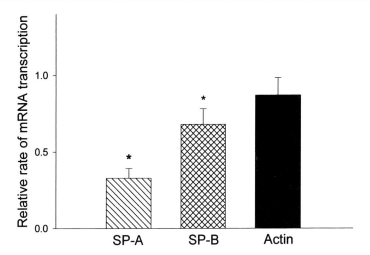

Fig. 6. Effects of insulin on SP-A, SP-B and actin gene transcription. H441 cells were treated with 2.5 μg/mL insulin for 24 h. Nuclear run-on transcription assays were then performed and the levels of SP-A, SP-B and actin gene transcription were determined. Data are the mean of seven to eight experiments. Control values were made equal to one for each gene and values for the insulin-treated condition were normalized to the controls in each experiment. Asterisks indicate a significant difference from control values (p < .05, paired *t* test). (From ref. *80*, with permission.)

transduction pathways are associated with activation of the insulin receptor, the ras/ mitogen-activated protein kinase pathway (MAPK) and the phosphatidylinositol 3-kinase pathway (PI 3-K) *(88)*. Nothing is known about the insulin signal transduction pathways that exist in the human fetal lung epithelial cell.

Insulin receptor binding capacity increases sixfold from day 15 to day 21 of gestation in fetal rat lung tissue while at the same time, the association constants for high- and low-affinity insulin binding sites remain unaltered *(89)*. In cultured rat fetal lung tissues, insulin receptors were downregulated to 50% of control levels in the presence of insulin for 24 h *(89)*. The insulin receptor binding capacity of fetal lung tissue obtained from fetuses of streptozotocin-induced diabetic pregnancies also increased during gestation; however, at 21 days of gestation, the levels of insulin receptor in fetuses of the diabetic mothers were 50% of control levels *(90)*. Mulay et al. *(91)* also reported lower specific insulin binding in membranes prepared from lung tissue of fetuses of diabetic rats when compared to binding in membranes from control fetuses. The combination of high glucose and insulin reduced specific insulin binding in fetal rat lung in vitro. High glucose and insulin also decreased insulin receptor mRNA levels and inhibited the tyrosine kinase activity of the insulin receptor. In addition, the combination of glucose and insulin diminished glucose uptake by fetal rat lung explants *(92)*. When added alone, however, neither glucose nor insulin affected insulin receptor tyrosine kinase activity or insulin receptor mRNA levels in the fetal rat lung explants *(92)*.

Studies of fetal rabbit lung also revealed a progressive increase in insulin binding activity during gestation, reaching a maximum at 29 d and declining by 30 d, reflecting a change in the number of insulin receptors in the tissue *(93)*. Type II cells isolated from fetal rabbit lungs contain two binding sites for insulin, with high and low affinity *(94)*. The binding affinity of the fetal rabbit lung insulin receptor did not change during gestation and was similar to that of the insulin receptor in adult lung tissue *(93)*. The number of insulin receptors in adult lung tissue was significantly lower than in lung tissue obtained from fetuses of 26–30 d gestational age *(93)*. Betamethasone treatment increased the number of insulin receptors in the fetal lung tissue 250% without changing their affinity *(93)*. Hypothyroidism, by contrast, decreased the number of insulin receptors by 70% compared to control fetuses *(93)*. Together, the data obtained in the rat and rabbit fetal lung are suggestive that insulin and the insulin receptor are present in the fetal type II cell and are involved in normal lung development.

## INSULIN, INSULIN RECEPTOR, INSULIN-LIKE GROWTH FACTOR, AND INSULIN-LIKE GROWTH FACTOR RECEPTOR GENE-DELETION MODELS

Analysis of gene-deletion models for the insulin, IGF-I, and IGF-II genes, as well as for their receptors may shed light on the role of these growth factors in lung development. Deletion of the insulin gene in mice results in growth retardation and multiple anomalies; however, specific effects on the lung have not been reported *(95)*. Insulin receptor-deficient mice are normal at birth, but develop postnatal growth retardation *(96,97)*. The normal prenatal development of the insulin receptor-deficient mice may be the result of compensatory interactions of insulin with the IGF-I receptor *(96,97)*. The phenotype of the insulin receptor gene-deleted mice differs markedly from humans with a homozygous mutated insulin receptor gene *(98)*. These individuals have impaired intrauterine development, hyperinsulinemia and fasting hypoglycemia, and die within the first year of life *(98)*. Humans with a mutated insulin receptor gene also suffer from repeated respiratory infections, data suggestive that there may be effects of this mutation on the lung *(98,99)*. IGF-I gene deletion in mice decreases their viability and severely impairs their growth *in utero*, data suggestive of the vital importance of IGF-I for normal prenatal growth *(100,101)*. IGF-I gene-deleted animals have been shown to have delayed lung development *(100)*. By contrast, IGF-II gene knockout animals are viable and healthy, but smaller than controls *(102)*. IGF-I receptor and IGF-II receptor gene-deleted animals are both characterized by delayed lung development *(101,103)*. The IGF-I receptor gene-deleted animals were growth-retarded at birth, whereas the IGF-II receptor gene deleted animals were macrosomic at birth *(101,103)*. A few clinical reports are suggestive that IGF-I and its receptor may also play an important role in lung development in the human. Severe intrauterine and postnatal growth retardation and mental delay were observed in an individual with homozygous partial deletion of the IGF-I gene; however, at 15y of age no abnormalities in the cardiovascular or respiratory systems were found *(104)*. In another report, loss of one copy of the IGF-I receptor gene resulted in delays in intrauterine growth and mental development complicated by respiratory distress syndrome after birth and lung hypoplasia *(105)*. These symptoms are typical for deletions of the distal long arm of chromosome 15, as well as ring chromosome 15 *(106–108)*. In aggregate, these data are suggestive that in the mouse, IGF-I and its receptors are required for normal mouse lung development and that the same may be true in the human. In addition, it seems that in the mouse, in the absence of a functional insulin receptor, insulin can act via the IGF-I receptor to facilitate intrauterine development of the fetus. In the human, defects in the insulin receptor seem to have more profound consequences on development.

## THE LUNG AND ADULT DIABETES

Pneumonia in patients with diabetes mellitus occurs with increased frequency and results in increased morbidity and mortality in this population *(109)*. Several pathogens have been frequently described as potentially causing severe pneumonia in diabetic patients, including *Staphylococcus aureus*, gram-negative organisms including *Pseudomonas*, fungi, *Streptococcus pneumoniae*, *Legionella*, and influenza *(109)*. SP-A has been shown to be involved in local defense mechanisms against many of these pathogens *(110)*. The link between diabetes mellitus and recurrent bacterial pneumonia has been examined by several in vitro studies. Abnormalities of phagocyte function and decreased intracellular leukocyte bacterial killing activity have been demonstrated in poorly controlled diabetics when compared to well-controlled diabetics and control subjects *(111,112)*. Depressed T-lymphocyte function and reduced chemotactic responses have also been implicated as a possible cause of the increased incidence of infections in diabetics *(113,114)*. With better metabolic control of diabetes and more effective antimicrobial agents, the incidence of pneumonia is not increased in diabetic patients when compared to those without diabetes *(115)*. Lung phospholipid and SP-A levels are abnormally regulated in animal models of diabetes *(116,117)*. SP-A levels have not been examined in lung tissue or bronchoalveolar lavage material from diabetic vs normal human patients. In light of the potential importance of this protein in local host defense mechanisms in the lung, it would be of great interest to conduct such a study.

Diabetic patients with increased hemoglobin $A_{1C}$ levels, a parameter suggestive of poor metabolic control, have been shown to have impaired pulmonary function *(118,119)*. Patients with advanced chronic obstructive pulmonary disease with concurrent diabetes mellitus have also been shown to have worse lung disease and outcomes *(120)*. In patients with cystic fibrosis, it was found that lung function declined concurrent with the development of diabetes and that insulin therapy improved their lung function *(121)*. In another study, a significant decline of pulmonary function, as reflected by a decline of forced vital capacity and forced expiratory volume in 1 s, was demonstrated in patients with diabetes mellitus when compared to control, nondiabetics *(122)*. The pathophysiology of the deleterious effects of diabetes on lung function are unknown. Based on studies in animal and human models however, it could be speculated that deficits in surfactant amount or composition could account for some of these observations.

The treatment of diabetes can include insulin administration, however, this requires frequent subcutaneous injections, and thus new modes of insulin administration are being studied. Heinemann and colleagues *(123)* have reported that inhaled insulin has a more rapid onset of action than subcutaneous insulin, with a sustained duration of action of 3 h. The dose required in this study was 99 Units of microcrystalline solid insulin and only 6–9% of the inhaled insulin was absorbed systemically from the respiratory mucosa *(123)*. A similar nebulized form of insulin therapy was effective in maintaining euglycemia in pediatric patients by Elliott et al. *(124)* with an absorption of 20–25% following a dose of 50 Units. It has been demonstrated that altering the velocity of aerosol administration improved the efficiency of insulin delivery to as high as 79%, and that a dose of 1 U/kg is effective in normalizing glucose levels in diabetic patients *(125)*. The long-term consequences of pulmonary exposure to aerosolized insulin are unknown. However, as discussed in this chapter, insulin, at high concentrations, may decrease the expression of two functionally important surfactant proteins, SP-A and SP-B, in the human lung. The volume of the epithelial lining fluid layer in the lung has been estimated to be approx 75 mL *(126)*. At an inhaled dose of 50 U of insulin, this would result in a concentration of approx 0.67 U/mL of insulin in the fluid bathing the alveolar epithelium, a concentration ten fold in excess of what has been shown to inhibit the production of human SP-A and SP-B in vitro. Based on these observations, we suggest that it will be important to determine that the use of inhaled insulin does not affect lung function.

## CONCLUSIONS

Newborns of gestational diabetic mothers have an increased risk of developing RDS and it has been hypothesized that their lung development is delayed. These infants tend to be macrosomic, hyperglycemic, and hyperinsulinemic. When the maternal diabetes is well-controlled, there is no longer an effect on fetal lung development. Several specific effects of maternal diabetes on fetal lung maturation have been documented. First, the fetus of the diabetic mother tends to have a normal L:S ratio, one that would be predictive of lung maturity in a nondiabetic pregnancy. Thus, in a diabetic pregnancy, a normal L:S ratio is not always predictive of lung maturity. Second, the levels of PG in amniotic fluid are decreased in diabetic pregnancies. A low or absent PG content in a diabetic pregnancy is associated with an increased risk of RDS. Third, the levels of SP-A, the major surfactant-associated protein, are decreased in amniotic fluid from diabetic pregnancies when compared to levels in nondiabetic pregnancies.

Fetuses in animal models of the diabetic pregnancy are generally characterized by hyperglycemia, hypoinsulinemia, and growth retardation. Except for hyperglycemia, these are not characteristics of the fetus of the human gestational diabetic pregnancy. Lung development is delayed in the fetuses of diabetic animals. The delay is apparent in the induction of both surfactant phospholipids and the surfactant-associated proteins. These results are suggestive that hyperglycemia decreases surfactant phospholipid synthesis and secretion and inhibits the induction of the surfactant-associated proteins in animal models of lung development.

It has been hypothesized that the hyperinsulinemia observed in the fetus of the diabetic human causes delayed lung development. In support of this concept, insulin inhibits the induction and accumulation of SP-A and SP-B in human fetal lung explants. Studies using a human lung epithelial cell line are suggestive that the effects of insulin occur at the transcriptional level. By contrast, it has been shown that insulin has no effect on surfactant PC synthesis or accumulation in human fetal lung explants maintained in vitro. These results, obtained using human in vitro models, are suggestive that the delayed lung development observed in the fetus of the diabetic woman may be related to a deficiency in the surfactant-associated proteins caused by high levels of insulin in the fetal circulation. Thus, while insulin and the insulin receptor probably play a role in normal lung development, the elevated serum levels of insulin observed in the fetus of the diabetic woman may delay specific aspects of human fetal lung maturation.

## ACKNOWLEDGMENT

This work was supported by NIH HDHL 50050. We thank Rose Marsh for her assistance in preparing the manuscript.

# REFERENCES

1. Robert MF, Neff RK, Hubbell JP, Taeusch, HW, Avery ME. Association between maternal diabetes and the respiratory distress syndrome in the newborn. N Engl J Med 1976;294:357–360.
2. Avery ME, Mead J. Surface properties in relation to aletectasis and hyaline membrane disease. Am J Dis Child 1959;97:517–523.
3. Wright JR, Clements JA. Metabolism and turnover of lung surfactant. Am Rev Respir Dis 1987; 136:426–444.
4. Pedersen J, Osler M. Hyperglycemia as the cause of characteristic features of the fetus and newborn diabetic mothers. Dan Med Bull 1961;8:78–83.
5. Tyrala EE. The infant of the diabetic mother. Obstet Gynecol Clin North Am 1996;23:221–241.
6. Gluck L, Kulovich MV. Lecithin/sphingomyelin ratios in amniotic fluid in normal and abnormal pregnancy. Am J Obstet Gynecol 1973;115:539–546.
7. Frantz ID III Epstein MF. Fetal lung development in pregnancies complicated by diabetes. In: Merkatz IR, Adam PAJ, eds. The diabetic pregnancy: a perinatal perspective ; New York: Grune & Stratton, 1979:227–233.
8. Mimouni F, Miodovnik M, Whitsett JA, Holroyde JC, Siddiqi TA, Tsang RC. Respiratory distress syndrome in infants of diabetic mothers in the 1980s: no direct adverse effect of maternal diabetes with modern management. Obstet Gynecol 1987;69:191–195.
9. Bradley R. Diabetic pregnancy. Hosp Med 1990;44:386–390.
10. Heding LG, Persson B, Stangenberg M. β cell function in newborn infants of diabetic mothers. Diabetologia 1980;19:427–432.
11. Sosenko IR, Kitzmiller JL, Loo SW, Blix P, Rubenstein AH, Gabbay KH. The infant of the diabetic mother. Correlation of increased cord C–peptide levels with macrosomia and hypoglycemia. N Engl J Med 1979;301:859–862.
12. Obenshain SS, Adam PAJ, King KC, Teramo K, Raivio KO, Raiha N, Schwartz R. Human fetal insulin response to sustained maternal hyperglycemia. N Engl J Med 1970;283:566–570.
13. Knip M, Lautala P, Leppaluoto J, Akerblom HK, Kouvalainen K. Relation of enteroinsular hormones at birth to macrosomia and neonatal hypoglycemia in infants of diabetic mothers. J Pediatr 1983; 103:603–611.
14. Isles TE, Dickon M, Farguhar JW. Glucose tolerance and plasma insulin in newborn infants of normal and diabetic mothers. Pediatr Res 1968;2:198–208.
15. Karlsson K Kjellmer I. The outcome of diabetic pregnancies in relation to the mother's blood sugar level. Am J Obstet Gynecol 1972;112:213–220.
16. Mallampalli RK, Acarregui MJ, Snyder JM. Differentiation of the alveolar epithelium in the fetal lung. In: McDonald JA, ed. Lung growth and development. New York: Marcel Dekker, 1997:119–162.
17. Gluck L, Kulovich MV, Borer RC Jr, Keidel WN. The interpretation and significance of the L/S ratio in amniotic fluid. Am J Obstet Gynecol 1974;120:142–155.
18. Whitfield CR, Sproule WB, Brudenell M. The amniotic fluid lecithin: sphingomyelin area ratio (LSAR) in pregnancies complicated by diabetes. J Obstet Gynecol Br Comw 1973;80:918–922.
19. Singh EJ, Mejia A, Zuspan FP. Studies of human amniotic fluid phospholipids in normal, diabetic and drug–abuse pregnancy. Am J Obstet Gynecol 1974;119:623–629.
20. Merola JC, Johnson LM, Bolognese RJ, Corson SL. Determination of fetal pulmonary maturity by amniotic fluid lecithin/sphingomyelin ratio and rapid shake test. Am J Obstet Gynecol 1974; 119:243–252.
21. Dyson D, Blake M, Cassady G. Amniotic fluid lecithin/sphingomyelin ratio in complicated pregnancies. Am J Obstet Gynecol 1975;122:772–781.
22. Skjæraasen J, Lindback T. Phospholipid concentrations in amniotic fluid from diabetic pregnant women. Acta Obstet Gynecol Scand 1976;55:225–232.
23. Cunningham MD, Desai NS, Thompson SA, Greene JM. Amniotic fluid phosphatidylglycerol in diabetic pregnancies. Am J Obstet Gynecol 1978;131:719–724.
24. Curet LB, Olson RW, Schneider JM, Zachman RD. Effects of diabetes mellitus on amniotic fluid L/S ratio and respiratory distress syndrome. Am J Obstet Gynecol 1979;135:10–13.
25. Kulovich MV, Gluck L. The lung profile II: complicated pregnancy. Am J Obstet Gynecol 1979; 135:64–70.
26. Hallman M, Teramo K. Amniotic fluid phospholipid profile as a predictor of fetal maturity in diabetic pregnancies. Obstet Gynecol 1979;54:703–707.

27. Tsai MY, Shultz EK, Nelson JA. Amniotic fluid phosphatidylglycerol in diabetic and control pregnant patients at different gestational lengths. Am J Obstet Gynecol 1984;149:388–392.

28. Farrell PM, Engle MJ, Curet LB, Perelman RH, Morrison JC. Saturated phospholipids in amniotic fluid of normal and diabetic pregnancies. Obstet Gynecol 1984;64:77–85.

29. Tydén O, Berne C, Eriksson UJ, Hansson U, Stangenberg M, Persson B. Fetal maturation in strictly controlled diabetic pregnancy. Diabetes Res 1984;1:131–134.

30. McMahan MJ, Mimouni F, Miodovnik M, Hull WM, Whitsett JA. Surfactant associated protein (SAP-35) in amniotic fluid from diabetic and non-diabetic pregnancies. Obstet Gynecol 1987;70: 94–98.

31. Curet LB, Tsao FH, Zachman RD, Olson RW, Henderson PA. Phosphatidylglycerol, lecithin/sphingomyelin ratio and respiratory distress syndrome in diabetic and non–diabetic pregnancies. Int J Obstet Gynecol 1989;30:105–108.

32. Snyder JM, Kwun JE, O'Brien JA, Rosenfeld CR, Odom MJ. The concentration of the 35-kDa surfactant apoprotein in amniotic fluid from normal and diabetic pregnancies. Pediatr Res 1988;24:728–734.

33. Piper JM, Samueloff A, Langer O. Outcome of amniotic fluid analysis and neonatal respiratory status in diabetic and non–diabetic pregnancies. J Reprod Med 1995;40:780–784.

34. Berkowitz K, Reyes C, Saadat P, Kjos SL. Fetal lung maturation: comparison of biochemical indices in gestational diabetic and nondiabetic pregnancies. J Reprod Med 1997;42:793–800.

35. Donald IR, Freeman RK, Goebelsmann U, Chan WH, Nakamura RM. Clinical experience with the amniotic fluid lecithin/sphingomyelin ratio .1. Antenatal prediction of pulmonary maturity. Am J Obstet Gynecol 1973;115:547–552.

36. Cruz AC, Buki WC, Birk SA, Spellacy WN. Respiratory distress syndrome with mature lecithin/spingomyelin ratios: diabetes mellitus and low Apgar scores. Am J Obstet Gynecol 1975;126:78–82.

37. Andrews AG, Brown JB, Jeffery PE, Horacek I. Amniotic fluid palmitic acid/stearic acid ratios. Lecithin/sphingomyelin ratios and palmitic acid concentrations in the assessment of fetal lung maturity in diabetic pregnancies. Br J Obstet Gynecol 1979;86:959–964.

38. Katyal SL, Amenta JS, Singh G, Silverman JA. Deficient lung surfactant apoproteins in amniotic fluid with mature phospholipid profile from diabetic pregnancies. Am J Obstet Gynecol 1984;148:42–53.

39. Hallman M, Kulovich M, Kirkpatrick E, Sugarman RG, Gluck L. Phosphatidylinositol and phosphatidylglycerol in amniotic fluid: indices of lung maturity. Am J Obstet Gynecol 1976;125:613–617.

40. Bleasdale JE, Mayberry MC, Quirk JG. Myo–inositol homeostasis in fetal rabbit lung. Biochem J 1982;206:43–52.

41. Weaver TE, Whitsett JA. Function and regulation of expression of pulmonary surfactant–associated proteins. Biochem J 1991;273:249–264.

42. Snyder JM, Mendelson CR. Insulin inhibits the accumulation of the major lung surfactant apoprotein in human fetal lung explants maintained in vitro. Endocrinology 1987;120:1250–1257.

43. King RJ, Ruch J, Gikas EG, Platzker AC, Creasy RK. Appearance of apoproteins of pulmonary surfactant in human amniotic fluid. Appl J Physiol 1975;39:735–741.

44. Smith BT, Giroud CJ, Robert M, Avery ME. Insulin antagonism of cortisol action on lecithin synthesis by cultured fetal lung cells. J Pediatr 1975;87:953–955.

45. Ballard PL. Hormonal regulation of pulmonary surfactant. Endocr Rev 1989;10:165–181.

46. Neufeld ND, Sevanian A, Barrett CT, Kaplan SA. Inhibition of surfactant production by insulin in fetal rabbit lung slices. Pediatr Res 1979;13:752–754.

47. Engle MJ, Langan SM, Sanders RL. The effects of insulin and hyperglycemia on surfactant phospholipid synthesis in organotypic cultures of type II pneumoncytes. Biochim Biophys Acta 1983;753:6–13.

48. Gross I, Smith GJ, Wilson CM, Maniscalco WM, Ingleson LD, Brehier A, Rooney SA. The influence of hormones on the biochemical development of fetal rat lung in organ culture. II. Insulin. Pediatr Res 1980;14:834–838.

49. Bourbon JR, Rieutort M, Engle MJ, Farrell PM. Utilization of glycogen for phospholipid synthesis in fetal rat lung. Biochim Biophys Acta 1982;712:382–389.

50. Mendelson CR, Johnston JM, MacDonald PC, Snyder JM. Multihormonal regulation of surfactant synthesis by human fetal lung in vitro. J Clin Endocrinol Metab 1981;53:307–317.

51. Snyder JM, Longmuir KJ, Johnston JM, Mendelson CR. Hormonal regulation of the synthesis of lamellar body phosphatidylglycerol and phosphatidylinositol in fetal lung tissue. Endocrinology 1983;112:1012–1018.

52. Hallman M, Wermer D, Epstein BL, Gluck L. Effects of maternal insulin or glucose infusion on the fetus: study on lung surfactant phospholipids, plasma myoinositol and fetal growth in the rabbit. Am J Obstet Gynecol 1982;142:877–882.

53. Levine DH. Hyperinsulinemia and decreased surfactant in fetal rabbits. Dev Pharmacol Ther 1985;8:284–291.

54. Pignol B, Bourbon J, Ktorza A, Marin L, Rieutort M, Tordet C. Lung maturation in the hyperinsulinemic rat fetus. Pediatr Res 1987;21:436–441.

55. Warburton D, Lew CD, Platzker AC. Primary hyperinsulinemia reduces surface active material flux in tracheal fluid of fetal lambs. Pediatr Res 1981;15:1422–1424.

56. Warburton D. Chronic hyperglycemia with secondary hyperinsulinemia inhibits the maturational response of fetal lamb lungs to cortisol. J Clin Invest 1983;72:433–440.

57. Rooney SA, Chu AJ, Gross I, Marino PA, Schwartz R, Seghal P, Singer DB, Susa JB, Warshaw JB, Wilson CM. Lung surfactant in the hyperinsulinemic fetal monkey. Lung 1983;161:313–317.

58. Bose CL, Manne DN, D'Ercole AJ, Lawson EE. Delayed fetal pulmonary maturation in a rabbit model of the diabetic pregnancy. J Clin Invest 1980;66:220–226.

59. Sosenko IR, Lawson EE, Demottag V, Frantz ID III. Functional delay in lung maturation in fetuses of diabetic rats. J Appl Physiol 1980;48:643–647.

60. Sosenko IR, Frantz ID III, Roberts RJ, Meyrick B. Morphologic distrubance of lung maturation in fetuses of alloxan diabetic rabbits. Am Rev Respir Dis 1980;122:687–695.

61. Sosenko IR, Hartig–Beecken I, Frantz ID III. Cortisol reversal of functional delay of lung maturation in fetuses of diabetic rabbits. J Appl Physiol 1980;49:971–974.

62. Bhavnani BR, Enhorning G, Ekelund L, Wallace D, Pan CC. Maternal diabetes and its effect on biochemical and functional development of rabbit fetal lung. Biochem Cell Biol 1988;66:396–404.

63. Epstein MF, Farrell PM, Chey RA. Fetal lung lecithin metabolism in the glucose–intolerant rhesus monkey pregnancy. Pediatrics 1976;57:722–728.

64. Tyden O, Berne C, Eriksson U. Lung maturation in fetuses of diabetic rats. Pediatr Res 1980; 14:1192–1195.

65. Tsai MY, Josephson MW, Brown DM. Fetal rat lung phosphatidylcholine synthesis in diabetic and normal pregnancies: a comparison of prenatal dexamethasone treatments. Biochim Biophys Acta 1981;664:174–181.

66. Mulay S, McNaughton L. Fetal lung development in streptozotocin–induced experimental diabetes: cytidylyl transferase activity, disaturated phosphatidylcholine and glycogen levels. Life Sci 1983;33:637–644.

67. Eriksson UJ, Tyden O, Berne C. Development of phosphatidyl glycerol biosynthesis in the lungs of fetuses of diabetic rats. Diabetologia 1983;24:202–206.

68. Eriksson UJ, Tyden O, Berne C. Glycogen content and lipid biosynthesis in the lungs of fetuses of diabetic rats. Biol Res Pregn 1983;4:103–106.

69. Gewolb IH, Rooney SA, Barrett C, Ingleson LD, Light D, Wilson CM, Walker Smith GJ, Gross I, Warshaw JB. Delayed pulmonary maturation in the fetus of the streptozotocin–diabetic rat. Exp Lung Res 1985;8:141–151.

70. Rotenberg M, Gewolb IH. Reversal of lung maturation delay in the fetus of the diabetic rat using triiodo–thyronine or dexamethasone. Biol Neonate 1993;64:318–324.

71. Bourbon JR, Pignol B, Marin L, Rieutort M, Tordet C. Maturation of fetal rat lung in diabetic pregnancies of graduated severity. Diabetes 1985;34:734–743.

72. Gewolb IH. High glucose causes delayed fetal lung maturation in vitro. Exp Lung Res 1993;19:619–630.

73. Gewolb IH. Effect of high glucose on fetal lung maturation at different times in gestation. Exp Lung Res 1996;22:201–211.

74. Gewolb IH, Torday JS. High glucose inhibits maturation of the fetal lung in vitro: morphometric analysis of lamellar bodies and fibroblast lipid inclusions. Lab Invest 1995;73:59–63.

75. Gewolb IH, O'Brien J. Surfactant secretion by type II pneumonocytes is inhibited by high glucose concentrations. Exp Lung Res 1997;23:245–255.

76. Dekowski SA, Snyder JM. Insulin regulation of messenger ribonucleic acid for the surfactant–associated proteins in human fetal lung in vitro. Endocrinology 1992;131:669–676.

77. Dekowski SA, Snyder JM. The combined effects of insulin and cortisol on surfactant protein mRNA levels. Pediatr Res 1995;38:513–521.

78. Katyal SL, Singh G, Locker J. Characterization of a second human pulmonary surfactant–associated protein SP–A gene. Am J Respir Cell Mol Biol 1992;6:446–452.

79. Kumar AR, Snyder JM. Differential regulation of SP–A1 and SP–A2 genes by cAMP, glucocorticoids and insulin. Am J Physiol 1998;274:L177–L185.

80. Miakotina OL, Dekowski SA, Snyder JM. Insulin inhibits surfactant protein A and B gene expression in the H441 cell line. Biochim Biophys Acta 1998;1442:60–70.

81. Guttentag SH, Phelps DS, Stenzel W, Warshaw JB, Floros J. Surfactant protein A expression is delayed in fetuses of streptozotocin–treated rats. Am J Physiol 1992;262:L489–L494.

82. Guttentag SH, Phelps DS, Warshaw JB, Floros J. Delayed hydrophobic surfactant protein SP-B, SP-C; expression in fetuses of streptozotocin–treated rats. Am J Respir Cell Mol Biol 1992;7:190–197.

83. Rayani HH, Warshaw JB, Floros J. Dexamethasone enhances surfactant protein gene expression in streptozotocin–induced immature rat lungs. Pediatr Res 1995;38:870–877.

84. Moglia BB Phelps DS. Changes in surfactant protein A mRNA levels in a rat model of insulin–treated diabetic pregnancy. Pediatr Res 1996;39:241–247.

85. Tavare JM, Siddle K. Mutational analysis of insulin receptor function: consensus and controversy. Biochim Biophys Acta 1993;1178:21–39.

86. Snyder JM, D'Ercole, AJ. Somatomedin C/insulin-like growth factor I production by human fetal lung tissue maintained in vitro. Exp Lung Res 1987;13:449–458.

87. Benito M, Valverde AM, Lorenzo M. IGF-I: a mitogen also involved in differentiation processes in mammalian cells. Int J Biochem Cell Biol 1996;28:499–510.

88. Saltiel AR. Diverse signaling pathways in the cellular actions of insulin. Am J Physiol 1996; 270:E375–E385.

89. Ulane RE, Graeber JE, Hansen JW, Liccini L, Cornblath M. Insulin receptors in the developing fetal lung. Life Sci 1982;31:3017–3022.

90. Ulane RE, Graeber JE, Steinherz RA. A comparison of insulin receptors in the developing fetal lung in normal and in streptozotocin–induced diabetic pregnancies. Pediatr Pulmonol 1985;1(3 Suppl):S86–S90.

91. Mulay S, Philip A, Solomon S. Influence of maternal diabetes on fetal rat development: alteration of insulin receptors in fetal liver and lung. J Endocrinol 1983;98:401–410.

92. Gewolb IH, O'Brien J, Palese TA, Phillip M. High glucose and insulin decrease fetal lung insulin receptor mRNA and tyrosine kinase activity in vitro Biochem Biophys Res Commun 1994; 202:694–700.

93. Devaskar SU, Ganguli S, Devaskar UP, Sperling MA. Glucocorticoids and hypothyroidism modulate development of fetal lung insulin receptors. Am J Physiol 1982;242:E384–E391.

94. Kaplan SA, Barrett CT, Scott ML, Whitson RH. Insulin receptors in fetal rabbit lung type II cells. Endocrinology 1984;114:2199–2204.

95. Duvillie B, Cordonnier N, Deltour L, Dandoy–Dron F, Itier JM, Monthioux E, Jami J, Joshi RL, Bucchini D. Phenotypic alterations in insulin–deficient mutant mice. Proc Natl Acad Sci 1997;94:5137–5140.

96. Accili D, Drago J, Lee EJ, Johnson MD, Cool MH, Salvatore P, Asico LD, Jose PA, Taylor SI, Westphal H. Early neonatal death in mice homozygous for a null allele of the insulin receptor gene. Nat Gen 1996;12:106–109.

97. Joshi RL, Lamothe B, Cordonnier N, Mesbah K, Monthioux E, Jami J, Bucchini D. Targeted disruption of the insulin receptor gene in the mouse results in neonatal lethality. EMBO J 1996;15:1542–1547.

98. Wertheimer E, Lu SP, Backeljauw PF, Davenport ML, Taylor SI. Homozygous deletion of the human insulin receptor gene results in leprechaunism. Nat Gen 1993;5:71–73.

99. Krook A, Brueton L, O'Rahilly S. Homozygous nonsense mutation in the insulin receptor gene in infant with leprechaunism. Lancet 1993;342:277–278.

100. Powell–Braxton L, Hollingshead P, Warburton C, Dowd M, Pitts–Meek S, Dalton D, Gillett N, Stewart TA. IGF–I is required for normal embryonic growth in mice. Genes Dev 1993;7:2609–2617.

101. Liu JP, Baker J, Perkins AS, Robertson EJ, Efstratiadis A. Mice carrying null mutations of the genes encoding insulin-like growth factor I (Igf-1) and type 1 IGF receptor (Igf1r). Cell 1993;75:59–72.

102. DeChiara TM, Robertson EJ, Efstratiadis A. Parental imprinting of the mouse insulin–like growth factor II gene. Cell 1991;64:849–859.

103. Wang ZQ, Fung MR, Barlow DP, Wagner EF. Regulation of embryonic growth and lysosomal targeting by the imprinted Igf2/Mpr gene. Nature 1994;372:464–467.

104. Woods KA, Camacho–Hubner C, Barter D, Clark AJ, Savage MO. Insulin–like growth factor I gene deletion causing intrauterine growth retardation and severe short stature. Acta Paediatr Suppl 1997;423:39–45.

105. Roback EW, Barakat AJ, Dev VG, Mbikay M, Chretien M, Butler MG. An infant with deletion of the distal long arm of chromosome 15 (q261—qter) and loss of insulin–like growth factor 1 receptor gene. Am J Med Gen 1991;38:74–79.
106. Siebler T, Lopaczynski W, Terry CL, Casella SJ, Munson P, De Leon DD, Phang L, Blakemore KJ, McEvoy RC, Kelley RI, Nissley P. Insulin–like growth factor 1 receptor expression and function in fibroblasts from two patients with deletion of the distal long arm of chromosome 15. J Clin Endocrinol Metabol 1995;80:3447–3457.
107. Tamura T, Tohma T, Ohta T, Soejima H, Harada N, Abe K, Niikawa N. Ring chromosome 15 involving deletion of the insulin–like growth factor 1 receptor gene in a patient with features of Silver–Russell syndrome. Clin Dysmorphol 1993;2:106–113.
108. Baba T, Kinoshita E, Matsumoto T, Yoshimoto M, Tsuji Y, Sasaoka K, Kamijo T. Decrease of insulin–like growth factor I receptor in patients with ring chromosome 15. Pediatr Res 1993;(33Suppl 5):S53.
109. Koziel H, Koziel MJ. Pulmonary complications of diabetes mellitus: pneumonia. Infect Dis Clin North Am 1995;9:65–96.
110. Crouch EC. Collectins and pulmonary host defense. Am J Respir Cell Mol Biol 1998;19:177–201.
111. Bagdade1 JD, Nelson KL, Bulger RJ. Reversible abnormalities of phagocytic function in poorly controlled diabetic patients. Am J Med Sci 1972;263:451–456.
112. Rayfield EJ, Ault MJ, Keusch GT. Infection and diabetes: the case for glucose control. Am J Med 1982;72:439–50.
113. Hill HR, Augustine NH, Rallison ML, Santos JI. Defective monocyte chemotactic responses in diabetes mellitus. J Clin Immunol 1983;3:70–77.
114. Saiki O, Negoro S, Tsuyuguchi I. Depressed immunological defense mechanisms in mice with experimentally induced diabetes. Infect Immun 1980;28:127–131.
115. Woodhead MA, MacFarlane JT, McCracken JS, Rose DH, Finch RG. Prospective study of the aetiology and outcome of pneumonia in the community. Lancet 1987;1:671–674.
116. Uhal BD, Longmore WJ. Altered phospholipid biosynthesis in type II pneumocytes isolated from streptozotocin–diabetic rats. Biochim Biophys Acta 1986;878:266–272 .
117. Sugahara K, Iyama K–I, Sano K, Morioka T. Overexpression of pulmonary surfactant apoprotein A mRNA in alveolar type II cells and nonciliated bronchiolar Clara; epithelial cells in streptozotocin-induced diabetic rats demonstrated by in situ hybridization. Am J Respir Cell Mol Biol 1992; 6:307–314.
118. Strojek K, Ziora D, Sroczynski JW, Oklek K. Pulmonary complication of type-1 (insulin-dependent) diabetic patients. Diabetology 1992;35:1173–1176.
119. Walton S, Byrd RR Jr, Fields CL, Ossorio MA, Roy TM. Abnormal pulmonary function and juvenile onset diabetes mellitus. Kentucky Med Assoc J 1994;92:101–104.
120. Antonelli IR, Fuso L, De Rosa M, Forastiere F, Rapiti E, Nardecchia B, Pistelli R. Co–morbidity contributes to predict mortality of patients with chronic obstructive pulmonary disease. Eur Respir J 1997;10:2794–2800.
121. Lanng S, Thorsteinsson B, Nerup J, Koch C. Influence of the development of diabetes mellitus on clinical status in patients with cystic fibrosis. Eur J Pediatr 1992;51:684–687.
122. Lange P, Groth S, Mortensen J, Appleyard M, Nyboe J, Schnohr P, Jensen G. Diabetes mellitus and ventilatory capacity: a five year follow–up study. Eur Resp J 1990;3:288–292.
123. Heinemann L, Traut T, Heise T. Time–action profile of inhaled insulin. Diabetic Med 1997;14:63–72.
124. Elliott RB, Edgar BW, Pilcher CC, Quested C, McMaster J. Parenteral absorption of insulin from the lung in diabetic children. Aust Pediatr J 1987;23:293–297.
125. Laube BL, Georgopoulos A, Adams III GK. Preliminary study of the efficacy of insulin aerosol delivered by oral inhalation in diabetic patient. JAMA 1993;269:2106–2109.
126. Effros RM. Permeability of the blood–gas barrier. In: Crystal RG, ed. The lung: scientific foundations. Philadelphia:Lippincott–Raven, 1997:1567–1580.

# 11

## The Insulin-like Growth Factor System and Lung

*Wayne A. Price, MD and Alan D. Stiles, MD*

The insulin-like growth factor (IGF) system is composed of two peptide growth factors, IGF-I and IGF-II, two cell-surface receptors, the type 1 and type 2 IGF receptors, and at least six binding proteins, IGFBP-1 to -6. The development of a comprehensive model of IGF system actions has been hampered by our incomplete understanding of the complex interactions both within the IGF system and with other hormones, growth factors, matrix components, and cytokines. However, there is strong evidence that the IGF system participates in lung development and various aspects of lung injury and repair.

## THE INSULIN-LIKE GROWTH FACTOR SYSTEM

### *Insulin-like Growth Factors, IGF-I and IGF-II*

#### IGF-I

Originally identified for its causative role in the sulfation of bone matrix, IGF-I has since been recognized as a peptide growth factor with significant impact on cell proliferation and differentiation *(1,2)*. IGF-I is encoded by a large complex gene located on human chromosome 12 spanning more than 95 kb, which contains four coding exons and at least two exons encoding 5' untranslated regions. The promoter region has been only partially characterized. Several transcriptional start sites, varying lengths of 3' untranslated regions, and multiple polyadenylation sites result in transcription of four major size RNA species ranging from 0.8 to 7.5 kb. The structure of the rat IGF-I gene and transcript sizes are similar to that seen in humans. The IGF-I protein is translated in a precursor form with a signal peptide and a carboxy-terminal extension that are cleaved to result in the mature 7.65 kD, 70 amino acid, basic peptide. IGF-I is structurally similar to insulin and shares almost 70% sequence homology with IGF-II.

The major determinants of IGF-I expression include developmental stage, cell type, trophic factors, and nutrition. IGF-I is widely expressed in both fetal and adult animals

From: *Contemporary Endocrinology: Endocrinology of the Lung: Development and Surfactant Synthesis*
Edited by: C. R. Mendelson © Humana Press Inc., Totowa, NJ

and is almost exclusively expressed in connective tissue and mesenchymal cells. IGF-I transcript abundance increases in the postnatal period and continues to be highly expressed throughout adult life. The presence of growth hormone or other trophic hormones, for example, estrogen in uterine tissue, are strongly correlated with IGF-I expression. In the fetus, placental lactogen, a growth hormone homolog, appears to stimulate IGF-I expression. The nutritional status of the organism is also a strong influence on IGF-I production *(3)*. In malnourished humans and animals, IGF-I tissue and serum concentrations fall, and return to normal as nutritional status improves. IGF-I expression also can be altered both in vitro and in vivo by inflammatory cytokines such as interleukin (IL)-1$\alpha$, IL-1$\beta$, IL-6 and tumor necrosis factor alpha (TNF-$\alpha$) *(4–6)*.

## IGF-II

IGF-II is a neutral peptide growth factor encoded by a 35-kb gene located on human chromosome 11 *(1,2)*. The IGF-II gene contains four characterized promoters and eight exons, three of which encode 5' untranslated regions. As with the IGF-I gene there are multiple transcripts ranging in size from 2.2 to 6.0 kb that result from use of different promoters and varying lengths of 5' untranslated region. The promoter selection and number of transcript sizes appear to be tissue and developmentally specific. The rat IGF-II gene differs from the human gene in having only three promoters, but results in a similar profile of transcripts by Northern analyses. IGF-II, like IGF-I, is translated as a precursor form with a signal peptide and carboxy-terminal extension. When these are cleaved, the mature 7.47 kD IGF-II peptide is 67 amino acids in length and is structurally similar to insulin.

Like IGF-I, IGF-II expression is also developmentally regulated. In humans and rodents, the expression of IGF-II is greater in the fetus than in the adult. There is little effect of growth hormone or nutrition on IGF-II expression, however, other trophic factors such as follicule-stimulating hormone and ACTH affect IGF-II expression in a tissue-specific manner. Unlike IGF-I, the cell types producing IGF-II vary with developmental stage, initially localizing to connective tissue and mesenchymal cells in early fetal stages, but later expressing in some epithelial cells.

## *Insulin-like Growth Factor Receptors*

Two cell surface receptors are components of the IGF system, the type 1 IGF receptor (IGF-1R) and the type 2 IGF receptor (IGF-2R, also known as the cation independent mannose-6-phosphate receptor). These receptors are widely distributed in tissues from all developmental stages and display structural similarity between humans and rodents.

## IGF-1R

The IGF-1R mediates the mitogenic and cell differentiation effects of IGF-I and IGF-II. The receptor is a heterotetramer composed of two identical $\alpha$ subunits (135 kD) and two $\beta$ subunits (90 kD) that possess tyrosine kinase activity *(7)*. Structurally homologous to the insulin receptor, the IGF-1R has greater binding affinities for IGF-I and IGF-II than for insulin. The two subunits of the IGF-1R are transcribed from a single gene located on human chromosome 15. This gene contains 21 exons and spans more than 100 kb. The $\alpha$ subunits are extracellular and contain the binding sites for the IGFs. Monoclonal antibodies specific to the $\alpha$ subunit of the IGF-1R block ligand binding to the receptor, preventing activation of the receptor, and its subsequent effects on DNA synthesis, cell differentiation, or cell survival. The membrane spanning $\beta$ subunit is linked to the $\alpha$ subunit by sulfhydryl bonds. IGF binding to the $\alpha$ subunit results in autophosphorylation of the $\beta$ subunit and receptor activation. The intracellular signaling pathways used by the IGF-1R are incompletely defined, although activation of the *Ras/* MAPK and PI-3 kinase pathways has been demonstrated in vitro *(7,8)*. Although the binding affinity of insulin for IGF-1R is reduced 100-fold compared to IGF-I, the mitogenic effects attributed to insulin in cell culture have been shown to be mediated through insulin binding to the IGF-1R. Virtually all cell types express IGF-1Rs throughout gestation and postnatal life. As with the IGFs, IGF-1R regulation is complex and includes developmental factors, nutrition, hormones and growth factors such as platelet-derived growth factor (PDGF) and fibroblast growth factor (FGF).

## IGF-2R

The IGF-2R is a single-chain glycosylated 270–300 kD polypeptide that binds IGF-II and lysosomal enzymes but has minimal affinity for IGF-I and does not bind insulin *(1)*. The human IGF-2R gene is located on the long arm of chromosome 6 and transcribes an mRNA of approx 9 kb. In mice, but not humans, the paternally derived allele is silenced through methylation *(9)*. The receptor protein is largely extracellular with short transmembrane and intracellular regions. The extracellular portion of the IGF-2R contains 15 repeat sequences with conserved cysteine residues and several glycosylation sites. There is no intrinsic protein kinase structure, although there are several phosphorylation sites in the cytosolic portion of the receptor. Biologic actions related to IGF binding to the IGF-2R remain uncertain. It is clear that this receptor is involved in transport of lysosomal enzymes to intracellular lysosomes and it also appears to transport bound IGF-II to lysosomes for degradation. Presently, there is no clear evidence that binding of IGFs by this receptor directly activates intracellular signaling pathways although there are several reports of biologic actions of IGF-II bound to this receptor *(1,2)*. There is an inverse relationship of IGF-II and lysosomal enzyme binding to the IGF-2R. This suggests that binding of lysosomal enzymes by the receptor may enhance IGF-II availability to the IGF-1R by increasing the unbound IGF-II in the local cellular environment. Conversely, local concentrations of extracellular lysosomal enzymes are increased by IGF-II binding by the receptor, contributing to breakdown of extracellular matrix and tissue remodeling. Cellular expression of the IGF-2R, like the IGF-1R, is widespread with some tissue specificity with greater expression in heart, muscle, lung, and kidney than liver and brain. In rats, the expression of the IGF-2R decreases postnatally in all tissues, paralleling the decrease in IGF-II expression.

## *IGF Binding Proteins*

IGFs in serum and extracellular fluids are complexed with a variety of IGFBPs. IGFBPs are produced by many tissues and are present in biologic fluids such as blood, lymph, urine, and others (Table 1). IGFBPs are characterized by their ability to bind IGFs and by common conserved cysteine regions in both the amino- and carboxy-terminal regions of the peptides. Six IGFBPs (IGFBP-1 to -6) bind IGFs with high affinity ($K_D$ less than $10^{-8}$ mol/L) and are well characterized *(10)*. Recently several similar proteins that bind IGFs with lower affinity have been described (IGFBP-7, -8, -9, and -10) *(11,12)*. Each IGFBP is derived from a distinct gene and each has unique structural characteristics (Table 1). IGFBPs in serum provide a rapidly accessible storage pool of IGFs and regulate the availability of the IGFs by controlling the clearance of circulating IGFs, and/or facilitating the transcapillary delivery of IGFs to specific tissues. IGFBPs in tissue may be locally produced or transported from serum and function to modulate IGF activity at the cell surface. The abundance of IGFBPs is highly regulated by developmental factors, hormonal environment, nutrition, IGF-I and – II, other growth factors (i.e. PDGF), and proinflammatory cytokines *(3,10,13–15)*.

Table 1
Structural and Functional Characteristics of IGFBPs

| IGFBP | MW (kDa) | Amino Acids | Structural features Chromosomal Location (Human) | Affect on IGF Bioactivity Action | IGF Affinity | IGF Independent | Present in |
|---|---|---|---|---|---|---|---|
| 1 | 25.3 | 234 | -RGD sequence -Phosphorylation -7p | Inhibition or potentiation | I = II | Yes | Amniotic fluid, serum, milk, urine, lymph, synovial fluid, interstitial fluid, seminal fluid |
| 2 | 31.4 | 289 | -RGD sequence -2q | Inhibition or potentiation | II > I | ND | CSF, serum, milk, urine, synovial fluid, interstitial fluid, lymph, follicular fluid, seminal fluid, amniotic fluid |
| 3 | 28.7 | 264 | -N-glycosylation -Phosphorylation -Binds heparin -7p | Inhibition or potentiation | I = II | Yes | Serum, follicular fluid, milk, urine, interstitial fluid, CSF, seminal fluid, synovial fluid, amniotic fluid |
| 4 | 26.0 | 237 | -N-glycosylation -2 extra cysteines -Binds heparin -17q | Inhibition | I = II | yes | Serum, follicular fluid, lymph, seminal fluid, synovial fluid, interstitial fluid |
| 5 | 28.5 | 252 | -Binds ECM, heparin, hydroxyapatite -O-glycosylation -Phosphorylation -2q | Potentiation | II > I | yes | Serum, CSF, seminal fluid |
| 6 | 22.8 | 216 | -O-glycosylation -2 less cysteines -12 | Inhibition | II > I | ND | CSF, serum, amniotic fluid |

ND, not determined: ECM, extracellular matrix.

## *Actions of the IGF System*

Originally, it was assumed that the IGFs acted primarily through endocrine mechanisms, being produced in the liver and transported to the sites of action via the circulation. It is now well documented that IGF system proteins are produced by multiple tissues where they function in an autocrine (produced by and then acting on the same cell) or paracrine (produced by one cell type and then acting on a neighboring cell) mechanisms. The local production and action of IGFs is recognized as a primary mechanism for IGF action in many tissues.

### MITOGENIC ACTIONS OF IGFs

The capacity of IGFs to stimulate cellular proliferation is well documented for many cell types *(1,2)*. As mitogens, the IGFs exert their actions in concert with other agents. In experiments using Balb/C 3T3 cells, IGF-I was shown to stimulate cell cycle progression, but only after cells were exposed to PDGF and epidermal growth factor (EGF). It was later shown that both of these growth factors increase IGF-1R expression. IGFs were found to act in mid to late G1 and were classified as "progression" factors. Either of the IGFs or insulin through binding with the IGF-1R serve the "progression" factor function. In cells lacking the IGF-1R, growth is slowed, and the cell cycle prolonged.

### IGF ACTIONS ON OTHER CELL FUNCTIONS

One of the earliest known functions of IGF-I, the capacity to stimulate extracellular matrix synthesis in skeletal tissue, was the basis for early IGF bioassays. The role of IGFs in extracellular matrix production has remained an area of intense study, particularly in connective tissue biology. IGFs also regulate cell differentiation and control specific cellular functions in other organs. For example, IGF-I induces differentiation of preadipocytes to adipocytes, myotube formation by myoblasts, and progesterone secretion by granulosa cells *(2)*.

More recently, investigators have characterized cell protective functions for the IGFs. In cell culture systems such as cultured oligodendrocytes, hematopoietic cells, fibroblasts, and human breast carcinoma cells, IGFs decrease programmed cell death (apoptosis) induced by various agents *(2,7)*. In vivo studies examining tissue injury, cell death, and the IGF system have focused on changes in the IGFs and IGFBPs with central nervous system hypoxic-ischemic injury *(16)*. Investigators using an adult rat model of hypoxic-ischemic brain injury found that brain IGFBP-5 expression was increased and IGFBP-4 decreased following a prolonged exposure to hypoxia. Because IGFBP-5 has been associated with augmentation of IGF actions, while IGFBP-4 seems to be a potent inhibitor of IGF actions, these findings suggest that IGFBPs may have a role in response to injury. In addition, adult rats treated with intrathecal IGF-I following hypoxic-ischemic brain injury had a reduction in infarction and neuronal loss *(17)*. Although mechanisms to account for these improvements in central nervous system injury have not been defined, the augmentation of in vitro cell survival by IGF-I suggests that it reduces the susceptibility of some cells to injury and necrosis following hypoxic–ischemic brain injury.

### IGFBP MODULATION OF IGF ACTIVITY

Accumulating evidence suggests that IGFBPs are a major posttranslational regulator of IGF activity in serum and tissues *(10)*. IGFBPs may inhibit or augment IGF activity depending on the specific IGFBPs present and their binding affinity for IGFs (Fig. 1).

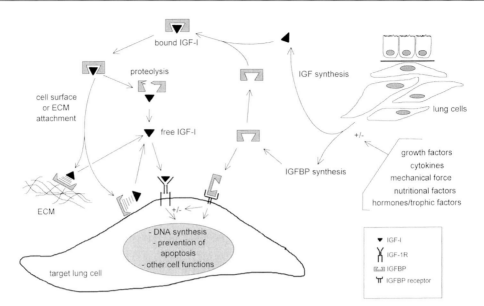

Fig. 1. Proposed mechanisms for IGF system action. IGFs and IGFBPs are synthesized and released into the pericellular space or are transported to sites of action via serum. Tightly bound IGFs are released from IGFBPs following IGFBP proteolysis or association of IGFBPs with ECM or cell surface proteoglycans. Free IGFs interact with the IGF-1R to influence cell proliferation, survival and/or other cell functions. IGFBPs also may directly interact with specific cell-surface receptors and/or influence IGF-1R signaling.

Soluble IGFBPs have a 10- to 40-fold higher affinity for IGFs than do IGF-1Rs and generally decrease IGF bioavailability. IGFs can be released from IGFBPs into the pericellular environment through the action of a variety of specific IGFBP proteases or following attachment of IGFBPs to the cell surface or ECM. IGFBPs bind to the cell surface through interaction with proteoglycans or through Arg-Gly-Asp (RGD) integrin binding sequences. IGFBPs bound to the cell surface or ECM have a lower affinity for IGFs and thus may augment IGF activity by facilitating delivery of IGFs to the IGF-1R or by promoting sustained, slow release of IGF and preventing IGF-induced IGF-1R downregulation. Another factor that alters the affinity of IGFBPs for IGF is phosphorylation. For example, phosphorylated IGFBP-1 has a high affinity for IGF-I and inhibits IGF-I action, while nonphosphorylated IGFBP-1 has a lower affinity for IGF-I and stimulates IGF-I action on cultured cells.

## DIRECT CELLULAR EFFECTS OF IGFBPS

Recently, direct effects of IGFBPs on the regulation of cell proliferation and apoptosis that are independent of IGFs and IGF-1R activation have been demonstrated (18,19). IGF-independent actions have been most clearly documented for IGFBP-3, -4, and -5 and may represent direct modulation of IGF-1R signaling by IGFBPs (20) or may be a result of interaction of IGFBPs with specific cell-surface IGFBP receptors (21–24).

## MODULATION OF IGFBP PRODUCTION
### BY OTHER GROWTH FACTORS, HORMONES, AND CYTOKINES

By modulating the activity of IGFs, or through direct IGF-independent activity, IGFBPs play a role in many processes that affect cellular proliferation and differentiation. It is becoming increasingly clear that hormones, proinflammatory cytokines, and peptide growth factors other than the IGFs regulate cell proliferation and differentiation by controlling IGFBP production, clearance, phosphorylation, localization, and/or proteolysis in a tissue and developmental-specific manner. For example, IGFBP production in bone is regulated by PTH, vitamin D, corticosteriods, inflammatory cytokines, and transforming growth factor-β (TGF-β) *(25–28)* and in reproductive cells by estrogens, activin A, LH, and FSH *(29–31)*. Experimental evidence suggests that changes in IGFBP production lead to altered cell proliferation. Retinoic acid and TGFβ each decrease DNA synthesis through downregulation of IGFBP-3 production *(21)*. Conversely, estradiol increases MCF-7 breast carcinoma cell DNA synthesis, in part, by suppressing IGFBP-5 production *(32)*. Thus, IGFBPs, by regulating IGF bioactivity or through direct cell action modulate cell proliferation or other cell functions in a rapid, cell-specific, and highly regulated manner. The multiple mechanisms involved in controlling IGFBP abundance facilitate tissue-specific IGFBP responses to various stimuli, including growth factors, hormones, or proinflammatory cytokines.

## THE INSULIN-LIKE GROWTH FACTOR SYSTEM AND THE LUNG

### Normal Lung Development and the IGF System

The earliest studies examining IGF system expression in lung demonstrated elaboration of immunoreactive IGF-I-like material by WI-38 cells, a human fetal lung-derived fibroblast line and by explants of fetal mouse and human lung *(33)*. These studies provided early support for the concept that IGF-I production was not limited to liver and that local IGF production, particularly in the fetus, could allow highly tissue-specific control of cell proliferation during organogenesis. Several approaches have been used to help determine the role of the IGF system in lung development, including descriptive studies of IGF expression and localization in the fetal and postnatal lung, study of cultured fetal lung cells, and development of transgenic models of altered IGF action.

#### EXPRESSION AND LOCALIZATION IN FETAL LUNG

Expression of IGF-I and –II transcripts has been documented in human *(34)*, mouse *(35)*, rat *(36-38)* and sheep *(39,40)* lung and in cells derived from lungs of other species *(41)*. Expression of the IGF-1R transcripts have been identified in lung from as early as embryonic day 13.5 in the rat *(42)* and day 12.5 in the mouse *(35)*, evidence that IGF-mediated cell proliferation occurs early in lung organogenesis. IGF and IGFBP mRNAs also have been documented throughout fetal lung development. The ontogeny of IGF system proteins has been most thoroughly studied in the rat. (*see* Table 2). IGF-I is expressed throughout fetal and adult life in lung with much higher IGF-I expression in fetal lung than in fetal liver *(43)*. As in other tissues, pulmonary IGF-II expression decreases postnatally. IGF-1R expression is increased in late fetal and postnatal life and IGF-2R expression decreases with advancing gestation. No IGFBP-1 expression is detectable in fetal or adult lung, however, IGFBP-2, -3, -4, -5, and -6 are expressed in a developmentally regulated manner, with IGFBP-6 detected only in adult lung. Results from human studies are similar, except that human fetal lung expresses IGFBP-6 *(44)*.

Localization of IGF transcripts in lung has been examined in fetal human, rat and mouse lungs. In the human fetus, *in situ* hybridization analyses localize IGF-I and –II mRNAs primarily to mesenchymal cells and connective tissue *(34)*, although more recent studies have also localized IGF-I *(45)* and IGF-II *(45,46)* to epithelial cells. Human fetal lung transcripts for IGFBP-4, -5, and -6 localize both to epithelium and

Table 2
Comparative Expression of IGFBPs During Rat Lung Development[a]

|          | Pseudoglandular E13-18 | Canalicular E18-19 | Saccular E20-D4 | Alveolar D5-21 | Adult |
|----------|------------------------|--------------------|-----------------|----------------|-------|
| IGF-I    | ++                     | ++                 | +++[b]          | +++            | +     |
| IGF-II   | +++                    | ++                 | +               | +              | –     |
| IGF-1R   | +                      | +                  | +++             | +++            | +++   |
| IGF-2R   | ++                     | +                  | +++             | Incomplete data | +    |
| IGFBP-1  | –                      | –                  | –               | –              | –     |
| IGFBP-2  | +++                    | +++                | +               | ++             | +     |
| IGFBP-3  | ++                     | ++                 | +++             | +++            | +     |
| IGFBP-4  | ++                     | ++                 | +++             | +++            | +     |
| IGFBP-5  | ++                     | +                  | +++             | +++            | +     |
| IGFBP-6  | –                      | –                  | +               | ++             | +++   |

[a] Plus signs represent relative expression for each transcript, not one transcript compared to another.
[b] There is a transient decrease in mRNA abundance for IGF-I during the midsaccular period to 1+.

mesenchyme in areas of active cellular proliferation *(47)*. Much more is known about the cellular localization of IGF system proteins in developing rat lung *(42,48–51)*. During the fetal period, IGF-I expression is confined to mesenchymal and connective tissues. Postnatally, IGF-I can also be identified in airway epithelium. IGF-II expression, initially localized to mesenchymal and connective tissues, is also present in airway epithelium as gestation progresses. Expression of the IGF-1R is widespread throughout gestation, but the IGF-2R is limited to mesenchyme and the medial layer of intrapulmonary vessels. IGFBP-2 expression is confined to proximal and distal airway epithelia and changes little with advancing gestation *(see* Table 3). IGFBP-3 and -5 are also expressed in proximal airway epithelium, but also in the interstitial and perivascular mesenchyme. The abundance of these IGFBP mRNAs increase as gestation progresses. IGFBP-4 expression is confined to interstitial mesenchyme and peaks in abundance on days 16 and 19. Similar patterns of IGFBP localization are found postnatally through the period of alveolarization with less prominent expression of IGFBP-2 and greater expression of IGFBP-4 and -5. In mouse, limited studies demonstrate a similar pattern of expression *(35)*.

Immunohistochemical localization of IGF-I, IGF-II, and IGFBPs suggest that IGFBPs may be a primary factor in IGF cellular localization during lung development. In human fetal lung, IGF peptides and IGFBP-1, -2, and -3 are associated with columnar epithelial cells of the airways *(52,53)*. The colocalization of the IGFBPs and IGF peptides in airway epithelium suggests that cell-associated IGFBPs bind and accumulate IGFs on the epithelial cell surface. In fetal rat lung, immunoreactive IGF-I localizes to airway epithelial cells as well as small vessels and capillaries within mesenchyme *(48,54)*. Immunoreactive IGF-II and IGFBP-2 colocalize on the apical surface of lung epithelia and in the mesenchyme *(48,54)*. Postnatally, there is abundant IGF-I and IGF-II localized to airway epithelium and mesenchyme and less in alveolar epithelium *(54)*. The abundance of both of these peptides decreases into adulthood. There is also epithelial-associated IGFBP-3 and -5 postnatally and localization of IGFBP-2 and -5 to airway smooth muscle cells (SMC) and blood vessels *(50)*. Adult animals show similar patterns of IGFBP localization with less IGFBP-2 present *(50,55)*.

Table 3
Localization of IGFBP Transcripts in Fetal Rat Lung by *In Situ* Hybridization Histochemistry

| | IGFBP-2 | IGFBP-3 | IGFBP-4 | IGFBP-5 |
|---|---|---|---|---|
| Pseudo-glandular E13–18 | All airway epithelium Mesenchyme : none | Airway epithelium Mesenchymal cells adjacent to blood vessels and airways | Epithelial cells : none Mesenchymal cells of interstitium | Proximal > distal airway epithelium Mesenchyme around primordial bronchi |
| Canalicular E18–19 | All airway epithelium Distal > proximal Mesenchyme : none | Epithelium of larger airways Mesenchymal cells around bronchovascular bundles | Epithelial cells : none Mesenchymal cells of interstitium Blood vessels | Proximal > distal airway epithelium and adjacent mesenchyme |
| Saccular E20–D4 | All airway epithelium Proximal > distal Mesenchyme : none | Epithelium of larger airways Mesenchymal cells around bronchovascular bundles | Epithelial cells : none Mesenchymal cells of interstitium Blood vessels | Proximal > distal airway epithelium and adjacent mesenchyme Adventitial layer of large vessels |
| Alveolar D5-D21 | Minimal to no expression | Airway epithelium Interstitium | Some epithelial cells Mesenchymal cells of interstitium Blood vessels | Airway epithelium Interstitium |
| Adult | Minimal to no expression | Bronchial epithelium Interstitium | Epithelium of large airways Mesenchymal cells of interstitium Blood vessels | Tracheal epithelium Interstitium |

These differing distribution patterns of IGF system proteins highlight the complex spatial and temporal regulation of the IGF system in lung . Several generalizations can be drawn from these descriptive studies. First, IGFBPs have wider protein distribution than mRNA expression, suggesting that each has paracrine affects on cells. It is also clear that IGFBPs are more highly regulated than IGFs or IGF receptors during development. Each IGFBP has a specific pattern of peak expression and localization, evidence that IGF system regulation is accomplished through changes in IGFBP production, localization and, clearance during organogenesis.

## CELL CULTURE

Much of the proposed role of the IGF system in lung development has been derived from studies of cultured lung cells. In early studies we used primary cultures of fetal rat lung epithelial cells and mesenchymal cells to examine the production of growth factors and their autocrine/paracrine mitogenic interactions. Neither fetal lung fibroblasts or epithelial cells required exogenous IGF-I to initiate DNA synthesis, suggesting that these cells produce IGF-I or -II that acts in an autocrine/paracrine fashion *(56)*. In support of this, several investigators, including our laboratory, reported that cultured WI-38 lung fibroblasts produce immunoreactive IGF-I, express IGF-1R, and increase cell proliferation in response to exogenous IGF-I *(57–59)*. In another effort to examine the autocrine/paracrine actions of IGF-I in these lung cells, we designed and used a specific IGF-I antisense oligodeoxynucleotide to inhibit IGF-I synthesis. The IGF-I antisense oligodeoxynucleotide reduced IGF-I in the conditioned medium from these cells and dramatically reduced DNA synthesis. DNA synthesis could be restored to normal with the addition of IGF-I to the medium. Similarly, in primary cultures of 19 day gestation fetal rat lung fibroblasts, we demonstrated that endogenous IGF-I production stimulated DNA synthesis via the IGF-1R *(60)*. We have also inhibited IGF-I production with antisense oligodeoxynucleotide using fetal rat lung fibroblasts with results that parallel those found with the WI-38 cells (W.A. Price and A.D. Stiles, *unpublished results*). These experiments provide strong evidence that IGF-I acts in an autocrine/paracrine fashion in lung cells and support the concept that local production and action of IGF-I is important during fetal lung development.

Studies examining IGFBP production by primary cultures of fetal lung epithelial cells and fibroblasts are consistent with the *in situ* hybridization studies of developing lung. IGFBP-2 is the predominant IGFBP secreted by epithelial cells and IGFBP-3 and -4 are the predominant fibroblast IGFBPs *(61)*. Abundance of IGFBPs is regulated by serum withdrawal and cell contact, suggesting that IGFBPs may be involved in regulating cell growth during density arrest and quiescence. Likewise, cell-specific changes are observed in IGFBP abundance in response to agents that alter lung cell growth and differentiation such as dexamethasone, retinoic acid, IGF-I, PDGF-BB, keratinocyte growth factor, basic FGF, and EGF *(15,61)*.

The IGFBPs produced by fetal lung cells may individually modulate the availability of IGF-I and IGF-II in culture based on the differing affinities of each IGFBP for IGF-I and IGF-II. In addition, IGFBP production by lung cells is differentially regulated by the IGFs. IGF-I stimulates IGFBP production by fetal rat lung fibroblasts and IGF-II does not do so *(61)*. Thus, the mitogenic activity of exogenous IGF-I, but not IGF-II, may be inhibited by the subsequent increase of IGFBP production by these cells, perhaps explaining the greater mitogenic response of these cells to added IGF-II *(62)*. Our findings with IGF-I antisense oligodeoxynucleotides suggest that endogenous IGF-I produced by the fetal lung fibroblast is mitogenically active in lung and is regulated by IGFBPs produced by lung cells *(59)*. Taken together, these findings may indicate that regulation of IGFBPs by other growth factors or cytokines is a mechanism by which these agents regulate lung cell proliferation during development. For example, in fetal rat lung, thinning of mesenchyme during the canalicular period of lung development is associated with decreased fetal lung fibroblast proliferation and increased PDGF-B mRNA expression. We have found that PDGF-BB stimulates IGFBP-4 production by mesenchymal cells derived from canalicular-stage lung *(15)* and IGFBP-4 inhibits DNA synthesis by these cells (unpublished results). Thus, elevated PDGF-B expression in fibroblasts during the canalicular period may increase local IGFBP-4 production and be a mechanism by which IGF-stimulated fibroblast proliferation is inhibited during acinar development.

Several studies suggest that IGF-I acts on lung epithelial cells also. Lung epithelium appears to have the capacity to bind and accumulate IGFs and IGF receptors localize to epithelial cells in lung. IGFBP-1 exhibits a pattern identical to that seen with the IGFs using immunohistochemical localization in fetal lung, suggesting that IGFBPs may be involved in the accumulation of IGFs by pulmonary epithelium *(63)*. These findings support a paracrine action of the IGFs in fetal lung, that is, IGFs act on airway epithelium, but are derived from nearby mesenchymal cells. Further support for this concept derives from our studies of adult canine tracheal epithelial cells in primary culture. We found that these cells synthesized functional IGF-1Rs capable of binding IGF-I with high affinity and that IGF-I binding to the IGF-1R stimulated DNA synthesis *(64)*. IGF-I also appears to act as a chemotactic agent for tracheal epithelial cells in culture *(65)*. These data suggest that IGF-I acts in a paracrine manner to enhance pulmonary epithelial cell proliferation and repopulation of the airway epithelial cells in postnatal trachea following airway injury.

The growth factor requirements for type 2 epithelial cells are of great interest because of the potential role of the type 2 cell as a stem cell for alveolar epithelium. In vitro, isolated distal fetal lung epithelial cells require insulin for maximal proliferation, presumably acting through the IGF-1R *(66)*. Growth arrest following serum withdrawal of SV-40 transformed type 2 epithelial cells, is associated with increased production and accumulation of IGFBP-2 in media, and increased expression of IGF-II and the IGF-2R *(67)*. With resumption of proliferation, each of these IGF system components rapidly decreases. Similarly, with glucocorticoid-mediated growth arrest of these cells, IGFBP-2 and IGF-II expression increase but IGF-2R expression is unchanged *(68)*. In vivo, the IGF-2R is present exclusively on type 1 alveolar cells within alveolar walls during alveolarization in the rat *(42)*, suggesting that the transformed type 2 cells have some type 1 cell characteristics. Taken together, these studies suggest that the IGF system participates in the transition of alveolar epithelial cells into and out of the cell cycle.

## TRANSGENIC MODELS

In a series of transgenic mouse experiments, lung development was indirectly examined using models that over-express IGF-I or have IGF-I, IGF-II or IGF-1R gene disruptions *(2)*. Mice that overexpress IGF-I under the control of the metallothionein promoter have somatic growth greater than littermate controls and lung sizes proportionate to body size. Conversely, mice with inactivated IGF-I genes are small (60% of normal) and have increased perinatal mortality with poorly inflated lungs at birth. On histologic examination, the lungs are atelectatic with increased cellularity, thick alveolar septae and poorly organized alveoli. No information concerning lung size was reported *(69)*. Animals with disruption of the active IGF-II gene were also growth retarded at birth and remained small postnatally, but are fertile and have no recognizable respiratory problems *(70)*. Mice with absent IGF-1R function die at birth with respiratory failure *(71)*. Morphologic analyses showed that there was no lung inflation in these mice, but immunostaining for "surfactant apoprotein" was normal. Severe muscle hypoplasia was present in these animals suggesting that the respiratory failure was a secondary phenomenon rather than a primary lung abnormality, however, no lung weights or morphologic analyses were performed. Taken together, these studies are consistent with IGF involvement in proportionate lung growth, but with the limited histologic examinations and lung growth data, it remains unclear whether the primary lung defects described are a direct result of absent IGF-I, -II or the IGF-1R. IGF-I or IGF-II also may act reciprocally in the absence of the other to support lung development. Information concerning other components of the IGF system in these animals is limited.

Using cogenic pair mice that are genetically identical except for a region of chromosome 17 that includes the IGF-2R gene, the IGF-2R has been implicated in lung development. Embryonic lung development proceeds at different rates in the two strains of mice, with the slower developing strain exhibiting higher levels of IGF-2R RNA and receptor protein *(72)*. Neither IGF-II nor IGF-I expression was reported in these animals. The investigators concluded that the development of these mice was delayed because IGF-II was bound by the increased IGF-2Rs and was unavailable to the IGF-1R, inhibiting the biologic effects of this growth factor and delaying lung development. These experiments emphasize the complexity of interactions within the IGF system and the potential importance of the IGF system proteins to fetal lung development.

### THE PULMONARY VASCULATURE AND THE IGF SYSTEM

Several lines of evidence from in vitro and in vivo studies support a role for the IGF system in vasculogenesis during development. IGFs and IGFBPs are localized to pulmonary vessels during development *(49,50)*. In vitro, IGF-I stimulates pulmonary artery vascular smooth muscle cell (SMC) and pericyte proliferation with neonatal cells showing greater responsiveness than adult cells *(73–75)*. IGFs also regulate production of connective tissue components such as elastin and collagen by pulmonary arterial SMC *(76)* and lung fibroblasts *(77)*. Vascular SMCs produce several species of IGFBPs *(78)* that are capable of modifying the mitogenic activity of IGF-I for SMCs *(79)*. These studies provide strong evidence that IGFs participate in the control of SMC proliferation and cell function in the pulmonary vascular bed and that these actions are modified by IGFBPs.

## *The IGF System During Pathologic Lung Processes or Altered Lung Growth*

### INFLAMMATORY CELLS OF THE LUNG AND THE IGF SYSTEM

IGF system proteins are expressed by macrophages and lymphocytes, cells involved in the inflammatory or immune response. Lung alveolar macrophages produce IGF-I, IGFBPs and IGF-1R *(80–83)*. The presence of IGF-1Rs on pulmonary macrophages is consistent with mitogenic autocrine/paracrine effects of macrophage-produced IGFs or IGFs produced by other lung cells on alveolar macrophages. Cultured lymphocytes express transcripts for IGF-1R , IGF-2R, IGFBP-2, and IGFBP-3 *(83)* and after stimulation with phytohemagglutinin, IGF-I, IGF-II, IGFBP-4, and IGFBP-5 also are expressed. Because macrophages and lymphocytes appear early in infection or inflammatory processes in lung, production of IGF-I and IGFBPs by macrophages and lymphocytes may be particularly important for delivery of these proteins to sites of injury or repair, supporting the concept that IGF system proteins derived from these cells may act in a paracrine fashion during lung inflammation or injury.

## PROINFLAMMATORY CYTOKINES

Among the proinflammatory mediators commonly encountered in lung injury or in response to airway hyperreactivity, IL-1α, IL-1β, IL-6, TNF-α, and leukotriene D4 are associated with changes in IGF system expression *(4,5,6,13,41,82)*. Leukotriene D4 is a proinflammatory eicosanoid that is associated with airway hyperreactivity and has a synergistic effect on IGF-stimulated proliferation of airway SMCs *(41)*. Accumulation of IGFBP-2 in airway SMC conditioned medium is decreased by leukotriene D4 because of increased proteolysis of IGFBP-2 . Because the addition of IGFBP-2 inhibits the mitogenic effects of IGF-I, reduction of IGFBP-2 may be a mechanism by which proinflammatory eicosanoids increase IGF-I mitogenic activity for airway smooth muscle cells and, thus, promote the airway cell hyperplasia associated with inflammatory conditions such as asthma. IL-1α, IL-1β, and TNF-α effects on the IGF system in lung have not been reported, although preliminary results from our laboratory demonstrate that IL-1β and TNF-α upregulate IGFBP-3 and -4 accumulation in fetal lung fibroblast conditioned medium (W.A. Price and A.D. Stiles, *unpublished results*). In cells from other tissues regulation of IGF system expression by these proinflammatory cytokines has been studied. Presently, the mechanism of IGF system regulation by the proinflammatory cytokines is dependent on the specific cell type where the interaction occurs. For example, chondrocyte exposure to IL-1β induces secretion of IGF-I and IGFBPs and increases IGF-1R on cell surfaces, but the changes are not associated with an increase in IGF-I transcript abundance and are not prostaglandin-dependent *(4)*. Likewise, TNF-α increases IGF-I expression by murine bone marrow derived macrophages, independent of PGE2 *(82)*. In contrast, mouse bone organ cultures increase steady state abundance of the 7.5 kb and 0.9 kb IGF-I transcripts and release greater amounts of IGF-I into culture medium after exposure to either IL-1α or IL-1β, but the effects are indirect, mediated in part by a prostaglandin (PGE1 or PGE2)-dependent mechanism *(5)*. Similarly, cytokines regulate IGFBPs through multiple mechanisms, including changes in transcription and altered protease activity *(13,14)*. It seems likely that proinflammatory cytokines in lung affect IGF system expression, but with the many cell types present in lung, effects may be heterogeneous because of the multiple mechanisms that may be involved.

## REGULATION OF THE IGF SYSTEM DURING ABNORMAL FETAL LUNG GROWTH

Several studies have examined changes in lung expression of IGF system components related to changes in the environment of the fetus or its lung. Fetal growth retardation induced by dexamethasone administration to pregnant rats results in decreased body weight, lung weight and lung DNA content *(85)*. Although no changes in lung IGF-I, IGF–II, or IGF-1R expression were found, IGFBP-1 expression in lung was increased fourfold. Intrauterine growth retardation secondary to maternal ethanol ingestion results in decreased IGF-II peptide release from fetal lung explants *(86)* and an increase in IGFBP-1 and IGFBP-2 expression in the fetal lung *(87)*. These findings suggest that local effects of IGF peptides in lung may be a result of decreased IGF-II production and/or increases in inhibitory IGFBPs. These findings also highlight the differences in regulation of IGF system protein in lung based on different mechanisms producing growth retardation.

The effects of mechanical factors on fetal lung expression of IGF-I and IGF-II have been examined in two studies. Tracheal obstruction in fetal sheep increases fetal lung DNA content and IGF-II expression, while fetal lung fluid drainage decreases lung DNA content and reduces IGF-II expression *(39)*. In another study using fetal sheep, tracheal ligation increased lung growth and IGF-I expression and decreased markers of epithelial cell differentiation and alveolar type 2 cell number *(40)*. Although the effects of IGF-I and -II on lung differentiation have not been studied systematically, these studies suggest that the IGF peptides participate in translating mechanical forces into signaling pathways that affect lung growth and may perhaps play a role in lung cell differentiation.

## HYPOXIA AND THE LUNG IGF SYSTEM

Hypoxic regulation of the lung IGF system is more apparent in postnatal than fetal animals. Fetal sheep subjected to long-term hypoxia secondary to reduction in maternal uterine blood flow have decreased fetal tissue DNA synthesis and no change in lung IGF-I or -II, although serum concentrations of IGFBP-1 are increased *(88)*. Increased serum IGFBP-1 may decrease the pool of IGF available for transport to tissues *(2)*. Whether this mechanism contributes to the reduced DNA synthesis found in this model is unknown. Postnatal exposure to hypoxia increases IGF-I and IGF-1R mRNA transcript abundance in lung *(89)*. Similar mRNA changes occur in the heart, but not liver, suggesting that hypoxia in postnatal animals regulates IGF-I and the IGF-1R in a tissue-specific manner. These tissue-specific responses of IGF-I and the IGF-1R to hypoxia may provide some benefit to the animal undergoing increased cardiopulmonary output, perhaps related to increased heart mass. Lung weights were unchanged in this experiment, suggesting that the increased IGF-I and IGF-1R expression in lung may be related to pulmonary vascular remodeling or other changes in a subpopulation of lung cells.

## HYPEROXIA AND THE LUNG IGF SYSTEM

Adult rats exposed to hyperoxia (85% oxygen) have increased immunoreactive IGF-I in their serum that is mitogenic for cultured pneumocytes and fibroblasts *(90)*, suggesting a role for serum IGF-I in the cell proliferation associated with hyperoxic lung injury. In this model, increased IGF-I protein is primarily immunolocalized to airway and alveolar epithelium and to a lesser degree to interstitial cells in the hyperoxic lung *(55)*. The epithelial distribution of IGF-I expression is in contrast to the findings in normal fetal lung where expression is limited to mesenchymal and connective tissues. IGF-1R is immunolocalized to peribronchial cells, perivascular cells, and endothelial cells early in the exposure period and is found with alveolar epithelial cells after 2 wk of exposure. These investigators speculated that the distribution of the IGF-1R supports a paracrine role for IGF-I in pulmonary hypertension, airway hyperreactivity, and late pneumocyte proliferation following oxygen exposure.

The IGF system has also been studied in neonatal rats exposed to hyperoxia. Newborn rats exposed to 60% oxygen for 2 weeks have increased lung weights, decreased lung volume, scattered areas of decreased DNA synthesis, and increased type 2 cell DNA synthesis. In this model, IGF-I and IGF-1R immunolocalize to areas of abnormal lung growth (parenchymal thickening) *(91)*, suggesting that IGF-I and the IGF-1R are involved in the dysplastic lung growth resulting from chronic hyperoxia exposure. Using another neonatal rat hyperoxia model where animals are exposed to 85–90% oxygen for up to 6 wk, our laboratory found increases in IGF-I and IGF-II expression *(92)*. *In situ* hybridization analyses showed that IGF-I expression was localized to mesenchymal cells, connective tissue and macrophages, while IGF-II, which normally has very low to undetectable expression in postnatal lung, was expressed by distal airway epithelial cells following hyperoxia, a pattern similar to that observed in fetal lung. Similarly, hyperoxic exposure of 3 wk-old rats enhances the growth of fibroblasts isolated from lung and their responsiveness to IGF-I *(93)*. These models support an autocrine/paracrine mechanism for action of IGF-I and IGF-II during the hyperoxic injury of lung in the neonatal animal.

Macrophages appear to be an important source of IGF-I in lung and may be important in the pathogenesis of oxygen injury. In a limited set of experiments, we used reverse transcription/polymerase chain reactions and/or *in situ* hybridization analyses to examine the expression of IGF system components in pulmonary macrophages isolated from rats after hyperoxia exposure for 3 d or untreated controls. Both groups of macrophages expressed IGF-I, IGF-1R, IGF-2R, IGFBP-1, -2, -3, -4, and -6, but not IGF-II or IGFBP-5 (W.A. Price and A.D. Stiles, *unpublished results*). We found no major changes in transcript abundance after oxygen exposure, but the number of pulmonary macrophages present in lavage fluid from hyperoxia exposed lung was substantially increased. These results suggest that the pulmonary macrophage may be a source of IGF-I and IGFBPs in lung during hyperoxic injury.

Cell culture studies examining hyperoxia and the IGF system in vitro have shown that exposure of SV-40 transformed type 2 cells to hyperoxia results in proliferation arrest, increased IGFBP-2 accumulation in media and increased IGFBP-2 expression *(94)*. These changes rapidly reverse with a return to normoxia. In these cells, transforming growth factor (TGF)-β expression also increases with hyperoxia. TGF-β is a potent stimulator of IGFBP-2 expression suggesting that there is a link between the expression of these proteins in hyperoxia and control of cell proliferation. These results support the idea that growth factors may mediate their effects on lung cell growth through regulation of IGFBPs.

## Pulmonary Fibrosis and the IGF System

There is growing evidence to implicate the IGF system in the pathogenesis of pulmonary fibrosis. Several studies suggest that alveolar fluid from patients with inflammatory lung disease contains IGF-I that is mitogenically active. Using a rat model of silica-induced lung injury, Chen et al. *(95)* demonstrated increased immunoreactive IGF-I concentrations in bronchoalveolar lavage fluid (BALF) with progressively longer exposure to silica. BALF from patients with systemic sclerosis was shown to be more potent in stimulating fibroblast proliferation than BALF from control patients, a response that was attenuated with neutralizing antibodies for IGF-I *(96)*.

Lung biopsies from patients with idiopathic pulmonary fibrosis demonstrate abundant IGF-I and IGFBP-3 expression in interstitial mesenchymal cells, epithelial cells and macrophages *(97)*. Of particular interest is the evidence of IGF-I production by macrophages because of the importance of the activated alveolar macrophage as a cellular mediator of fibrotic lung disease. Macrophages isolated from lungs of patients with pulmonary fibrosis or various animal models of pulmonary fibrosis express IGF-I, IGF-1R, and IGFBP-3 *(95–99)*. Studies of cultured macrophages isolated from patients with idiopathic pulmonary fibrosis have shown increased IGFBP-3 but no change in IGF-I production compared to macrophages from control patients *(97)*, although the number of macrophages expressing these growth factors is greater from patients with idiopathic pulmonary fibrosis or sarcoidosis *(100)*.

These findings suggest that macrophages are a primary source of IGF-I and IGFBPs during pulmonary fibrosis. IGF-I, derived from pulmonary macrophages or other cell types, may act via the IGF-1R receptor to enhance macrophage proliferation or possibly affect other cell functions of the macrophages. IGF-I may also be active on nearby cells such as epithelial cells, fibroblasts, or smooth muscle cells. Cultured pulmonary fibroblasts have been shown to increase collagen formation with IGF-I *(77)* and IGF-I produced by postnatal airway epithelial cells is mitogenically active for cultured pulmonary fibroblasts *(101)*. Because IGFBP-3 may augment IGF-I mitogenic activity, increased production of IGFBPs may be an important mechanism for increasing IGF-I mitogenic activity on pulmonary cells during the fibrotic process.

Other factors are likely to modulate IGF system activity during lung injury. Proinflammatory cytokines are important mediators in the pathogenesis of inflammation and lung injury and growth factors such as PDGF *(100)* and TGF-α *(98)* are expressed in lungs with pulmonary fibrosis. Both of these growth factors and various proinflammatory cytokines are known to regulate IGF system proteins in lung as well as other cell types *(6,14,15)*. Regulation of IGFBPs by growth factors and cytokines is a major mechanism by which these factors modulate IGF-I activity *(21,32)* and may influence the proliferative response of lung cells to inflammation *(32)*.

With our present understanding of the actions of IGF system proteins and the information available concerning pulmonary fibrosis processes, it seems likely that IGF-I, IGF-1R, and IGFBP-3 (and possibly other IGFBPs) actively participate in both the development and chronic state of fibrotic lung disorders. Experimental results are consistent with autocrine/paracrine IGF-I activity during the pulmonary fibrosis and remodeling processes with modulation of the IGF-I bioactivity by IGFBPs. As with other organs, there are multiple influences on IGF system bioactivity, including cellular growth factors and cytokines, intercellular interactions, and environmental factors.

## LUNG CANCER AND THE IGF SYSTEM

The mitogenic actions of the IGFs have led investigators to explore the potential role of these growth factors in neoplastic processes. One of the earliest associations of the IGF system with lung tumors was the demonstration of increased immunoreactive IGF-I in primary human lung tumor biopsy specimens *(102)*. The content of IGF-I in the neoplastic tissue was shown to be 3 to 7 times greater than in the normal adjacent lung tissue. Various lung cancer cells produce immunoreactive IGF-I, express IGF-1R and mitogenically respond to exogenous IGF-I and IGF-II. Nakanishi et al. *(103)* found that adenocarcinoma (A549, SK-LU-1, Ca-Lu-6) and squamous cell carcinoma cell lines (Ca-Lu-1, and SK-Mes-1) produce measurable immunoreactive IGF-I, demonstrate IGF-1R binding, and respond to IGF-I with cell proliferation that may be abolished with IGF-1R antibody. Ankrapp et al. *(104)* was unable to measure IGF-I in lung cancer cell conditioned medium of some of the same cell lines. Inconsistencies such as these have been observed with other cell types and my result from differences in sample handling, sample preparation, or the method used for IGF-I measurement.

Many primary lung cancers express the IGF-1R, with squamous cell carcinomas exhibiting the most prominent expression *(105)*. Of 42 non-small cell lung cancer (NSCLC) and small cell lung cancer (SCLC) cell lines 41 expressed IGF-1R in two separate studies *(106,107)*. The presence of the IGF-1R may be of pathophysiologic significance for both tumor growth and metastasis *(7)*. Nude mice injected with lung cancer cells transfected with an IGF-1R antisense plasmid to decrease IGF-1R expression have prolonged survival compared to mice injected with cells with unaltered IGF-1R expression *(108)*. In addition, lung carcinoma cells with decreased IGF-1R expression do not respond to IGF-I in vitro and have a greatly reduced metastatic potential *(109)*.

Other investigators have examined the production of IGFBPs by lung tumor cell lines. SCLC cell lines primarily produce IGFBP-2 *(110–112)* and NSCLC cell lines produce a variety of IGFBPs *(113)*. Reeve et al. *(111)* studied the binding of radiolabeled IGF-I to the cell membrane of various SCLC and NSCLC cell lines and found that IGF-I primarily binds to IGFBP-2 on the surface of SCLC cells but binds to the IGF-1R for NSCLC cells, which have less membrane-associated IGFBP-2 . They speculated that IGFBPs on the surface of the SCLC cells may serve as a reservoir for IGF-I that may compete with the IGF-1R for IGF-I binding. As with normal lung cells, IGFBP production by lung cancer cells is regulated by IGF-I. Incubation of various NSCLC cells with IGF-I increases release of membrane associated IGFBP-3 and increases proteolysis of IGFBP-4 *(113,114)*.

These findings suggest that the IGF system participates in the pathogenesis of lung cancer growth and metastasis with IGF-I autocrine/paracrine effects mediated by the IGF-1R and modulated by IGFBPs.

## PNEUMONECTOMY AND THE IGF SYSTEM

Compensatory growth of the lung after pneumonectomy has been recognized for many years, but the causative mechanisms of the accelerated growth are incompletely understood. Evidence of cell proliferation and hypertrophy suggest that growth factors such as IGFs may be involved. In support of this, kidney tissue concentrations of IGF-I increase with compensatory growth *(115)*. Likewise, lung tissue concentrations of IGF protein were shown to be increased during early compensatory growth following pneumonectomy *(116)*. BALF obtained from lungs undergoing compensatory growth following pneumonectomy was found to contain increased IGF-I concentrations *(117)*. The predominate cell type in the BALF from the postpneumonectomy model at the time of increased IGF-I concentrations was macrophages, a possible source of IGF-I in lung *(80,82)*. Our studies of IGF system expression postpneumonectomy found no increase in IGF-I mRNA expression in the first week following pneumonectomy in 6-wk-old male rats, nor changes in tissue or serum concentrations of IGF-I *(118)* in contrast to earlier reports. We also found that lungs from animals undergoing pneumonectomy had greatly reduced IGF-II expression on the first postoperative day compared to sham-operated animals and small changes in transcript abundance for IGFBPs-2 through -6 were noted, but were not felt to be of physiologic significance. Based on these findings, we concluded that the changes observed in the lung IGF system transcripts do not likely represent a major contribution to postpneumonectomy lung growth. The findings leading to our conclusion should not be misinterpreted to indicate that the IGF system does not participate in postpneumonectomy lung growth, but rather that intrinsic lung production of the IGF system proteins likely play an interactive role with other growth promoting factors in the lung or derived from serum during the process and are not necessarily directive in the process.

## THE PULMONARY HYPERTENSION AND THE IGF SYSTEM

The pathogenesis of pulmonary hypertension is complex. Two of the pathologic hallmarks of pulmonary hypertension are SMC hypertrophy and/or hyperplasia and excessive ECM deposition. Given the role of IGFs in both of these processes, it is not surprising that IGFs have been implicated in the pathogenesis of pulmonary hypertension in the neonate and adult. IGF-I appears to play a major role in the mitogenic and hypertrophic response of vascular SMCs to various stimuli including vascular load, growth factors and hypoxia, all of which may contribute to the pathogenesis of pulmonary hypertension *(119)*. For example, IGF-I stimulates pulmonary artery SMC proliferation, a response that is enhanced in cells derived from animals exposed to hypoxia *(120)* . In addition to promoting mitogenesis, IGFs stimulate elastin and collagen synthesis in pulmonary vascular walls *(76,121)* and may contribute to ECM deposition. Endothelial cell IGFBP production is also regulated by hypoxia *(122)*, suggesting a mechanism by which endothelial cells may modulate the activity of IGF on nearby cells. Pulmonary hypertension is also associated with various inflammatory diseases of the lung. Inflammatory cytokines can directly stimulate IGF-I production by endothelial cells *(123)*. Also, reactive oxygen species, produced in response to proinflammatory cytokines, are capable of stimulating IGF-I synthesis and decreasing production of inhibitory IGFBP-4 by vascular SMCs *(124)*. In addition, a role for IGF-I in the control of vascular tone has been proposed based on studies showing that IGF-I regulates production of nitric oxide by cultured endothelial cells *(125)*. Taken together, these studies suggest several mechanisms by which IGFs may promote SMC proliferation, ECM production, and/or changes in vascular tone and contribute to the pathogenesis of pulmonary hypertension.

## SUMMARY

Despite accumulating evidence of the IGF system's importance in lung, the role of these proteins remains incompletely understood. The presence of the IGFs at critical stages of lung development and in the mature lung argues for an important role of the IGF system in lung development and maintenance. Furthermore, the effects of the IGFs on cell survival, the production of components of the IGF system by inflammatory cells, and the alterations in IGF system expression by proinflammatory mediators are areas of investigation that are incomplete, but are of potential importance in treating or preventing lung disease.

## ACKNOWLEDGMENTS

This work was supported by grants from the National Institutes of Health (HL55581;WAP and HL19171 SCOR; ADS).

## REFERENCES

1. Stewart CEH, Rotwein P. Growth, differentiation, and survival: multiple physiological functions for insulin-like growth factors. Physiol Rev 1996;76:1005–1026.
2. Jones JI, Clemmons DR. Insulin-like growth factors and their binding proteins: biological actions. Endocr Rev 1995;16:3–34.
3. Underwood LE. Nutritional regulation of IGF-I and IGFBPs. J Pediatr Endocrinol Metab 1996;9(Suppl 3):303–312.
4. Matsumoto T, Tsukazaki T, Enomoto H, Iwasaki K, Yamashita S. Effects of interleukin-1β on insulin-like growth factor-I autocrine/paracrine axis in cultured rat articular chondrocytes. Ann Rheum Dis 1994;53:128–133.
5. Linkhart TA, MacCharles DC. Interleukin-1 stimulates release of insulin-like growth factor-I from neonatal mouse calvaria by a prostaglandin synthesis-dependent mechanism. Endocrinology 1992;131:2297–2305.

6. Franchimont N, Gangji V, Durant D, Canalis E. Interleukin-6 with its soluble receptor enhances the expression of insulin-like growth factor-I in osteoblasts. Endocrinology 1997;138:5248–5255.

7. Rubin R, Baserga R. Insulin-like growth factor-I receptor – Its role in cell proliferation, apoptosis, and tumorigenicity. Lab Invest 1995;73:311–331.

8. Sepp–Lorenzino L. Structure and function of the insulin-like growth factor I receptor. Breast Cancer Res Treat 1998;47:235–253.

9. Riesewijk AM, Schepens MT, Welch TR, Van den Berg–Loonen EM, Mariman EM, Ropers HH, Kalscheuer VM. Maternal-specific methylation of the human IGF2R gene is not accompanied by allele-specific transcription. Genomics 1996;31:158–166.

10. Clemmons DR. Insulin-like growth factor binding proteins and their role in controlling IGF actions. Cytokine Growth Factor Rev 1997;8:45–62.

11. Oh Y. IGF-independent regulation of breast cancer growth by IGF binding proteins. Breast Cancer Res Treat 1998;47:283–293.

12. Kim HS, Nagalla SR, Oh Y, Wilson E, Roberts CTJ, Rosenfeld RG. Identification of a family of low-affinity insulin-like growth factor binding proteins (IGFBPs): characterization of connective tissue growth factor as a member of the IGFBP superfamily. Proc Natl Acad Sci USA 1997;94:12981–12986.

13. Olney RC, Wilson DM, Mohtai M, Fielder PJ, Smith RL. Interleukin-1 and tumor necrosis factor-alpha increase insulin-like growth factor-binding protein-3 (IGFBP-3) production and IGFBP-3 protease activity in human articular chondrocytes. J Endocrinol 1995;146:279–286.

14. Scharla SH, Strong DD, Mohan S, Chevalley T, Linkhart TA. Effect of tumor necrosis factor-a on the expression of insulin-like growth factor I and insulin-like growth factor binding protein 4 in mouse osteoblasts. Acta Endocrinol (Copenh) 1994;131:293–301.

15. Price WA. Peptide growth factors regulate insulin-like growth factor binding protein production by fetal rat lung fibroblasts. Am J Respir Cell Mol Biol. 1998;20:332–341.

16. Guan J, Williams C, Gunning M, Mallard C and Gluckman P. The effects of IGF-1 treatment after hypoxic-ischemic brain injury in adult rats. J Cereb Blood Flow Metab 1993;13:609–616.

17. Beilharz EJ, Klempt ND, Klempt M, Sirimanne E, Dragunow M, Gluckman PD. Differential expression of insulin-like growth factor binding proteins.IGFBP-4 and -5 mRNA in the rat brain after transient hypoxic-ischemic injury. Mol Brain Res 1993;18:209–215.

18. Rajah R, Valentinis B, Cohen P. Insulin like growth factor (IGF)-binding protein-3 induces apoptosis and mediates the effects of transforming growth factor-β1 on programmed cell death through a p53- and IGF-independent mechanism. J Biol Chem 1997;272:12181–12188.

19. Oh Y, Müller HL, Lamson G, Rosenfeld RG. Insulin-like growth factor (IGF)-independent action of IGF-binding protein-3 in Hs578T human breast cancer cells. Cell surface binding and growth inhibition. J Biol Chem 1993;268:14964–14971.

20. Mohseni–Zadeh S, Binoux M. Insulin-like growth factor.IGF binding protein-3 interacts with the type 1 IGF receptor, reducing the affinity of the receptor for its ligand: an alternative mechanism in the regulation of IGF action. Endocrinology 1997;138:5645–5648.

21. Gucev ZS, Oh Y, Kelley KM, Rosenfeld RG. Insulin-like growth factor binding protein 3 mediates retinoic acid- and transforming growth factor β2-induced growth inhibition in human breast cancer cells. Cancer Res 1996;56:1545–1550.

22. Singh P, Dai B, Dhruva B, Widen SG. Episomal expression of sense and antisense insulin-like growth factor (IGF)-binding protein-4 complementary DNA alters the mitogenic response of a human colon cancer cell line.HT-29; by mechanisms that are independent of and dependent upon IGF-I. Cancer Res 1994;54:6563–6570.

23. Andress DL. Insulin-like growth factor-binding protein-5 (IGFBP-5) stimulates phosphorylation of the IGFBP-5 receptor. Am J Physiol Endocrinol Metab 1998;274:E744–E750.

24. Oh Y, Müller HL, Pham H, Rosenfeld RG. Demonstration of receptors for insulin-like growth factor binding protein-3 on Hs578T human breast cancer cells. J Biol Chem 1993;268:26045–26048.

25. Scharla SH, Strong DD, Rosen C, Mohan S, Holick M, Baylink DJ, Linkhart TA. 1,25-Dihydroxyvitamin D$_3$ increases secretion of insulin-like growth factor binding protein-4 (IGFBP-4) by human osteoblast-like cells in vitro and elevates IGFBP-4 serum levels in vivo. J Clin Endocrinol Metab 1993;77:1190–1197.

26. Okazaki, R, Riggs BL, Conover CA. Glucocorticoid regulation of insulin-like growth factor– binding protein expression in normal human osteoblast-like cells. Endocrinology 1994;134:126–132.

27. DiBattista JA, Doré S, Morin N, Abribat T. Prostaglandin E$_2$ up-regulates insulin-like growth factor binding protein-3 expression and synthesis in human articular chondrocytes by a c-AMP-independent pathway: role of calcium and protein kinase A and C. J Cell Biochem 1996;63:320–333.

28. Gabbitas B, Canalis E. Growth factor regulation of insulin-like growth factor binding protein-6 expression in osteoblasts. J Cell Biochem 1997;66:77–86.

29. Grimes RW, Samaras SE, Barber JA, Shimasaki S, Ling N. Gonadotropin and cAMP modulation of IGF binding protein. Am J Physiol 1992;262:E497–E503.

30. Liu X-J, Malkowski M, Guo Y, Erickson GF, Shimasaki S, Ling N. Development of specific antibodies to rat insulin-like growth factor-binding proteins (IGFBP-2 to -6): analysis of IGFBP production by rat granulosa cells. Endocrinology 1993;132:1176–1183.

31. Cataldo NA, Fujimoto VY, Jaffe RB. Interferon-gamma and activin A promote insulin-like growth factor-binding protein-2 and -4 accumulation by human luteinizing granulosa cells, and interferon–gamma promotes their apoptosis. J Clin Endocrinol Metab 1998;83:179–186.

32. Huynh H, Yang XF, Pollak M. A role for insulin-like growth factor binding protein 5 in the antiproliferative action of the antiestrogen ICI 182780. Cell Growth Differ 1996;7:1501–1506.

33. Stiles AD, D'Ercole AJ. The insulin-like growth factors and the lung. Am J Respir Cell Mol Biol 1990;3:93–100.

34. Han VK, D'Ercole AJ, Lund PK. Cellular localization of somatomedin (insulin-like growth factor) messenger RNA in the human fetus. Science 1987;236:193–197.

35. Schuller AG, Van NJ, Beukenholdt RW, Zwarthoff EC, Drop SL. IGF, type I IGF receptor and IGF–binding protein mRNA expression in the developing mouse lung. J Mol Endocrinol 1995;14:349–355.

36. Lund PK, Moats–Staats BM, Hynes MA, Simmons JG, Jansen M, D'Ercole AJ, Van Wyk JJ. Somatomedin-C/insulin-like growth factor-I and insulin-like growth factor-II mRNAs in rat fetal and adult tissues. J Biol Chem 1986;261:14539–14544.

37. Davenport ML, D'Ercole AJ, Azizkhan JC, Lund PK. Somatomedin-C/insulin-like growth factor I.Sm-C/IGF-I; and insulin-like growth factor II (IGF-II) mRNAs during lung development in the rat. Exp Lung Res 1988;14:607–618.

38. Brown AL, Graham DE, Nissley SP, Hill DJ, Strain AJ, Rechler MM. Developmental regulation of insulin-like growth factor II mRNA in different rat tissues. J Biol Chem 1986;261:13144–13150.

39. Hooper SB, Han VKM, Harding R. Changes in lung expansion alter pulmonary DNA synthesis and IGF-II gene expression in fetal sheep. Am J Physiol Lung Cell Mol Physiol 1993;265:L403–L409.

40. Joe P, Wallen LD, Chapin CJ, Lee CH, Allen L, Han VKM, Dobbs LG, Hawgood S, Kitterman JA. Effects of mechanical factors on growth and maturation of the lung in fetal sheep. Am J Physiol Lung Cell Mol Physiol 1997;272:L95–L105.

41. Cohen P, Noveral JP, Bhala A, Nunn SE, Herrick DJ, Grunstein MM. Leukotriene $D_4$ facilitates airway smooth muscle cell proliferation via modulation of the IGF axis. Am J Physiol Lung Cell Mol Physiol 1995;269:L151–L157.

42. Maitre B, Clement A, Williams MC, Brody JS. Expression of insulin-like growth factor receptors 1 and 2 in the developing lung and their relation to epithelial cell differentiation. Am J Respir Cell Mol Biol 1995;13:262–270.

43. Batchelor DC, Hutchins AM, Klempt M, Skinner SJM. Developmental changes in the expression patterns of IGFs, type 1 IGF receptor and IGF-binding proteins-2 and -4 in perinatal rat lung. J Mol Endocrinol 1995;15:105–115.

44. Han, VKM, Matsell, DG, Delhanty, PJD, Hill, DJ, Shimasaki, S and Nygard, K.1996; IGF-binding protein mRNAs in the human fetus: Tissue and cellular distribution of developmental expression HormRes 45, 160–166.

45. Lallemand AV, Ruocco SM, Joly PM, Gaillard DA. In vivo localization of the insulin-like growth factors I and II (IGF-I and IGF-II) gene expression during human lung development. Int J Dev Biol 1995;39:529–537.

46. Birnbacher R, Amann G, Breitschopf H, Lassmann H, Suchanek G, Heinz-Erian P. Cellular localization of insulin-like growth factor II mRNA in the human fetus and the placenta: detection with a digoxigenin-labeled cRNA probe and immunocytochemistry. Pediatr Res 1998;43:614–620.

47. Delhanty PJ, Hill DJ, Shimasaki S, Han VK. Insulin-like growth factor binding protein-4, -5 and -6 mRNAs in the human fetus: localization to sites of growth and differentiation? Growth Regulation 1993;3:8–11.

48. Klempt M, Hutchins A-M, Gluckman PD, Skinner SJM. IGF binding protein-2 gene expression and the location of IGF-I and IGF-II in fetal rat lung. Development 1992;115:765–772.

49. Retsch–Bogart GZ, Moats–Staats BM, Howard K, D'Ercole AJ, Stiles AD. Cellular localization of messenger RNAs for insulin-like growth factors (IGFs), their receptors and binding proteins during fetal rat lung development. Am J Respir Cell Mol Biol 1996;14:61–69.

50. Wallen LD, Myint W, Nygard K, Shimasaki S, Clemmons DR, Han VM. Cellular distribution of insulin-like growth factor binding protein mRNAs and peptides during rat lung development. J Endocrinol 1997;155:313–327.

51. Wallen LD, Han VKM. Spatial and temporal distribution of insulin-like growth factors I and II during development of rat lung. Am J Physiol Lung Cell Mol Physiol 1994;267:L531–L542.

52. Han VK, Hill DJ, Strain AJ, Towle AC, Lauder JM, Underwood LE, D'Ercole AJ. Identification of somatomedin/insulin-like growth factor immunoreactive cells in the human fetus. Pediatr Res 1987;22:245–249.

53. Hill DJ, Clemmons DR. Similar distribution of insulin-like growth factor binding proteins-1,-2,-3 in human fetal tissues. Growth Factors 1992;6:315–326.

54. Wallen LD, Han VKM. Spatial and temporal distribution of insulin-like growth factors I and II during development of rat lung. Am J Physiol 1994;267:L531–L542.

55. Han RNN, Han VKM, Buch S, Freeman BA, Post M, Tanswell AK. Insulin-like growth factor-I and type I insulin-like growth factor receptor in 85% $O_2$-exposed rat lung. Am J Physiol Lung Cell Mol Physiol 1996;271:L139–L149.

56. Stiles AD, Smith BT, Post M. Reciprocal autocrine and paracrine regulation of growth of mesenchymal and alveolar epithelial cells from fetal lung. Exp Lung Res 1986;11:165–177.

57. Atkinson PR, Weidman ER, Bhaumick B, Bala RM. Release of somatomedin-like activity by cultured WI-38 human fibroblasts. Endocrinology 1980;106:2006–2012.

58. Phillips PD, Pignolo RJ, Cristofalo VJ. Insulin-like growth factor-I: specific binding to high and low affinity sites and mitogenic action throughout the life span of WI-38 cells. J Cell Physiol 1987;133:135–143.

59. Moats-Staats BM, Retsch-Bogart GZ, Price WA, Jarvis HW, D'Ercole AJ, Stiles AD. Insulin-like growth factor-I (IGF-I) antisense oligodeoxynucleotide mediated inhibition of DNA synthesis by WI-38 cells: evidence for autocrine actions of IGF-I. Mol Endocrinol 1993;7:171–180.

60. Stiles AD, Moats-Staats BM. Production and action of insulin-like growth factor I/somatomedin-C in primary cultures of fetal lung fibroblasts. Am J Respir Cell Mol Biol 1989;1:21–26.

61. Price WA, Moats-Staats BM, D'Ercole AJ, Stiles AD. Insulin-like growth factor binding protein production by fetal lung cells. Am J Respir Cell Mol Biol 1993;8:425–432.

62. Fraslon C, Bourbon JR. Comparison of effects of epidermal and insulin-like growth factors, gastrin releasing peptide and retinoic acid on fetal lung cell growth and maturation in vitro. Biochim Biophys Acta Lipids Lipid Metab 1992;1123:65–75.

63. Hill DJ, Clemmons DR, Wilson S, Han VK, Strain AJ, Milner RD. Immunological distribution of one form of insulin-like growth factor (IGF)-binding protein and IGF peptides in human fetal tissues. J Mol Endocrinol 1989;2:31–38.

64. Retsch-Bogart GZ, Stiles AD, Moats-Staats BM, Van Scott MR, Boucher RC, D'Ercole AJ. Canine tracheal epithelial cells express the type 1 insulin-like growth factor receptor and proliferate in response to insulin-like growth factor I. Am J Respir Cell Mol Biol 1990;3:227–234.

65. Shoji S, Ertl RF, Linder J, Koizumi S, Duckworth WC, Rennard SI. Bronchial epithelial cells respond to insulin and insulin-like growth factor-I as a chemoattractant Am J Resp Cell Mol Biol 1990;2:553–557.

66. Deterding RR, Jacoby CR, Shannon JM. Acidic fibroblast growth factor and keratinocyte growth factor stimulate fetal rat pulmonary epithelial growth. Am J Physiol Lung Cell Mol Physiol 1996;271:L495–L505.

67. Mouhieddine OB, Cazals V, Maitre B, Le Bouc Y, Chadelat K, Clement A. Insulin-like growth factor-II (IGF-II), type 2 IGF receptor, and IGF-binding protein-2 gene expression in rat lung alveolar epithelial cells: Relation to proliferation. Endocrinology 1994;135:83–91.

68. Mouhieddine OB, Cazals V, Kuto E, Le Bouc Y, Clement A. Glucocorticoid-induced growth arrest of lung alveolar epithelial cells is associated with increased production of insulin-like growth factor binding protein-2. Endocrinology 1996;137:287–295.

69. Powell–Braxton L, Hollingshead P, Warburton C, Dowd M, Pitts–Meek S, Dalton D, Gillett N, Stewart TA. IGF–I is required for normal embryonic growth in mice. Genes Dev 1993;7:2609–2617.

70. DeChiara TM, Efstratiadis A, Robertson EJ. A growth–deficiency phenotype in heterozygous mice carrying an insulin-like growth factor II gene disrupted by targeting. Nature 1990;345:78–80.

71. Liu J-P, Baker J, Perkins AS, Robertson EJ, Efstratiadis A. Mice carrying null mutations of the genes encoding insulin– like growth factor I (Igf-1) and type 1 IGF receptor (Igf1r). Cell 1993;75:59–72.

72. Melnick M, Chen HM, Rich KA, Jaskoll T. Developmental expression of insulin-like growth factor II receptor (IGF-IIR) in congenic mouse embryonic lungs: Correlation between IGF-IIR mRNA and protein levels and heterochronic lung development. Mol Reprod Dev 1996;44:159–170.

73. Dempsey EC, Badesch DB, Dobyns EL, Stenmark KR. Enhanced growth capacity of neonatal pulmonary artery smooth muscle cells in vitro: Dependence on cell size, time from birth, insulin-like growth factor I, and auto-activation of protein kinase C. J Cell Physiol 1994;160:469–481.

74. Dempsey EC, Stenmark KR, McMurtry IF, O'Brien RF, Voelkel NF, Badesch DB. Insulin-like growth factor I and protein kinase C activation stimulate pulmonary artery smooth muscle cell proliferation through separate but synergistic pathways. J Cell Physiol 1990;144:159–165.

75. Davies P, Patton W. Peripheral and central vascular smooth muscle cells from rat lung exhibit different cytoskeletal protein profiles but similar growth factor requirements. J Cell Physiol 1994;159:399–406.

76. Badesch DB, Lee PDK, Parks WC, Stenmark KR. Insulin-like growth factor I stimulates elastin synthesis by bovine pulmonary arterial smooth muscle cells. Biochem Biophys Res Commun 1989;160:382–387.

77. Goldstein RH, Poliks CF, Pilch PF, Smith BD, Fine A. Stimulation of collagen formation by insulin and insulin-like growth factor I in cultures of human lung fibroblasts. Endocrinology 1989;124:964–970.

78. Boes M, Booth BA, Dake BL, Moser DR, Bar RS. Insulin-like growth factor binding protein production by bovine and human vascular smooth muscle cells: production of insulin-like growth factor binding protein-6 by human smooth muscle. Endocrinology 1996;137:5357–5363.

79. Imai Y, Busby WHJ, Smith CE, Clarke JB, Garmong AJ, Horwitz GD, Rees C, Clemmons DR. Protease-resistant form of insulin-like growth factor-binding protein 5 is an inhibitor of insulin-like growth factor-I actions on porcine smooth muscle cells in culture. J Clin Invest 1997;100:2596–2605.

80. Rom WN, Basset P, Fells GA, Nukiwa T, Trapnell BC, Crystal RG. Alveolar macrophages release an insulin-like growth factor I-type molecule. J Clin Invest 1988;82:1685–1693.

81. Nagaoka I, Trapnell BC, Crystal RG. Regulation of insulin-like growth factor I gene expression in the human macrophage-like cell line U937. J Clin Invest 1990;85:448–455.

82. Noble PW, Lake FR, Henson PM, Riches DWH. Hyaluronate activation of CD44 induces insulin-like growth factor-1 expression by a tumor necrosis factor-$\alpha$-dependent mechanism in murine macrophages. J Clin Invest 1993;91:2368–2377.

83. Nyman T, Pekonen F. The expression of insulin-like growth factors and their binding proteins in normal human lymphocytes. Acta Endocrinol (Copenh) 1993;128:168–172.

84. Rajah R, Nunn SE, Herrick DJ, Grunstein MM, Cohen P. Leukotriene $D_4$ induces MMP-1, which functions as an IGFBP protease in human airway smooth muscle cells. Am J Physiol Lung Cell Mol Physiol 1996;271:L1014–L1022.

85. Price WA, Stiles AD, Moats–Staats BM, D'Ercole AJ. Gene expression of insulin-like growth factors (IGFs), the type 1 IGF receptor, and IGF-binding proteins in dexamethasone-induced fetal growth retardation. Endocrinology 1992;130:1424–1432.

86. Mauceri HJ, Lee W–H, Conway S. Effect of ethanol on insulin-like growth factor-II release from fetal organs. Alcoholism (NY) 1994;18:35–41.

87. Fatayerji N, Engelmann GL, Myers T, Handa RJ. In utero exposure to ethanol alters mRNA for insulin-like growth factors and insulin-like growth factor-binding proteins in placenta and lung of fetal rats. Alcohol Clin Exp Res 1996;20:4–100.

88. McLellan KC, Hooper SB, Bocking AD, Delhanty PJD, Phillips ID, Hill DJ, Han VKM. Prolonged hypoxia induced by the reduction of maternal uterine blood flow alters insulin-like growth factor-binding protein-1 (IGFBP-1) and IGFBP-2 gene expression in the ovine fetus. Endocrinology 1992;131:1619–1628.

89. Moromisato DY, Moromisato MY, Zanconato S, Roberts CT Jr, Brasel JA, Cooper DM. Effect of hypoxia on lung, heart, and liver insulin-like growth factor-I gene and receptor expression in the newborn rat. Crit Care Med 1996;24:919–924.

90. Tanswell AK, Han RN, Buch SJ, Fraher LJ. Circulating factors that modify lung cell DNA synthesis following exposure to inhaled oxidants III Effects of plasma on lung pneumocyte and fibroblast DNA synthesis following exposure of adult rats to 85% oxygen. Exp Lung Res 1991;17:869–886.

91. Han RNN, Buch S, Tseu I, Young J, Christie NA, Frndova H, Lye SJ, Post M, Tanswell AK. Changes in structure, mechanics, and insulin-like growth factor-related gene expression in the lungs of newborn rats exposed to air or 60% oxygen. Pediatr Res 1996;39:921–929.

92. Veness-Meehan KA, Moats-Staats BM, Price WA, Stiles AD. Re-emergence of a fetal pattern of insulin-like growth factor expression during hyperoxic rat lung injury. Am J Respir Cell Mol Biol 1997;16:538–548.

93. Kelleher MD, Naureckas ET, Solway J, Hershenson MB. In vivo hyperoxic exposure increases cultured lung fibroblast proliferation and c-Ha-ras expression. Am J Respir Cell Mol Biol 1995;12:19–26.

94. Cazals V, Mouhieddine B, Maitre B, Le Bouc Y, Chadelat K, Brody JS, Clement A. Insulin-like growth factors, their binding proteins, and transforming growth factor-$\beta$ 1 in oxidant-arrested lung alveolar epithelial cells. J Biol Chem 1994;269:14111–14117.

95.  Chen F, Deng HY, Ding GF, Houng DW, Deng YL, Long ZZ. Excessive production of insulin-like growth factor-I by silicotic rat alveolar macrophages. APMIS 1994;102:581–588.

96.  Harrison NK, Cambrey AD, Myers AR, Southcott AM, Black CM, Du Bois RM, Laurent GJ, McAnulty RJ. Insulin-like growth factor-I is partially responsible for fibroblast proliferation induced by bronchoalveolar lavage fluid from patients with systemic sclerosis. Clin Sci 1994;86:141–148.

97.  Aston C, Jagirdar J, Lee TC, Hur T, Hintz RL, Rom WN. Enhanced insulin-like growth factor molecules in idiopathic pulmonary fibrosis. Am J Respir Crit Care Med 1995;151:1597–1603.

98.  Lee TC, Gold LI, Reibman J, Aston C, Begin R, Rom WN, Jagirdar J. Immunohistochemical localization of transforming growth factor-beta and insulin-like growth factor-I in asbestosis in the sheep model. Int Arch Occup Environ Health 1997;69:157–164.

99.  Melloni B, Lesur O, Bouhadiba T, Cantin A, Bégin R. Partial characterization of the proliferative activity for fetal lung epithelial cells produced by silica-exposed alveolar macrophages. J Leukoc Biol 1994;55:574–580.

100.  Homma S, Nagaoka I, Abe H, Takahashi K, Seyama K, Nukiwa T, Kira S. Localization of platelet-derived growth factor and insulin-like growth factor I in the fibrotic lung. Am J Respir Crit Care Med 1995;152:2084–2089.

101.  Cambrey AD, Kwon OJ, Gray AJ, Harrison NK, Yacoub M, Barnes PJ, Laurent GJ, Chung KF. Insulin-like growth factor I is a major fibroblast mitogen produced by primary cultures of human airway epithelial cells. Clin Sci 1995;89:611–617.

102.  Minuto F, Del Monte P, Barreca A. Evidence for increased somatomedin–C/insulin-like growth factor I content in primary human lung tumors. Cancer Res 1986;46:985–988.

103.  Nakanishi Y, Mulshine JL, Kasprzyk PG, Natale RB, Maneckjee R, Avis I, Treston AM, Gazdar AF, Minna JD, Cuttitta F. Insulin-like growth factor I can mediate autocrine proliferation of small cell lung cancer cell lines in vitro. J Clin Inv 1988;82:354–359.

104.  Ankrapp DP, Bevan DR. Insulin-like growth factor-I and human lung fibroblast-derived insulin-like growth factor-I stimulate the proliferation of human lung carcinoma cells in vitro. Cancer Res 1993;53:3399–3404.

105.  Kaiser U, Schardt C, Brandscheidt D, Wollmer E, Havemann K. Expression of insulin-like growth factor receptors I and II in normal human lung and in lung cancer. J Cancer Res Clin Oncol 1993;119:665–668.

106.  Rotsch M, Maasberg M, Erbil C, Jaques G, Worsch U, Havemann K. Characterization of insulin-like growth factor I receptors and growth effects in human lung cancer cell lines. J Cancer Res Clin Oncol 1992;118:502–508.

107.  Quinn KA, Treston AM, Unsworth EJ, Miller MJ, Vos M, Grimley C, Battey J, Mulshine JL, Cuttitta F. Insulin-like growth factor expression in human cancer cell lines. J Biol Chem 1996;271:11,477–11,483.

108.  Lee CT, Wu S, Gabrilovich D, Chen HL, Nadaf-Rahrov S, Ciernik IF, Carbone DP. Antitumor effects of an adenovirus expressing antisense insulin-like growth factor I receptor on human lung cancer cell lines. Cancer Res 1996;56:3038–3041.

109.  Long L, Rubin R, Baserga R, Brodt P. Loss of the metastatic phenotype in murine carcinoma cells expressing an antisense RNA to the insulin-like growth factor receptor. Cancer Res 1995;55:1006–1009.

110.  Reeve JG, Brinkman A, Hughes S, Mitchell J, Schwander J, Bleehen NM. Expression of insulin-like growth factor (IGF) and IGF binding protein genes in human lung tumor cell lines. J Natl Cancer Inst 1992;84:628–634.

111.  Reeve JG, Morgan J, Schwander J, Bleehen NM. Role for membrane and secreted insulin-like growth factor-binding protein-2 in the regulation of insulin-like growth factor action in lung tumors. Cancer Res 1993;53:4680–4685.

112.  Kiefer P, Jaques G, Schoneberger J, Heinrich G, Havemann K. Insulin-like growth factor binding protein expression in human small cell lung cancer cell lines. Exp Cell Res 1991;192:414–417.

113.  Noll K, Wegmann BR, Havemann K, Jaques G. Insulin-like growth factors stimulate the release of insulin-like growth factor-binding protein-3 (IGFBP-3) and degradation of IGFBP-4 in nonsmall cell lung cancer cell lines. J Clin Endocrinol Metab 1996;81:2653–2662.

114.  Price WA, Moats-Staats BM, Stiles AD. Insulin-like growth factor-I (IGF-I) regulates IGFBP-3 and IGFBP-4 by multiple mechanisms in A549 human adenocarcinoma cells. Am J Respir Cell Mol Biol 1995;13:466–476.

115.  Stiles AD, Sosenko IR, D'Ercole AJ, Smith BT. Relation of kidney tissue somatomedin-C/insulin-like growth factor I to postnephrectomy renal growth in the rat. Endocrinology 1985;117:2397–2401.

116.  Khadempour MH, Ofulue AF, Sekhon HS, Cherukupalli KM, Thurlbeck WM. Changes of growth hormone, somatomedin C, and bombesin following pneumonectomy. Exp Lung Res 1992;18:421–432.

117. McAnulty RJ, Guerreiro D, Cambrey AD, Laurent GJ. Growth factor activity in the lung during compensatory growth after pneumonectomy: evidence of a role for IGF-1. Eur Respir J 1992;5:739–747.
118. Price WA, Moats-Staats BM, Sekhon HS, Chrzanowska BL, Thurlbeck WM, Stiles AD. Expression of the insulin-like growth factor system in postpneumonectomy lung growth. Exp Lung Res 1998;24:203–217.
119. Delafontaine P. Insulin-like growth factor I and its binding proteins in the cardiovascular system. Cardiovasc Res 1995;30:825–834.
120. Xu Y, Stenmark KR, Das M, Walchak SJ, Ruff LJ, Dempsey EC. Pulmonary artery smooth muscle cells from chronically hypoxic neonatal calves retain fetal-like and acquire new growth properties. Am J Physiol 1997;273:L234–L245.
121. Morin FC, Stenmark KR. Persistent pulmonary hypertension of the newborn. Am J Respir Crit Care Med 1995;151:2010–2032.
122. Tucci M, Nygard K, Tanswell BV, Farber HW, Hill DJ, Han VM. Modulation of insulin-like growth factor (IGF) and IGF binding protein biosynthesis by hypoxia in cultured vascular endothelial cells. J Endocrinol 1998;157:13–24.
123. Glazebrook H, Hatch T, Brindle NJ. Regulation of insulin-like growth factor-1 expression in vascular endothelial cells by the inflammatory cytokine interleukin-1. J Vasc Res 1998;35:143–149.
124. Delafontaine P, Ku L. Reactive oxygen species stimulate insulin-like growth factor I synthesis in vascular smooth muscle cells. Cardiovasc Res 1997;33:216–222.
125. Muniyappa R, Walsh MF, Rangi JS, Zayas RM Standley PR, Ram JL, Sowers JR. Insulin like growth factor 1 increases vascular smooth muscle nitric oxide production. Life Sci 1997;61:925–931.

# 12

## Platelet-Derived Growth Factor and Lung Development

*Nicholas J. Cartel and Martin Post, PhD*

### CONTENTS

## PLATELET-DERIVED GROWTH FACTOR: AN INTRODUCTION

Platelet-derived growth factor (PDGF) is a potent stimulant of connective-tissue cell proliferation and migration. PDGF is a dimer composed of two highly homologous peptide chains, A and B, joined by disulfide bonds. Three different forms of PDGF exist in vivo: PDGF-AA, PDGF-AB, and PDGF-BB. The three isoforms of PDGF differ in their functional properties as well as in their secretory behavior *(1)*. The A-chain and B-chain precursors both contain signal sequences that allow PDGF-AA and PDGF-AB to be rapidly secreted from their producer cell. A 24-kD form of PDGF-BB remains, to a large extent, associated with the producer cell, and relatively small amounts of the 30-kD PDGF-BB are secreted *(2,3)*. Homodimeric isoforms of PDGF are widely

From: *Contemporary Endocrinology: Endocrinology of the Lung: Development and Surfactant Synthesis*
Edited by: C. R. Mendelson © Humana Press Inc., Totowa, NJ

expressed by normal cell lines and tissue. As mentioned, PDGF is well recognized to be a potent mitogen for cells of mesenchymal origin, but recent findings have shown that it may also induce growth of some specialized epithelial cells *(4)*, capillary endothelial cells *(5)*, and some types of white blood cells *(6)*. In analogy with the different PDGF chains, two different high-affinity PDGF receptors, α and β, are expressed by many cell types *(7)*. The PDGF receptor is a representative of a class of receptor tyrosine kinases distinct from other receptors because the catalytic domain is split by an intervening stretch of approx 100 amino acids, and the extracellular region is organized into immunoglobulinlike repeats *(8)*. PDGF-BB can bind to both PDGF α- and β-receptors, whereas PDGF-AA binds only the α-receptor *(9)*. Upon binding of a PDGF dimer to its receptor, two appropriate PDGF receptor subunits are brought together, and a number of specific tyrosine residues on the receptor subunits are phosphorylated *(10)*. This receptor tyrosine autophosphorylation is manifested as a transphosphorylation between the two receptor dimers. There are 16 known autophosphorylated tyrosine residues in the β-receptor for PDGF. One site is a conserved tyrosine residue localized inside the kinase domain ($Tyr^{857}$). Mutation of this residue to a phenylalanine residue gives a receptor with a lowered kinase activity, suggesting that phosphorylation of $Tyr^{857}$ is important for activation of the kinase *(11)*. A total of 11 of the 15 tyrosine residues in the noncatalytic part of the receptor are phosphorylated. Mapping data of phosphorylated residues on the α-receptor are less well characterized *(12)*. The receptor tyrosine phosphorylation creates binding sites for several molecules that interact with specific phosphotyrosines through their SH2 (src homology 2) domains *(13)*. The SH2 domain proteins that interact with the PDGF β-receptor fall into two categories: (i) molecules with enzymatic or other activity, and (ii) adaptor molecules which serve to connect the receptor with other molecules *(14)*. Phospholipase Cγ (PLCγ), Ras GTPase-activating protein (Ras-GAP), the regulatory subunit of phosphatidylinositol 3-kinase (p85 of PI 3-kinase), growth factor receptor-bound protein 2 (GRB2), the tyrosine-specific phosphatase Syp, Src homology and collagen protein (Shc), and members of the Src family have been found to bind specific phosphotyrosines in the activated PDGF β-receptor *(15)*. Receptor dimerization and the subsequent receptor autophosphorylation and tyrosine-kinase activation are required for transduction of the signals leading to proliferation and migration *(16)*. The ability of homo- and heterodimers of PDGF to induce mitogenesis and migration depends on both the PDGF dimer present and the relative numbers of the two different PDGF receptor subunits on the responding cell *(17)*. There is considerable cross-talk between different signaling pathways and stimulatory and inhibitory signals often are initiated in parallel *(18–20)*.

Apart from being potent mitogens, the PDGF isoforms may induce several other critical functions. It acts as a potent chemoattractant for a number of cells and induces gene expression of cell matrix-related molecules such as fibronectin, collagen, and glycosaminoglycans *(21)*.

## FETAL LUNG DEVELOPMENT AND THE INVOLVEMENT
## OF PLATELET-DERIVED GROWTH FACTOR

Growth of the mammalian fetal lung, in preparation for air breathing after birth, occurs in three well-described stages: the *pseudoglandular stage* of airway development, the *canalicular stage* during which the respiratory portion of the lung is developed and where there is increasing vascularization of the mesenchyme, and the *saccular stage* of increased differentiation of the respiratory region *(22)*. Mesenchymal–epithelial interactions play an important role in lung morphogenesis. During the embryonic period, the mesenchyme directs and controls lung epithelial budding and branching. Fibroblast–epithelial interactions also play a role in lung maturation at late fetal gestation *(23)*. Fibroblasts from the pseudoglandular stage of lung development stimulate epithelial cell proliferation, whereas fibroblasts from the saccular stage promote epithelial cell differentiation. The developmental switch from proliferation to differentiation seems to be controlled by both cell types. Upon partial characterization, in 1986, it was evident that the growth-promoting activity elaborated by the fibroblasts is a PDGF-like molecule *(24)*. Since then it has been unequivocally demonstrated that the fetal lung produces PDGF molecules, and herein we review the potential role of PDGFs and their cognate receptors during fetal lung development.

## PLATELET-DERIVED GROWTH FACTOR AND PLATELET-DERIVED GROWTH FACTOR RECEPTOR EXPRESSION DURING LUNG DEVELOPMENT

Both homodimers of PDGF (AA and BB) and both PDGF receptors ($\alpha$ and $\beta$) are present in early embryonic rat lung *(25–29)*. The content of both PDGF proteins decreases with advancing gestation *(25)*. Molecular analyses of fetal rat lung mRNA reveals a positive relationship between mRNA expression of PDGF, but not its receptors, and that of growth related genes histone 3 and DNA polymerase $\alpha$ at late fetal gestation *(30)*. The peak of DNA synthesis, based on histone 3 and DNA polymerase $\alpha$ expression, occurs during the canalicular stage of rat lung development on days 19 and 20 of gestation. Expression of message for PDGF-A and PDGF-B chains is low during the pseudoglandular stage on day 18, peaks during the canalicular stage on days 19 and 20, then falls again during the saccular stage at days 21 and 22 of gestation. The peaks of steady-state mRNA for PDGF-A chain and PDGF-B chain during the canalicular stage of lung development suggest a specific role for PDGF at this stage, during which the saccular epithelium becomes recognized and vascularization occurs *(22)*. At late gestation, lung fibroblasts express the PDGF B-chain and $\beta$-receptor genes *(31)*. Fibroblasts also express the PDGF-A-chain throughout late fetal gestation, although the message levels are low and do not change with advancing gestation. Lung fibroblasts at late gestation do not express the $\alpha$-receptor *(31,32)*. Fetal rat lung epithelial cells transcribe all the PDGF-related genes and translate the PDGF-A and PDGF-B mRNAs into protein *(33)*. Message levels for PDGF B-chain of fetal lung epithelial cells increase with advancing gestation *(33)*, whereas those of fetal lung fibroblasts decline *(31)*. The developmental increase in PDGF-B chain mRNA in epithelial cells is due to a greater rate of transcription *(33)*. Although the developmental expression pattern of PDGF-B of the individual cells does not mimic that of the whole fetal lung, it is likely that the changing lung cell populations at late fetal gestation influences the PDGF-B expression pattern in vivo. Similar to what occurs in the whole fetal rat lung, epithelial cells express the PDGF-A chain throughout late fetal gestation. The number of PDGF-A transcripts decline in epithelial cells with advancing gestation due to a decrease in RNA stability *(33)*. As mentioned earlier, PDGF-A expression by fetal lung fibroblasts does not change during gestation. In common with whole fetal rat lung, PDGF $\beta$-receptor gene in lung fibroblasts is expressed at a constant level throughout late fetal gestation. By contrast, message levels for PDGF β-receptor decline in epithelial cells with advancing gestation *(31)*. It is worthwhile to mention that there is a steep decline in PDGF β-receptor mRNA levels of whole fetal lung just before birth *(31)*. Similar to what occurs in the whole fetal rat lung, PDGF α-receptor expression by fetal lung epithelial cells increases during the canalicular stage of lung development *(33)*. Although it is oversimplistic to discuss gene expression in whole fetal lung in the context of two cell types, it appears that both fibroblasts and epithelial cells are major determinants of the developmental expression pattern of PDGF-related genes in lung.

## PLATELET-DERIVED GROWTH FACTOR
## AND LUNG BRANCHING MORPHOGENESIS

Branching morphogenesis of many organs, including lung, takes place in response to epithelial–mesenchymal tissue interactions *(34,35)*. The molecular signals guiding branching morphogenesis are largely unknown. As branching morphogenesis involves cell proliferation, migration, and differentiation, the ontogenic sequence of these events in early lung organogenesis needs to be well coordinated. Polypeptide growth factors, such as PDGF, are believed to play a vital role in a number of these cellular processes. Expression studies have implicated PDGF and its receptors in epithelial-to-mesenchyme signaling *(36,37)*. In early lung development, PDGF receptors are mostly expressed in mesenchymal cells *(27,29)* while expression of PDGF homodimers, AA and BB, is confined to the epithelium *(26,27,38)*. The physiologic role of PDGF in embryonic lung development has been partly delineated by in vitro and genetic approaches.

Translation arrest of endogenous PDGF-BB in embryonic lung explants with antisense PDGF-B oligonucleotides results in smaller lungs and a decrease in DNA synthesis *(28)*. The number of terminal buds and the degree of branching is not significantly affected by antisense PDGF-B treatment *(28)*. The inhibitory effect of antisense PDGF-B on DNA synthesis is reversed by the addition of exogenous PDGF-BB but not PDGF-AA. Incubation of lung explants with PDGF-BB neutralizing antibodies also results in an inhibition of DNA synthesis that can be overcome with exogenous PDGF-BB. The epithelial component of the antisense-treated lungs is specifically reduced, both in mass and DNA labeling index.

The PDGF-B null phenotype in mice is embryonic lethal but shows no abnormal lung branching morphogenesis *(39)*. At late gestation, homozygous mutant mice develop general hemorrhaging and edema. Although these genetic data suggest that PDGF-BB is not involved in regulating early lung branching, it is possible that maternal and/or placental leakage of PDGF-BB in amniotic fluid *(39)* or duplication by PDGF-AA or other members of the PDGF superfamily mask the early developmental defects in the PDGF-B-deficient mice.

Inhibition of PDGF-AA translation in vitro with antisense PDGF-A oligonucleotides results in smaller, less branched lungs *(27)*. Antisense PDGF-A treatment also reduces DNA synthesis and, consequently, lung size. Exogenous PDGF-AA, but not PDGF-BB, attenuates the inhibitory effect of antisense PDGF-A on early lung branching and size. Incubation of explants with neutralizing PDGF-AA antibodies also reduces DNA synthesis and early branching morphogenesis. These results are compatible with PDGF-AA influencing early lung branching. Since PDGF-AA only binds to the PDGF α-receptor, data acquired with antisense PDGF-A suggest that PDGF mediates its effect on early lung branching via the PDGF α-receptor. Exogenous PDGF-BB, which also binds to the PDGF α-receptor, did not overcome the inhibitory effect of antisense PDGF-AA *(27)*. As PDGF β-receptors appear to be more abundant in fetal lung than α-receptors *(26)*, it is possible that the exogenous PDGF-BB was mostly bound to the PDGF β-receptor. Alternatively, PDGF-AA and PDGF-BB may elicit different responses when bound to the PDGF α-receptor. It has been suggested that the high-affinity binding sites for PDGF-AA and PDGF-BB in the extracellular domain of the α-receptor are not structurally coincident *(40)*.

A mouse PDGF-A null allele is homozygous lethal, with two distinct restriction points, one prenatally before E10 and one postnatally *(41)*. The lung phenotype of PDGF-A null embryos dying before day 10.5 has not been clearly determined and, thus, it is not known whether PDGF-A is involved in the early formation of the lung. Postnatally surviving PDGF-A-deficient mice develop lung emphysema secondary to the failure of alveolar septation. PDGF α-receptor positive cells in the lung, which localize with alveolar smooth muscle cell progenitors are specifically absent in PDGF-A null mutants *(42)*. Proposed functions of the alveolar smooth muscle cells must consider their close proximity to septal deposits of tropoelastin, and, as such, it is suggested that the alveolar smooth muscle cells are the source of septal elastin *(43)* and that elastin plays a role in alveogenesis *(44)*. The phenotype of the PDGF-A null mice provides information concerning the function of alveolar smooth muscle cells. The specific lack of these alveolar smooth muscle cells, but not of bronchial or vascular smooth muscle or lung fibroblasts, suggests that these cell types have, in part, separate ontogeny. Demonstration of a scattered subpopulation of PDGF α-receptor-positive cells in the peripheral lung parenchyma of the late gestational mouse embryo, which is missing in the corresponding PDGF-A null embryo, implicates these cells as the precursors of the alveolar smooth muscle cells. As the abundance and distribution of these cells corresponds to the distribution of the mature alveolar smooth muscle cells, it may be considered that these two cell types are identical. Moreover, the specific loss of parenchymal elastin fibers in PDGF-AA null mice argues that the alveolar smooth muscle cells constitute the major source of such fibers. Furthermore, the lack of alveolar septa in the PDGF-A null lungs suggests a crucial role for the alveolar smooth muscle cells in alveolar septal formation and, consequently, in alveogenesis *(41)*. Taken together, the genetic data demonstrate that PDGF-AA is crucial for alveolar smooth muscle cell ontogeny *(41)* and alveogenesis *(42)* (*see* chapter 14 for further discussion).

## PLATELET-DERIVED GROWTH FACTOR RECEPTORS AND LUNG DEVELOPMENT

Treatment of embryonic lung explants with antisense PDGF α-receptor oligonucleotide inhibits lung growth and branching *(29)*. PDGF-BB but not PDGF-AA partially attenuates the inhibitory effect of antisense α-receptor on lung growth. By contrast, PDGF-BB does not overcome the inhibitory effect on early lung branching. This finding suggests that the β-receptor cannot replace this biologic role of the α-receptor in early lung development. Inhibition of PDGF β-receptor signaling with antisense PDGF β-receptor treatment results in smaller lungs but no reduction in lung branching. Both PDGF isoforms restore embryonic lung growth when added to antisense β-receptor-treated explants, suggesting that the α-receptor can transduce similar mitogenic signals as the β-receptor in early lung development. These data suggest that PDGF-BB stimulation of both receptors leads to lung growth, whereas PDGF-AA stimulation of the α-receptor induces transduction pathways that lead lung branching. Therefore, it is likely that distinct intracellular signaling pathways are initiated by PDGF binding to each type of PDGF receptor that lead to either growth or branching. Whether both receptors are present on the same cell or separate mesenchymal cells remains to be established.

The patch *(Ph)* mice, which are homozygous for a large deletion encompassing the PDGF α-receptor locus, die at early postimplantation to midgestational stages *(45–48)*. Although the defective tissues in patch homozygotes normally express PDGF α-receptor, it is possible that part of the patch phenotype reflects the loss, or misexpression, of other genes, such as c-kit *(49)*. The mutants have compromised mesenchymal cell compartments and generalized connective tissue deficiencies indicating a crucial role for PDGF-A signaling via the PDGF α-receptor. The antisense α-receptor oligonucleotide selectively reduces the epithelial cell mass in lung explants and, to a lesser extent, the mesenchyme, similar to the effect of antisense PDGF-A oligonucleotides, which resembles the results collected from PDGF α-receptor null experiments *(50)*. Mutant mice deficient in the PDGF α-receptor gene die during embryonic development and exhibit severe developmental defects. The phenotype of the α-receptor mutant mice differs from that of the PDGF-A mutant mice. However, early lung development proceeds normally in the α-receptor null mutants. The PDGF β-receptor null phenotype is also lethal and displays similar phenotypes as the PDGF-B-deficient mice, most notedly, hemorrhaging *(39,50)*. However, the data from these knockout studies differ from the antisense experiments. Both antisense PDGF-B and PDGF β-receptor oligonucleotides inhibit fetal lung growth. These data indicate that there may be cross-talk between the two receptors after ligand stimulation and that in the PDGF β-receptor knockout situation there may be disinhibition that results in PDGF α-receptor signaling due to the combinatorial effects of all PDGF ligands (AA, AB, and BB), which compensates for the lack of PDGF β-receptor signaling and its effects on lung growth. In the PDGF-B knockout, signaling through the PDGF α-receptor may acquire new mechanisms of transduction enabling growth to some degree.

Certainly, in vivo compensatory mechanisms must be considered when addressing results collected from knockout studies compared to in vitro antisense oligonucleotide studies.

## EFFECTS OF OTHER GROWTH FACTORS ON PLATELET-DERIVED GROWTH FACTOR RECEPTORS

Although PDGF α-receptors are not detectable in unstimulated rat lung fibroblasts by [$^{125}$I]PDGF-AA binding, the number of receptors is upregulated several-fold following interleukin-1β treatment, resulting in a marked increase in the mitogenic and chemotactic effects elicited by all three PDGF isoforms *(51)*. Even when upregulated, however, the cell-surface rat lung fibroblast PDGF α-receptor is still relatively low in number (approx 30 fmol/million cells) when compared to the PDGF β-receptor (approx 200 fmol/million cells). The PDGF α-receptor may serve as a regulator for the PDGF isoforms to transduce the most potent mitogenic and chemotactic signals *(52)*, which are necessary in lung development and injury. Conversely, TGFβ1 downregulates the PDGF α-receptor on rat and human lung fibroblasts *(53)*. TGFβ1 downregulates PDGF α-receptor gene expression, which is accompanied a decrease in cell-surface PDGF α-receptor. TGFβ1 treatment does not alter the rate of PDGF α-receptor mRNA degradation following the inhibition of transcription using actinomycin D. Thus, TGFβ1-induced downregulation of the PDGF α-receptor gene is not due to an increase in the rate of PDGF α-receptor mRNA degradation. [$^{125}$I]PDGF-AB binding sites are downregulated approximately 25%, and the number of [$^{125}$I]PDGF-BB binding sites is not changed by TGFβ1 treatment, indicating that the PDGF β-receptor was not affected. TGFβ1 reduces the mitogenic and chemotactic response to PDGF-AA by > 90%, whereas the biologic response to PDGF-AB and PDGF-BB are inhibited 50% to 80%, respectively (52).

The gestational period and the varied regulation and expression of numerous growth factors and cytokines must be addressed in order to begin to analyze the biologic consequence upon the PDGF isoforms and their cognate receptors during development. The involvement of multiple growth factors in branching morphogenesis may explain the observation that blocking the function of PDGF-AA alone did not completely inhibit early lung branching.

## ELEVATED OXYGEN
## AND PLATELET-DERIVED GROWTH FACTOR IN LUNG

Sustained inhalation of an elevated concentration of $O_2$ is believed to cause lung injury and to contribute to the pulmonary fibrosis observed in both human adults (54,55) and infants (56) requiring chronic respiratory support. A variety of animal models have been developed for studies of $O_2$-mediated lung injury (57), of which the young adult rat exposed to 85% $O_2$ for intervals up to 2 wk (58). This concentration of $O_2$ is associated with an increase of pulmonary antioxidant enzymes (58) and tolerance to the lethal effects of $O_2$, which are not observed with greater (58) or lesser (59) $O_2$ concentrations. Despite tolerance to the lethal effects of 85% $O_2$, the lung suffers diffuse pulmonary injury. After 7 d of exposure to 85% $O_2$ the total cell number has been reported to increase by 82%, with a 102% increase in type II pneumocytes, a 273% increase in interstitial cells, and a 41% reduction in the number of endothelial cells (58).

Morphometric analyses conducted with an animal model (58), have demonstrated increased whole-lung DNA synthesis, as interpreted from histone H3 gene expression, at 6 and 14 d subsequent to exposure at 85% $O_2$. There is a parallel reduction of whole-lung RNA toward control values by 14 d of exposure to 85% $O_2$ (60).

Type II cell and fibroblast proliferative response, observed with $O_2$ exposure and a variety of other lung injuries, is believed to be mediated through polypeptide growth factors (61,62). A modest increase of PDGF-B chain gene expression has been observed at 4 and 6 d of exposure to 85% $O_2$ (63) that may be lung derived, since lungs of rats exposed to 85% $O_2$ have increased expression of PDGF-BB mRNA from 3 to 7 d following the onset of exposure (64). Nuclear runoff analysis demonstrates that this increase of PDGF-BB chain mRNA reflects a true increase of transcription, and Western blot analysis suggests that this increased PDGF-B chain mRNA is translated into increased PDGF-B chain synthesis (60). Although it is difficult to exclude a contribution from platelets trapped in the $O_2$-exposed lung, the probable source is a primary lung cell, since an increase at 3 d of exposure precedes the phagocyte influx observed in the course of this lung injury (58).

The lack of any change in PDGF-AA chain gene expression over the course of the exposure period indicates that the PDGF-AA chain may not be involved in the proliferative response to 85% $O_2$ (60).

Immunocytochemical localization studies are compatible with the hypothesis that PDGF-BB is produced by one subset of lung fibroblasts that then acts in a paracrine, or juxtacrine, fashion against another subset of fibroblasts. It is hypothesized that the early pulmonary fibroblast hyperplasia observed following exposure to 85% $O_2$ is mediated by increased PDGF-BB chain gene expression and may also be mediated by changes in PDGF β-receptor gene expression *(60)* reinforcing the effect of PDGF-BB in lung growth over PDGF-AA.

## CHEMOTAXIS
## AND PLATELET-DERIVED GROWTH FACTOR IN LUNG

PDGF are potent chemoattractants and mitogens for fibroblasts *(65–68)* and smooth muscle cells *(69,70)* that function as mediators in development and tissue repair. Alteration of the PDGF receptor system could be important in enhancing the mitogenic and chemotactic potential of lung fibroblasts during pulmonary fibrogenesis. Pretreatment of fibroblasts with interleukin-1β increases chemotaxis to all three PDGF isoforms. As discussed earlier, interleukin-1β pretreatment markedly increases the number of PDGF α-receptors but does not change the number of β-receptors *(51)*. Neomycin, a cationic aminoglycoside antibiotic *(71)*, has been used as a blocking agent for PDGF-AA binding to the PDGF α-receptor *(72)*, was used as a PDGF α-receptor antagonist and completely blocked [$^{125}$I] PDGF-AA binding and PDGF-AA-induced chemotaxis. The binding affinity of [$^{125}$I] PDGF-AB and [$^{125}$I]PDGF-BB was increased two- to threefold by neomycin, and chemotaxis to PDGF-AB and PDGF-BB was enhanced. The data indicates that neomycin increases PDGF-BB-induced chemotaxis by increasing the binding affinity of PDGF-BB to PDGF α-receptor. These results define a role for the PDGF α-receptor as a regulatory receptor subtype that is necessary for PDGF isoforms to exert maximal chemotaxis *(73)*, which may have a role in branching morphogenesis in the developing lung.

## EXTRACELLULAR MATRIX
## AND PLATELET-DERIVED GROWTH FACTOR IN LUNG

The extracellular matrix (ECM) is composed of four major classes of macromolecules. The collagens *(74,75)*, structural glycoproteins (76–80), proteoglycans *(81–83)*, and, as previously discussed, elastin *(84,85)*, collectively comprise the ECM of animal cells.

It has been demonstrated that fibroblast procollagen synthesis is not increased at concentrations of PDGF isoforms that are maximally mitogenic *(86)*. These data suggest that other growth factors and/or other cell types are likely involved in the stimulation of fibroblast procollagen synthesis and deposition that is observed in fibroproliferative disorders of the lung. To this end, it has been demonstrated that intratracheal, but not intravenous, injection of PDGF-BB causes transient proliferation of pulmonary mesenchymal and epithelial cells accompanied by collagen deposition *(87)*. PDGF-BB-induced fibroblast proliferation and collagen fibrosis is mainly localized in the peribrochial and perivascular areas, with relative sparing of the alveolar septa, and has been described as comparable to early pathologic changes in a pulmonary fibrosis model *(88)*.

Fibronectin is a structural glycoprotein *(81)* that has been demonstrated to play a role in growth regulation, differentiation, and migration *(89)*. Data have demonstrated that PDGF-BB can greatly enhance colony number and formation in fibroblasts obtained from fibrotic lung or from neonatal lung tissue under anchorage-independent growth conditions as compared with fibroblasts from normal adult lung tissue *(90)*. Observed increases in fibronectin deposition and expression of the fibronectin receptor subsequent to PDGF-BB stimulation has been hypothesized to serve a role in the anchorage of the growing colony to the ECM *(91,92)* and demonstrates that an increase in ECM molecule expression is an important component in growth and fibrosis.

Proteoglycans are a class of substances that consist of specific types of polysaccharide chains attached covalently to a core protein. These polysaccharides, termed glycosaminoglycans (GAGs), consist of *N*-sulfidrylglucosamine or *N*-acetylglucosamine or *N*-acetylgalactosamine residues alternating in glycosidic linkages with glucuronic acid, iduronic acid, or galactose residues to form unbranched polysaccharide chains *(81,93)*. GAGs bind to other matrix components, cell adhesion molecules, and growth factors *(94–98)*. These properties suggest that GAGs may mediate, at least in part, cell adhesion, branching, tissue remodeling, cell differentiation, and cell proliferation during fetal lung development *(95)*. As lung morphogenesis is in part regulated by the ECM and cytokines may indirectly control lung development via modulation of the ECM, the effect of different PDGF isoforms on the synthesis of GAGs by fetal rat lung cells has been investigated *(99)*. The data, as shall be presented forthwith, have elucidated significant developmental properties of the lung. Independent of gestational age, PDGF-BB, but not PDGF-AA or PDGF-AB, stimulated GAG synthesis of fetal lung fibroblasts. By contrast, GAG synthesis by epithelial cells was not affected by any of the PDGF isoforms. The relative proportion of the individual GAG molecules was not altered by PDGF-BB exposure. Actinomycin D and cycloheximide did not abrogate the PDGF-BB effect, suggesting that no new RNA or protein synthesis is required. The proteoglycan synthesis blocker, β-D-xyloside, also did not inhibit the PDGF-BB action on fibroblast GAG synthesis. These data suggest that the effect of PDGF on GAG synthesis is cell type- and isoform-specific and is most likely a direct effect on the GAG chain elongation enzymes *(99)*.

Neither TGF-$\beta_1$, EGF, IGF-I, nor bFGF stimulated GAG synthesis of fetal lung cells. However, it is possible that higher concentrations give different results. TGF-$\beta_1$ has also been shown to stimulate hyaluronan synthesis in human embryonic lung fibroblasts *(100)*. PDGF-BB augmented the synthesis of all individual GAG types measured, however, in contrast to TGF$\beta_1$ *(101)*, PDGF-BB did not alter the proportion of total GAGs and did not affect the distribution of individual GAGs between medium and cell layer *(102)*.

The finding that staurosporine, and not genistein, abrogated the PDGF-BB stimulatory effect on GAG synthesis suggests that the PDGF-BB effect is mediated via a PDGF receptor *(103)*. These results are consistent with the finding that PDGF β-receptors are more important than PDGF α-receptors in mediating the stimulatory effect of PDGF on hyaluronan synthesis by fibroblasts *(104)*. In keeping with the concept that PDGF-BB may activate or stabilize the chain-elongation enzymes was the finding that cycloheximide decreased total GAG formation but did not inhibit the PDGF-BB effect of increased GAG formation *(99)*. Moreover, PDGF-BB also enhanced $^{35}SO_4$ incorporation into the small, soluble proteoglycan biglycan without affecting biglycan's core protein mRNA expression *(105)*. As PDGF-BB seems to be localized to the epithelium during lung development *(25)*, there is an indication that PDGF-BB modulation of fibroblast GAG and proteoglycan production may involve mesenchymal–epithelial interactions.

PDGF-BB-stimulated GAG synthesis was abrogated by tyrphostin 9, a PDGF receptor-associated tyrosine kinase inhibitor, implying that the stimulatory effect is mediated via the PDGF β-receptor *(105)*. Furthermore, PDGF-BB stimulation triggered PDGF β-receptor-associated P13K activity. Both PDGF-BB-induced P13K activation and GAG synthesis were abolished by the P13K inhibitors, wortmannin and LY-294002. These data suggest that P13K is a downstream mediator of PDGF-BB-stimulated GAG synthesis in fetal rat lung fibroblasts and that phosphatidylinositol 3,4,5-trisphosphate ($PIP_3$) accumulation is essential for this cell response *(105)*. $PIP_3$ may be involved in regulating the transport of proteoglycans through the Golgi complex by activating and stabilizing Rab proteins, thereby affecting the elongation and/or sulfation of GAGs linked to proteoglycan core proteins.

Although receptor-associated P13K activity was stimulated by PDGF-BB, PDGF β-receptor failed to relay a mitogenic signal in fetal rat lung fibroblasts *(105)*. These data suggest that the mitogenic response of cells to PDGF depends on many variables, which may include receptor density and receptor isoform on the cell surface and the sum of intracellular signals arising from activated PDGF β-receptors. It has been found that embryonic rat lung fibroblasts (day 13) respond mitogenically to PDGF-BB *(28)*, implying that the PDGF-BB signal in the same cell type is transduced in different physiologic responses depending on gestation and/or differentiation *(105)*.

## MECHANICAL STRETCH
## AND PLATELET-DERIVED GROWTH FACTOR IN LUNG

It has been hypothesized that fetal breathing movements are essential for normal lung growth *in utero*. This premise was examined by employing the effect of mechanical stretch on proliferation of mixed fetal rat lung cells maintained in an organotypic culture *(106)*. Mechanical stretch (5% elongation, 60 cycles/min for 15 min each hour) of fetal lung cells, cultured in a three-dimensional environment provided by Gelfoam sponges, increased DNA synthesis *(106)* and the mRNA levels of PDGF-B and PDGF β-receptor *(107)*. Both PDGF-BB and PDGF β-receptor proteins were increased after intermittent strain *(107)*. Antisense PDGF-B and PDGF β-receptor oligonucleotides abolished the stretch-enhanced DNA synthesis and cell growth *(107)*. A neutralizing PDGF-BB antibody also attenuated stretch-induced DNA synthesis. Furthermore, the stretch-induced stimulatory effect on DNA synthesis of fetal lung cells was blocked by tyrphostin 9, a PDGF receptor-associated tyrosine kinase inhibitor, but not by its inactive structural analog tyrphostin 1. These results suggest that physical forces such as fetal breathing movements regulate fetal lung cell growth by controlling PDGF-B and PDGF β-receptor gene expression *(107)*.

## SUMMARY

PDGF and PDGF receptors are critical components that contribute to the responses cells will elicit during lung organogenesis. Translation arrest of endogenous PDGF-BB or PDGF β-receptor results in smaller lungs and a decrease in DNA synthesis, whereas translation arrest of PDGF-AA or PDGF α-receptor results in smaller, less branched lungs. The PDGF-B null phenotype is embryonic lethal but does not exhibit abnormal lung branching morphogenesis. However, the PDGF-A null phenotype is characterized by a lack of PDGF α-receptor-positive (smooth muscle) cells in the lung. The loss of PDGF α-receptor positive cells results in the loss of parenchymal elastin fibers and suggests an important role in alveolar septal formation and alveogenesis. Furthermore, the absence of PDGF α-receptor positive cells in PDGF-A null mutants suggests a

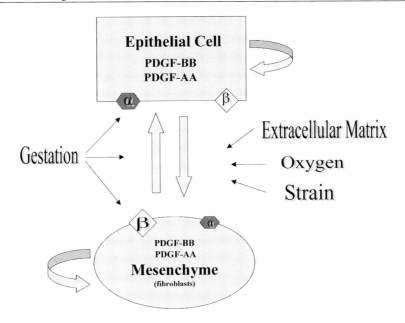

Fig. 1. Schematic summary of PDGF expression and action in fetal lung cells.

stimulatory role for PDGF-AA on the PDGF α-receptor. The PDGF α-receptor null mutant is lethal resulting in compromised mesenchymal cell compartments supporting the critical role for PDGF-A signaling via the PDGF α-receptor. The PDGF α-receptor is also important as a regulator for PDGF isoforms to exert maximal chemotaxis. The PDGF β-receptor null mutant is also lethal and displays similar phenotypes as the PDGF-B null mutant. Pulmonary fibroblast hyperplasia, observed following to 85% $O_2$, is considered to be mediated by an increase in PDGF-BB chain gene expression and may also be mediated by an increase in PDGF β-receptor gene expression. Fetal breathing movements modeled in culture through mechanical stretch of fetal lung cells also leads to an increase in DNA synthesis as well as the mRNA levels for PDGF-B and PDGF β-receptor. Glycosaminoglycans are upregulated in cultured lung fibroblasts after mechanical stretch or PDGF-BB treatment and have been suggested to mediate cell adhesion, branching, tissue remodeling, cell differentiation and cell proliferation during fetal lung development through the PI3K signal transduction pathway. Other extracellular matrix molecules, such as fibronectin and collagen family members, have also been implicated in fetal lung growth and development subsequent to PDGF-BB stimulation. Thus, environmental factors such as physical forces and oxygen may influence proper lung development by regulating PDGF/PDGFR expression. More research is warranted to address mesenchymal–epithelial interactions and the corresponding signal transduction cascades that underlie the responses to PDGF, other growth factors, oxidative status and/or mechanical forces (Fig. 1).

## ACKNOWLEDGMENTS

Our work is supported by a Group Grant from the Medical Research Council of Canada. Nicholas Cartel is a recipient of a Doctoral Research Award from the Medical Research Council of Canada.

# REFERENCES

1. Heldin C-H, Westermark B. Platelet-derived growth factor: mechanism of action and possible in vivo function. Cell Regulation 1990;1:555–566.
2. Ostman A, Rall L, Hammacher A, Wormstead MA, Coit D, Valenzuela P, Betsholtz C, Westermark B, Heldin C–H. Synthesis and assembly of a functionally active recombinant platelet–derived growth factor AB heterodimer. J Biol Chem 1988;263:16,202–16,208.
3. Robbins KC, Leal F, Pierce JH, Aaronson SA. The v-sis/PDGF-2 transforming gene product localizes to cell membranes but is not a secretory membrane. EMBO J 1985;4:1783–1792.
4. Duel F. Polypeptide growth factors: roles in normal and abnormal cell growth. Annu Rev Cell Biol 1987;3:443–492.
5. Delwiche F, Raines E, Powell J, Ross R, Adamson J. Platelet-derived growth factor enhances in vitro erythropoiesis via stimulation of mesenchymal cells. J Clin Invest 1985;76:137–142.
6. Ross R. Platelet-derived growth factor. Lancet 1989;1:1179–1182.
7. Hart CE, Forstrom JW, Kelly JD, Seifert RA, Smith RA, Ross R, Murray MJ, Bowen-Pope DF. Two classes of PDGF receptor recognize different isoforms of PDGF. Science 1988;240:1529–1531.
8. Yarden Y, Ullrich A. Molecular analysis of signal transduction by growth factors. Biochemistry 1988;27:3113–3119.
9. Ullrich A, Schlessinger J. Signal transduction by receptors with tyrosine kinase activity. Cell 1990;61:203–212.
10. Kazlauskas A, Cooper JA. Autophosphorylation of the PDGF receptor in the kinase insert region regulates interactions with cell proteins. Cell 1989;58:1121–1133.
11. Fantl WJ, Escobedo JA, Williams LT. Mutations of the platelet-derived growth factor receptor that cause a loss of ligand-induced conformational change, subtle changes in kinase activity, and impaired ability to stimulate DNA synthesis. Mol Cell Biol 1989;9:4473–4478.
12. Heldin CH. Simultaneous induction of stimulatory and inhibitory signals by PDGF. FEBS Lett 1997;410:17–21.
13. Pawson T, Gish GD. SH2 and SH3 domains: from structure to function. Cell 1992;71:359–362.
14. Mori S, Ronnstrand L, Yokote K, Engstrom A, Courtneidge SA, Claesson-Welsh L, Heldin CH. Identification of two juxtamembrane autophosphorylation sites in the PDGF beta-receptor; involvement in the interaction with Src family tyrosine kinases. EMBO J 1993;12:2257–2264.
15. Bornfeldt KE, Raines EW, Graves LM, Skinner MP, Krebs EG, Ross R. Platelet-derived growth facto: distinct signal transduction pathways associated with migration versus proliferation. Ann NY Acad Sci 1995;766:416–430.
16. Seifert RA, Hart CE, Phillips PE, Forstrom JW, Ross R, Murray MJ, Bowen-Pope DF. Two different subunits associate to create isoform-specific platelet-derived growth factor receptors. J Biol Chem 1989;264:8771–8778.
17. Ferns GA, Sprugel KH, Seifert RA, Bowen–Pope DF, Kelly JD, Murray M, Raines EW, Ross R. Relative platelet-derived growth factor receptor subunit expression determines cell migration to different dimeric forms of PDGF. Growth Factors 1990;3:315–324.
18. Graves LM, Bornfeldt KE, Raines EW, Potts BC, Macdonald SG, Ross R, Krebs EG. Protein kinase A antagonizes platelet-derived growth factor-induced signaling by mitogen-activated protein kinase in human arterial smooth muscle cells. Proc Natl Acad Sci USA 1993;90:10,300–10,304.
19. Wu J, Dent P, Jelinek T, Wolfman A, Weber MJ, Sturgill TW. Inhibition of the EGF-activated MAP kinase signaling pathway by adenosine 3',5'-monophosphate. Science 1993;262:1065–1069.
20. Cook SJ, McCormick F. Inhibition by cAMP of Ras-dependent activation of Raf. Science 1993;262:1069–1072.
21. Martin GR, Sank AC. In: Sporn MB, Roberts AB, eds. Peptide growth factors and their receptors, Vol 2. Berlin: Springer-Verlag, 1989:463–467
22. Meyrick B, Reid LM. In: Hodson WA, ed. Lung biology in health and disease, development of the lung, Vol 6. New York:Marcel Dekker, 1977:135–214.
23. Caniggia I, Tseu I, Han RN, Smith BT, Tanswell K, Post M. Spatial and temporal differences in fibroblast behavior in fetal rat lung. Am J Physiol 1991;261:L424–433.
24. Stiles AD, Smith BT, Post M. Reciprocal autocrine and paracrine regulation of growth of mesenchymal and alveolar epithelial cells from fetal lung. Exp Lung Res 1986;11:165–177.
25. Han RN, Mawdsley C, Souza P, Tanswell AK, Post M. Platelet–derived growth factors and growth-related genes in rat lung. III. Immunolocalization during fetal development. Pediatr Res 1992;31:323–329.

26. Han RN, Liu J, Tanswell AK, Post M. Ontogeny of platelet-derived growth factor receptor in fetal rat lung. Microsc Res Tech 1993;26:381–388.

27. Souza P, Kuliszewski M, Wang J, Tseu I, Tanswell AK, Post M. PDGF-AA and its receptor influence early lung branching via an epithelial-mesenchymal interaction. Development 1995;121:2559–2567.

28. Souza P, Sedlackova L, Kuliszewski M, Wang J, Liu J, Tseu I, Liu M, Tanswell AK, Post M. Antisense oligodeoxynucleotides targeting PDGF-B mRNA inhibit cell proliferation during embryonic rat lung development. Development 1994;120:2163–2173.

29. Souza P, Tanswell AK, Post M. Different roles for PDGF-alpha and -beta receptors in embryonic lung development. Am J Respir Cell Mol Biol 1996;15:551–562.

30. Buch S, Jones C, Sweezey N, Tanswell K, Post M. Platelet-derived growth factor and growth-related genes in rat lung. I. Developmental expression. Am J Respir Cell Mol Biol 1991;5:371–376.

31. Buch S, Jones C, Liu J, Han RN, Tanswell AK, Post M. Differential regulation of platelet-derived growth factor genes in fetal rat lung fibroblasts. Exp Cell Res 1994;211:142–149.

32. Caniggia I, Liu J, Han R, Buch S, Funa K, Tanswell K, Post M. Fetal lung epithelial cells express receptors for platelet-derived growth factor. Am J Respir Cell Mol Biol 1993;9:54–63.

33. Buch S, Jassal D, Cannigia I, Edelson J, Han R, Liu J, Tanswell K, Post M. Ontogeny and regulation of platelet-derived growth factor gene expression in distal fetal rat lung epithelial cells. Am J Respir Cell Mol Biol 1994;11:251–161.

34. Rudnick, D. Developmental capacities of the chick lung in chorioallantoic grafts. J Exp Zool 1933;66:125–153.

35. Wessels, NK. Mammalian lung development: interactions in formation and morphogenesis of tracheal buds. J Exp Zool 1979;175:445–460.

36. Holmgren L, Glaser A, Pfeifer-Ohlsson S, Ohlsson R. Angiogenesis during human extraembryonic development involves the spatiotemporal control of PDGF ligand and receptor gene expression. Development 1991;113:749–754.

37. Orr–Urtreger A, Lonai P. Platelet-derived growth factor-A and its receptor are expressed in separate, but adjacent cell layers of the mouse embryo. Development 1992;115:1045–1058.

38. Mercola M, Wang CY, Kelly J, Brownlee C, Jackson-Grusby L, Stiles C, Bowen-Pope D. Selective expression of PDGF A and its receptor during early mouse embryogenesis. Dev Biol 1990;138:114–122.

39. Leveen P, Pekny M, Gebre-Medhin S, Swolin B, Larsson E, Betsholtz C. Mice deficient for PDGF B show renal, cardiovascular, and hematological abnormalities. Genes Dev 1994;8:1875–8187.

40. Heideran MA, Yu JH, Jensen RA, Pierce JH, Aaronson, SA. A deletion in the extracellular domain of the (platelet-derived growth factor (PDGF) receptor differentially impairs PDGF-AA and PDGF-BB affinities. J Biol Chem 1992;267:2884–2887.

41. Bostrom H, Willetts K, Pekny M, Leveen P, Lindahl P, Hedstrand H, Pekna M, Hellstrom M, Gebre-Medhin S, Schalling M, Nilsson M, Kurland S, Tornell J, Heath JK, Betsholtz C. PDGF-A signaling is a critical event in lung alveolar myofibroblast development and alveogenesis. Cell 1996;85:863–873.

42. Lindahl P, Karlsson L, Hellstrom M, Gebre-Medhin S, Willetts K, Heath JK, Betsholtz C. Alveogenesis failure in PDGF-A-deficient mice is coupled to lack of distal spreading of alveolar smooth muscle cell progenitors during lung development. Development 1997;124:3943–3953.

43. Noguchi A, Reddy R, Kursar JD, Parks WC, Mecham RP. Smooth muscle isoactin and elastin in fetal bovine lung. Exp Lung Res 1989;15:537–552.

44. Emery JL. The post natal development of the human lung and its implications for lung pathology. Respiration 1970;27:41–50.

45. Gruneberg H, Truslove GM. Two closely linked genes of the mouse. Genet Res 1960;1;69–90.

46. Morrison-Graham K, Schatteman GC, Bork T, Bowen-Pope DF, Weston JA. A PDGF receptor mutation in the mouse (Patch) perturbs the development of a non-neuronal subset of neural crest-derived cells. Development 1992;115:133–142.

47. Orr-Urtreger A, Bedford MT, Do MS, Eisenbach L, Lonai P. Developmental expression of the alpha receptor for platelet-derived growth factor, which is deleted in the embryonic lethal Patch mutation. Development 1992;115:289–303.

48. Schatteman GC, Morrison-Graham K, van Koppen A, Weston JA, Bowen-Pope DF. Regulation and role of PDGF receptor alpha-subunit expression during embryogenesis. Development 1992;115:123–131.

49. Duttlinger R, Manova K, Berrozpe G, Chu TY, DeLeon V, Timokhina I, Chaganti RSK, Zelenetz AD, Bachvarova RF, Besmer P. The Wsh and Ph mutations effect the c-kit expression profile: c-kit misexpression in embryogenesis impairs melanogenesis in Wsh and Ph mutant mice. Proc Natl Acad Sci USA 1995;92;3754–3758.

50. Soriano P. Abnormal kidney development and hematological disorders in PDGF beta-receptor mutant mice. Genes Dev 1994;8:1888–1896.

51. Lindroos PM, Coin PG, Osornio-Vargas AR, Bonner J. Interleukin 1 beta (IL-1 beta) and the IL-1 beta-alpha 2-macroglobulin complex upregulate the platelet-derived growth factor alpha-receptor on rat pulmonary fibroblasts. Am J Respir Cell Mol Biol 1995;13:455–465.

52. Bonner JC, Goodell AL, Coin PG, Brody AR. Chrysotile asbestos upregulates gene expression and production of alpha–receptors for platelet–derived growth factor (PDGF–AA) on rat lung fibroblasts. J Clin Invest 1993;92:425–430.

53. Bonner JC, Badgett A, Lindroos PM, Osornio-Vargas AR. Transforming growth factor beta 1 downregulates the platelet-derived growth factor alpha-receptor subtype on human lung fibroblasts in vitro. Am J Respir Cell Mol Biol 1995;13:496–505.

54. Gould VE, Tosco R, Wheelis RF, Gould NS, Kapanci Y. Oxygen pneumonitis in man: ultrastructural observations on the development of alveolar lesions. Lab Invest 1972;26:499–508.

55. Katzenstein AL, Bloor CM, Leibow AA. Diffuse alveolar damage: the role of oxygen, shock, and related factors. Am J Pathol 1976;85:209–228.

56. Edwards DK, Dyer WM, Northway WH Jr. Twelve years' experience with bronchopulmonary dysplasia. Pediatrics 1977;59:839–846.

57. Ballantyne JD. In: Pathology of oxygen toxicity. New York: Academic Press, 1982:82–109.

58. Crapo JD, Barry BE, Foscue HA, Shelburne J. Structural and biochemical changes in rat lungs occurring during exposures to lethal and adaptive doses of oxygen. Am Rev Respir Dis 980;122:123–143.

59. Hayatdavoudi G, O'Neil JJ, Barry BE, Freeman BA, Crapo JD. Pulmonary injury in rats following continuous exposure to 60% $O_2$ for 7 days. J Appl Physiol 1981;51:1220–1231.

60. Han RN, Buch S, Freeman BA, Post M, Tanswell AK. Platelet-derived growth factor and growth-related genes in rat lung. II. Effect of exposure to 85% $O_2$. Am J Physiol 1992;262:L140–146.

61. Kelley J. Cytokines of the lung. Am Rev Respir Dis 1990;141:765–788.

62. King RJ, Jones MB, Minoo P. Regulation of lung cell proliferation by polypeptide growth factors. Am J Physiol 1989;257:L23–L38.

63. Tanswell AK, Han RN, Buch SJ, Fraher LJ. Circulating factors that modify lung cell DNA synthesis following exposure to inhaled oxidants. III. Effects of plasma on lung pneumocyte and fibroblast DNA synthesis following exposure of adult rats to 85% oxygen. Exp Lung Res 1991;17:869–886.

64. Fabisiak JP, Evans JN, Kelley J. Increased expression of PDGF-B (c-sis) mRNA in rat lung precedes DNA synthesis and tissue repair during chronic hyperoxia. Am J Respir Cell Mol Biol 1989;1:181–189.

65. Ross R, Raines EW, Bowen-Pope DF. The biology of platelet-derived growth factor. Cell 1986;46:155–169.

66. Seppa H, Grotendorst G, Seppa S, Schiffmann E, Martin GR. Platelet-derived growth factor in chemotactic for fibroblasts. J Cell Biol 1982;92:584–588.

67. Osornio-Vargas AR, Bonner JC, Badgett A, Brody AR. Rat alveolar macrophage-derived platelet-derived growth factor is chemotactic for rat lung fibroblasts. Am J Respir Cell Mol Biol 1990;3:595–602.

68. Bonner JC, Osornio-Vargas AR, Badgett A, Brody AR. Differential proliferation of rat lung fibroblasts induced by the platelet-derived growth factor-AA, -AB, and -BB isoforms secreted by rat alveolar macrophages. Am J Respir Cell Mol Biol 1991;5:539–547.

69. Grotendorst GR, Chang T, Seppa HE, Kleinman HK, Martin GR. Platelet-derived growth factor is a chemoattractant for vascular smooth muscle cells. J Cell Physiol 1982;113:261–266.

70. Sjolund M, Hedin U, Sejersen T, Heldin CH, Thyberg J. Arterial smooth muscle cells express platelet-derived growth factor (PDGF) A chain mRNA, secrete a PDGF-like mitogen, and bind exogenous PDGF in a phenotype- and growth state-dependent manner. J Cell Biol 1988;106:403–413.

71. Carney DH, Scott DL, Gordon EA, LaBelle EF. Phosphoinositides in mitogenesis: neomycin inhibits thrombin-stimulated phosphoinositide turnover and initiation of cell proliferation. Cell 1985;42:479–488.

72. Vassbotn FS, Ostman A, Siegbahn A, Holmsen H, Heldin CH. Neomycin is a platelet-derived growth factor (PDGF) antagonist that allows discrimination of PDGF alpha- and beta-receptor signals in cells expressing both receptor types. J Biol Chem 1992;267:15,635–15,641.

73. Osornio-Vargas AR, Lindroos PM, Coin PG, Badgett A, Hernandez-Rodriguez NA, Bonner JC. Maximal PDGF-induced lung fibroblast chemotaxis requires PDGF receptor-alpha. Am J Physiol 1996;271:L93–L99.

74. Burgeson RE, Nimni ME. Collagen types: molecular structure and tissue distribution. Clin Orthop 1992;282:250–272.

75. Li K, Christiano AM, Copeland NG, Gilbert DJ, Chu ML, Jenkins NA, Uitto J. cDNA cloning and chromosomal mapping of the mouse type VII collagen gene (Col7a1): evidence for rapid evolutionary divergence of the gene. Genomics 1993;16:733–739.

76. Martinez-Hernandez A, Amenta PS. The basement membrane in pathology. Lab Invest 1983; 48:656–677.

77. Ruoslahti E. Fibronectin and its receptors. Annu Rev Biochem 1988;57:375–413.

78. Martin GR, Timpl R, Kuhn K. Basement membrane proteins: molecular structure and function. Adv Protein Chem 1988;39:1–50.

79. Tryggvason K. The laminin family. Curr Opin Cell Biol 1993;5:877–82.

80. Erickson HP. Tenascin-C, tenascin-R and tenascin-X: a family of talented proteins in search of functions. Curr Opin Cell Biol 1993;5:869–876.

81. Ruoslahti E. Structure and biology of proteoglycans. Annu Rev Cell Biol 1988;4:229–255.

82. Kjellen L, Lindahl U. Proteoglycans: structures and interactions. Annu Rev Biochem 1991; 60:443–475.

83. Hassell JR, Kimura JH, Hascall VC. Proteoglycan core protein families. Annu Rev Biochem 1986;55:539–567.

84. Sakai LY, Keene DR, Engvall E. Fibrillin, a new 350-kD glycoprotein, is a component of extracellular microfibrils. J Cell Biol 1986;103:2499–2509.

85. Rosenbloom J, Abrams WR, Mecham R. Extracellular matrix 4: the elastic fiber. FASEB J 1993;7:1208–1218.

86. Clark JG, Madtes DK, Raghu G. Effects of platelet-derived growth factor isoforms on human lung fibroblast proliferation and procollagen gene expression. Exp Lung Res 1993;19:327–344.

87. Yi ES, Lee H, Yin S, Piguet P, Sarosi I, Kaufmann S, Tarpley J, Wang NS, Ulich TR. Platelet-derived growth factor causes pulmonary cell proliferation and collagen deposition in vivo. Am J Pathol 1996;149:539–548.

88. Zhang K, Rekhter MD, Gordon D, Phan SH. Myofibroblasts and their role in lung collagen gene expression during pulmonary fibrosis: a combined immunohistochemical and in situ hybridization study. Am J Pathol 1994;145:114–125.

89. Hynes RO, George EL, Georges EN, Guan JL, Rayburn H, Yang JT. Toward a genetic analysis of cell–matrix adhesion. Cold Spring Harbor Symp Quant Biol 1992;57:249–258.

90. Torry DJ, Richards CD, Podor TJ, Gauldie J. Anchorage- independent colony growth of pulmonary fibroblasts derived from fibrotic human lung tissue. J Clin Invest 1994;93:1525–1532.

91. Grinnell F, Toda K, Takashima A. Activation of keratinocyte fibronectin receptor function during cutaneous wound healing. J Cell Sci Suppl 1987;8:199–209.

92. Clark AF. Fibronectin matrix deposition and fibronectin receptor expression in healing and normal skin. J Invest Dermatol 1990;94:128–134.

93. Silbert JE, Sugumaran G. Intracellular membranes in the synthesis, transport, and metabolism of proteoglycans. Biochim Biophys Acta 1995;1241:371–384.

94. Roberts CR, Burke AK. Remodelling of the extracellular matrix in asthma: proteoglycan synthesis and degradation. Can Respir J 1998;5:48–50.

95. Sannes PL, Burch KK, Khosla J, McCarthy KJ, Couchman JR. Immunohistochemical localization of chondroitin sulfate, chondroitin sulfate proteoglycan, heparan sulfate proteoglycan, entactin, and laminin in basement membranes of postnatal developing and adult rat lungs. Am J Respir Cell Mol Biol 1993;8:245–251.

96. Guzowski DE, Blau H, Bienskowski RS. Extracellular Matrix. In: Scarpelli E, ed. pulmonary physiology of the fetus, newborn, child and adolescent. Philadelphia: Lea and Febiger, 1990:83–105.

97. Smith CI, Webster EH, Nathanson MA, Searls RL, Hilfer SR. Altered patterns of proteoglycan deposition during maturation of the fetal mouse lung. Cell Differ Dev 1990;32:83–96.

98. Juul SE, Kinsella MG, Wight TN, Hodson WA. Alterations in nonhuman primate (M. nemestrina) lung proteoglycans during normal development and acute hyaline membrane disease. Am J Respir Cell Mol Biol 1993;8:299–310.

99. Caniggia I, Post M. Differential effect of platelet-derived growth factor on glycosaminoglycan synthesis by fetal rat lung cells. Am J Physiol 1992;263:L495–L500.

100. Westergren-Thorsson G, Persson S, Isaksson A, Onnervik PO, Malmstrom A, Fransson LA. L-Iduronate-rich glycosaminoglycans inhibit growth of normal fibroblasts independently of serum or added growth factors. Exp Cell Res 1993;206:93–99.

101. Dubaybo BA, Thet LA. Effect of transforming growth factor beta on synthesis of glycosaminoglycans by human lung fibroblasts. Exp Lung Res 1990;16:389–403.

102. Caniggia I, Tanswell K, Post M. Temporal and spatial differences in glycosaminoglycan synthesis by fetal lung fibroblasts. Exp Cell Res 1992;202:252–258.

103. Secrist JP, Sehgal I, Powis G, Abraham RT. Preferential inhibition of the platelet-derived growth factor receptor tyrosine kinase by staurosporine. J Biol Chem 1990;265:20,394– 20,400.

104. Heldin P, Laurent TC, Heldin CH. Effect of growth factors on hyaluronan synthesis in cultured human fibroblasts. Biochem J 1989;258:919–922.

105. Liu J, Fitzli D, Liu M, Tseu I, Caniggia I, Rotin D, Post M. PDGF-induced glycosaminoglycan synthesis is mediated via phosphatidylinositol 3-kinase. Am J Physiol 1998;274:L702–L713.

106. Liu M, Skinner SJM, Xu J, Han RNN, Tanswell AK, Post M. Stimulation of fetal rat lung cell proliferation in vitro by mechanical stretch. Am J Physiol 1992;263:L376–L383.

107. Liu M, Liu J, Buch S, Tanswell AK, Post M. Antisense oligonucleotides for PDGF-B and its receptor inhibit mechanical strain-induced fetal lung cell growth. Am J Physiol 1995;269:L178–L184.

# 13

# Transforming Growth Factor-β Receptor Signaling and Lung Development

## Yun Zhao, MD, PhD

### Contents

Lung organogenesis starts as a simple foregut bud encroaching on surrounding mesenchyme *(1,2)*. Interactions between epithelium and mesenchyme are essential to the induction and morphogenesis of the lung. The transforming growth factor-beta (TGF-β) family of regulatory peptides plays a central role during lung development as one important group of highly conserved cytokines with demonstrated pleiotropic effects on their own biosynthesis, mesenchymal mitogenesis and epithelial differentiation *(3)*. Emphasis in this chapter is placed on current knowledge regarding TGF-β, its receptors, and TGF-β receptor-mediated signal transduction during lung development.

## TRANSFORMING GROWTH FACTOR-BETA FAMILY

The TGF-β superfamily consists of a large group of multifunctional regulatory polypeptides that can be classified into four subfamilies: the TGF-βs, activins/inhibins, Müllerian inhibiting substance/anti-Müllerian hormone (MIS/AMH), and the decapenta-

From: *Contemporary Endocrinology: Endocrinology of the Lung: Development and Surfactant Synthesis*
Edited by: C. R. Mendelson © Humana Press Inc., Totowa, NJ

plegic/Vg-related factors including the bone morphogenetic proteins (BMP) *(3,4)*. This supergene family includes about 40 members that can act as growth and differentiation signals in developmental events.

TGF-β was initially identified by its ability to promote anchorage-independent growth and a transformed phenotype in nontumorigenic mesenchymal cells *(5)*. TGF-β activities are represented by a subfamily of closely related isoforms TGF-β1, TGF-β2, TGF-β3, TGF-β4, and TGF-β5 *(3)*. Three of the isoforms, TGF-β1, TGF-β2, and TGF-β3, with an amino acid identity of 64% to 82%, are from human and other mammalian sources. The three TGF-β isoforms exhibit the same cellular effects but with distinct potencies in most cultured cells. Two isoforms, TGF-β4 and TGF-β5, have been identified in chicken and *Xenopus laevis*. All TGF-βs are synthesized as precursor molecules approx 400 amino acids in length. An amino-terminal hydrophobic signal targets the precursor to the secretory pathway. A *N*-glycosylated prodomain may assist in folding, dimerization, and regulation of factor activity. The precursor protein is usually cleaved at a dibasic or RXXR site to release a mature bioactive carboxy-terminal domain (mature TGF-β) and a latency-associated peptide (LAP). The actual signaling molecule is made up of disulfide-linked hetero- or homodimers of 25 kDa of the carboxy-terminal segment *(6)*.

## CELLULAR SOURCES
## OF TRANSFORMING GROWTH FACTOR-BETA IN THE LUNG

TGF-β is an autocrine/paracrine/endocrine growth factor. A wide variety of lung-derived cell types include epithelial cells and mesenchymal cell fibroblasts and smooth muscle cells secrete various TGF-β activity in the lung. Lung fibroblasts express all three isoforms including TGF-β1, TGF-β2, and TGF-β3, whereas epithelial cells appear to synthesize only TGF-β1 and TGF-β3 *(7,8)*. Macrophages release primarily TGF-β1 activity. Lymphocytes, neutrophils, and endothelial cells also produce significant amounts of TGF-β. TGF-β is able to autoregulate its own production in human lung fibroblasts *(9)*, which suggests that a positive autocrine feedback signal cascade occurs in the pulmonary interstitium.

The widespread expression of TGF-β in the lung agrees with its autocrine or paracrine roles in regulating cellular growth, differentiation, immune defense, and matrix protein production *(10)*. The endocrine circulation of TGF-β may be also involved in lung development. It has been found that TGF-β1 is transferred both transplacentally and through the maternal milk from heterozygous mothers to fetuses and neonates, which contributed, in part, to a lack of a perinatal phenotype in TGF-β1 null mice *(11)*.

TGF-β is released from cells in a latent form consisting of the mature growth factor associated with an amino-terminal propeptide and a cysteine-rich latent TGF-β binding protein (LTBP). LTBP has features in common with extracellular matrix proteins, and targets latent TGF-β to the matrix *(12,13)*. Activation of latent TGF-β can be accomplished in vitro by denaturing treatments, plasmin digestion, ionizing radiation, and interaction with thrombospondin. The mechanisms by which latent TGF-β is activated physiologically, however, are not well understood. The extracellular inactive form of TGF-β is colocalized with fibronectin, types I and II collagen and proteoglycans along ducts and in crotches of epithelial branches in the developing lung when branching morphogenesis and tissue stabilization occur *(14)*.

# BIOLOGICAL ACTIVITIES
# OF TRANSFORMING GROWTH FACTOR-BETA ON LUNG CELLS

TGF-β elicits a multiplicity of effects in various lung-derived cell types after release from inactive complexes. TGF-β can act as either a positive or a negative regulator of cell division depending on cell type and culture conditions *(15)*. TGF-β usually acts as a mitogenic factor for mesenchyme-derived cells such as fibroblasts and osteoblasts. TGF-β augments the action of epidermal growth factor on human lung fibroblasts *(16)*, but blocks the stimulatory effect of TGF-α or epidermal growth factor in neonatal rabbit type II alveolar epithelial cells *(17)*.

TGF-β acts as a powerful growth inhibitor of cells of epithelial and endothelial origin *(18)*. TGF-β is able to modulate not only cell proliferation but also cell differentiation. The effects of TGF-β on differentiation are variable. TGF-β induces squamous differentiation of human and rabbit lung epithelial cells *(19,20)*, and reduces mitotic activity and increases the percent of mucus-secreting gobletlike cell types of a human lung adenocarcinoma growing in male athymic mice *(21)*.

Cell–extracellular matrix interactions are one class of important mechanisms that direct lung development or repair of lung injury *(22,23)*. TGF-β is a cytokine with a profound effect on extracellular matrix production. TGF-β increases the synthesis of extracellular matrix components such as types I, III, and V collagens without affecting the proportion of collagen types in fibroblasts cultured from human lung *(16,24,25)*. It has been shown that TGF-β increases elastin production in rat lung fibroblasts *(26,27)*, leading to a dramatic increase in the steady-state level of elastin mRNA by a posttranscriptional mechanism *(28)*. TGF-β increases tenascin expression in rat fetal lung explant tissues *(29)*. TGF-β stimulates the expression of fibronectin in human lung fibroblasts *(30)* and in type II cells *(31)*. TGF-β induces selectively the expression of proteoglycan I, but does not change the level of proteoglycan II in human embryonic lung fibroblasts *(32)*. Furthermore, TGF-β modulates the pattern of extracellular matrix by increasing the synthesis of inhibitors of extracellular matrix degrading enzymes such as plasminogen activator inhibitor-I and urokinase-type plasminogen activator *(33,34)*.

TGF-β controls not only cell proliferation, cell differentiation, and matrix deposition but also expression of various genes associated with lung development. TGF-β decreases cyclin A mRNA levels in control embryonic lung explants, and TGF-β type II receptor antisense oligodeoxynucleotides prevents the downregulation of cyclin and stimulates embryonic mouse lung branching morphogenesis in culture *(35)*. TGF-β has been shown to decrease surfactant protein C expression in type II cells *(31,36)*. TGF-β enhances type II transglutaminase activity in undifferentiated human bronchial epithelial cells but does not increase type I transglutaminase, two early markers of squamous differentiation *(37)*. TGF-β modulates β-adrenergic receptor number and function in cultured human tracheal smooth muscle cells *(38)*. In fibroblasts cultured from human lung, TGF-β downregulates the platelet-derived growth factor-alpha-receptor subtype *(39)*, and activates a $H_2O_2$-generating NADH oxidase and induces the release of $H_2O_2$ *(40)*.

# LUNG DEVELOPMENT IN MICE
# LACKING TRANSFORMING GROWTH FACTOR-BETA

All three TGF-β isoforms are expressed during lung development, but there is a distinct temporal difference among TGF-β1, TGF-β2, and TGF-β3 expression. A low level of TGF-β1 was expressed at early gestational days when the same samples had high expression of TGF-β2 and TGF-β3. The apparent high expression at early developmental stages of TGF-β3 and TGF-β2 compared to TGF-β1 raises interesting possibilities for different or unique roles of each of the TGF-βs in lung development. Direct experimental evidence of functional roles of each TGF-β in the regulation of processes concerning lung development and pathologic lung physiology has been provided by in vivo models that involve the target disruption or overexpression of TGF-β genes.

Homologous recombinant knockouts of TGF-β1, TGF-β2, and TGF-β3 have been successfully performed (41–43). The recombinant knockout mice deficient in TGF-β1 do not have a conspicuous lung phenotype but have an immune cell dysfunction. There occurs postnatally excessive inflammatory responses and a fatal proliferation of lymphocytes into several organs, including the lung. Maternal TGF-β1 has been found in TGF-β1 null pups, which might rescue TGF-β1-deficient animals from embryonic and postnatal lethalities (11). Overexpression of TGF-β1 in the developing respiratory epithelium of transgenic mice inhibits lung sacculation and epithelial cell differentiation in vivo, indicating a role for TGF-β1 in lung morphogenesis and differentiation (44).

TGF-β2 null mice exhibit a wide range of developmental defects and perinatal mortality (42). TGF-β2 knockout mice show postnatal defects in the conducting airways of the lung but have no gross morphologic defects in prenatal lungs. The TGF-β3 knockout, in contrast to the TGF-β1 and TGF-β2 knockouts, produced a profound inhibition of lung development and was lethal at birth because of respiratory insufficiency (43). The phenotypes of TGF-β2 and TGF-β3 knockout mice suggest important roles in mesenchymal–epithelial interactions and extracellular matrix production.

## TRANSFORMING GROWTH FACTOR-BETA RECEPTORS

The cellular effects of TGF-β are mediated through binding to a variety of transmembrane proteins on cell surfaces (45). Several different types of putative receptors for TGF-β, including three distinct size classes, termed type I (53–55 kDa), type II (70–80 kDa), and type III (a 300-kDa proteoglycan with a 120-kDa core protein), have been identified by affinity labeling and crosslinking of TGF-β to cell surface proteins (45). Crosslinking of TGF-β to fetal lung fibroblasts or adult lung fibroblasts revealed three species of receptors with apparent molecular weights of 60, 85, and 280 kDa (46). It has been shown that receptors for TGF-β on rat lung fibroblasts have higher affinity for TGF-β1 than for TGF-β2 (47). Studies based on TGF-β nonresponsive mutant cell lines suggest that the type I and type II receptors are essential for TGF-β signal transduction, whereas the type III receptor appears to be a modifier of the TGF-β signal and is dispensable for TGF-β signaling (48–50). Cells not expressing the type III receptor respond to TGF-β, and cells that express the type III receptor, but not the type I or II TGF-β receptor, do not respond to TGF-β.

The type III receptor, also called β-glycan, is a membrane-anchored proteoglycan (51,52). The amino acid sequence of β-glycan includes an amino-terminal signal peptide, a large extracellular domain, a transmembrane region and a carboxyl-terminal cytoplasmic domain. The short and highly conserved cytoplasmic domain has no apparent signal motif.

Molecular cloning of cDNAs of TGF-β type I and type II receptors has shown that both types belong to a novel family of transmembrane serine/threonine kinases with structural homology to Daf-1, the first member of this family that was isolated from the *Caenorhabiditis elegans* (53). The structure of type I and type II receptors comprises a small extracellular domain, a single transmembrane segment, and an intracellular region with a serine–threonine kinase domain. The schematic structure of TGF-β type I and type II receptors is shown in Fig. 1. Type I receptors share several highly conserved structural features not found in the type II receptors, including the juxtamembrane GS box (or type I box), the EIF box, the RIKKT box, a shorter extracellular domain, and they lack a serine–threonine-rich tail *(54,55)*.

A series of type I and type II serine–threonine kinase receptors have been identified from mammals, *C. elegans* and *Drosophila*. Based on sequence similarities, the type I and type II receptors form two distinct subfamilies in the serine–threonine kinase receptor family (Table 1). The type I receptor subfamily, also known as activin receptor-like kinases (ALK), includes TβRI/ALK5/R4 *(56,57)*, ActR-I/ALK2/R1 *(58,59)*, ActR-1B/ALK-4/R2 *(60,61)*, Atr-1 *(62)*, BMPR-1A/ALK3 *(63)*, BMPR-1B/ALK6 *(63)*, ALK1/TSR-1 *(60)*, Sax *(64)*, Daf-1 *(53)* and C14 *(65)*. Although three type I receptors including TβRI/ALK5, ActR-1/ALK-2, and BMPR-1A/ALK3, are able to bind TGF-β, only Tβ RI/ALK-5 has been shown to mediate TGF-β-dependent signal transduction. ALK-2 and ALK-4 are activin type I receptors, and ALK-3 and ALK-6 are BMP type I receptors. The ligand for ALK-1 remains to be identified. The type II receptor subfamily includes TβRII *(55)*, ActRII *(66)*, ActRIIB *(67,68)*, Atr-II *(69)*, BMPRII *(70,71)*, AMHRII *(65,72)* and Daf-4 *(73)*. Three type II receptors including ActR-II, ActRIIB and Atr-II are activin type II receptors. TβRII, BMPRII and AMHR are type II receptors for TGF-β, BMP and MIS, respectively.

## SIGNALING MECHANISMS
## OF TRANSFORMING GROWTH FACTOR-BETA RECEPTORS

Proteins in the TGF-β family exert their effects by interacting with their type I and type II serine–threonine kinase receptors. A complex of TβRI and TβRII but not the individual components, mediates TGF-β signal transduction *(56,74)*. In the absence of TGF-β, TβRII forms homooligomers and exits on cell surface as a constitutively active kinase *(75,76)*. TβRII is able to recognize and bind TGF-β, whereas the type I receptor is not. Once type II receptor binds to TGF-β, the TβRI recognizes the signaling complex of TGF-β and type II receptor and is recruited into the complex. In the heteromeric receptor complex, several serine and threonine residues in the GS domain of TGF-β type I receptor are phosphorylated by TβRII. Upon being activated as the downstream signaling substrate of type II receptor kinase, the TβRI acts as an effector of TGF-β response and propagates the signal. Recent studies revealed that Mothers Against dpp (MAD) in *Drosophila* and its homologs are essential intracellular signaling components of the TGF-β superfamily *(77,78)*. Smad2 and 3 are phosphorylated by TβRI upon ligand binding, form a heteromer with Smad4, and then translocate into the nucleus, which is required for efficient TGF-β signal transduction *(79)*. The known or proposed features of the TGF-β signal transduction pathway are summarized in Fig. 2.

The cytoplasmic domain of type II and type I receptor is a functional serine–threonine kinase that is essential for signaling activity. The truncated derivatives of TβRII and TβRI that lacked the cytoplasmic serine–threonine kinase domain have been shown to act as dominant-negative inhibitors of TGF-β signal transduction. Expression of a truncated TβRII lacking the intracellular kinase domain suppresses inhibition of cell proliferation and secretion of extracellular matrix protein plasminogen activator inhibitor I and fibronectin induced by TGF-β in mink lung epithelial cell lines *(80)*, TGF-β induced

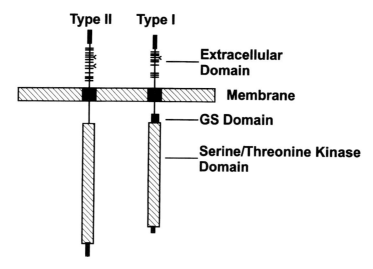

Fig. 1. Schematic representation of the signal transducing TGF-β receptors on cell surfaces.

transcriptional activation of specific genes in neonatal cardiac myocytes *(81)*, and TGF-β-induced mitogenic action and extracellular matrix production in lung fibroblasts *(46,46a)*.

## TRANSFORMING GROWTH FACTOR-BETA RECEPTOR-INTERACTING PROTEINS

To elucidate the intracellular signaling cascades of TGF-β, considerable efforts have been concentrated on the identification and characterization of the signaling components that interact with TβRII and TβRI and serve as substrates for serine–threonine kinase receptors. Using the cytoplasmic domains of the type I or type II receptors as bait, FKBP12 and farnesyl-protein transferase-α subunit (FT-α) have been identified as type I receptor interacting proteins, whereas a WD-repeat containing protein named TGF-β receptor interacting protein-1 (TRIP-1) as type II receptor-associated protein *(82,83)*.

FKBP12 is a ubiquitously expressed 12 kDa cytosolic protein that serves as a cellular receptor for various natural and synthetic immunosuppressive drugs such as FK506 and rapamycin *(84,85)*. FKBP12 interacts with the cytoplasmic domain of the type I receptor and restrains TGF-β signal transduction by binding to TβRI and inhibiting phosphorylation of TβRI by TβRII *(82)*.

Interaction between TβRI and FT-α was observed both in a yeast two-hybrid system and in mammalian cells. FT-α is a cytoplasmic interactor for phosphorylated TβRI and is phosphorylated and released from its binding site on the type I receptor upon ligand binding with TβRII *(83)*. However, farnesyl transferase activity is dispensable for TGF-β signaling of growth inhibitory and transcriptional responses and the interaction between TβRI and FT-α does not affect the known functions of these two proteins *(86)*.

TRIP-1 contains five WD repeats that may mediate various protein–protein interactions. Interaction of TRIP-1 with TβRII induces TRIP-1 phosphorylation on serine and threonine by TβRII kinase activity, but the functional significance of TRIP-1 in TGF-β signaling is unknown *(87)*. Although there is no concrete evidence that FKBP12, FT-

Table 1
Serine–Theonine Kinase Receptors for the TGF-β Family

| Receptor | Other Designation | Ligands |
|---|---|---|
| Type I Receptor | | |
| TβRI | ALK5,R4,RPK2 | TGF-βs |
| ActRI | ALK2,Tsk7L,R1,SKR1 | Activins |
| ActRIB | ALK4,R2, | Activins |
| Atr-1 | | Activins,BMPs |
| BMPR-IA | ALK3,BRK-1 | BMPs |
| BMPR-IB | ALK6,RPK-1 | BMPs |
| ALK1 | TSR-1,R3 | Unknown |
| Sax | | Dpp (BMP) |
| Daf-1 | | Unknown |
| C-14 | | Unknown |
| Type II Receptor | | |
| TβRII | | TGF-βs |
| ActRII | | Activins |
| ActRIIB | | Activins |
| Atr-II | | Activins |
| BMPR-II | | BMPs |
| AMHR-II | MISRII | AMH/MIS |

α and TRIP-1 are essential downstream components of TGF-β signal transduction pathway, they may play regulatory roles in TGF-β signaling.

A member of the mitogen-activated protein kinase kinase kinase (MAPKKK) family, TGF-β activated kinase 1 (TAK1), has been identified as a mediator in the signaling pathway of TGF-β superfamily (88). TAK1 participates in regulation of transcription by TGF-β. Furthermore, kinase activity of TAK1 was stimulated in response to TGF-β and bone morphogenetic protein. Two novel proteins, termed TAB1 and TAB2 (for TAK1 binding protein), interact with TAK1(89). The importance of TAK1, TAB1, and TAB2 in the TGF-β signal transduction pathway remains to be defined.

## MAD-RELATED PROTEINS IN TRANSFORMING
## GROWTH FACTOR-BETA SIGNALING PATHWAYS

A remarkable breakthrough in TGF-β signaling comes from genetic analysis of decapentaplegic (dpp) signaling pathway in *Drosophila (78)*. Genetic screening in *Drosophila* revealed that Mothers Against dpp (MAD) plays an important role in the intracellular signal transduction of the serine–threonine kinase receptors for the TGF-β superfamily *(77,78)*. Three *Caenorhabditis elegans* genes, sma-2, sma-3, and sma-4 were identified subsequently as MAD homologs *(90)*. Several homologs of MAD have now been identified in vertebrates, including human, mouse, rat, and Xenopus *(91)*. The members of these newly identified intracellular signaling components of the TGF-β superfamily were referred as Smad proteins, the term coined from Sma and MAD. Smad proteins are 40-to 70-kD intracellular proteins that share a highly conserved amino-terminal MH1 domain (for MAD homology 1), a conserved carboxyl-terminal MH2 domain, and an intervening nonconserved region (Fig. 3).

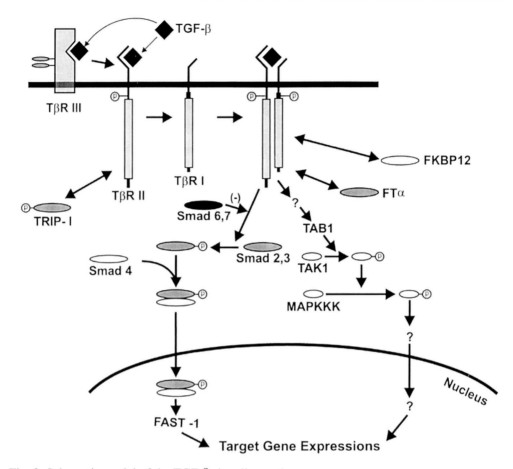

Fig. 2. Schematic model of the TGF-β signaling pathway.

Smads fall into three classes based on structural and functional characteristics (Table 2). The class I Smads include Smad1, Smad2, Smad3, and Smad5. They are direct substrates of specific serine–threonine kinase receptors and act in a pathway-restricted fashion. The class II Smads participate in TGF-β signaling by associating with class I Smads. Smad4 is the only member in vertebrates that has been identified in this subfamily. Smad6 and Smad7 belong to the class III Smads, which inhibit signaling by antagonizing the function of the other two classes of Smads.

Smad1, Smad2, Smad3, and Smad5 are ligand-specific. Smad2 and Smad3 are highly similar in their structure. They are activated by TβRI/ALK5 and ActR-IB/ALK4 and mediate signaling by TGF-β and activin (92,93). Smad1 and Smad5 are substrates of BMPR-1A/ALK3 and BMPR-1B/ALK6 and transduce signals from bone morphogenetic proteins. The pathway-restricted Smads are phosphorylated by type I serine–threonine receptor kinases. Smad4 diverges structurally from the members of the pathway-restricted Smads and functions as a commom-mediator for transcriptional activation (94). Smad4 forms heteromeric complexes with Smad2 and Smad3 after TGF-β or activin stimulation and with Smad1 and Smad5 in response to bone morphogenetic proteins, and then translocates into the nucleus where they form a complex with FAST-1 that requires these three components to activate transcription (95,96).

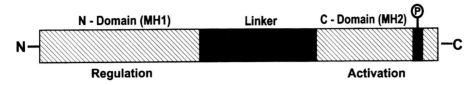

Fig. 3. Schematic illustration of the general structure of Smads.

Smad6 and Smad7 are distantly related to other Smad proteins *(97–99)*, and they function as inhibitors of signaling by pathway-restricted Smads. Smad6 and Smad7 interact with the activated type I receptor, thereby blocking the association, phosphorylation, and activation of pathway-restricted Smads.

It is clear that the Smad family is important for TGF-β signaling. However, our understanding of how TGF-β mediates multiple signals such as cell proliferation, cell differentiation, growth inhibition, apoptosis, extracelluar matrix production and gene transcription, is still incomplete. New TGF-β signaling components and cascades are expected to be uncovered and characterized in the future.

## EXPRESSION OF TRANSFORMING GROWTH FACTOR-BETA RECEPTORS DURING LUNG DEVELOPMENT

TβRI and TβRII are the only signaling receptors identified for TGF-β. Both TβRI and TβRII are present during lung development. Expression of the TβRII and TβRI is temporally and spatially regulated during rat lung development *(100,100a)*. TβRII mRNA was expressed in rat fetal lung tissue early in development, increased as development proceeded, reached maximal concentration postnatally, and then decreased to the adult level. The pattern of TβRI expression during lung development was distinct from that of TβRII. Expression of TβRI increased with a peak shortly before the time of birth and then declined as lung development proceeded.

The TβRII gene was expressed in the mesenchymal tissue and in the epithelial lining of the developing airway. TβRII mRNA was also observed in the adventitial layer of small blood vessels. Expression of the TβRII gene in the developing airway epithelium occurred along a proximal–distal gradient. The intensity of the TβRII hybridization signal paralleled the differentiation of the airway epithelium *(100)*.

The distribution of TβRI in developing lung overlapped the localization of TβRII. TβRI mRNA was expressed by the cells of the interstitium, the airway epithelium and the blood vessels during lung development. Expression of both type I and type II receptors is altered in pathologic conditions *(101)*.

In addition to TβRI and TβRII, other type I and type II serine–threonine kinase receptors are also found in the lung. Two cDNA sequences encoding serine–threonine kinase domains of type I and type II (bTSR1 and bTSR2) were identified in baboon lung by sequencing analysis *(102)*. Both bTSR1 and bTSR2 were expressed throughout embryonic lung development and in adult lungs. The expressions of bTSR1 and bTSR2 were developmentally regulated and each had a distinct expression pattern. Furthermore, the expressions of bTSR1 and bTSR2 in fetal baboon lung were altered by oxygen exposure. Two type I serine–threonine kinase receptors, ALK-1 and ALK-4, were also present in the lung *(103,104)*. ALK-1 was expressed in pulmonary blood vessels with a higher level of gene expression in endothelium than in adjacent smooth muscle, whereas

Table 2
Smad Family

| Designation | Signaling Specificity |
|---|---|
| Pathway-restricted Smads | |
| ⌈ Smad 2 | TGF-β |
| ⌊ Smad 3 | Activin |
| | |
| ⌈ Smad 1 | BMP |
| ⌊ Smad 5 | |
| | |
| Common-partner Smad | |
| Smad 4 | All |
| | |
| Inhibitory Smads | |
| ⌈ Smad 6 | All |
| ⌊ Smad 7 | |

the activin type IB receptor ALK-4 is expressed in putative developing airways. The expression pattern of ALK-1 and ALK-4 differs from that of TβRI. The expression of TβRI was found to be ubiquitous in the lung.

Inhibition of TGF-β receptor expression during development has been reported in two in vitro models. Inhibition by addition of antisense oligodeoxynucleotides stimulated embryonic mouse lung branching morphogenesis in culture *(35)*. Recently, an adenoviral vector carrying a nonfunctional TGF-β type II receptor mutant was introduced into embryonic mouse lung in culture and this model also showed a stimulated branching of the conducting airways *(105)*.

## ACKNOWLEDGMENTS

This work was supported by grants from the American Lung Association, the Department of Veterans Affairs and the National Institutes of Health. The author would like to thank Dr. S. L. Young for his critical reading of the manuscript.

## REFERENCES

1. Spooner BS, Wessells NK. Mammalian lung development: interactions in primordium formation and bronchial morphogenesis. J Exp Zool 1970;175:445–54.
2. Ten Have-Opbroek AA. Lung development in the mouse embryo. Exp Lung Res 1991;17:111–30.
3. Massague J. The transforming growth factor-beta family. Annu Rev Cell Biol 1990;6:597–641.
4. Kingsley DM. The TGF-beta superfamily: new members, new receptors, and new genetic tests of function in different organisms. Genes Dev 1994;8:133–46.
5. Roberts AB, Anzano MA, Lamb LC, Smith JM, Sporn MB. New class of transforming growth factors potentiated by epidermal growth factor: isolation from non-neoplastic tissues. Proc Natl Acad Sci USA 1981;78:5339–5343.
6. Cheifetz S, Weatherbee JA, Tsang ML, et al. The transforming growth factor-beta system, a complex pattern of cross-reactive ligands and receptors. Cell 1987;48:409–415.
7. de Bortoli C, Chailley-Heu B, Bourbon JR. Production of transforming growth factor (TGF) beta by fetal lung cells. Biol Cell 1995;84:215–218.
8. Pelton RW, Johnson MD, Perkett EA, Gold LI, Moses HL. Expression of transforming growth factor-beta 1, -beta 2, and -beta 3 mRNA and protein in the murine lung. Am J Respir Cell Mol Biol 1991;5:522–530.

9. Kelley J, Shull S, Walsh JJ, Cutroneo KR, Absher M. Auto-induction of transforming growth factor-beta in human lung fibroblasts. Am J Respir Cell Mol Biol 1993;8:417–424.

10. Coker RK, Laurent GJ, Shahzeidi S, et al. Diverse cellular TGF-beta 1 and TGF- beta 3 gene expression in normal human and murine lung. Eur Respir J 1996;9:2501–2507.

11. Letterio JJ, Geiser AG, Kulkarni AB, Roche NS, Sporn MB, Roberts AB. Maternal rescue of transforming growth factor–beta 1 null mice. Science 1994;264:1936–1938.

12. Taipale J, Miyazono K, Heldin CH, Keski-Oja J. Latent transforming growth factor-beta 1 associates to fibroblast extracellular matrix via latent TGF-beta binding protein. J Cell Biol 1994;124:171–181.

13. Miyazono K, Olofsson A, Colosetti P, Heldin CH. A role of the latent TGF-beta 1-binding protein in the assembly and secretion of TGF-beta 1. EMBO J 1991;10:1091–1101.

14. Heine UI, Munoz EF, Flanders KC, Roberts AB, Sporn MB. Colocalization of TGF-beta 1 and collagen I and III, fibronectin and glycosaminoglycans during lung branching morphogenesis. Development 1990;109:29–36.

15. Sporn MB, Roberts AB. Peptide growth factors are multifunctional. Nature 1988;332:217–219.

16. Fine A, Goldstein RH. The effect of transforming growth factor-beta on cell proliferation and collagen formation by lung fibroblasts. J Biol Chem 1987;262:3897–3902.

17. Ryan RM, Mineo-Kuhn MM, Kramer CM, Finkelstein JN. Growth factors alter neonatal type II alveolar epithelial cell proliferation. Am J Physiol 1994;266:L17–22.

18. Masui T, Wakefield LM, Lechner JF, LaVeck MA, Sporn MB, Harris CC. Type beta transforming growth factor is the primary differentiation-inducing serum factor for normal human bronchial epithelial cells. Proc Natl Acad Sci USA 1986;83:2438–2442.

19. Jetten AM, Vollberg TM, Nervi C, George MD. Positive and negative regulation of proliferation and differentiation in tracheobronchial epithelial cells. Am Rev Respir Dis 1990;142:S36–S39.

20. Pfeifer AM, Lechner JF, Masui T, Reddel RR, Mark GE, Harris CC. Control of growth and squamous differentiation in normal human bronchial epithelial cells by chemical and biological modifiers and transferred genes. Environ Health Perspect 1989;80:209–220.

21. Twardzik DR, Ranchalis JE, McPherson JM, et al. Inhibition and promotion of differentiated-like phenotype of a human lung carcinoma in athymic mice by natural and recombinant forms of transforming growth factor-beta. J Natl Cancer Inst 1989;81:1182–1185.

22. Hay ED. Extracellular matrix, cell skeletons, and embryonic development. Am J Med Genet 1989;34:14–29.

23. McGowan SE. Extracellular matrix and the regulation of lung development and repair. FASEB J 1992;6:2895–2904.

24. Raghu G, Masta S, Meyers D, Narayanan AS. Collagen synthesis by normal and fibrotic human lung fibroblasts and the effect of transforming growth factor-beta. Am Rev Respir Dis 1989;140:95–100.

25. Fine A, Poliks CF, Smith BD, Goldstein RH. The accumulation of type I collagen mRNAs in human embryonic lung fibroblasts stimulated by transforming growth factor-beta. Connect Tissue Res 1990;24:237–247.

26. McGowan SE, McNamer R. Transforming growth factor–beta increases elastin production by neonatal rat lung fibroblasts. Am J Respir Cell Mol Biol 1990;3:369–376.

27. McGowan SE, Jackson SK, Olson PJ, Parekh T, Gold LI. Exogenous and endogenous transforming growth factors-beta influence elastin gene expression in cultured lung fibroblasts. Am J Respir Cell Mol Biol 1997;17:25–35.

28. Kucich U, Rosenbloom JC, Abrams WR, Bashir MM, Rosenbloom J. Stabilization of elastin mRNA by TGF-beta: initial characterization of signaling pathway. [See Comments]. Am J Respir Cell Mol Biol 1997;17:10–16.

29. Zhao Y, Young SL. TGF-beta regulates expression of tenascin alternative-splicing isoforms in fetal rat lung. Am J Physiol 1995;268:L173–L180.

30. Roberts CJ, Birkenmeier TM, McQuillan JJ, et al. Transforming growth factor beta stimulates the expression of fibronectin and of both subunits of the human fibronectin receptor by cultured human lung fibroblasts. J Biol Chem 1988;263:4586–4592.

31. Maniscalco WM, Sinkin RA, Watkins RH, Campbell MH. Transforming growth factor-beta 1 modulates type II cell fibronectin and surfactant protein C expression. Am J Physiol 1994;267:L569–L577.

32. Romaris M, Heredia A, Molist A, Bassols A. Differential effect of transforming growth factor beta on proteoglycan synthesis in human embryonic lung fibroblasts. Biochim Biophys Acta 1991;1093:229–233.

33. Lund LR, Riccio A, Andreasen PA, et al. Transforming growth factor-beta is a strong and fast acting positive regulator of the level of type-1 plasminogen activator inhibitor mRNA in WI-38 human lung fibroblasts. EMBO J 1987;6:1281–1286.

34. Gerwin BI, Keski-Oja J, Seddon M, Lechner JF, Harris CC. TGF-beta 1 modulation of urokinase and PAI-1 expression in human bronchial epithelial cells. Am J Physiol 1990;259:L262–L269.

35. Zhao J, Bu D, Lee M, Slavkin HC, Hall FL, Warburton D. Abrogation of transforming growth factor-beta type II receptor stimulates embryonic mouse lung branching morphogenesis in culture. Dev Biol 1996;180:242–257.

36. Whitsett JA, Weaver TE, Lieberman MA, Clark JC, Daugherty C. Differential effects of epidermal growth factor and transforming growth factor-beta on synthesis of Mr = 35,000 surfactant-associated protein in fetal lung. J Biol Chem 1987;262:7908–7913.

37. Vollberg TM, George MD, Nervi C, Jetten AM. Regulation of type I and type II transglutaminase in normal human bronchial epithelial and lung carcinoma cells. Am J Respir Cell Mol Biol 1992;7:10–18.

38. Nogami M, Romberger DJ, Rennard SI, Toews ML. TGF-beta 1 modulates beta-adrenergic receptor number and function in cultured human tracheal smooth muscle cells. Am J Physiol 1994; 266:L187–L191.

39. Bonner JC, Badgett A, Lindroos PM, Osornio-Vargas AR. Transforming growth factor beta 1 downregulates the platelet-derived growth factor alpha–receptor subtype on human lung fibroblasts in vitro. Am J Respir Cell Mol Biol 1995;13:496–505.

40. Thannickal VJ, Fanburg BL. Activation of an H2O2-generating NADH oxidase in human lung fibroblasts by transforming growth factor beta 1. J Biol Chem 1995;270:30,334–30,338.

41. Geiser AG, Letterio JJ, Kulkarni AB, Karlsson S, Roberts AB, Sporn MB. Transforming growth factor beta 1 (TGF-beta 1) controls expression of major histocompatibility genes in the postnatal mouse: aberrant histocompatibility antigen expression in the pathogenesis of the TGF-beta 1 null mouse phenotype. Proc Natl Acad Sci USA 1993;90:9944–9948.

42. Sanford LP, Ormsby I, Gittenberger-de Groot AC, et al. TGFbeta2 knockout mice have multiple developmental defects that are non-overlapping with other TGFbeta knockout phenotypes. Development 1997;124:2659–2670.

43. Kaartinen V, Voncken JW, Shuler C, et al. Abnormal lung development and cleft palate in mice lacking TGF-beta 3 indicates defects of epithelial–mesenchymal interaction. Nat Genet 1995;11:415–421.

44. Zhou L, Dey CR, Wert SE, Whitsett JA. Arrested lung morphogenesis in transgenic mice bearing an SP-C-TGF-beta 1 chimeric gene. Dev Biol 1996;175:227–238.

45. Massague J. Receptors for the TGF-beta family. Cell 1992;69:1067–1070.

46. Zhao Y, Young SL. Requirement of transforming growth factor-beta (TGF-beta) type II receptor for TGF-beta-induced proliferation and growth inhibition. J Biol Chem 1996;271:2369–2372.

46a. Zhao, Y. Transforming growth factor-beta (TGF-beta) type I and type II receptors are both required for TGF-beta-mediated extracellular matrix production in lung fibroblasts. Mol Cell Endocrinol 1999;150:91-97.

47. Kalter VG, Brody AR. Receptors for transforming growth factor-beta (TGF-beta) on rat lung fibroblasts have higher affinity for TGF-beta 1 than for TGF-beta 2. Am J Respir Cell Mol Biol 1991;4:397–407.

48. Laiho M, Weis MB, Massague J. Concomitant loss of transforming growth factor (TGF)–beta receptor types I and II in TGF-beta-resistant cell mutants implicates both receptor types in signal transduction. J Biol Chem 1990;265:18518–18524.

49. Boyd FT, Massague J. Transforming growth factor-beta inhibition of epithelial cell proliferation linked to the expression of a 53-kDa membrane receptor. J Biol Chem 1989;264:2272–2278.

50. Morello JP, Plamondon J, Meyrick B, Hoover R, MD OC-M. Transforming growth factor-beta receptor expression on endothelial cells: heterogeneity of type III receptor expression. J Cell Physiol 1995;165:201–211.

51. Wang XF, Lin HY, Ng-Eaton E, Downward J, Lodish HF, Weinberg RA. Expression cloning and characterization of the TGF-beta type III receptor. Cell 1991;67:797–805.

52. Lopez-Casillas F, Cheifetz S, Doody J, Andres JL, Lane WS, Massague J. Structure and expression of the membrane proteoglycan betaglycan, a component of the TGF-beta receptor system. Cell 1991;67:785–795.

53. Georgi LL, Albert PS, Riddle DL. daf-1, a C. elegans gene controlling dauer larva development, encodes a novel receptor protein kinase. Cell 1990;61:635–645.

54. Ebner R, Chen RH, Shum L, et al. Cloning of a type I TGF-beta receptor and its effect on TGF-beta binding to the type II receptor. Science 1993;260:1344–1348.

55. Lin HY, Wang XF, Ng-Eaton E, Weinberg RA, Lodish HF. Expression cloning of the TGF-beta type II receptor, a functional transmembrane serine/threonine kinase [published erratum appears in Cell 1992 Sep 18;70(6):following 1068]. Cell 1992;68:775–785.

56. Franzen P, ten Dijke P, Ichijo H, et al. Cloning of a TGF beta type I receptor that forms a heteromeric complex with the TGF beta type II receptor. Cell 1993;75:681–692.

57. Yamashita H, ten Dijke P, Franzen P, Miyazono K, Heldin CH. Formation of hetero-oligomeric complexes of type I and type II receptors for transforming growth factor–beta. J Biol Chem 1994;269:20172–20178.

58. Attisano L, Carcamo J, Ventura F, Weis FM, Massague J, Wrana JL. Identification of human activin and TGF beta type I receptors that form heteromeric kinase complexes with type II receptors. Cell 1993;75:671–680.

59. Yamashita H, ten Dijke P, Huylebroeck D, et al. Osteogenic protein-1 binds to activin type II receptors and induces certain activin-like effects. J Cell Biol 1995;130:217–226.

60. ten Dijke P, Ichijo H, Franzen P, et al. Activin receptor-like kinases: a novel subclass of cell-surface receptors with predicted serine/threonine kinase activity. Oncogene 1993;8:2879–2887.

61. Carcamo J, Weis FM, Ventura F, et al. Type I receptors specify growth-inhibitory and transcriptional responses to transforming growth factor beta and activin. Mol Cell Biol 1994;14:3810–3821.

62. Wrana JL, Tran H, Attisano L, et al. Two distinct transmembrane serine/threonine kinases from Drosophila melanogaster form an activin receptor complex. Mol Cell Biol 1994;14:944–950.

63. ten Dijke P, Yamashita H, Sampath TK, et al. Identification of type I receptors for osteogenic protein-1 and bone morphogenetic protein-4. J Biol Chem 1994;269:16985–16988.

64. Xie T, Finelli AL, Padgett RW. The Drosophila saxophone gene: a serine-threonine kinase receptor of the TGF-beta superfamily. Science 1994;263:1756–1759.

65. Baarends WM, van Helmond MJ, Post M, et al. A novel member of the transmembrane serine/threonine kinase receptor family is specifically expressed in the gonads and in mesenchymal cells adjacent to the mullerian duct. Development 1994;120:189–197.

66. Mathews LS, Vale WW. Expression cloning of an activin receptor, a predicted transmembrane serine kinase. Cell 1991;65:973–982.

67. Attisano L, Wrana JL, Cheifetz S, Massague J. Novel activin receptors: distinct genes and alternative mRNA splicing generate a repertoire of serine/threonine kinase receptors. Cell 1992;68:97–108.

68. Mathews LS, Vale WW, Kintner CR. Cloning of a second type of activin receptor and functional characterization in Xenopus embryos. Science 1992;255:1702–1705.

69. Childs SR, Wrana JL, Arora K, Attisano L, MB OC, Massague J. Identification of a Drosophila activin receptor. Proc Natl Acad Sci USA 1993;90:9475–9479.

70. Liu F, Ventura F, Doody J, Massague J. Human type II receptor for bone morphogenic proteins (BMPs): extension of the two-kinase receptor model to the BMPs. Mol Cell Biol 1995;15:3479–3486.

71. Nohno T, Ishikawa T, Saito T, et al. Identification of a human type II receptor for bone morphogenetic protein-4 that forms differential heteromeric complexes with bone morphogenetic protein type I receptors. J Biol Chem 1995;270:22522–22526.

72. di Clemente N, Wilson C, Faure E, et al. Cloning, expression, and alternative splicing of the receptor for anti-Mullerian hormone. Mol Endocrinol 1994;8:1006–1020.

73. Estevez M, Attisano L, Wrana JL, Albert PS, Massague J, Riddle DL. The daf-4 gene encodes a bone morphogenetic protein receptor controlling C. elegans dauer larva development. Nature 1993; 365:644–649.

74. Wrana JL, Attisano L, Wieser R, Ventura F, Massague J. Mechanism of activation of the TGF-beta receptor. Nature 1994;370:341–347.

75. Henis YI, Moustakas A, Lin HY, Lodish HF. The types II and III transforming growth factor-beta receptors form homo-oligomers. J Cell Biol 1994;126:139–154.

76. Chen RH, Derynck R. Homomeric interactions between type II transforming growth factor-beta receptors. J Biol Chem 1994;269:22868–22874.

77. Raftery LA, Twombly V, Wharton K, Gelbart WM. Genetic screens to identify elements of the decapentaplegic signaling pathway in Drosophila. Genetics 1995;139:241–254.

78. Sekelsky JJ, Newfeld SJ, Raftery LA, Chartoff EH, Gelbart WM. Genetic characterization and cloning of mothers against dpp, a gene required for decapentaplegic function in Drosophila melanogaster. Genetics 1995;139:1347–1358.

79. Nakao A, Imamura T, Souchelnytskyi S, et al. TGF-beta receptor-mediated signalling through Smad2, Smad3 and Smad4. EMBO J 1997;16:5353–5362.

80. Wieser R, Attisano L, Wrana JL, Massague J. Signaling activity of transforming growth factor beta type II receptors lacking specific domains in the cytoplasmic region. Mol Cell Biol 1993; 13:7239–7247.

81. Brand T, MacLellan WR, Schneider MD. A dominant–negative receptor for type beta transforming growth factors created by deletion of the kinase domain. J Biol Chem 1993;268:11,500–11,503.

82. Chen YG, Liu F, Massague J. Mechanism of TGFbeta receptor inhibition by FKBP12. EMBO J 1997;16:3866–3876.

83. Wang T, Danielson PD, Li BY, Shah PC, Kim SD, Donahoe PK. The p21(RAS) farnesyltransferase alpha subunit in TGF-beta and activin signaling. Science 1996;271:1120–1122.

84. Abraham RT, Wiederrecht GJ. Immunopharmacology of rapamycin. Annu Rev Immunol 1996; 14:483–510.

85. Sabatini DM, Erdjument-Bromage H, Lui M, Tempst P, Snyder SH. RAFT1: a mammalian protein that binds to FKBP12 in a rapamycin-dependent fashion and is homologous to yeast TORs. Cell 1994;78:35–43.

86. Ventura F, Liu F, Doody J, Massague J. Interaction of transforming growth factor-beta receptor I with farnesyl-protein transferase-alpha in yeast and mammalian cells. J Biol Chem 1996;271:13931–13934.

87. Chen RH, Miettinen PJ, Maruoka EM, Choy L, Derynck R. A WD-domain protein that is associated with and phosphorylated by the type II TGF-beta receptor. Nature 1995;377:548–552.

88. Yamaguchi K, Shirakabe K, Shibuya H, et al. Identification of a member of the MAPKKK family as a potential mediator of TGF-beta signal transduction. Science 1995;270:2008–2011.

89. Shibuya H, Yamaguchi K, Shirakabe K, et al. TAB1: an activator of the TAK1 MAPKKK in TGF-beta signal transduction. Science 1996;272:1179–1182.

90. Savage C, Das P, Finelli AL, et al. Caenorhabditis elegans genes sma-2, sma-3, and sma-4 define a conserved family of transforming growth factor beta pathway components. Proc Natl Acad Sci USA 1996;93:790–794.

91. Eppert K, Scherer SW, Ozcelik H, et al. MADR2 maps to 18q21 and encodes a TGFbeta-regulated MAD-related protein that is functionally mutated in colorectal carcinoma. Cell 1996;86:543–552.

92. Macias–Silva M, Abdollah S, Hoodless PA, Pirone R, Attisano L, Wrana JL. MADR2 is a substrate of the TGFbeta receptor and its phosphorylation is required for nuclear accumulation and signaling. Cell 1996;87:1215–1224.

93. Zhang Y, Feng X, We R, Derynck R. Receptor-associated Mad homologues synergize as effectors of the TGF-beta response. Nature 1996;383:168–172.

94. Zhang Y, Musci T, Derynck R. The tumor suppressor Smad4/DPC 4 as a central mediator of Smad function. Curr Biol 1997;7:270–276.

95. Liu F, Pouponnot C, Massague J. Dual role of the Smad4/DPC4 tumor suppressor in TGFbeta-inducible transcriptional complexes. Genes Dev 1997;11:3157–3167.

96. Zhou S, Zawel L, Lengauer C, Kinzler KW, Vogelstein B. Characterization of human FAST-1, a TGF beta and activin signal transducer. Mol Cell 1998;2:121–127.

97. Imamura T, Takase M, Nishihara A, et al. Smad6 inhibits signalling by the TGF-beta superfamily [see comments]. Nature 1997;389:622–626.

98. Nakao A, Afrakhte M, Moren A, et al. Identification of Smad7, a TGFbeta-inducible antagonist of TGF-beta signaling. [See Comments]. Nature 1997;389:631–635.

99. Hayashi H, Abdollah S, Qiu Y, et al. The MAD-related protein Smad7 associates with the TGFbeta receptor and functions as an antagonist of TGFbeta signaling. Cell 1997;89:1165–1173.

100. Zhao Y, Young SL. Expression of transforming growth factor-beta type II receptor in rat lung is regulated during development. Am J Physiol 1995;269:L419–L426.

100a. Zhao Y, Young SL, Silbajoris R. (Expression of TGF-beta type I receptor is distinct from that of type II receptor during lung development. Mol Biol Cell 1999;10s:274a.

101. Zhao Y, Gilmore BJ, Young SL. Expression of transforming growth factor-beta receptors during hyperoxia-induced lung injury and repair. Am J Physiol 1997;273:L355–L362.

102. Zhao Y, Silbajoris R, Young SL. Identification and developmental expression of two activin receptors in baboon lung. Biochem Biophys Res Commun 1996;229:50–57.

103. Roelen BA, van Rooijen MA, Mummery CL. Expression of ALK-1, a type 1 serine/threonine kinase receptor, coincides with sites of vasculogenesis and angiogenesis in early mouse development. Dev Dyn 1997;209:418–430.

104. Panchenko MP, Williams MC, Brody JS, Yu Q. Type I receptor serine–threonine kinase preferentially expressed in pulmonary blood vessels. Am J Physiol 1996;270:L547–L558.

105. Zhao J, Sime PJ, Bringas P, Jr., Gauldie J, Warburton D. Epithelium-specific adenoviral transfer of a dominant–negative mutant TGF-beta type II receptor stimulates embryonic lung branching morphogenesis in culture and potentiates EGF and PDGF-AA. Mech Dev 1998;72:89–100.

# 14

## Transgenic Mouse Models for the Study of Growth Factor Signaling During Lung Morphogenesis

*Jeffrey A. Whitsett,* MD *and*
*Thomas R. Korfhagen,* MD, PHD

**CONTENTS**

## LUNG MORPHOGENESIS IN THE DEVELOPING MOUSE

Formation of the lung begins with an outpouching of endodermal tissue from the lateral esophageal laryngeal sulcus at approx 9 d postconception in the mouse. The endodermal-derived cells form the trachea and mainstem bronchi, and the esophagus separates from the trachea during the early embryonic period of lung morphogenesis.

From: *Contemporary Endocrinology: Endocrinology of the Lung: Development and Surfactant Synthesis*
Edited by: C. R. Mendelson © Humana Press Inc., Totowa, NJ

Endodermal tissue grows into the splanchnic mesenchyme and undergoes stereotypic dichotomous branching to form the bronchioles and acinar structures characteristic of mammalian lung. The columnar epithelial cells lining the endodermally derived tubules remain relatively undifferentiated until day 13–14 pc, when the conducting airways are virtually complete. Pulmonary vessels form along the airways to produce the highly vascularized capillary bed of the pulmonary vasculature. The splanchnic mesenchyme differentiates to form vascular, lymphatic, and stroma tissues that are distinct in proximal, as compared to peripheral, regions of the lung. Cell differentiation, expansion of the airspaces, and thinning of the splanchnic mesenchyme precedes birth. Successful adaptation to air breathing following birth requires production of pulmonary surfactant by type II epithelial cells, clearance of lung liquid, and continued growth of the gas exchange surface. Angiogenesis and vasculogenesis generate the extensive capillary network that forms during alveolarization. Thus, the orderly growth and differentiation of numerous cell types is required for the formation of the lung, and is thought to be mediated by tightly controlled paracrine signaling that occurs between the respiratory epithelium and the underlying mesenchyme.

## TRANSCRIPTIONAL CONTROL OF LUNG DEVELOPMENT

Formation of the foregut endoderm and further commitment of endodermal cells to form respiratory epithelial cell lineages are under the control of a number of diverse families of transcription factors that regulate gene expression in target cells. Thyroid transcription factor 1 (TTF-1) is a 38-kDa polypeptide member of the Nkx homeodomain containing transcription factors (1). TTF-1 is first detected in subsets of endodermal cells in the thyroid and pulmonary primordia at approximately 9 d pc, and is expressed in subsets of epithelial cells in both conducting and peripheral airways of the developing lung (2). TTF-1 binds to and regulates the transcription of both the thyroid and pulmonary specific genes products, including surfactant proteins A, B, C, and CCSP (3–7). Gene targeting of the TTF-1 gene causes thyroid agenesis and marked pulmonary hypoplasia with associated absence of distal respiratory epithelium and lack of the expression of TTF-1 target genes (8) (Fig. 1). The TTF-1 gene is regulated by both HNF-3β (9), a transcriptional protein of the forkhead family of the winged helix proteins, and GATA-6 (10), a leucine zipper containing DNA binding protein. HNF-3β is critical for the formation of the node patterning and formation of the foregut (11,12), being coexpressed with TTF-1 in the developing avian (13), murine (14), and human lung (15). GATA-6 activates TTF-1 gene transcription and is required for commitment of progenitor cells to form respiratory tubules (10,16). Thus, interactions among these families of transcription factors are likely critical to the proliferation and differentiation of foregut endodermal cells, ultimately producing the respiratory epithelium. Although the signaling pathways inducing the transcriptional machinery controlling lung cell differentiation are unknown at present, there is increasing evidence that the splanchnic mesenchyme provides information critical to the process of lung morphogenesis.

## ROLE OF GROWTH FACTOR PRODUCTION
## BY THE PULMONARY MESENCHYME IN LUNG MORPHOGENESIS

The requirement of mesenchymal signals for the growth and branching of the endodermally derived lung buds has been well established in vitro. Dissection of the splanchnic mesen-

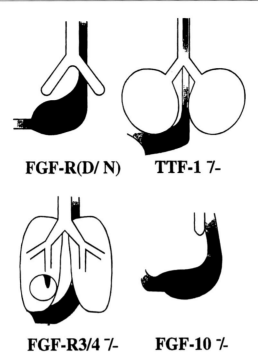

**FGF-R(D/ N)        TTF-1 7-**

**FGF-R3/4 7-        FGF-10 7-**

Fig. 1. Abnormal lung morphogenesis in mice with targeted gene inactivation. Transgenic mice expressing a mutated form of FGF-RIIb (FGF-R D/N) in distal epithelial cells developed normal trachea and
mainstem bronchi but no distal lung structures *(36)*. Mice homozygous for a null mutation of the TTF-
1 gene (TTF-1 –/–) developed normal trachea and bronchi ending in large saccules*(8)*. Normal distal lung
structures were absent. Mice homozygous for null mutations in FGF-R3 and 4 (FGF-R3/4 –/–) developed
abnormal, emphysematous alveoli despite persistent and increased elastin production*(27)*. Mice homozygous for a null mutation in the FGF-10 gene failed to develop any lung structures beyond the trachea*(38)*.
Lung structures are depicted as open structures while the esophagus and stomach, included for reference,
are depicted as filled-in structures.

chyme from the lung buds renders them unable to either proliferate or undergo dichotomous
branching in vivo *(17)*. Coculture of tracheal endoderm with mesenchyme from the peripheral embryonic lung results in ectopic branching, proliferation, and differentiation of cells
with features characteristic of the peripheral airway (e.g., SP-C expression) *(18)*. On the
contrary, tracheal mesenchyme inhibits branching of distal respiratory tubules *(19)*. The
information provided by paracrine signaling between epithelium and mesenchyme is required for the proper cell commitment, differentiation, proliferation, and/or migration of
progenitor cells of the lung.

## ROLE OF FIBROBLAST GROWTH FACTOR SIGNALING
## IN LUNG MORPHOGENESIS

The temporospatial pattern of expression of fibroblast growth factors (FGFs) and their
receptors (FGFRs), and their ability to provide signals directing cell proliferation and
differentiation in numerous developing organ systems, has provided strong support for
their involvement in lung morphogenesis. Likewise, recent studies implicating both
FGFs and FGFRs in tracheal morphogenesis in *Drosophila* supports the conservation of

FGF signaling in the formation of lung in other organisms *(20,21)*. For example, deletion of FGF causes marked abnormalities in the tracheal system in *Drosophila*, termed *branchless* that is associated with abnormal migration of tracheal cells in the developing tracheal tubules *(20)*. Likewise, mutations in an FGF receptor homolog causes the *breathless* phenotype in *Drosophila (21)*.

There are presently at least 18 distinct FGFs identified in mammalian species that mediate cell proliferation, migration and differentiation in various organs. The activity of FGFs is mediated by binding to four known receptors, FGFRs (FGFR1, FGFR2, FGFR3, FGFR4, and their splice variants). These receptors share extracellular IgG-like domains, a single membrane spanning domain, and an intracellular tyrosine kinase-containing domain. The receptors form heterodimers or homodimers following ligand binding, and, subsequently, the cytoplasmic domain is phosphorylated to activate signal transduction within the cell. Both FGFs and FGFRs are expressed in distinct temporospatial patterns in the developing mammalian lung *(22)*. FGF-1, FGF-7, FGF-10, and FGF-18 have been identified in developing lung, being expressed in distinct patterns primarily in mesenchymal tissues *(23–26)*. While FGF signaling has been widely implicated in the regulation of mammalian organogenesis, analysis of the role of specific organ development is complicated by both early embryonic lethality in null mutations, for example, FGFR1, FGF-4, FGF-8, and FGFR2, and functional redundancy, as observed in FGF-7, FGFR3, and FGF-4 null mice in vivo *(27)*. Nevertheless, experiments using antisense oligonucleotides, neutralizing antibodies, tissue recombinants, as well as the addition of FGFs or FGF-coated beads to organ culture and cells, support their role in epithelial–mesenchymal signaling during organogenesis of the lung and other organs *(28–31)*.

## DOMINANT-NEGATIVE DELETION
## OF FIBROBLAST GROWTH FACTOR SIGNALING
## IN THE LUNG IN VIVO

Deletion mutation of the cytoplasmic domain of FGFRs generates a molecule that binds and competes for ligands (FGFs) and forms heterodimers with wild-type FGF receptors in the membrane, but fails to complete the phosphorylation-dependent signal transduction required for the function of the receptor. Thus, expression of high levels of an FGFR mutant receptor creates a dominant-negative receptor that inhibits signaling through wild-type receptors. Such dominant-negative FGF receptors have been used to uncover the role of FGF signaling in various developing organs, including skin *(32)*, gastrulation in *Xenopus (33)*, the lens *(34)*, breast *(35)*, and lung *(36)*.

A dominant-negative FGFRIIb isoform was expressed in the lungs of transgenic mice under control of the surfactant protein C promoter *(36)*. The human SP-C promoter element directs expression of genes in the highly organ-specific manner, beginning on day 9.5–10 of gestation, and continuing postnatally in the peripheral cells of the developing respiratory tubules *(37)*. Postnatally, the SP-C promoter is active in the peripheral bronchioles, acini and in alveolar type II cells. Transgenic mice bearing the SP-C-FGFRIIb dominant-negative isoforms all succumbed from respiratory failure at birth; pathologic findings in these mice were confined to the lungs *(36)*. The respiratory tract consisted of intact tracheal and bronchial tubes, but there was a complete lack of peripheral lung parenchyma in these mice (Fig. 1). While the remaining respiratory tubules were lined by ciliated and Clara cells, the latter expressing CCSP (a Clara cell nonciliated secretory cell marker), markers of peripheral lung cells (e.g., SP-C) were entirely lacking, as were vascular and other stromal tissues, demonstrating the requirement of endoderm for maintenance and differentiation of lung stroma. These studies demonstrate a critical role of FGF signaling in lung morphogenesis. Since the FGF dominant-negative receptor is likely to block various FGF ligands, by dimerizing with various FGFR isoforms, it is unclear from this study whether lung morphogenesis is dependent on specific or redundant functions of specific FGFs and FGF receptors.

## DELETION OF FIBROBLAST GROWTH FACTOR-10, BUT NOT FIBROBLAST GROWTH FACTOR-7, BLOCKS LUNG ORGANOGENESIS

FGF-10 is expressed in the mesenchyme of both lung and limb buds *(25)*. Min et al. *(38)* generated mice bearing a null mutation in FGF-10, demonstrating a dramatic phenotype that lacked both limbs and lungs at birth. Lungs in the FGF-10 (–/–) mice were completely absent; however, trachea with cartilaginous rings, lined by ciliated and goblet cells, was observed in the remaining upper tracheal tissue (Fig. 1). Thus, endodermal cells committed to lung cell lineages required for tracheal formation do not require FGF-10. However, formation of bronchi and peripheral lung tissues absolutely require FGF-10. The findings in the FGF-10 –/– mice is similar to the phenotype seen in FGFRIIb dominant-negative mice that lacked peripheral lung tissues, but differ in the presence of mainstem bronchi in SP-C-FGFRIIb dominant-negative model, likely related to the lack of expression of the dominant-negative FGF receptor in the subset of cells that forms trachea and mainstem bronchi, as is typical of the SP-C promoter *(37)*. In contrast to findings in FGF-10 (–/–) mice, targeted deletion of FGF-7 failed to alter lung or other organ morphogenesis, demonstrating the likely functional redundancy of the FGF-7 signaling *(39)*. Abnormalities in the FGF-7 (–/–) mice were confined to alterations in hair structure.

## EFFECTS OF FIBROBLAST GROWTH FACTOR-7 IN VIVO

FGF-7 is a powerful mitogen for a number of epithelial cells in liver, breast, lung, and other tissues. Intratracheal administration of FGF-7 in the adult mouse causes marked mitotic activity and proliferation of both conducting airway, and alveolar type II cells *(40)*. Preadministration of FGF-7 before lung injury, protects the lung from injury, supporting the potential role of FGF-7 in repair *(41)*. Expression of FGF-7 under control of the SP-C promoter in transgenic mice caused large cystadenomatoid malformations in the fetal lung. The marked swelling of pulmonary tissues resulted in embryonic lethality at approximately E-15 to E-16 *(42)*. Thus missexpression of FGF-7 in the lungs of transgenic mice caused disruption of branching morphogenesis and cyst formation with histologic features virtually identical to those seen in human infants with cystadenomatoid malformations. Cyst formation induced by FGF-7 was associated with increased chloride secretion that was mediated by non-CFTR-dependent chloride channels *(43)*. FGF-7 caused cell proliferation, enhanced the expression of SP-C and induced morphologic features characteristic of type II epithelial cells when added to isolated respiratory epithelial cells in vitro *(29)*. Taken together, both in vivo and in vitro experiments, support the concept that the precise temporospatial patterning of FGF expression is critical for proper branching morphogenesis and cell differentiation in the developing lung. In vitro effects of FGF-7 appear to be distinct from those of FGF-10. Cardosa et al.

*(44)* placed FGF-7 or FGF-10 containing beads within embryonic lung tissue in explant culture, demonstrating that the effects of each FGF on cell proliferation and morphogenesis were distinct. FGF-10-coated beads caused migration of epithelial cells to the source of FGF, while FGF-7 caused proliferation and distention of peripheral tubules.

The precise FGFs and FGF receptor(s), influencing various aspects of lung morphogenesis, remain to be clarified. However, there is ample evidence for distinct roles of various FGF-Rs in lung morphogenesis. Gene targeting of either FGF-R3 or FGF-R4 did not alter lung morphogenesis; however, significant abnormalities in alveolarization were noted in doubly homozygous FGF-R3/FGF-R4 mutant mice (Fig. 1). The development of emphysema in the FGF-R3/FGF-R4 mutant mice was associated with persistent expression of elastin mRNA and increased elastin staining in lung parenchyma *(27)*. Since many FGFs, including FGF-1, FGF-9, FGF-10, and FGF-18, are also expressed in the lung, knowledge of the precise sites, regulation of expression, and signaling pathways mediating the actions of the FGFs is likely to be critical to understanding the process of lung morphogenesis and offers the potential for developing new therapies for various pulmonary disorders.

## PLATELET-DERIVED GROWTH FACTORS AND ALVEOLOGENESIS

### *PDGF-A and-B*

Platelet-derived Growth Factors (PDGF's) are encoded by two distinct genes, A and B. PDGF-A and PDGF-B form homo- or heterodimers that bind and activate one of two receptor tyrosine kinases, PDGF receptor $\alpha$ or $\beta$ (PDGFR$\alpha$ or PDGFR$\beta$). PDGF-A and PDGFR$\alpha$ are expressed in a variety of tissues of developing vertebrates *(45,46)*. To decipher biologic function of PDGFs in vivo, null mutant mice were generated by gene targeting. Mice carrying a null mutation in the PDGF-B chain gene develop cardiovascular, hematologic, and renal anomalies *(47)* but do not have abnormalities in the lung. By contrast, mice bearing a null mutation in the PDGF-A chain gene develop lung abnormalities associated with alterations of alveologenesis (see Chapter 12 for further discussion).

### *PDGF-A (–/–) mice*

The PDGF-A gene was mutated by a targeting construct deleting exon 4, removing $NH_2$-teminal regions essential for its bioactivity. While heterozygous PDGF-A-deleted mice were normal, half of the expected homozygous null mice died before embryonic day 10, indicating that in certain mouse strains, the embryos die before lung development. Approximately 50% of the null mutants died postnatally, with no survivors being detected after 6 wk of age. Null PDGF-A mutant mice were smaller than age-matched littermates. Lungs appeared hyperinflated with evidence of emphysema (Fig. 2). The right ventricle of the heart was enlarged, consistent with cor pulmonale, probably secondary to the pulmonary disease *(46)*. Fetal lungs from PDGF-A null mutant mice were histologically indistinguishable from heterozygous littermates. However, null mouse lungs had emphysema associated with lack of secondary septation. Lungs of null mutants had a profound deficiency of alveolar $\alpha$ smooth muscle actin expressing myofibroblasts and were deficient in elastin fibers. Bronchial and vascular smooth muscle cells appeared normal, indicating that the lung defect in PDGF-A-targeted mice was specific to the lung parenchyma. The deficiency of elastin was attributed to a lack of tropoelastin synthesis in the alveolus *(46)*.

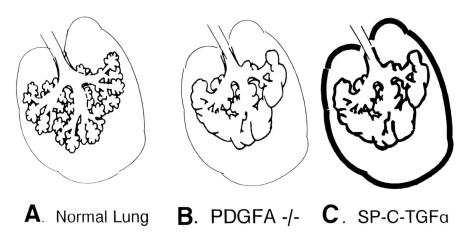

**A**. Normal Lung    **B**. PDGFA -/-    **C**. SP-C-TGFα

Fig. 2. Growth factor-associated emphysema. (**A**) Normal lung structures. (**B**) Mice homozygous for a null mutation of the PDGF-A gene develop emphysema during alveologenesis due to lack of elastin deposition and formation of secondary septal *(46,48)*. (**C**) Mice bearing a transgene causing overexpression of TGF-α develop emphysema and fibrosis during postnatal alveologenesis *(66,67)*. A single bronchus and alveoli surrounded by pleura are depicted. Thickened alveoli and pleura represent fibrosis (panel C).

PDGF-A is produced by the developing respiratory epithelium and binds to the PDGFRα receptor expressed on mesenchymal cells, that surround epithelial buds during the pseudoglandular and canalicular phases of lung development. Postnatally, during alveologenesis, the expression of PDGFRα mRNA decreases in the prospective alveoli, while tropoelastin synthesis increases. The PDGFRα expressing mesenchymal cells are thought to give rise to the tropoelastin producing alveolar smooth muscle cells. Elastin forms a framework required for the formation of secondary septae critical to alveologenesis. In the PDGF-A (–/–) mice, the PDGFRα– expressing cells fail to proliferate, and alveolar smooth muscle cells fail to develop. Tropoelastin synthesis and elastin deposition are blocked, causing failure of formation of secondary septae, disrupting alveologenesis, and causing emphysema *(48)*. Thus, PDGF-A gene-targeted mice revealed a previously unknown role for PDGF-A in determining proliferation and migration of developing alveolar smooth muscle cells that play a critical role in alveologenesis.

## EPIDERMAL GROWTH FACTOR RECEPTOR SIGNALING AND LUNG MORPHOGENESIS

Transforming growth factor-alpha (TGF-α) is a member of the epidermal growth factor family of peptides that bind and activate the epidermal growth factor receptor (EGF-R). Epidermal growth factor peptides are expressed in a variety of tissues including the lung. TGF-α, epidermal growth factor (EGF), and EGF-R are expressed in the lung *(49,50)*. TGF-α is produced in airway epithelial cells, macrophages and some fibroblasts in the pre- and postnatal lung and was identified in respiratory epithelial cells in lungs from infants with bronchopulmonary dysplasia *(50)*. Intratracheal delivery of bleomycin to rat lungs increased TGF-α and EGF-R expression in vivo *(51)*. Furthermore, isolated lung fibroblasts produced TGF-α in response to hyperoxia and isolated alveolar macrophages produced TGF-α in response to bacterial endotoxin *(52,53)*. Increased TGF-α was detected following asbestos injury *(54)*, and increased TGF-α and EGF and the EGF-R were observed following naphthalene-induced injury in mice *(55)*. Thus the epidermal growth factor family of peptides appears to play a role in the complex responses of the lung to injury.

## ROLE OF EPIDERMAL GROWTH FACTOR RECEPTOR IN LUNG MORPHOGENESIS

The role of epidermal growth factor peptides in lung development remains somewhat controversial. Warburton et al. *(56)* reported that EGF enhanced branching morphogenesis of explanted fetal mouse lungs. By contrast, Ganser et al. *(57)* observed decreased branching of fetal mouse lungs exposed to TGF-α. Administration of EGF to fetal rhesus monkeys intraperitoneally or in the amniotic fluid decreased type II cell content of glycogen, and increased lamellar bodies and surfactant protein-A without increasing lung growth *(58)*. Increased proliferation of freshly isolated type II cells was observed in the presence of EGF or TGF-α *(59)*.

Lung development was studied in EGF-R null mutant mice generated by targeted gene inactivation; however, abnormalities in EGF-R gene-targeted mice were strongly influenced by genetic background *(60)*. In the CF-1 strain, EGF-R (–/–) mice died by stage E 7.5 to 8.5. CF-1-EGF-R (–/–) embryos had abnormal inner cell masses and no distinct endoderm. In the 129SV strain, embryos survived to at least E 12.5 to 13.6, but none of the embryos survived to birth. In CD-1 outbred stains, 16% of the EGF-R (–/–) mice survived to term, but no survival was observed beyond 3 wk of age. Abnormalities were observed in numerous organs, including the brain, colon, kidneys, hair, and tongue. However, lungs of EGF-R null mutant mice were morphologically indistinguishable from normal E18.5 littermates. Differences were not detected in the cellular distribution of surfactant protein B (SP-B) or proproteins for SP-B or SP-C. Sibilia and Wagner *(61)* also generated null mutations of the EGF-R and noted that inbred strains died during early development. Defects were detected in whisker formation, hair follicles, and corneal differentiation. Pups surviving to P20 were dehydrated and appeared to suffer from a wasting syndrome. In contrast to Threadgill et al. *(60)*, Sibilia and Wagner detected poorly aerated lungs that appeared immature. Miettinen et al. *(62)* also generated null mutations of the EGF-R using gene inactivation. Defects were detected in hair follicles, fungiform papillae, and skin. Intestinal defects were detected in growth-restricted EGF-R null mutant mice, including decreased sized intestinal villi and hemorrhagic, distended bowel. Lungs of EGF-R (–/–) mice that survived postnatally, contained collapsed alveoli, and decreased staining for the surfactant proteins SP-C or SP-A. Miettenen et al. *(63)* also reported that branching of lungs from fetal EGF-R (–/–) mice was reduced in explant culture in vitro.

## WA-1 AND WA-2 MUTANT MICE

Wa-2 mice bear a spontaneous point mutation in the EGF-R (wa-2), that caused decreased, but not complete absence of EGF-R signaling *(64,65)*. Survival, breeding and lung histology were unaltered in wa-2/wa-2 mice. However, nursing mothers had impaired lactation causing malnutrition of some of the pups. Likewise, no abnormalities in lung formation were observed in wa-1/wa-1 mice that lack TGF-α. Thus the effects of altered EGF-R signaling on mouse development in vivo varies among mouse strains and may be influenced by the extent of EGF-R activity. While inbred strains of EGF-R (–/– mice die) in the embryonic period, outbred strains of mice develop kidney, skin, and intestinal defects. Lung abnormalities have not been detected in all EGF-R (–/–) strains.

# INCREASED EXPRESSION
# OF TRANSFORMING GROWTH FACTOR-ALPHA
# CAUSES PULMONARY EMPHYSEMA IN TRANSGENIC MICE

To further assess the role of TGF-$\alpha$ in lung injury and repair in vivo, transgenic mice were generated in which human TGF-$\alpha$ was expressed in distal respiratory epithelial cells under control of the 3.7-kb human SP-C promoter/enhancer sequences (66,67). In this model, human TGF-$\alpha$ mRNA was detected primarily in type II epithelial cells. Lungs of SP-C-TGF-$\alpha$ mice were markedly emphysematous, and extensive fibrotic lesions were observed adjacent to blood vessels and on pleural surfaces (Fig. 2). The extent of pulmonary abnormalities varies with the level of expression of TGF-$\alpha$ in various transgenic lines.

## BITRANSGENIC MICE [SP-C-TGF-A X WA-2 (–/–) OR SP-C-EGF-R-M]

To identify the cellular signaling pathways mediating the TGF-$\alpha$ induced pulmonary lesions, SP-C-TGF-$\alpha$ transgenic mice were bred into wa-2/wa-2 mice and into mice expressing a dominant/negative EGF-R mutation in the distal respiratory epithelium. In the wa-2/wa-2 mice, reduced EGF-R signaling occurs in all cell types. In the SP-C-EGF-R-M mice, a truncated EGF-R (EGF-R-M), lacking a portion of the intracytoplasmic domain, forms heterodimers with wild-type EGF receptors creating a dominant/negative receptor. Since the heterodimers do not cause phosphorylation of the intracytoplasmic domain, signal transduction of the wild-type EGF-R in respiratory epithelial cells is inhibited. The mutated EGF receptor was expressed selectively in the lung epithelium under control of the SP-C promoter, reducing signaling from EGF related polypeptides in respiratory epithelial cells, while maintaining EGF-R signaling in other cell types. TGF-$\alpha$ dependent changes in lung morphogenesis were ameliorated when the SP-C-TGF-$\alpha$ transgene was bred into either wa-2/wa-2 mice or SP-C-EGF-R-M mice, indicating that TGF-$\alpha$ receptor signaling in respiratory epithelial cells mediates TGF-$\alpha$ induced lung remodeling (68) likely via an autocrine-paracrine dependent mechanism (Fig. 3).

# TRANSFORMING GROWTH FACTOR-ALPHA
# PROTECTS ADULT LUNGS FROM INJURY

Although expression of TGF-$\alpha$ in the lungs of transgenic mice caused lung remodelling during postnatal alveologenesis, recent studies in adult SP-C-TGF-$\alpha$ mice demonstrated a marked protective effect of TGF-$\alpha$ during pulmonary inflammation (69). SP-C-TGF-$\alpha$ transgenic mice had improved survival after exposure to ultrafine Teflon particles that cause acute oxidant injury in the lung.

# SUMMARY OF STUDIES
# ON THE EPIDERMAL GROWTH FACTOR PEPTIDE FAMILY

Epidermal growth factor peptides are produced by respiratory epithelial cells or fibroblasts during development and in response to lung injury. Disruption of EGF-R signaling in the mouse had variable effects on perinatal lung function and lung morphogenesis, being strongly influenced by the genetic strain. Prolonged expression of TGF-$\alpha$ during postnatal alveologenesis caused severe emphysema and pulmonary fibrosis. The finding that TGF-$\alpha$ induced abnormalities in lung morphogenesis were blocked by an inhibitory EGF-R expressed in respiratory epithelial cells, supports the presence of an autocrine–

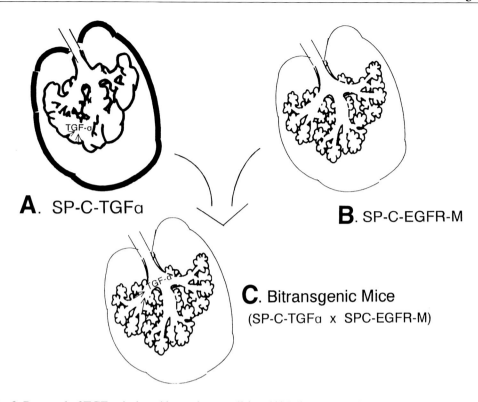

**A**. SP-C-TGFα

**B**. SP-C-EGFR-M

**C**. Bitransgenic Mice
(SP-C-TGFα x SPC-EGFR-M)

Fig. 3. Reversal of TGF-α induced lung abnormalities. (**A**) Mice expressing the TGF-α transgene develop emphysema and fibrosis *(66,67)*. (**B**) Mice expressing a dominant-negative mutation of the EGF-R in type II cells form normal lung structures *(68)*. (**C**) Bitransgenic mice overexpressing TGF-α and the dominant negative EGF-R, do not develop pulmonary abnormalities *(68)*. The bitransgenic mice demonstrate that EGF-R signaling in type II cells in critical to cause TGF-α induced lung abnormalities. A single bronchus and alveoli surrounded by pleura are depicted. Overexpression of TGF-α by the SP-C-TGF-α transgene is depicted by TGF-α in the alveoli.

paracrine loop, in which growth factor binding to the respiratory epithelial cells influences the process or alveolarization of repair after injury.

## ACKNOWLEDGMENTS

This work was supported by the National Institutes of Health HL56387 (SCOR), the Cystic Fibrosis Foundation Research and Development Program, and HL58795 (T.R.K.).

## REFERENCES

1. Guazzi S, Lonigro R, Pintonello L, Boncielli E, Di Lauro R, Mavilio F. The thyroid transcription factor-1 gene is a candidate target for regulation by Hox proteins. EMBO J 1994;13:3339–3347.
2. Lazzaro D, Price M, De Felice M, DiLauro R. The transcription factor TTF-1 is expressed at the onset of thyroid and lung morphogenesis and in restricted regions of the foetal brain. Development 1991;113:1093–1104.
3. Francis-Lang H, Price M, Polycarpou-Schwarz M, DiLauro R. Cell-type-specific expression of the rat thyroperoxidase promoter indicates common mechanisms for thyroid-specific gene expression. Mol Cell Biol 1992;12:576–588.
4. Bruno MD, Bohinski RJ, Huelsman KM, Whitsett JA, Korfhagen TR. Lung cell specific expression of the murine surfactant protein A gene is mediated by interactions between the SP-A promoter and thyroid transcription factor-1. J Biol Chem 1995;270:6531–6536.

5. Bohinski RJ, DiLauro R, Whitsett JA. The lung–specific surfactant protein B gene promoter is a target for thyroid transcription factor 1 and hepatocyte nuclear factor 3 indicating common factors for organ-specific gene expression along the foregut axis. Mol Cell Biol 1994;14:5671–5681.

6. Kelly SE, Bachurski CJ, Burhans MS, Glasser SW. Transcription of the lung-specific surfactant protein C gene is mediated by thyroid transcription factor-1. J Biol Chem 1996;271:6881–6888.

7. Zhang L, Whitsett JA, Stripp BR. Regulation of Clara cell secretory protein gene transcription by thyroid transcription factor-1. Biochim Biophys Acta 1997;1350:359–367.

8. Kimura S, Hara Y, Pineau T, Fernandez-Salguero P, Fox C H, Ward JM, Gonzalez FJ. The T/ebp null mouse: thyroid specific enhancer-binding protein is essential for the organogenesis of the thyroid lung ventral forebrain and pituitary. Gene Develop 1996;10:60–69.

9. Ikeda K, Clark JC, Shaw-White JR, Stahlman MT, Boutell CJ, Whitsett JA. Gene structure and expression of human thyroid transcription factor–1 in respiratory epithelial cells. J Biol Chem 1995;270:8108–8114.

10. Shaw-White JR, Bruno MD, Whitsett JA. GATA-6 activates transcription of thyroid transcription factor-1. J Biol Chem 1999;274:2658–2664.

11. Ang SL, Rossant J. HNF-3β is essential for node and notochord formation in mouse development. Cell 1994;78:561–574.

12. Weinstein DC, Ruiz I, Altaba A, Chen WS, Hoodless P, Prezioso VR, Jessell TM, Darnell JE. The winged-helix transcription factor HNF-3 beta is required for notochord development in the mouse embryo. Cell 1994;78:575–588.

13. Zeng X, Yutzey KE, Whitsett JA. Thyroid transcription factor-1 hepatocyte nuclear factor-3β and surfactant protein A and B in the developing chick lung. J Anat 1998;193:399–408.

14. Zhou L, Lim L, Costa RH, Whitsett JA. Thyroid transcription factor-1, hepatocyte nuclear factor-3β, surfactant protein B, C, and Clara cell secretory protein in developing mouse lung. J Histochem Cytochem 1996;44:1183–1193.

15. Stahlman MT, Gray ME, Whitsett JA. Temporal-spatial distribution of hepatocyte nuclear factor-3β in developing human lung and other foregut derivatives. J Histochem Cytochem 1998;46:955–962.

16. Morrisey EE, Tang Z, Sigrist K, Lu MM, Jiang F, Ip HS, Parmacek MS. GATA6 regulates HNF4 and is required for differentiation of visceral endoderm in the mouse embryo. Genes Dev 1998; 12:3579–3590.

17. Wessells NK. Mammalian lung development: interactions in formation and morphogenesis of tracheal buds. J Exp Zool 1970;175:455–466.

18. Shannon JM. Induction of alveolar type II cell differentiation in fetal tracheal epithelium by grafted distal lung mesenchyme. Dev Biol 1994;166:600–614.

19. Shannon JM, Nielsen LD, Gebb SA, Randell SH. Mesenchyme specifies epithelial differentiation in reciprocal recombinants of embryonic lung and trachea. Dev Dyn 1998;212:482–494.

20. Sutherland D, Samakoulis C, Krasnow MA. branchless encodes a Drosophila Fgf homolog that controls tracheal migration and the pattern of branching. Cell 1996;87:1091–1101.

21. Klambt C, Glazer L, Shilo B. breathless a Drosophila FGF receptor homolog is essential for migration of tracheal and specific midline glial cells. Genes Dev 1992;6:1668–1678.

22. Hogan BLM, Yingling JM. Epithelial/mesenchymal interactions and branching morphogenesis of the lung. Curr Opin Gene Dev 1998;8:481–486.

23. Fu Y, Spirito P, Yu Z, Biro S, Sasse J, Lei J, Ferrans VJ, Epstein SE, Casscells W. Acidic fibroblast growth factor in the developing rat embryo. J Cell Biol 1991;114:1261–1273.

24. Finch PW, Cunha GR, Rubin JS, Wong J, Ron D. Pattern of keratinocyte growth factor and keratinocyte growth factor receptors during mouse fetal development suggests a role in mediating morphogenic mesenchymal–epithelial interactions. Dev Dyn 1995;203:223–240.

25. Bellusci S, Grindley J, Emoto H, Itoh N, Hogan BLM. Fibroblast growth factor 10 (FGF10) and branching morphogenesis in the embryonic mouse lung. Development 1997;124:4867–4878.

26. Hu MC, Qiu WR, Wang Y, Hill D, Ring BD, Scully S, Bolon B, DeRose M, Luethy R, Simonet WS, Arakawa T, Danilenko DM. FGF-18 a novel member of the fibroblast growth factor family stimulates hepatic and intestinal proliferation. Mol Cell Biol 1998;18:6063–6074.

27. Weinstein M, Xu X, Ohyama K, Deng CX. FGF-R-3 and FGF-R-4 function cooperatively to direct alveogenesis in murine lung. Development 1998;125:3615–3623.

28. Shannon JM, Deterding RR. Epithelial–mesenchymal interactions in lung development. In: McDonald JA, ed. Lung growth and development. New York: Marcel Dekker,1997:81–118.

29. Deterding RR, Jacoby CR, Shannon JM. Acidic fibroblast growth factor and keratinocyte growth factor stimulate fetal rat pulmonary epithelial growth. Am J Physiol 1996;271:L495–L505.

30. Nogawa H, Itoh A. Branching morphogenesis of embryonic mouse lung epithelium in mesenchyme free cultures. Development 1995;121:1015–1022.
31. Cardoso W, Itoh A, Nogawa H, Mason J, Brody JS. FGF-1 and FGF-7 induce distinct patterns of growth and differentiation in embryonic lung epithelium. Dev Dyn 1997;208:398–405.
32. Werner S, Smola H, Liao X, Longaker MT, Kreig T, Hofschneider PH, Williams LT. The function of KGF in morphogenesis of epithelium and re-epithelialization of wounds. Science 1994;266:819–822.
33. Amaya E, Musci TJ, Kirschner MW. Expression of a dominant negative mutant of the FGF receptor disrupts mesoderm formation in Xenopus embryos. Cell 1991;66:257–270.
34. Robinson ML, MacMillan LA, Thompson JA, Overbeck PA. Expression of a truncated FGF receptor results in defective lens development in transgenic mice. Development 1995;121:3959–3967.
35. Jackson D, Bresnick J, Rosewell I, Crafton T, Paulson R, Stamp G, Dickson C. Fibroblast growth factor receptor signaling has a role in lobuloalveolar development of the mammary gland. J Cell Sc 1997;110:1261–1268.
36. Peters K, Werner S, Liao X, Wert S, Whitsett J, Williams L. Targeted expression of a dominant negative FGF receptor blocks branching morphogenesis and epithelial differentiation of the mouse lung. EMBO J 1994;13:3296–3301.
37. Wert SE, Glasser SW, Korfhagen TR, Whitsett JA. Transcriptional elements from the human SP-C gene direct expression in the primordial respiratory epithelium of transgenic mice. Dev Biol 1993;156:426–443.
38. Min H, Danilenko DM, Scully SA, Bolon B, Ring BD, Tarpley JE, DeRose M, Simonet WS. Fgf-10 is required for both limb and lung development and exhibits striking functional similarity to Drosophila branchless. Genes Dev 1998;12:3156–3161.
39. Guo L, Degentein L, Fuchs E. Keratinocyte growth factor is required for hair development but not for wound healing. Genes Dev 1996;10:165–175.
40. Ulich TR, Yi ES, Longmuir K, Yin S, Biltz R, Morris CF, Housley RM, Pierce GF. Keratinocyte growth factor is a growth factor for type II pneumocytes in vivo. J Clin Invest 1994;93:1298–1306.
41. Panos RJ, Rubin JS, Aaronson SA, Mason RJ. Keratinocyte growth factor and hepatocyte growth factor/scatter factor are heparin-binding growth factors for alveolar type II cells in fibroblast-conditioned medium. J Clin Invest 1993;92:969–977.
42. Simonet WS, DeRose ML, Bucay N, Nguyen HQ, Wert SE, Zhou L, Ulich TR, Thomason A, Danilenko DM, Whitsett JA. Pulmonary malformation in transgenic mice expressing human keratinocyte growth factor in the lung. Proc Natl Acad Sci USA 1995;92:12,461–12,465.
43. Zhou L, Graef RW, McCray PB, Simonet WS, Whitsett JA. Keratinocyte growth factor stimulates CFTR-independent fluid secretion in the fetal lung in vitro. Am J Physiol 1996;271:L987–L994.
44. Park WY, Miranda B, Lebeche D, Hashimoto G, Cardoso WV. FGF-10 is a chemotactic factor for distal epithelial buds during lung development. Dev Biol 1998;201:125–134.
45. Orr-Urtreger A, Lonai P. Platelet-derived growth factor-A and its receptor are expressed in separate but adjacent cell layers of the mouse embryo. Development 1992;115:1045–1058.
46. Boström H, Willetts K, Pekny M, Levéen P, Lindahl P, Hedstrand H, Pekna M, Hellström M, Gebre-Medhin S, Schalling M, Nilsson M, Kurland S, Törnell J, Heath JK, Betsholtz C. PDGF-A signaling is a critical event in lung alveolar myofibroblast development and alveogenesis Cell 1996;85:863–873.
47. Leveen P, Pekny M, Gebre-Medhin S, Swolin B, Larsson E, Betsholtz C. Mice deficient for PDGF B show renal cardiovascular and hematological abnormalities. Genes Dev 1994;8:1875–1887.
48. Lindahl P, Karlsson L, Hellstrom M, Gebre-Medhin S, Willetts K, Heath JK, Betsholtz C. Alveogenesis failure in PDGF-A-deficient mice is coupled to lack of distal spreading of alveolar smooth muscle cell progenitors during lung development. Development 1997;124:3943–3953.
49. Ruocco S, Lallemand A, Tournier JM, Gaillard D. Expression and localization of epidermal growth factor, transforming growth factor-α, and localization of their common receptor in fetal human lung development. Pediatr Res 1996;39:448–455.
50. Strandjord TP, Clark JG, Guralnick DE, Madtes DK. Immunolocalization of transforming growth factor-α, epidermal growth factor (EGF), and EGF-receptor in normal and injured developing human lung. Pediatr Res 1995;38:851–856.
51. Madtes DK, Busby HK, Strandjord TP, Clark JG. Expression of transforming growth factor-α and epidermal growth factor receptor is increased following bleomycin-induced lung injury in rats. Am J Respir Cell Mol Biol 1994;11:540–551.
52. Vivekananda J, Lin A, Coalson JJ, King RJ. Acute inflammatory injury in the lung precipitated by oxidant stress induces fibroblasts to synthesize and release transforming growth factor-α J Biol Chem 1994;269:25,057–25,061.

53. Madtes DK, Raines EW, Sakariassen KS, Assoian RK, Sporn MB, Bell GI, Ross R. Induction of transforming growth factor-alpha in activated human alveolar macrophages. Cell 1988;53:285–293.

54. Liu JY, Morris GF, Lei WH, Conti M, Brody AR. Up–regulated expression of transforming growth factor α in the bronchiolar–alveolar duct regions of asbestos-exposed rats. Am J Pathol 1996;149:205–217.

55. Van Winkle LS, Isaac JM, Plopper CG. Distribution of epidermal growth factor receptor and ligands during bronchiolar epithelial repair from naphthalene-induced Clara cell injury in the mouse. Am J Pathol 1997;151:443–459.

56. Warburton D, Seth C, Shum L, Horcher PG, Hall FL, Werb Z, Slavkin HC. Epigenetic role of epidermal growth factor expression and signalling in embryonic mouse lung morphogenesis. Dev Biol 1992;149:123–133.

57. Ganser GL, Stricklin GP, Matrisian L. EGF and TGFα influence in vitro lung development by the induction of matrix-degrading mettaloproteinases. Int J Dev Biol 1991;35:453–461.

58. Plopper CG, St George JA, Reed LC, Nishio SJ, Weir AJ, Edwards L, Tarcantal AF, Pinkerton KE, Styne D, Merritt TA, Whitsett JA, George-Nascimento C. Acceleration of alveolar type II cell differentiation in the fetal Rhesus monkey lung by administration of epidermal growth factor. Am J Respir Physiol 1992;262:L313–L321.

59. Ryan RM, Mineo-Kuhn MM, Kramer CM, Finkelstein JN. Growth factors alter neonatal type II alveolar epithelial cell proliferation. Am J Physiol 1994;266:L17–L22.

60. Threadgill DW, Dlugosz AA, Hansen LA, Tennenbaum T, Lichti U, Yee D, LaMantia C, Mourton T, Herrup K, Harris RC, Barnard JA, Yuspa SH, Coffey RJ, Magnuson T. Targeted disruption of mouse EGF receptor: effect of genetic background on mutant phenotype. Science 1995;269:230–238.

61. Sibilia M, Wagner EF. Strain-dependent epithelial defects in mice lacking the EGF receptor. Science 1995;269:234–238.

62. Miettinen PJ, Berger JE, Menses J, Phung Y, Pedersen RA, Werb Z, Derynck R. Epithelial immaturity and multiorgan failure in mice lacking epithelial growth factor receptor. Nature 1995;376:337–341.

63. Miettinen PJ, Warburton D, Bu D, Zhao J–S, Berger JE, Minoo P, Koivisto T, Allen L, Dobbs L, Werb Z, Derynck R. Impaired lung branching morphogenesis in the absence of functional EGF receptor. Dev Biol 1997;186:224–236.

64. Fowler KJ, Walker F, Alexander W, Hibbs ML, Nice EC, Bohmer RM, Mann GB, Thumwood C, Maglitto R, Danks JA, Chetty R, Burgess AW, Dunn AR. A mutation in the epidermal growth factor receptor in waved-2 mice has a profound effect on receptor biochemistry that results in impaired lactation. Proc Natl Acad Sci USA 1995;92:1465–1469.

65. Luetteke NC, Phillips HK, Qiu TH, Copeland NG, Earp HS, Jenkins NA, Lee DC. The mouse waved-2 phenotype results from a point mutation in the EGF receptor tyrosine kinase. Genes Dev 1994;8:399–413.

66. Korfhagen TR, Swantz RJ, Wert SE, McCarty JM, Kerlakian CB, Glasser SW, Whitsett JA. Respiratory epithelial cell expression of human transforming growth factor-α induces lung fibrosis in transgenic mice. J Clin Invest 1994;93:1691–1699.

67. Hardie WD, Bruno MD, Huelsman KM, Iwamoto HS, Carrigan PE, Leikauf GD, Whitsett JA, Korfhagen TR. Postnatal lung function and morphology in transgenic mice expressing transforming growth factor α. Am J Pathol 1997;151:1075–1083.

68. Hardie WD, Kerlakian CB, Bruno MD, Huelsman KM, Wert SE, Glasser SW, Whitsett JA, Korfhagen TR. Reversal of lung lesions in transgenic transforming growth factor α mice by expression of mutant epidermal growth factor receptor. Am J Respir Cell Mol Biol 1996;15:499–508.

69. Hardie WD, Prows DR, Leikauf GD, Korfhagen TR. Attenuation of acute lung injury in transgenic mice expressing human transforming growth factor-alpha. Am J Physiol 1999;277:L1045–L1050.

# 15

# Parathyroid Hormone-Related Protein

## *Lewis P. Rubin, MD, and John S. Torday, PhD*

## INTRODUCTION

In 1987, a second member of the parathyroid hormone (PTH) family, PTH-related protein (PTHrP), was identified and cloned *(1)*. PTHrP is produced in many normal fetal *(2–11)* and adult *(7,12–19)* tissues, including several endocrine tissues, cartilage and bone, heart, vascular and other smooth muscle, skin, central nervous system, liver, kidney, and lung. The cell types that produce PTHrP encompass all three embryonic

From: *Contemporary Endocrinology: Endocrinology of the Lung: Development and Surfactant Synthesis*
Edited by: C. R. Mendelson © Humana Press Inc., Totowa, NJ

germ layers and the extraembryonic trophectoderm. The PTHrP gene is expressed in certain mesenchymal cells, but production of the protein typically is restricted to the epithelium of organs, while its receptor is often expressed in adjacent mesenchyme. During the past decade, investigations of PTHrP structure and functions have provided insights into new and novel actions of the PTH/PTHrP family leading to an appreciation of these molecules as important developmental and physiologic regulators. Although investigation of the functional significance of PTHrP gene expression in the lung has only recently begun in earnest, current evidence supports roles for the protein regulating pulmonary function, differentiation, and growth.

## PARATHYROID HORMONE AND PARATHYROID HORMONE-RELATED PROTEIN: STRUCTURAL AND FUNCTIONAL RELATIONSHIPS

PTH is the principal hormonal regulator of calcium homeostasis in birds and mammals. By contrast, under physiologic conditions, PTHrP appears to act principally as a paracrine, autocrine, and intracrine factor. Overproduction of the protein by tumors, including all major lung cancer cell types (20–22) and, occasionally, benign tumors (23), led to the discovery of this second PTH family member. In this setting, PTHrP exerts classical endocrine effects on bone and kidney and induces the common paraneoplastic syndrome of humoral hypercalcemia of malignancy (HHM) (24,25). HHM is a frequent complication of squamous cell carcinoma of the lung and contributes substantially to morbidity and mortality of that disease. Fuller Albright first described HHM during a 1941 Massachusetts General Hospital clinical pathologic conference (26) in a discussion of a hypercalcemic and hypophosphatemic patient who had renal carcinoma and only a single bone metastasis. The systemic calcium and phosphate derangements resolved after irradiation of the tumor, prompting Albright's proposal that the renal carcinoma secreted either PTH or a humoral PTH-like substance.

The biochemical similarities between primary hyperparathyroidism and HHM include hypercalcemia, hypophosphatemia (resulting from a reduced renal phosphate threshold), and increased nephrogenous adenosine 3',5'-cyclic monophosphate (cAMP) excretion (a hallmark of ligand interaction with proximal tubular PTH receptors) (27). In distinction from hyperparathyroidism, HHM patients show higher fractional calcium excretion, reduced circulating 1,25-dihydroxyvitamin D levels and, on bone histomorphometry, osteoclastic bone resorption with decreased osteoblastic activity, that is, bone formation "uncoupled" from bone resorption (28). These differences, as well as the findings that immunoreactive PTH (29) is suppressed in HHM and that the tumors lack detectable PTH mRNA (30), stimulated the search for a distinct molecule that could mimic certain PTH actions. Guided by sensitive in vitro bioassays, several research groups successfully purified a tumor-derived adenylyl cyclase-stimulating HHM factor from conditioned medium of a human lung squamous carcinoma cell line (BEN) (31) and renal carcinoma cells (32,33). Shortly afterward, cDNA clones that encode PTHrP were identified from lung (1) and renal (34,35) carcinomas. Over several years, the alternative names "PTH-like protein," "HHM factor," and "human hypercalcemia factor" have been discarded in favor of the designation PTHrP.

As predicted, circulating PTHrP is markedly elevated in HHM (22,36–39). The causal relationship between PTHrP and hypercalcemia has been demonstrated by the activity of PTHrP neutralizing antibodies reversing the hypercalcemia induced in animals by transplanted human tumor cells *(40)*. When administered subcutaneously to humans, amino-terminal PTHrP [PTHrP(1–36)] increases circulating immunoreactive PTHrP(1–36) levels, reduces serum phosphorus and the renal phosphorus threshold, increases fractional calcium and nephrogenous cAMP excretion, and increases circulating 1,25-dihydroxyvitamin D *(41)*.

As disclosed by molecular cloning, the amino acid sequences of PTH and PTHrP are homologous only at the amino terminus, where 8 of the first 13 amino acid residues in human PTH and PTHrP are identical (Fig. 1). This homologous domain bridges the molecular region critical for activation of the PTH receptor. Beyond this region, the primary sequences of PTH and PTHrP have little in common. However, although the receptor binding domains of PTH and PTHrP (amino acids 14–34) are dissimilar, both peptides share a common secondary structure α-helical binding domain which permits each ligand to bind with similar affinities to a common receptor.

Compared to the 84-amino acid peptide circulating PTH, mature human PTHrP is translated as three isoforms of 139, 141, and 173 amino acids having identical sequences through amino acid 139. Alternative RNA splicing of the PTHrP gene gives rise to 3' heterogeneity, which results in the several mRNAs encoding the differing carboxy-terminal peptide isoforms. A common 36 amino acid amino-terminal prepropeptide in translated PTHrP is cleaved intracellularly, via proprotein convertase (furin) and pro-teasomal degradation pathways common to many secretory proteins *(42,43)*. The amino PTHrP acid sequence from residues 140–173 is derived from exon 5, which is present in the human gene but not in the rodent or chicken gene. This isoform appears to be specific to humans and, possibly, to closely related primates. The relative secretory rates and physiologic importance of the PTHrP isoforms have not yet been elucidated *(44,45)*.

Human PTHrP is encoded by a single-copy gene located on chromosome 12p12.1–p11.2 *(34)* in an analogous chromosomal position to the PTH gene on chromosome 11 *(46)*. The identical organizational pattern of the central portion of the PTH and PTHrP genes (comprising PTHrP exons 2–4 and the respective introns), the amino-terminal region amino acid and nucleotide homologies, and the relatedness of the genes flanking the mammalian PTH and PTHrP genes all point to a common evolutionary origin through a gene duplication event.

In phylogeny, the parathyroid glands first appear in tetrapods, coincident with the transition from an aquatic to terrestrial environment and the evolution of the internal skeleton as a calcium store. More primitive vertebrates and invertebrates, although lacking recognizable parathyroid cells, express neural PTH or PTH-like peptides *(47)*. In addition, the only known site in mammals of extraparathyroidal PTH mRNA expression is the central nervous system *(48,49)*. Therefore, it may be inferred that parathyroidal PTH evolved from an ancestral neuropeptide. Similarly, PTHrP also is an evolutionarily ancient gene product which has fundamental functions (including neuroendocrine) in vertebrates *(50,51)*.

Although the *PTH* gene is a model of genomic simplicity, the PTHrP gene has a much more complicated organization. The human PTHrP gene spans more than 13 kb and includes three spatially distinct promoters, a 5'-flanking silencer, and nine exons *(52,53)*, only two of which are invariantly represented in PTHrP transcripts. The genomic organization reveals how the multiple human PTHrP RNA transcripts arise by the use of multiple transcription start sites with differently sized 5'-untranslated sequences and by alternative splicing of exons encoding the different 3'-coding region sequences. PTHrP

PTHrP

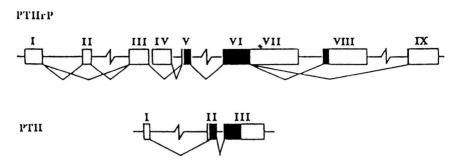

Fig. 1. Genomic organization pf PTHrP and PTH.

transcription is regulated by upstream and downstream TATA promoters (designated P1 and P3) and a GC-rich promotor (P2). Human PTHrP mRNAs contain either exon 6 [PTHrP(1–139)], exon 8 [PTHrP(1–141)], or exon 7 [PTHrP(1–173)]. As yet, little information is available about cell-specific expression of the three PTHrP mRNAs encoding the three human PTHrP isoforms (45,54–56).

The 3'-untranslated regions of the several PTHrP mRNAs also contain AUUUA-rich "instability" sequences associated with mRNA degradation and commonly found in growth factor, cytokine and immediate-early response gene transcripts. PTHrP gene expression is induced by serum and cycloheximide, features common to the regulation of early response genes (57,58). PTHrP mRNA half-lives are about 30 min to 3 h, suggesting that mRNA stability as well as transcriptional rate may be important points for physiologic regulation.

The probable evolution of PTH and PTHrP from neural peptides also bears on the organization of translated PTHrP as a classical "neuroendocrine"-type polyprotein. The full-length PTHrP polyhormone sequence undergoes extensive post-translational endoproteolytic processing to yield a series of mature secretory forms of the protein (44,59) (Fig. 2). Each secreted daughter peptide presumably has its own receptor(s). PTHrP-producing cells secrete an amino-terminal peptide, PTHrP(1–36), and longer amino-terminal forms (60). A separately secreted mid-region peptide beginning with amino acid 38 and having a mass of approx 7 kDa has been identified (45,59,61). Carboxy-terminal peptides recognized by PTHrP(109–138) antibodies are detectable in the circulation (37,45,62,63), although some carboxy-terminal fragments may be generated extracellularly. These various region-specific peptides generally correspond to the fragments predicted from the locations of di- and polybasic putative cleavage sites along the full-length PTHrP amino acid sequence. This pattern of posttranslational cleavage by prohormone convertases is characteristic of neuroendocrine polyproteins such as proopiomelanocortin, which is the precursor of ACTH, endorphin peptides and melanocyte-stimulating hormones.

At the time of this review, PTHrP is unique in that it is produced both by neuroendocrine cell types and by constitutively secreting cell types. Using immunohistochemical and perifusion techniques, Plawner et al. (64) demonstrated that all three PTHrP daughter peptides are secreted via secretory granules in neuroendocrine cells, but

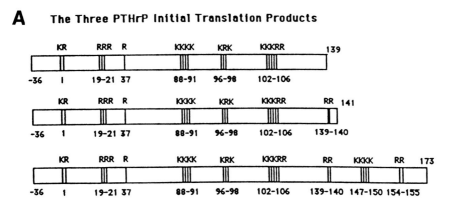

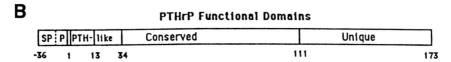

Fig. 2. Three initial PTHrP isoforms (**A**) and functional domains (**B**) of PTHrP. The three human PTHrP isoforms are identical from amino acids –36 to + 139 and are rich in di- and multibase residues. (Adapted from ref. *44*, with permission.)

PTHrP expression in nonneuroendocrine cells defaults to a constitutive pathway, similar to the secretion of cytokines and growth factors.

Several distinct physiologic actions have been localized to specific regions of the full-length PTHrP sequence or to the respective secreted region-specific daughter peptides. Amino-terminal PTHrP exhibits classical PTH-like actions in calcium and phosphorus metabolism and, along with PTH, is a cardiac inotrope *(65)*. The midmolecule region of PTHrP is responsible for transplacental calcium transport from mother to fetus against a concentration gradient *(66,67)* allowing the fetus in late pregnancy to develop with sufficient mineral for bone growth and an ambient mild hypercalcemia *(68)*. Carboxy-terminal PTHrPs [e.g., PTHrP(107–139)] have inhibitory effects on osteoclastic bone resorption, an action which is opposed to amino-terminal PTHrP and PTH. Consequently, this sequence has been termed "osteostatin" *(69,70)*.

Immunocytochemical and molecular studies recently have implicated certain actions of PTHrP as "intracrine", that is, following translation PTHrP may travel directly into the nucleus or nucleolus (71–73). A midmolecule, highly basic nuclear targeting sequence (NTS) which is homologous to NTSs identified within human retroviral (human immunodeficiency type 1 and human T-cell leukemia virus type 1) regulatory proteins targets PTHrP to the nucleolar site where ribonucleoprotein complexes form in vivo. Intracrine activities of PTHrP, independent of PTHrP daughter peptide actions as ligands for specific cell surface receptors, may be responsible for certain of the peptide effects on cell cycle progression and apoptosis *(72,73)*.

# PARATHYROID HORMONE-RELATED
# PROTEIN RECEPTOR BIOLOGY

Identity and conformational homology of the corresponding amino-terminal domains of PTH and PTHrP permit both molecules to interact with a common receptor *(74–76)* equipotently on a molar basis, for example, in pulmonary fibroblasts *(77)*. This PTH/PTHrP receptor initially was cloned from rat osteoblastic and opossum renal cell cDNA libraries. It is a 585 amino acid, seven-transmembrane domain, G protein-coupled receptor *(74,75,78)* which localizes to human chromosome region 3p21.1–p22 and the syntenous mouse and rat chromosomes *(79,80)*. The receptor transcripts are expressed in the classic PTH target organs associated with calcium homeostasis, namely, bone and kidney, as well as in numerous other organs. Binding of PTH and PTHrP to this common receptor results in adenylyl cyclase-dependent and phospholipase C-dependent signaling, generating cAMP and inositol polyphosphate/diacylglycerol/cytosolic calcium second messengers, respectively. Like other G protein-linked, adenylyl cyclase-activating receptors, stimulation of receptor-dependent intracellular cAMP levels induces homologous downregulation of the PTH/PTHrP receptor *(81)*.

The PTHrP receptor gene extends over 22 kb and contains at least 15 exons and alternative 3' sequences that permit differential cleavage and polyadenylation of the transcript *(82)*. Expression of the mammalian PTH/PTHrP receptor is controlled by at least three promoters, two of which appear to be ubiquitously expressed, and one which may be selectively active in kidney *(83,84)*. The major (rat) transcript in most tissues is 2.3–2.5 kb in size, but several larger and smaller tissue-specific mRNA species can be detected *(85)*. The single 2.3-kb human PTH/PTHrP receptor transcript is expressed principally in kidney, placenta, liver, and lung *(86)*. In amphibian embryonal and larval development, two nonallelic functional PTH/PTHrP receptor isoforms are expressed, both of them abundantly in lung *(87)*.

Based on sequence homology, the PTH/PTHrP receptor is a member of a distinct, newly characterized subfamily of class II G protein-coupled receptors *(88)* that includes receptors for secretin, calcitonin, growth hormone-releasing hormone, vasoactive intestinal peptide type 1, gastrin-inhibitory polypeptide, glucagon, glucagonlike peptide 1, corticotropin-releasing factor, and pituitary adenylate cyclase activating peptide 1. The sequence similarities of these "secretin receptor family" members may allow cross-reactivity with their respective ligands *(89)* in a manner akin to the pleiotropy of cytokine families, although significant heterologous ligand–receptor binding at physiologic concentrations of ligand has not been demonstrated.

Like PTHrP, the PTH/PTHrP receptor is also expressed widely, in this case principally in mesenchymal cells of many organs, often adjacent to cells producing PTHrP *(85,90,91)*. The view that the PTH/PTHrP receptor mediates many of the developmental functions of PTHrP is supported by the findings of similar phenotypes of the growth plates *(92)*, breast tissue *(91)*, and lung *(93)* in PTHrP(–/–) and PTH/PTHrP receptor (–/–) mice. Deletion of the murine gene for the PTH/PTHrP receptor by homologous recombination also causes midgestation fetal death *(92)*, a phenotype that is not seen in PTHrP(–/–) mice, perhaps because of compensatory effects of maternal PTHrP or fetal PTH.

In 1995, Usdin et al. *(94–96)* identified a second seven-transmembrane domain G protein-coupled receptor that *selectively* recognizes amino-terminal PTH. This receptor, designated the PTH2 receptor (PTHR2), by sequence identity criteria also is a member of the receptor subfamily structurally related to the secretin. The PTH2 receptor sequence most resembles the PTH/PTHrP receptor (51% overall amino acid identity). The PTHR2 gene is expressed in brain, endothelium, and vascular smooth muscle, pancreas, testis, placenta, and lung *(94,95)*. In the lung, PTH2 receptor mRNA is detected by *in situ* hybridization both in bronchi and in the parenchyma *(95)*. These findings suggest that the PTH2 receptor may be responsible for certain PTH effects in several organ systems. Currently, the relevance of PTH2 receptor-dependent signaling to lung development and physiology remains to be determined.

The physiologic and pharmacologic evidence suggests that PTH *(97)* and PTHrP *(98)* activate specific receptors for their respective carboxy-terminal (PTH and PTHrP) or midmolecule (PTHrP) peptide sequences. At the time of this review, these proteins have not been identified.

## PARATHYROID HORMONE-RELATED PROTEIN AS A DEVELOPMENTAL REGULATORY MOLECULE

Aside from the notable exception of HHM, circulating levels of PTHrP are considerably lower than the levels of PTH, and it is doubtful that PTHrP plays a major *endocrine* role in maintenance of extrauterine calcium homeostasis in mammals. The relevance of circulating PTHrP levels during pregnancy *(99)*, in postpartum maternal calcium metabolism *(100,101)*, and in the fetus remains controversial. The common observation that novel tumor products often are fetal proteins and findings that embryonic and fetal PTHrP gene expression is widespread have motivated investigations of the developmental functions of this complex protein.

During murine postimplantation development, PTHrP mRNA is detected in the trophoblast, maternal epithelial cells of the antimesometrial crypt and cells of the inner zone of the decidua adjacent to the implanted embryo. Nowak et al. *(102)* recently showed that TGF-β stimulates mouse blastocyst outgrowth, in part, through increasing endogenous production of PTHrP. Parietal endoderm formation, one of the first differentiation processes during murine development, is regulated by a paracrine mechanism involving PTHrP-expressing trophoblast cells and extra-embryonal endoderm cells that express the PTH/PTHrP receptor *(90,103–105)*. In murine development, this process is separable into two distinct stages in which retinoic acid initiates differentiation of pluripotent stem cells into a cell type with characteristics of primitive endoderm, followed by expression of PTHrP and the PTH/PTHrP receptor, which mediates further differentiation into parietal endoderm, including foregut structures. Differentiation along an alternative pathway, to visceral endoderm, fails to stimulate receptor expression *(104)* and receptor mRNA signal gradually ebbs in visceral endoderm after day 7.5 *(90)*. From day 11.5 onward, PTHrP mRNA is detected in neural structures, choroid plexus, epithelial cells of the lung, heart, dermis and sites of endochondral bone formation *(105)*.

The phenotypes of mice overexpressing a PTHrP transgene *(13,106,107)* or homozygous *(67,93,108–111)* or heterozygous *(112)* for a disrupted PTHrP allele provide further evidence that PTHrP is an important developmental regulatory protein in skin and skin appendages, placenta, bone, teeth, mammary gland, and lung. Targeted, tissue-specific overexpression of PTHrP in breast or skin interferes with branching morphogenesis in developing mammary glands *(107)* and with normal hair follicle development *(106)*, respectively. Similarly, studies of the biologic actions of PTHrP in cultured keratinocytes and in SKH-1 hairless mice *(113,114)* strongly suggest that the protein regulates epidermal and hair follicle growth. Kaiser et al. *(113)* inhibited endogenous PTHrP production in a transformed keratinocyte line using antisense RNA, thereby inhibiting expression of maturation-specific keratinocyte markers and implicating endogenous PTHrP in keratinocyte differentiation.

PTHrP is expressed in placenta *(11,115)*. In humans, PTHrP is secreted by amnion cells and may play a role in onset of uterine contractions *(6)* and, possibly, in the maintenance of fetal epithelia exposed to amniotic fluid, for example, skin and gastrointestinal tract. In lactating mammary tissue, PTHrP is vectorially secreted into milk in concentrations at least 10,000-fold greater than its serum concentration *(36)*. It is speculative at this point whether PTHrP functions in maintenance of the neonatal intestinal tract and postprandial mesenteric perfusion.

The role of PTHrP as a developmental regulator has so far been examined most extensively in skeletal tissues. PTHrP is a bifunctional modulator of chondrogenesis and some of its actions are exerted via a mechanism distinct from the recognized signaling pathways linked to the PTH/PTHrP receptor *(116)*. Chondrocyte differentiation, necessary for skeletal morphogenesis, is regulated by a conserved family of Hedgehog secreted proteins *(117)*. Indian hedgehog (Ihh) induces PTHrP as a critical second signal in periarticular perichondrium. PTHrP interacts with its receptor in prehypertrophic chondrocytes of cartilage, mediating the effects of Ihh through formation of a negative feedback loop that modulates the rate of chondrocyte differentiation *(92,110)*.

The essential role of PTHrP in skeletal morphogenesis, which is clear from the severe skeletal dysplasias of PTHrP(–/–) and PTH/PTHrP receptor(–/–) mice *(92,108,109)*, has led to the identification of PTHrP signaling mutants in the pathogenesis of human chondrodystrophies. Expression of activating mutations of the PTH/PTHrP receptor is responsible for the Murk Jansen type of metaphyseal chondrodysplasia *(118)*. The pathogenetic role of the mutant PTH/PTHrP receptor is apparent from the indistinguishable abnormal growth plate maturation and biochemical findings (hypercalcemia, hypophosphatemia, increased renal excretion of phosphate, and cAMP) seen in hyperparathyroidism and the constitutively activated Jansen PTH/PTHrP receptor phenotype. Inactivating mutations of the PTH/PTHrP receptor *(119–121)* have been demonstrated in Blomstrand chondrodysplasia, also a rare lethal disorder, characterized by advanced endochondral bone maturation, short limbs, polyhydramnios, hydrops fetalis, facial anomalies, and increased bone density *(122)*. The skeletal abnormalities caused by absence of functional PTH/PTHrP receptors are the mirror image of those observed in Jansen chondrodysplasia.

The physiologic functions of PTHrP in pulmonary development have not been yet examined as thoroughly. This chapter reviews several actions of PTHrP that have demonstrated or potential relevance to lung, specifically, regulation of tissue growth and differentiation, pulmonary surfactant synthesis, smooth muscle (vascular and airway) tone, transepithelial calcium transport, and tumor biology.

# PULMONARY EXPRESSION OF PARATHYROID HORMONE-RELATED PROTEIN AND THE PARATHYROID HORMONE/PARATHYROID HORMONE-RELATED PROTEIN RECEPTOR

Among endodermal derivatives in the developing rat, the highest levels of PTHrP mRNA expression occur in lung on day 15.5 of the 21-d rat gestation *(5)*. Pulmonary PTHrP production is highly cell type- and developmental stage-specific and becomes prominent by days 13–15 *(4,5,8,10)*, during the glandular stage of lung development. The protein is detected first in the undifferentiated lung bud epithelium and later, in canalicular and saccular stage lung, in epithelial progenitor cells of the alveoli, that is, type II pneumocytes *(123)*, and bronchioles, that is, Clara cells *(5,124)*. Lung epithelial PTHrP expression also peaks shortly before birth *(3–5,125)*, cotemporal with the phase of accelerated surfactant production. In the human fetus, by 8 wk PTHrP immunoreactivity is widespread throughout the branching airway epithelium and is transiently detectable in mesenchyme. It is uncertain whether this PTHrP immunoreactivity noted in early fetal lung mesenchyme represents peptide targeted to these sites from adjacent epithelium or locally produced. With increasing gestation, PTHrP immunoreactivity becomes progressively more focal, localizing in clusters of epithelial cells *(3,14,125)* and in adult lung *(126,127)*. Production and secretion of PTHrP have been demonstrated in cultured rat adult *(123)* and fetal type II cells *(128)* and the A549 and H441 pulmonary epithelial cell lines *(128,129)*. The protein also is detectable in tracheal aspirates of newborn infants *(130)*.

Pulmonary PTH/PTHrP receptors are localized to the adepithelial mesenchyme *(10)* adjacent to sites of PTHrP synthesis. Receptor mRNA is detected in the fetal rat lung mesenchyme from day 10.5 and it is highly expressed by days 15–16 *(90)*. PTH/PTHrP receptor mRNA signal density diminishes with increasing distance from the epithelial boundary *(10,90)*.

The pattern of focal epithelial PTHrP expression and diffuse receptor mRNA expression in the adjacent mesenchyme is paralleled in skin, intestine and several other organs, where the relative expression levels of PTHrP and its receptor also are often inversely correlated within the tissue or in certain locales along a border of apposition. This tight coupling of ligand and receptor expression would seem to imply either feedback downregulation of the receptor or precise coordinate regulation of the two genes during the course of fetal development *(10)*.

The "hand-in-glove" expression pattern of ligand and receptor is a distinguishing feature of paracrine regulators of lung maturation, such as epidermal growth factor, hepatocyte growth factor, tumor necrosis factor-$\alpha$, and the fibroblast growth factors *(131)*, and suggests that PTHrP may be a patterning or differentiation factor during pulmonary development. An inductive paracrine mechanism for PTHrP action in lung development and physiology predicts PTHrP binding to PTH/PTHrP receptors on fibroblasts and cross-talk between type II cells and alveolar fibroblasts. In this scheme, alveolar epithelial cells produce factors (including PTHrP) that modulate fibroblast function; perialveolar fibroblasts, in turn, produce factors that modulate epithelial functions (including the production of PTHrP) in a classic spatiotemporal sequence (Fig. 3). This description is based on current experimental data regarding the interaction between *amino-terminal* PTHrP and the cognate PTH/PTHrP receptor. In addition, as may occur during tooth development *(132)*, pulmonary PTHrP probably undergoes post-translational processing, the resultant products acting as paracrine or autocrine regulators of cell division and maturation or of local vascular dilatation during alveolarization.

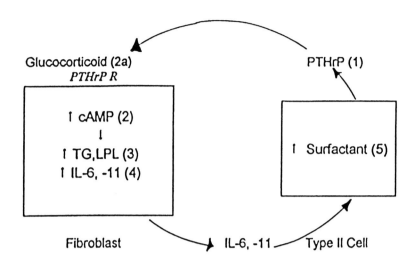

Fig. 3. Panacrine model of parathyroid hormone-related protein (PTHrP)-regulated type II cell maturation: (1) type II cells increase PTHrP expression in response to fluid distention and mechanical deformation; (2) PTHrP binds to mesenchymal PTHrP receptors and, synergistically with glucocorticoid (2a), triggers intracellular second messenger pathways, stimulates (3) triglyceride (TG) uptake via increased fibroblast lipoprotein lipase (LPL) activity, and (4) stimulates production of specific cytokines; (5) secretion of PTHrP-inducible mesenchymal molecules (such as IL-6, IL-11) stimulates type II cell surfactant phospholipid and surfactant-associated protein production, thereby completing paracrine loop. (From ref. *128*, with permission.)

## REGULATION OF PARATHYROID HORMONE-RELATED PROTEIN AND PARATHYROID HORMONE-RELATED PROTEIN RECEPTOR EXPRESSION

Like immediate-early response genes, PTHrP mRNA is induced by growth factors, serum and cyclohexamide *(133)*. In a variety of cell types, PTHrP mRNA expression and immunoreactive PTHrP are stimulated by treatment with insulin-like growth factor (IGF) I and II, insulin, epidermal growth factor (EGF) and transforming growth factor (TGF)-$\alpha$, TGF-$\beta$1, interleukin (IL)-1$\beta$, IL-6, tumor necrosis factor (TNF)-$\alpha$, and prolactin *(134–140)*. EGF stimulation of PTHrP expression is complex *(55,141)* and involves increased gene transcription, principally from the P1 and GC-rich P2 promoters, and enhanced expression of more stable PTHrP mRNA species containing two of the alternative 3' exons (VII or VIII). It is expected that similar regulatory complexity is involved in other PTHrP-inducible pathways. In several organs, TGF-$\beta$ functions as a paracrine or autocrine positive regulator of PTHrP production *(142–145)*.

PTHrP expression and secretion in rat type II cells *(123)*, lung epithelial tumor lines *(146)* and other cell types is principally regulated by PKC-dependent, cAMP-independent pathways. In lung, upregulation of PTHrP production by cytokines and products of inflammatory cells, such as interleukins, TNF-$\alpha$ and IGF I may be important. Inflammatory mediators also have been proposed as stimulators of PTHrP production by pulmonary sarcoid macrophages *(147)*.

The two principal identified negative regulators of PTHrP expression in all cell types and species examined are glucocorticoid and 1,25-dihydroxyvitamin D *(52,136,138, 148–152)*. Their principal mode of action is to decrease PTHrP gene transcription rate.

Regulation of the PTH/PTHrP receptor mRNA appears to follow a reciprocal pattern to regulation of PTHrP. Receptor gene expression is downregulated by TGF-β *(153,154)*, TNF-α, and retinoic acid *(155)* and is upregulated by dexamethasone *(156)*. It is anticipated that these regulators of lung development, that is, PTHrP, glucocorticoids, TGF-β and accessory molecules, participate in complex feedback loops during lung morphogenesis and response to lung injury.

## PARATHYROID HORMONE-RELATED PROTEIN AS AN INDUCER OF ALVEOLAR CYTODIFFERENTIATION AND PULMONARY SURFACTANT PRODUCTION

Biological actions of PTHrP in lung were first demonstrated by Rubin et al. *(77)*, who showed that PTH*(1–34)* and PTHrP*(1–34)* produced time- and dose-dependent increases in surfactant phospholipid production in rat fetal type II cells in vitro by epithelial-mesenchymal interactions. These peptides stimulated receptor-dependent accumulations of cAMP and inositol polyphosphates in isolated alveolar fibroblasts but not in purified preparations of alveolar epithelial cells. The presence of fibroblasts as cell cocultures or tissue explants was required for PTHrP-stimulated surfactant synthesis. Recently, Speziale et al. *(130)* examined tracheal aspirate PTHrP in intubated newborn infants. Tracheal aspirate concentrations of the protein were correlated with pulmonary maturation of preterm newborns and were low in infants with hyaline membrane disease, or surfactant deficiency *(130)*.

In the developing lung, paracrine/juxtacrine signals between rudimentary epithelial cells and surrounding mesenchymal cells are crucial for airway branching and air sac cytodifferentiation *(131,156–158)*. PTHrP stimulates mesenchymal production of several growth factors and cytokines relevant to pulmonary epithelial differentiation and surfactant production, including IGF I *(159)*, keratinocyte growth factor *(160)*, IL-6 and IL-11 *(161)*, thereby closing the inductive paracrine loop (Fig. 3).

The pulmonary expression of PTHrP may influence commitment to a mature type II cell phenotype by autocrine as well as paracrine mechanisms. Studies by Hastings et al. *(129)* determined that adult rat type II cells and A549 cells increase secretion of saturated phosphatidylcholine after exposure to PTHrP*(1–34)*. The conflicting results with those obtained in fetal rat type II cells *(77)* may reflect either cell type or methodological differences.

To study the physiologic roles of PTHrP in intact organisms, Karaplis et al. *(108)* disrupted the murine PTHrP gene and generated a mouse strain deficient in PTHrP. Mice heterozygous (haplodeficient, +/–) for the disrupted PTHrP allele appear phenotypically indistinguishable from wild type (+/+) litter mates at birth, but PTHrP homozygous null mutants (–/–) have a distinctive chondrodystrophy. The null (PTHrP knockout) neonates usually die within 30 min after birth of uncertain causes but occasional mice survive for 12 to 36 h *(93)*. Although the lungs of PTHrP(–/–) newborn mice were originally thought to be structurally normal, albeit small *(108)*, ablation of PTHrP expression causes structural and functional defects in alveolar epithelial and mesenchymal development and interferes with surfactant synthesis.

Lungs removed from spontaneously delivered PTHrP(–/–) animals are smaller, denser, and more compact than are lungs from normal litter mates and they do not float *(93)*. In lung tissue from PTHrP(–/–) animals that survive for several hours, there is accumulation of eosinophilic intraalveolar material which is immunoreactive for surfactant-associated proteins and resembles hyaline membranes, the histologic marker of neonatal respiratory distress syndrome in humans. These lungs differ from the hypoplastic lungs of other murine chondrodystrophies, in which maturation takes place on schedule *(162,163)*, despite thoracic constriction.

PTHrP(–/–) lung tissue *in situ* as well as embryonic lung (days 13.5–14.5) maintained in serumless organ culture for five days showed decreased incorporation of [$^3$H]choline chloride into saturated phosphatidylcholine. By contrast, PTHrP(–/–) lung buds similarly cultured for several days demonstrated no significantly impaired expression of the mRNAs for surfactant-associated proteins SP-A, SP-B or SP-C *(93)*. This discordance between delayed surfactant phospholipid synthesis and normal surfactant protein gene expression is unusual but is consistent with observations that regulation of surfactant-associated gene expression, phospholipid synthesis, and lamellar body formation may be subject to different controls *(164,165)*. The finding that PTHrP promotes specific aspects of surfactant synthesis warrants further investigation.

In terms of lung architecture, disruption of the PTHrP gene in mice also is associated with persistence until birth of a primitive-appearing, compact lung containing acini lined with glycogen-rich, cuboidal epithelial cells, few or no lamellar bodies and sparse endoplasmic reticulum. Like the impairment of surfactant phospholipid synthesis, certain structural defects in PTHrP(–/–) lung at least partly result from lack of pulmonary production of PTHrP per se since embryonic lungs maintained for several days ex vivo also exhibit impaired type II cell differentiation. It may be relevant that PTHrP(–/–) *(109)* and PTH/PTHrP receptor(–/–) *(76)* mice have increased glycogen deposition in chondrocytes, perhaps suggesting a wider role for PTHrP action in glycogen metabolism.

Ablation of the PTHrP gene in mice also perturbs epithelial-mesenchymal cell relationships in the pulmonary septae. PTHrP(–/–) newborn lungs lack the basement membrane discontinuities and epithelial foot processes extending from cuboidal epithelial cells to underlying interstitial cells that are maximal in the perinatal period, coincident with the appearance of lamellar bodies and surfactant synthesis *(157,166)*, as well as during lung injury and repair *(167)*. These gaps may allow direct mesenchymal–epithelial interaction and be important for PTHrP juxtacrine signaling, growth control, and surfactant synthesis.

A role for PTHrP in regulation of branching morphogenesis in the lung has not yet been explored. In the murine mammary gland, the protein plays a critical functional role during embryonic development by regulating epithelial–mesenchymal communications that guide the initial round of branching morphogenesis *(91)*. The ability of PTHrP to support embryonic mammary development appears to depend on receptor-mediated activation by amino-terminal PTHrP, since the mammary gland phenotypes of PTHrP(–/–) and PTH/PTHrP receptor(–/–) mice are similar *(91)*. Overexpression of PTHrP in mammary tissue of transgenic mice similarly impairs branching morphogenesis during sexual maturity and early pregnancy *(107)*. Hu et al. *(168)* recently demonstrated that PTHrP*(1–34)* increases rHOX expression in osteoblasts *(168)*. This rat homeobox gene has a known function in bronchial differentiation, prompting the speculation that PTHrP might modulate pulmonary branching via actions on effector morphogens. Similarly, it is reasonable to assume that the chondrocyte differentiation pathway of Hedgehog activation of PTHrP expression is not unique to that cell type. Epithelially derived Sonic hedgehog is another regulator of branching morphogenesis in the lung *(169)*.

Recently, expression of a constitutively active PTH/PTHrP receptor targeted to the growth plate by the rat $\alpha1(II)$ collagen promoter has corrected the major skeletal abnormalities of PTHrP(–/–) mice and allowed their survival for several months *(170)*. These "rescued" PTHrP(–/–) mice should prove useful for studying the role of PTHrP in postnatal organ development.

## PARATHYROID HORMONE-RELATED PROTEIN AND PARACRINE INDUCTION OF ALVEOLAR LIPOFIBROBLAST DIFFERENTIATION

A remarkable feature of PTHrP(–/–) lung is an abundance of abnormal lipid-laden interstitial cells *(93)*. Based on lipid content, pulmonary interstitial cells may be divided into "lipid interstitial cells" (or lipofibroblasts) and a nonlipid interstitial cell population, which lacks the characteristic lipid droplets and is located more peripherally in the alveolar septum *(172–174)*. Differentiation of interstitial cells into lipofibroblasts is dependent on exposure to alveolar epithelial paracrine factors *(171)*. The perialveolar lipofibroblasts maximally accumulate triglyceride (TG) just before the appearance of surfactant-containing lamellar bodies in neighboring type II cells *(175,176)* as well as following alveolar injury, consistent with a functional role in surfactant synthesis. This hypothesis has been tested by Torday et al. *(176,177)*, who showed in mixed cell culture systems that tagged pulmonary fibroblast TG is transferred to type II cells and incorporated into surfactant phospholipids. Subsequent in vitro studies of rat fetal lung cells showed that PTHrP and glucocorticoid both stimulate TG uptake by pulmonary fibroblasts, but PTHrP specifically enhances TG transfer to type II cells *(160,171)*. One may infer that alveolar lipofibroblasts, like adipocytes, serve specialized functions for the synthesis and storage of TGs and for their mobilization and transport to other cells. The profusion of lipid droplet-packed fibroblasts in PTHrP(–/–) murine lung, in turn, might indicate a defect in lipid trafficking between these cells and neighboring type II cells. Fibroblasts and adipocytes are among the very few cell types that have not been reported to produce PTHrP. On the other hand, both cell types are targets for PTHrP actions *(77,178–180)*.

The responsiveness of fetal lung fibroblasts to glucocorticoid and PTHrP appears to be differentially programmed. Dexamethasone administered to the pregnant rat can augment preexisting features of fetal lung fibroblast phenotype, such as TG uptake *(177)* and glucocorticoid receptor activity *(181)* but not induce these activities before the point in gestation when they ordinarily increase. PTHrP stimulates functional lipofibroblast activity in the rat fetus at least 2 to 3 d (J.S. Torday, *unpublished observations*) before the time when normal maturation can be induced in response to exposure to exogenous glucocorticoids. These findings suggest one mechanism that could account for why antenatal glucocorticoid therapy in human pregnancy does not clearly decrease the incidence of respiratory distress syndrome (RDS) in extremely preterm infants born at 24–28 wk gestation, although it does reduce the severity of the disease *(182)*.

The molecular mechanisms by which pulmonary epithelial PTHrP regulates lipofibroblast function are not established. PTHrP stimulates pulmonary fibroblast lipoprotein lipase protein and activity (L.P. Rubin and J.S. Torday, *unpublished observations*), an early marker of adipocyte differentiation. Torday et al. *(171)* also recently determined that adipose differentiation-related protein (ADRP) expression is activated during the process of pulmonary lipofibroblast maturation and showed that

ADRP mRNA and protein are stimulated by PTHrP. ADRP is a novel 50-kDa membrane-associated protein whose mRNA levels are induced rapidly and maximally upon triggering adipocyte differentiation. ADRP also is expressed in a variety of adipogenic and steroidogenic tissues and cultured cell lines, where it localizes to the surface of neutral lipid storage droplets *(183,184)*. ADRP coating of lipofibroblast TG droplets appears to be required for their exocytosis, similar to ADRP function in steroidogenic cells. Induction of ADRP and, possibly, other adipogenic differentiation molecules may mediate PTHrP-regulated neutral lipid trafficking in the alveolus.

## PARATHYROID HORMONE-RELATED PROTEIN AS A TRANSDUCER OF MECHANICAL FORCES IN DEVELOPING LUNG

Distension of lung tissue in vivo promotes septal thinning and precocious appearance of surfactant in type II cells *(185,186)* and mechanical deformation of pulmonary epithelial cells promotes differentiation in vitro *(124,187)*. It is expected that these developmental changes are mediated by the induction of genes whose expression can be regulated by mechanical forces.

Mechanical stretch and pulsatility have potent inductive effects on PTHrP mRNA and protein production. This phenomenon was first discovered by Thiede et al. *(2)*, who determined that PTHrP expression was induced in rat myometrium by intrauterine occupancy. Stretch, organ distention, or induced muscle contractility (deformation) variously increase PTHrP production in urinary bladder *(188,189)*, avian oviduct *(190)*, amnion *(6)*, vascular smooth muscle *(191)*, the gastrointestinal tract *(192)*, and, presumably, cardiac atrial myocytes *(17)*. Glucocorticoids, which decrease PTHrP gene transcription, may modulate stretch induction of PTHrP in smooth muscle. In rat gastric smooth muscle, for example, muscle activity caused by distention only increases PTHrP expression if serum corticosterone is suppressed by pretreatment with metyrapone, an inhibitor of 11 β-hydroxylation *(192)*.

Pulmonary epithelial PTHrP mRNA and protein also are induced by mechanical forces *(128,174,193)*. Mechanical stretching of rat fetal lung fibroblasts in monolayer culture increases PTH/PTHrP receptor activity and responsiveness to ligand *(128)*, suggesting that stretching couples PTHrP expression with receptor-mediated effects in the distended alveolar wall. Manipulation of cultured pulmonary epithelial cells and whole fetal lungs suggests that induction of pulmonary PTHrP gene expression may be more dependent on a cyclical deformation than a static continuous stretch or distention *(124)*. This finding contrasts to stretch-dependent induction of the protein in uterine smooth muscle *(16)* and urinary bladder *(188)*, where the greater the urinary volume within the bladder at any moment, the higher the level of PTHrP expression.

As Fig. 3 illustrates, in developing lung, PTHrP appears to be both a differentiation factor and a transducer of those mechanical forces which promote lung maturation. In the lung, PTHrP and its upstream (e.g., retinoic acid, Hedgehog proteins) or downstream (e.g., cAMP, hox proteins) effectors in the developing alveolus may act as "morphogens," in Alan Turing's original sense *(194)*, that is, molecules whose function is establishment of inhomogeneity, that is, spontaneous pattern organization. To define a factor as a morphogen, it is necessary to demonstrate that it has a direct effect on target cells and that it affects the development of target cells in a *concentration-dependent* manner. Models of "morphogenetic reaction–diffusion systems" *(195–199)* have been an attractive theoretical basis for explaining pattern formation in the embryo during organogenesis, despite an absence, until recently, of experimental validation of their predictive power.

In mechanochemical morphogenetic models, the roles of mechanical strain and local calcium release are similar to the long-range inhibitor and the short-range activator originally postulated in the Turing models. Although the resulting mathematical equations differ in detail, the resulting eigen-function patterns are the same *(198, 200–202)*. The mechanical instability provided by cyclic deformation and fluid distension of the developing alveolus might serve as and interact with other morphogenetic functions for which Turing's chemical instability and other reaction–diffusion systems have been proposed. According to this framework, diffusion-driven instability engendered by hormonally and mechanically induced PTHrP and PTH/PTHrP receptor expression, and asymmetric tissue gradients of PTHrP or PTHrP-stimulated cAMP *(203)* could serve as morphogenetic Turing couples. Such models suggest experimental strategies and require analysis of the concentration- and distance-dependent effects of PTHrP on alveolar histogenesis.

## LUNG VASCULAR TONE AND VASCULOGENESIS

The hypotensive and vasodilatory actions of PTH, first described in 1925, have been topics of extensive investigation *(204)*. The discovery of PTHrP was followed by the determination that this protein has similar (nanomolar) effects on vascular tone *(111)*. The relaxation of smooth induced muscle by the addition of exogenous PTHrP has been observed in virtually all smooth muscle beds examined. Regional arterial systems seem to be affected differentially, and these regional differences may be species-specific *(111)*.

The smooth muscle dilatory properties reside in the amino-terminal fragments of PTH and PTHrP *(205)* and are, at least in part, mediated by cAMP-dependent inhibition of voltage-dependent L-type calcium channels, which prevents entry of extracellular calcium and causes vasorelaxation *(206)*. Although smooth muscle cells express the PTH/PTHrP receptor *(207)*, which is coupled via different G proteins to adenylyl cyclase *and* phospholipase C, receptor activation in smooth muscle cells apparently does not influence basal levels of cytosolic calcium *(188,208)* or inositol phosphates, even when recombinant receptor is overexpressed in these cells *(209)*. This finding concurs with observations that increments in cytosolic calcium mediate the actions of numerous vasoconstrictors, including angiotensin II, norepinephrine, and endothelin-1. Selective use of one of the two PTHrP receptor-coupled signal transduction pathways presents an interesting puzzle. There is precedent for this phenomonon in the structually related calcitonin receptor, for which selective activation of one or the other pathway in renal cells is cell cycle-dependent *(210)*. PTHrP signaling exclusively through phospholipase C-dependent pathways also occurs in some other cell types, notably keratinocytes *(98)*, but it is unclear whether these cell types signal through the bifunctional PTH/PTHrP receptor.

PTHrP mRNA induction by mechanical stretch can be demonstrated by balloon distention of the aorta *(191)* and cyclic stretching of vascular smooth muscle cells in culture *(18)*. The mechanical induction of PTHrP resulting in smooth muscle relaxation is adapted to accommodate volume or flow in the organ or tissue in question. In cardiac muscle, the PTHrP expression is greatest in atrial myocytes *(114,211)*, that is, in the heart chambers which are more compliant than ventricles to volume distention. In some atrial cells, PTHrP is coexpressed with atrial natriuretic peptide and packaged in secretory vesicles. These observations suggest a possible role for the protein in the cardiovascular system as the calcium counterpart for the atrial natriuretic–sodium regulatory axis *(11,211)*.

In the vasculature, both arterial smooth muscle cells *(212)* and endothelial cells *(213)* express the PTHrP and PTH/PTHrP receptor. The effects of PTHrP on relaxing vascular tone can be demonstrated in regionally perfused arterial beds and in isolated smooth muscle strips and cell preparations and do not require the presence of endothelium. However, vascular endothelial PTHrP produced, for example, in response to cytokines, may modulate local vascular function. For example, incubation of simian virus 40-transformed rat lung vascular endothelial cells with PTHrP(1–34) reduces thrombin-stimulated endothelin-1 expression *(213)*. Although central PTHrP effects on blood pressure have been proposed *(214)*, PTHrP appears princpally to be a local (autocrine, paracrine) regulator of vascular tone *(215–217)*. For example, systemic hypertension induced in Sprague-Dawley rats by angiotension II infusion and salt loading increases cardiovascular expression of PTHrP *(205)*, and this pathway is impaired in the mutant spontaneously hypertensive rat (SHR) strain *(218)*.

The role of PTH and PTHrP in *pulmonary* vasodilatation and modulation of the vasoconstrictive effects of other agents is currently under investigation. Gao and Raj *(219)* have reported that PTHrP caused receptor-mediated relaxation of fetal and neonatal lamb isolated pulmonary arteries and veins when the vascular rings were preconstricted with endothelin-1. PTHrP had no effect on the tone of bronchial rings preconstricted with acetylcholine. These initial data point to a role of the protein in the perinatal period, at least, as a specific dilator for pulmonary vessels but not for airways.

One pertinent observation is that PTHrP(1–34) inhibits serum and platelet-derived growth factor-BB-induced migration and proliferation of vascular smooth muscle cells via receptor-dependent mechanisms *(220)*. It is not known yet whether this finding might be relevant to the pathogenesis of pulmonary hypertension. A role for PTHrP in pulmonary vasculogenesis also may help to explain certain PTHrP-mediated effects on alveolar cytodifferentiation, since the type I cell phenotype is promoted by capillary growth, whether through loss of epithelial contact with the fibroblast and its products, or through effects of endothelial matrix *(157)*.

## PARATHYROID HORMONE-RELATED PROTEIN REGULATION OF CELL GROWTH AND SURVIVAL

Mitogenic actions of PTHrP have been demonstrated in several cell types that express the protein *(116,221,222)*. The rapid (within 5 min) serum stimulation of PTHrP gene expression *(57)*, a feature shared with growth factor-regulated early response genes, raises the possibility that PTHrP contributes to the early mitogenic response of lung cells to growth factor stimulation. Lam et al. *(222)* have examined the relationship of PTHrP to the cell cycle. In a human keratinocyte cell line (HaCat), PTHrP expression was greatest in actively dividing cells when cells were in S and G2 + M phases of the cell cycle and was lowest in quiescent G1 cells. Mitogen stimulation of PTHrP mRNA expression was dependent on the cells being in G1. In cells released from a G2 + M block by addition of serum, PTHrP expression increased coincident with cell progression into G1. Furthermore, immunoreactive PTHrP was localized to the nucleolus in quiescent cells, but was redistributed to the cytoplasm when cells were actively dividing. These findings implicate an autocrine role for PTHrP in the G1 response to mitogens and during cell division, when its expression is high and it is relocated from the nucleolus to the cytoplasm.

PTHrP is an endogenous *anti*proliferative factor in keratinocytes, a property that resides in the PTH-like amino-terminal 1–34 fragment *(222a)*. Other investigations determined that carboxy-terminal 107–111 and 107–139 PTHrP fragments also inhibit proliferation of cycling keratinocytes and stimulate DNA synthesis and proliferation of quiescent keratinocytes, respectively, via a PKC-dependent pathway *(223)*. Clearly, the effects of various PTHrP daughter proteins and peptide regions modulating cell division are complex and will require further investigation using asynchronous and synchronized cultured, nontransformed cell types.

Hastings et al. *(224)* have shown that PTHrP(1–36) activity inhibits rat adult type II cell proliferation by autocrine mechanisms. Inhibition or depletion of PTHrP activity stimulates proliferation. These findings suggest that stretch-induced PTHrP gene expression in the late gestational fetal lung may be important for the observed peripartum decrease in alveolar cell growth. The further implications for growth control in pulmonary PTHrP producing and target cells have not yet been investigated.

A newly established role for PTHrP is cellular protection from apoptosis. In several cell types, the protein is involved in an autocrine loop promoting cell survival *(72,225)*, in part, by increasing expression of the antiapoptotic protein, Bcl-2 *(226)*. PTHrP inhibition of chondrocyte apoptosis requires nucleolar translocation *(72)*.

Hastings et al. *(227)* have reported that intratracheal instillation of PTHrP neutralizing antibodies in adult rats promoted type II cell apoptosis marked by increases in DNA fragmentation, caspase 3 activity and production of the proapoptotic protein, Bax. Exogenous PTHrP(67–86) blocked the apoptosis induced by this reduction in endogenous PTHrP action. Similarly, the PTHrP(–/–) lung shows a marked increase in alveolar epithelial cells having ultrastructural characteristics of apoptosis. Increased chondrocyte apoptosis (DNA fragmentation and decreased Bcl-2 mRNA expression) has previously been observed in these mutant mice *(228,229)*. These observations suggest that different PTHrP peptides may independently regulate type II cell proliferation and cell death.

## PARATHYROID HORMONE-RELATED PROTEIN
## AND TRANSEPITHELIAL CALCIUM TRANSPORT

Examples of tissues or organs for which there is at least circumstantial evidence for PTHrP-mediated epithelial calcium transport include the distal nephron, mammary epithelium, placenta, and the shell gland (distal oviduct) of the chicken (reviewed in ref. *111*). Late in mammalian development, calcium transport into the presumptive airspace may be important for surfactant stabilization in preparation for birth *(230)*.

## PARATHYROID HORMONE-RELATED PROTEIN
## AND LUNG CARCINOMA

Although the paraneoplastic syndrome of HHM is most closely associated with squamous carcinoma of the lung, virtually all lung tumor types may express PTHrP, including adenocarcinomas and neuroendocrine tumors (small cell lung carcinomas and carcinoids). Correlation of tumor type and serum calcium levels indicates that PTHrP secretion by nonsquamous cell lung carcinomas is often insufficient to induce hypercalcemia *(21)*. Ectopic tumoral production of PTH, on the contrary, is exceedingly rare *(231)*.

The selective tumor-associated induction of *PTHrP* gene expression in neoplastic transformation remains largely unexplained. A potential molecular mechanism underlying the frequent amplified expression of PTHrP in tumors relates to oncogene activation of the *PTHrP* gene. Oncogene (H-ras and v-src)-transformed cell lines show an increased rate of *PTHrP* gene transcription and the PTHrP gene appears to be a downstream target for ras and src *(232,233)*. In the BEN squamous cell lung carcinoma line from which PTHrP originally was cloned, chromosomal *in situ* hybridization indicates that the PTHrP locus on chromosome 12 is amplified 30-fold, and the adjacent KRAS2 oncogene locus is coamplified 14-fold *(234)*.

The role of epigenetic mechanisms in overexpression of the *PTHrP* gene is uncertain *(235)*. In BEN cells, methylation of the CpG dinucleotide islands in the 5' region of the PTHrP gene does not prevent expression via any of the three PTHrP gene promoters *(236)*, despite the frequent association of CpG island methylation with inhibition of gene transcription.

PTHrP probably stimulates tumor growth, in part, via autocrine mitogen actions. This growth phenomenon has been demonstrated in BEN cells, seemingly as part of an autocrine loop involving TGF-α *(237)*. PTHrP(1–34) is an autocrine growth factor in several cultured cell lines *(221,237)*. Hidaka et al. *(238)* have proposed that accelerated production of PTHrP may be associated with tumor progression. The cell cycle control of PTHrP mRNA expression, observed in normal keratinocytes and smooth muscle cells, is lost in squamous tumor cells *(222,234)*, suggesting that PTHrP effects on proliferation are dysregulated in cancers. The effects of PTHrP promoting vasodilatation and vasculogenesis probably are important consequences of high tumoral levels of expression of this protein.

## CONCLUSIONS

PTHrP, originally associated with paraneoplastic phenomena in lung cancer, has recently been recognized as a regulator of lung development and remodeling. the protein is a transducer for certain effects of mechanical forces in pulmonary tissues. Among the several modes of PTHrP action (endocrine, paracrine/juxtacrine, autocrine, intracrine), paracrine activities of amino-terminal PTHrP involving mesenchymal PTH/PTHrP receptors have received most attention. The findings in lung are similar to experimental studies of mammary epithelial cell PTHrP and mesenchymal PTH/PTHrP receptor *(25)*, and enamel organ PTHrP and dental mesenchymal PTH/PTHrP receptor *(239)*, and indicate that the ligand and receptor represent functional epithelial/mesenchymal signaling circuits during morphogenesis. The current experimental evidence, then, supports the hypothesis that PTHrP is a regulator of programmed epithelial cytodifferentiation in the distal airway. Further investigation undoubtedly will uncover new and unanticipated functions for this fascinating and complex family of peptides.

## ACKNOWLEDGMENTS

We thank Regina Allen for assistance with the preparation of the manuscript. This work was supported by NIH grants HL55268 and HD11343 and by the American Heart Association.

# REFERENCES

1. Suva LJ, Winslow GA, Wettenhall REH, Hammonds RG, Moseley JM, Diefenbach-Jagger H, Rodda CP, Kemp BE, Rodriguez H, Chen EY, Hudson PJ, Martin TJ, Wood WI. A parathyroid hormone-related protein implicated in malignant hypercalcemia: cloning and expression. Science 1987;237:893–896.
2. Thiede MA, Daifotis AG, Weir EC, Brines ML, Burtis WJ, Ikeda K, Dreyer BE, Garfield RE, Broadus AE. Intrauterine occupancy controls expression of the parathyroid hormone-related peptide gene in preterm rat myometrium. Proc Natl Acad Sci USA 1990;87:6969–6973.
3. Moniz C, Burton PBJ, Malik AN, Dixit M, Banga JP, Nicolaides K, Quirke P, Knight DE, McGregor AM. Parathyroid hormone-related peptide in normal fetal development. J Mol Endocrinol 1990;5:259–266.
4. Campos RV, Asa SL, Drucker DL. Immunocytochemical localization of parathyroid hormone-like peptide in the rat fetus. Cancer Res 1991;51:6351–6357.
5. Senior PV, Heath DA, Beck F. Expression of parathyroid hormone-related protein mRNA in the rat before birth: demonstration by hybridization histochemistry.J Mol Endocrinol 1991;6:281–290.
6. Ferguson JE 2d Gorman JV, Bruns DE, Weir EC, Burtis WJ, Martin TJ, Bruns ME. Abundant expression of parathyroid hormone-related protein in human amnion and its association with labor. Proc Natl Acad Sci USA 1992;89:8384–8388.
7. Bui TD, Shallal A, Malik AN, al-Mahdawi S, Moscoso G, Bailey ME, Burton PB, Moniz C. Parathyroid hormone related peptide gene expression in human fetal and adult heart. Cardiovasc Res 1993;27:1204–1208.
8. Burton PJB, Moniz P, Quirke P, Malik A, Bui TD, Juppner H, Segre GV, Knight DE. Parathyroid hormone-related peptide: expression in fetal and neonatal development. J Pathol 1992;167:291–296.
9. Dunne FP, Ratcliffe WA, Mansour P, Heath DA. Parathyroid hormone related protein (PTHrP) gene expression in fetal and extra-embryonic tissue of early pregnancy. Hum Reprod 1994;9:149–156.
10. Lee K, Deeds JD, Segre GV. Expression of parathyroid hormone-related peptide and its receptor messenger ribonucleic acids during fetal development of rats. Endocrinology 1995;136:453–463.
11. Deftos LJ, Burton DW, Pinar H, Rubin LP. Neoplastic hormone-producing cells of the placenta produce and secrete parathyroid hormone-related protein: studies by immunohistology immunoassay and polymerase chain reaction. Lab Invest 1994;71:847–852.
12. Merendino JJ, Jr, Insogna KL, Milstone LM, Broadus AE, Stewart AF. A parathyroid hormone-like protein from cultured human keratinocytes. Science 1986;231:388–390.
13. Weir EC, Philbrick WM, Amling M, Neff L A, Baron R, Broadus AE. Targeted overexpression of parathyroid hormone-related peptide in chondrocytes causes chondrodysplasia and delayed endochondral bone formation. Proc Natl Acad Sci USA 1996;93:10,240–10,245.
14. Kramer S, Reynolds FH, Jr, Castillo M, Valenzuela DM, Thorikay M, Sorvillo JM. Immunological identification and distribution of parathyroid hormone-related protein polypeptides in normal and malignant tissues. Endocrinology 1991;128:1927–1937.
15. Hongo T, Kupfer J Enomoto H, Sharifi B, Giannella-Neto D, Forrester JS, Singer FR, Goltzman D, Hendy GN, Pirola C. Abundant expression of parathyroid hormone-related protein in primary rat aortic smooth muscle cells accompanies serum-induced proliferation. J Clin Invest 1991;88:1841–1847.
16. Daifotis AG, Weir EC, Dreyer BE, Broadus AE. Stretch-induced parathyroid hormone-related peptide gene expression in the rat uterus. J Biol Chem 1992;267:23,455–23,458.
17. Deftos LJ, Burton DW, Brandt DW. Parathyroid hormone-like protein is a secretory product of atrial myocytes. J Clin Invest 1993;92:727–735.
18. Noda M, Katoh T, Takuwa N, Kumada M, Kurokawa K, Takuwa Y. Synergistic stimulation of parathyroid hormone-related peptide gene expression by mechanical stretch and angiotensin II in aortic smooth muscle cells. J Biol Chem 1994;269:17911–17917.
19. Thiede MA, Rodan GA. Expression of a calcium–mobilizing parathyroid hormone-related peptide in lactating mammary tissue. Science 1988;242:278–280.
20. Brandt DW, Burton DW, Gazdar AF, Oie HE, Deftos LJ. All major lung cancer cell types produce parathyroid hormone-like protein: heterogeneity assessed by high performance liquid chromatography.Endocrinology 1991;129:2466–2470.
21. Davidson LA, Black M, Carey FA, Logue F, McNicol AM. Lung tumours immunoreactive for parathyroid hormone related peptide: analysis of serum calcium lavels and tumour type. J Pathol 1996;178:398–401.
22. Takai E, Yano T, Iguchi H, Fukuyama Y, Yokoyama H, Asoh H, Ichinose Y. Tumor-induced hypercalcemia and parathyroid hormone-related protein in lung carcinoma. Cancer 1996;78:1384–1387.

23. Knecht TP, Behling CA, Burton DW, Glass CK, Deftos LJ. The humoral hypercalcemia of benignancy. A newly appreciated syndrome. Am J Clin Pathol 1996;105:487–492.

24. Wysolmerski JJ, Broadus AE. Hypercalcemia of malignancy – the central role of parathyroid hormone-related protein. Annu Rev Med 1994;45:189–200.

25. Dunbar ME, Wysolmerski JJ, Broadus AE. Parathyroid hormone-related protein: from hypercalcemia of malignancy to developmental regulatory molecule. Am J Med Sci 1996;312:287–294.

26. Mallory TB. Case records of the Massachusetts General Hospital: case #27461. N Engl J Med 1941;225:789–791.

27. Stewart AF, Horst R, Deftos LJ, Cadman EC, Lang R, Broadus AE. Biochemical evaluation of patients with cancer–associated hypercalcemia: evidence for humoral and non–humoral groups. N Engl J Med 1980;303:1377–1383.

28. Stewart AF, Vignery A, Silverglate A, Ravin ND, LiVolsi V, Broadus AE, Baron R. Quantitative bone histomorphometry in humoral hypercalcemia of malignancy. J Clin Endocrinol Metab 1982; 55:219–227.

29. Nussbaum S, Zahradnik RJ, Lavigne JR, Brennan GL, Nozawa-Ung K, Kim LY, Keutmann HT, Wang CA, Potts JT Jr, Segre GV. Highly sensitive two-site immunoradiometric assay of parathyrin and its clinical utility in evaluating patients with hypercalcemia. Clin Chem 1987;33:1364–1367.

30. Simpson EL, Mundy GR, D'Souza SM, Ibbotson KL, Bockman R, Jacobs JW. Absence of PTH mRNA in non-parathyroid tumors associated with hypercalcemia of malignancy. N Engl J Med 1983;309:325–330.

31. Moseley JM, Kubota M, Diefenbach–Jagger H, Wettenhall RE, Kemp BE, Suva LJ, Rodda CP, Ebeling PR, Hudson PJ, Zajac JD. Parathyroid hormone-related protein purified from a human lung cancer cell line. Proc Natl Acad Sci USA 1987;84:5048–5052.

32. Strewler GJ, Stern PH, Jacobs JW, Evelott J, Klein RF, Leung SC, Rosenblatt M, Nissenson RA. Parathyroid hormone-like protein from human renal carcinoma cells.: structural and functional homology with parathyroid hormone. J Clin Invest 1987;80:1803–1807.

33. Stewart AF, Wu T, Goumas D, Burtis WJ, Broadus AE. N-terminal amino acid sequence of two novel tumor-derived adenylate cyclase stimulating proteins: identification of parathyroid hormone-like and parathyroid-unlike domains. Biochem Biophys Res Commun 1987;146:672–678.

34. Mangin M, Webb AC, Dreyer B.E, Posillico JT, Ikeda K, Weir EC, Stewart AF, Bander NH, Milstone L, Barton DE, Franke U, Broadus AE. Identification of a cDNA encoding a parathyroid hormone-like protein from a human tumor associated with humoral hypercalcemia of malignancy. Proc Natl Acad Sci USA 1988;85:597–601.

35. Thiede MA, Strewler GJ, Nissenson RA, Rosenblatt M, Rodan GA. Human renal carcinoma expresses two messages encoding a parathyroid hormone-like peptide: evidence for the alternative splicing of a single-copy gene. Proc Natl Acad Sci USA 1988;85:4605–4609.

36. Budayr AA, Nissenson RA, Klein RF, Pun KK, Clark OH, Diep D, Arnaud CD, Strewler GJ. Increased serum levels of a parathyroid hormone-like protein in malignancy-associated hypercalcemia. Ann Intern Med 1989;111:807–812.

37. Burtis WJ, Brady TG, Orloff JJ, Ersbak JB, Warrell RP, Jr, Olson BR, Wu TL, Mitnick ME, Broadus AE, Stewart AF. Immunochemical characterization of circulating parathyroid hormone-related protein in patients with humoral hypercalcemia of cancer. N Engl J Med 1990;322:1106–1112.

38. Ratcliffe WA, Norbury S, Heath DA, Ratcliffe JG. Development and validation of parathyrin-related protein in unextracted plasma Clin Chem 1991;37:678–685.

39. Budayr AA, Zysset E, Jenzer A, Thiebaud D, Ammann P, Rizzoli P, Jaquet-Muller F, Bonjour JP, Gertz B, Burckhardt P, Halloran BP, Nissenson RA, Strewler GJ. Effects of treatment of malignancy-associated hypercalcemia on serum parathyroid hormone-related protein. J Bone Miner Res 1994;9:521–526.

40. Kukreja SC, Shevrin DH, Wimbiscus SA, Ebeling PR, Danks JA, Rodda CP, Wood WI, Martin TJ. Antibodies to parathyroid hormone-related protein lower serum calcium in athymic mouse models of malignancy associated hypercalcemia due to human tumors. J Clin Invest 1988;82:1798–1802.

41. Henry JG, Mitnick M, Dann PR, Stewart AF. Parathyroid hormone-related protein–(1–36) is biologically active when administered subcutaneously to humans. J Clin Endocrinol Metab 1996; 82:900–906.

42. Hendy GN, Bennett HPJ, Gibbs BF, Lazure C, Day R, Seidah NG. Proparathyroid hormone is preferentially cleaved to parathyroid hormone by the prohormone convertase farin. A mass spectrometric study. J Biol Chem 1995;270:9517–9525.

43. Meerovitch K, Wing S, Goltzman D. Proparathyroid hormone-related protein is associated with the chaperone protein BiP and undergoes proteasome-mediated cleavage. J Biol Chem 1998; 273:21,025–21,030.

44. Orloff JJ, Reddy D, de Papp AE, Yang KH, Soifer NE, Stewart AF. Parathyroid hormone-related protein as a prohormone: posttranslational processing and receptor interactions. Endocr Rev 1994;15:40–60.

45. Yang KH, dePapp AE, Soifer NE, Dreyer BE, Wu TL, Porter SE, Bellantoni M, Burtis WJ, Insogna KL, Broadus AE. Parathyroid hormone-related protein: evidence for isoform- and tissue-specific posttranslational processing. Biochemistry 1994;33:7460–7469.

46. Mallette LE. Parathyroid hormone and parathyroid hormone-related protein as polyhormones: evolutionary aspects and non-classical actions. In: Bilezikian JP, Levine MA, Marcus R, eds. The parathyroids. New York: Lippincott-Raven Press, 1994:171–184.

47. Harvey S, Wang R. Parathyroid hormone and neural calcium regulation: phylogenetic perspectives. In: Dacke C, Danks J, Caple I, Flik G, eds. The comparative endocrinology of calcium regulation. Bristol, UK: Journal of Endocrinology Ltd, 1996:3–15.

48. Fraser RA, Kronenberg HM, Pang PKT, Harvey S. Parathyroid hormone mRNA in the rat hypothalamus. Endocrinology 1990;127:2517–2522.

49. Nutley MT, Parimi SA, Harvey S. Sequence analysis of hypothalamic parathyroid hormone messenger ribonucleic acid. Endocrinology 1995;136:5600–5607.

50. Devlin AJ, Danks JA, Faulkner MK, Power DM, Canario AV, Martin TJ, Ingleton PM. Immunochemical detection of parathyroid hormone-related protein in the saccus vasculosus of a teleost fish. Gen Comp Endocrinol 1996;101:83–90.

51. Danks JA, Trivett MK, Power DM, Canario AV, Martin TJ, Ingleton PM. Parathyroid hormone-related protein in lower vertebrates. Clin Exp Pharmacol Physiol 1998;25:750–752.

52. Ikeda K, Lu C, Weir EC, Mangin M, Broadus AE. Transcriptional regulation of parathyroid hormone-like peptide gene by glucocorticoids and vitamin D in a human C-cell line. J Biol Chem 1989;264: 15,743–15,746.

53. Mangin M, Ikeda K, Dreyer BE, Broadus AE. Isolation and characterization of the human parathyroid hormone-like peptide gene. Proc Natl Acad Sci USA 1989;86:2408–2412.

54. Brandt DW, Bruns ME, Bruns DE, Ferguson JEII Burton DW, Deftos LJ. The parathyroid hormone-related protein (PTHrP) gene preferentially utilizes a GC-rich promotor and the PTHrP 1–139 coding pathway in normal human amnion. Biochem Biophys Res Commun 1992;189:938–943.

55. Heath JK, Southby J, Fukomoto S, O'Keefe LM, Martin TJ, Gillespie MT. Epidermal growth factor-stimulated parathyroid hormone-related protein expression involves increased gene transcription and mRNA stability. Biochem J 1995;307:159–167.

56. Campos RV, Zhang L, Drucker DJ. Differential expression of RNA transcripts encoding unique carboxy–terminal sequences of the human parathyroid hormone-related peptide. Mol Endocrinol 1994;8:1656–1666.

57. Allinson ET, Drucker DJ. Parathyroid hormone-like peptide shares features with members of the early response gene family: rapid induction by serum growth factors and cycloheximide. Cancer Res 1992;52:3103–3109.

58. Falzon M. Serum stimulation of parathyroid hormone-related peptide gene expression in ROS 17/2.8 osteosarcoma cells through transcriptional and posttranscriptional mechanisms. Endocrinology 1996;137:3681–3688.

59. Philbrick WM, Wysolmerski JJ, Galbraith S, Holt E, Orloff JJ, Yang KH, Vasavada RC, Weir EC, Broadus AE, Stewart AF. Defining the roles of parathyroid hormone-related protein in normal physiology. Physiol Rev 1996;76:127–173.

60. Bowden SJ, Hughes SV, Ratcliffe WA. Molecular forms of parathyroid hormone-related protein in tumours and biological fluids. Clin Endocrinol 1993;38:287–294.

61. Soifer NE, Dee KE, Insogna KL, Burtis WJ, Matovcik LM, Wu TL, Milstone LM, Broadus AE, Philbrick WM, Stewart AF. Parathyroid hormone-related protein: evidence for secretion of a novel mid-region fragment by three different cell types. J Biol Chem 1992;267:18236–18243.

62. Orloff JJ, Soifer NE, Fodero JP, Dann P, Burtis WJ. Accumulation of carboxy–terminal fragments of parathyroid hormone-related protein in renal failure. Kidney Int 1993;43:1371–1376.

63. Burtis WJ, Dann P, Gaich GA, Soifer NE. A high abundance midregion species of parathyroid hormone-related protein: immunological and chromatographic characterization in plasma. J Clin Endocrinol Metab 1994;78:317–322.

64. Plawner LL, Philbrick WM, Burtis WJ, Broadus AE, Stewart AF. Cell type-specific secretion of parathyroid hormone-related protein via the regulated versus the constitutive secretory pathway. J Biol Chem 1995;270:14078–14084.

65. Ogine K, Burkhoff D, Bilezikian JP. The hemodynamic basis for the cardiac effects of parathyroid hormone . PTH; and PTH-related protein. Endocrinology 1995;136:3024–3030.

66. Care AD, Abbas SK, Pickard DW, Barri M, Drinkhill M, Findlay JB, White IR, Caple IW. Stimulation of ovine placental transport of calcium and magnesium by mid-molecule fragments of human parathyroid hormone-related protein. Exp Physiol 1990;75:605–608.

67. Kovacs CS, Lanske B, Hunzelman JL, Guo J, Karaplis AC, Kronenberg HM. Parathyroid hormone-related peptide (PTHrP) regulates fetal–placental calcium transport through a receptor distinct from the PTH/PTHrP receptor. Proc Natl Acad Sci USA 1996;93:15,233–15,238.

68. Rubin LP, Posillico JT, Anast CS, Brown EM. Circulating levels of biologically active and immunoreactive intact parathyroid hormone in human newborns. Pediatr Res 1991;29:201–207.

69. Fenton AJ, Kemp BE, Hammonds RG, Mitchelhill K, Martin TJ, Nicholson GC. A potent inhibitor of osteoclastic bone resorption within a highly conserved pentapeptide region of PTHr (107–111). Endocrinology 1991;129:3424–3426.

70. Zheng MH, McCaughan HB, Papadimitriou JM, Nicholson GC, Wood DJ. Tartrate resistant acid phosphatase activity in rat cultured osteoclasts is inhibited by a carboxyl terminal peptide (osteostatin) from parathyroid hormone-related protein. J Cell Biochem 1994;54:145–153.

71. Kaiser SM, Laneuville P, Bernier SM, Rhim JS, Kremer R, Goltzman D. Enhanced growth of a human keratinocyte line by antisense RNA for PTHrP. J Biol Chem 1992;267:13,623–13,628.

72. Henderson JE, Amizuka N, Warshawsky H, Biasotto D, Lanske BM, Goltzman D, Karaplis AC. Nucleolar localization of parathyroid hormone-related peptide enhances survival of chondrocytes under conditions that promote apoptotic cell death. Mol Cell Biol 1995;15:4064–4075.

73. Nguyen MT, Karaplis AC. The nucleus: a target site for parathyroid hormone-related peptide (PTHrP) action. J Cell Biochem 1998;70:193–199.

74. Juppner H, Abou-Samra AB, Freeman M, Kong XF, Schipani E, Richards J, Kolakowski LF Jr, Hock J, Potts JT Jr, Kronenberg HM, Segre GV. A G protein-linked receptor for parathyroid hormone and parathyroid hormone-related peptide. Science 1991;254:1024–1026.

75. Abou-Samra AB, Juppner H, Force T, Freeman MW, Kong XF, Schipani E, Urena P, Richards J, Bonventre JV, Potts JT Jr, Kronenberg HM, Segre GV. Expression cloning of a receptor for parathyroid hormone and parathyroid hormone-related peptide from rat osteoblast-like cells: a single receptor stimulates intracellular accumulation of both cAMP and inositol triphosphates and increases intracellular free calcium. Proc Natl Acad Sci USA 1992;89:2732–2736.

76. Lanske B, Divieti P, Kovacs CS, Pirro A, Landis WJ, Krane SM, Bringhurst PR, Kronenberg HM. The parathyroid hormone (PTH)/PTH-related peptide receptor mediates actions of both ligands in murine bone. Endocrinology 1998;139: 5194–5204.

77. Rubin LP, Kifor, O, Hua J, Brown EM, Torday JS. 1994; Parathyroid hormone (PTH) and PTH-related protein stimulate surfactant phospholipid synthesis in rat fetal lung apparently by a mesenchymal–epithelial mechanism. Biochim Biophys Acta 1998;1223:91–100.

78. Kronenberg HM, Lanske B, Kovacs CS, Chung UI, Lee K, Segre GV, Schipani E, Juppner H. Functional analysis of the PTH/PTHrP network of ligands and receptors. Recent Prog Horm Res 1998;53:283–301.

79. Gelbert L, Schipani E, Juppner H, Abou–Samra AB, Segre GV, Naylor S, Drabkin H, Heath H 3rd. Chromosomal localization of the parathyroid hormone/parathyroid hormone-related protein receptor gene to human chromosome 3p21.1–p24.2. J Clin Endocrinol Metab 1994;79:1046–1048.

80. Pausova Z, Bourdon J, Clayton D, Mattei MG, Seldin MJ, Janicic N, Riviere M, Szpirer J, Levan G, Szpirer C, Goltzman D, Hendy GN. Cloning of a parathyroid hormone/parathyroid hormone-related peptide receptor (PTHR) cDNA from a rat osteosarcoma (UMR 106) cell line: chromosomal assignment of the gene in the human mouse and rat genomes. Genomics 1994;20:20–26.

81. Fukayama S, Schipani E, Juppner H, Lanske B, Kronenberg HM, Abou–Samra AB, Bringhurst FR. Role of protein kinase-A in homologous down-regulation of parathyroid hormone (PTH)/PTH-related peptide receptor messenger ribonucleic acid in human osteoblast-like SaOS-2 cells. Endocrinology 1994;134:1851–1858.

82. Kong XF, Schipani E, Lanske B, Joun H, Karperien M, Defize LH, Juppner H, Potts JT Jr, Segre GV, Kronenberg HM. The rat mouse and human genes encoding the receptor for parathyroid hormone and parathyroid hormone-related peptide are highly homologous. Biochem Biophys Res Commun 1994;201:1290–1299.

83. Bettoun JD, Minagawa M, Kwan MY, Lee HS, Yasuda T, Hendy GN, Goltzman D, White JH. Cloning and characterization of the promotor regions of the human parathyroid hormone (PTH)/PTH-related peptide receptor gene: analysis of deoxyribonucleic acid from normal subjects and patients with pseudohypoparathyroidism type 1b. J Clin Endocrinol Metab 1997;82:1031–1040.
84. Bettoun JD, Minagawa M, Hendy GN, Alpert LC, Goodyer CG, Goltzman D, White JH. Developmental upregulation of human parathyroid hormone . (PTH)/PTH-related peptide receptor gene expression from conserved and human-specific promotors. J Clin Invest 1998; 102:958–967.
85. Urena P, Kong XF, Abou-Samra AB, Juppner H, Kronenberg HM, Potts JT Jr, Segre GV. Parathyroid hormone (PTH)/PTH-related peptide receptor messenger ribonucleic acids are widely distributed in rat tissues. Endocrinology 1993;133:617–623.
86. Adams AE, Pines M, Nakamoto C, Behar V, Yang QM, Bessalle R, Chorev M, Rosenblatt M, Levine MA, Suva LJ. Probing the bimolecular interactions of parathyroid hormone and the human parathyroid hormone/parathyroid hormone-related protein receptor. 2. Cloning, characterization, and photoaffinity labeling of the recombinant human receptor. Biochemistry 1995;34:10,553–10,559.
87. Bergwitz C, Klein P, Kohno H, Forman SA, Lee K, Rubin D, Juppner H. Identification functional characterization and developmental expression of two nonallelic parathyroid hormone (PTH)/PTH-related peptide receptor isoforms in Xanopus laevis (Daudin). Endocrinology 1998;139:723–732.
88. Juppner H. Molecular cloning and characterization of a parathyroid hormone/parathyroid hormone-related peptide receptor: a member of an ancient family of G protein–coupled receptors. Curr Opin Nephrol Hypertension 1994;3:371–378.
89. Botella A, Rekik M, Delvaux M, Davicco MJ, Barlet JP, Frexinos J, Bueno L. Parathyroid hormone (PTH) and PTH-related peptide induce relaxation of smooth muscle cells from guinea pig ileum: interaction with vasoactive intestinal peptide receptors. Endocrinology 1994;135:2160–2167.
90. Karperien M, van Dijk TB, Hoeijmakers T, Cremers F, Abou-Samra AB, Boonstra J, de Laat SW, Defize LH. Expression pattern of parathyroid hormone/parathyroid hormone-related peptide receptor mRNA in mouse preimplantation embryo indicates involvement in multiple developmental processes. Mech Dev 1994;47:29–42.
91. Wysolmerski JJ, Philbrick WM, Dunbar ME, Lanske B, Kronenberg H, Broadus AE. Rescue of the parathyroid hormone-related protein knockout mouse demonstrates that parathyroid hormone-related protein is essential for mammary gland development. Development 1998;125:1285–1294.
92. Lanske B, Karaplis AC, Leek Luz A, Vertkamp A, Pirro A, Karperien M, Defize LHK, Ho C, Mulligan RC, Abou–Samra AB, Juppner H, Segre GV, Kronenberg HM. PTH/PTHrP receptor in early development and Indian hedgehog-related bone growth. Science 1996;273:663–666.
93. Rubin LP, Kovacs CS, Pinar H, DePaepe ME, Tsai S.–W, Torday JS, Kronenberg HM. Arrested pulmonary alveolar cytodifferentiation and defective surfactant synthesis in mice missing the gene for parathyroid hormone-related protein. J Cell Biol 2000;149: in press.
94. Usdin TB, Gruber C, Bonner TI. Identification and functional expression of a receptor selectively recognizing parathyroid hormone the PTH2 receptor. J Biol Chem 1995;270:15,455–15,458.
95. Usdin TB, Bonner TI, Harta G, Mezey E. Distribution of parathyroid hormone-2 receptor messenger ribonucleic acid in rat. Endocrinology 1996;137:4285–4297.
96. Usdin TB, Modi W, Bonner TI. Assignment of the human PTH2 receptor gene (PTHR2) to chromosome 2q33 by fluorescence in situ hybridization. Genomics 1996;37:140–141.
97. Inomata N, Akiyama M, Kubota A, Juppner H. Characterization of a novel PTH-receptor with specificity for the carboxy–terminal region of PTH (1–84). Endocrinology 1995;136:4732–4740.
98. Orloff JJ, Kats J, Urena P, Schipani E, Vasavada RC, Philbrick WM, Behal A, Abou-Samra AB, Segre GV, Juppner H. Further evidence for a novel receptor for amino–terminal PTHrP on keratinocytes and squamous cell lines. Endocrinology 1995;136:3016–3023.
99. Bertelloni S, Baroncelli GI, Pelletti A, Battini R, Saggese G. Parathyroid hormone-related potein in healthy pregnant women. Calcif Tisues Intl 1994;54:195–197.
100.Dobnig H, Kainer F, Stepan V, Winter R, Lipp R, Schaffer M, Kahr, A, Nocnik S, Patterer G, Leb G. Elevated parathyroid hormone-related peptide levels after human gestation: relationship to changes in bone and mineral metabolism. J Clin Endocrinol Metab 1995;80:3699–3707.
101.Sowers MF, Hollis BW, Shapiro B, Randolph J, Janney CA, Zhang D, Schork A, Crutchfield M, Stanczyk F, Russell-Aulet M. Elevated parathyroid hormone-related peptide associated with lactation and bone density loss. JAMA 1996;276:549–554.
102.Nowak RA, Haimovici F, Biggers JD, Erbach GT. Transforming growth factor-beta stimulates blastocyst outgrowth through a mechanism involving parathyroid hormone-related protein. Biol Reprod 1999;60:85–93.

103.Chan SDH, Strewler GH, King KL, Nissenson RA. Expression of a parathyroid hormone-like protein and its receptor during differentiation of embryonal carcinoma cells. Mol Endocrinol 1990; l4:638–646.

104.Van de Stolpe A, Karperien M, Loewik CWGM, Juppner H, Segre GV, Abou-Samra AB, de Laat SW, Defize LHK. Parathyroid hormone-related peptide as an endogenous inducer of parietal endoderm differentiation. J Cell Biol 1993;120:235–243.

105.Karperien M, Lanser P, de Laat SW, Boonstra J, Defize LH. Parathyroid hormone related peptide mRNA expression during murine development: evidence for involvement in multiple differentiation processes. Int J Dev Biol 1996;40:599–608.

106.Wysolmerski JJ, Broadus AE, Zhou J, Fuchs E, Milstone LM, Philbrick WM. Overexpression of parathyroid hormone-related peptide in the skin of transgenic mice interferes with hair follicle development. Proc Natl Acad Sci USA 1994;91:1133–1137.

107.Wysolmerski JJ, McCaughern-Carucci JF, Daifotis AG, Broadus AE, Philbrick WM. Overexpression of parathyroid hormone-related protein or parathyroid hormone in transgenic mice impairs branching morphogenesis during mammary gland development. Development 1995;121:3539–3547.

108.Karaplis AC, Luz A, Glowacki J, Bronson RT, Tybulewicz VL, Kronenberg HM, Mulligan RC. Lethal skeletal dysplasia from targeted disruption of the parathyroid hormone-related peptide gene. Genes Dev 1994;8:277–289.

109.Amizuka N, Warshawsky H, Henderson JE, Goltzman D, Karaplis AC. Parathyroid hormone-related peptide-depleted mice show abnormal epiphyseal cartilage development and altered endochondral bone formation. J Cell Biol 1994;126:1611–1623.

110.Vortkamp A, Lee K, Lanske B, Segre GV, Kronenberg HM, Tabin CJ. Regulation of the rate of cartilage differentiation by Indian hedgehog and PTH-related protein. Science 1996;273:613–622.

111.Philbrick WM, Dreyer BE, Nakchbandi IA, Karaplis AC. Parathyroid hormone-related protein is required for tooth eruption. Proc Natl Acad Sci USA 1998;95:11,846–11,851.

112.Amizuka N, Karaplis AC, Henderson JE, Warshawsky H, Lipman ML, Matsuki Y, Ejiri S, Tanaka M, Izumi N, Ozawa H, Goltzman D. Haploinsufficiency of parathyroid hormone-related peptide (PTHrP) results in abnormal postnatal bone development. Dev Biol 1996;175:166–176.

113.Kaiser SM, Sebag, M, Rhim JS, Kremer R, Goltzman D. Antisense-mediated inhibition of parathyroid hormone-related peptide production in a keratinocyte cell line impedes differentiation. Mol Endocrinol 1994;8:139–147.

114.Holick MF, Ray S, Chen TC, Tian X, Persons KS. A parathyroid hormone antagonist stimulates epidermal proliferation and hair growth in mice. Proc Natl Acad Sci USA 1994;91:8014–8016.

115.Emly JF, Gregory J, Bowden SJ, Ahmed A, Whittle MJ, Rushton DI, Ratcliffe WA. Immunohistochemical localization of parathyroid hormone-related protein (PTHrP) in human term placenta and membranes. Placenta 1994;15:653–660.

116.Henderson JE, He B, Goltzman D, Karaplis AC. Constitutive expression of parathyroid hormone-related peptide (PTHrP) stimulates growth and inhibits differentiation of CFK2 chondrocytes. J Cell Physiol 1996;169:33–41.

117.Johnson RL, Scott MP. New players and puzzles in the Hedgehog signaling pathway. Curr Opin Genet Dev 1998;8:450–456.

118.Schipani E, Langman CB, Parfitt AM, Jensen GS, Kikuchi S, Kooh SW, Cole WG, Juppner H. Constitutively activated receptors for parathyroid hormone and parathyroid hormone-related peptide in Jansen's metaphyseal chondrodysplasia. N Engl J Med 1996;335:708–714.

119.Jobert AS, Zhang P, Couvineau A, Bonaventure J, Roume J, Le Merrer M, Silve C. Absence of functional receptors for parathyroid hormone and parathyroid hormone-related peptide in Blomstrand chondrodysplasia. J Clin Invest 1998;102:34–40.

120.Zhang P, Joubert AS, Couvineau A, Silve C. A homozygous inactivating mutation in the parathyroid hormone/parathyroid hormone-related peptide receptor causing Blomstrand chondrodysplasia. J Clin Endocrinol Metab 1998;83:3365–3368.

121. Karaplis AC, He B, Nguyen MT, Young ID, Semeraro D, Ozawa H, Amizuka N. Inactivating mutation in the human parathyroid hormone receptor type 1 gene in Blomstrand chondrodysplasia. Endocrinology 1998;139:5255–5258.

122.Loshkajian A, Roume J, Stanescu V, Delezoide AL, Stampf F, Maroteaux P. Familial Blomstrand chondrodysplasia with advanced skeletal maturation: further delineation. Am J Med Genet 1997;22:283–288.

123.Hastings RH, Duong H, Burton DW, Deftos LJ. Alveolar epithelial cells express and secrete parathyroid hormone-related protein. Am J Respir Cell Mol Biol 1994;11:701–706.

124.Sanchez-Esteban J, Tsai SW, Sang J, Qin J, Torday JS, Rubin LP. Effects of mechanical forces on lung-specific gene expression. Am J Med Sci 1998;316:200–204.

125. Moseley JM, Hayman JA, Danks JA, Alcorn D, Grill V, Southby J, Horton MA. Immunohistochemical detection of parathyroid hormone-related protein in human fetal epithelia. J Clin Endocrinol Metab 1991;73:478–484.

126. Ichinose Y, Iguchi H, Ohta M, Katakami H. Establishment of a lung cancer cell line producing parathyroid hormone-related protein. Cancer Lett 1993;74:119–124.

127. Kitazawa S, Fukase M, Kitazawa R, Takenaka A, Gotoh A, Fujita T, Maeda S. Immunohistologic evaluation of parathyroid hormone-related protein in human lung cancer and normal tissue with a newly developed monoclonal antibody. Cancer 1991;67:984–989.

128. Torday JS, Sanchez-Esteban J, Rubin LP. The physiologic role of fluid deformation in fetal lung development. Am J Med Sci 1998;316:205–208.

129. Hastings RH, Summers-Torres D, Cheung TC, Ditmer LS, Petrin EM, Burton DW, Spragg RG, Li J, Deftos LJ. Parathyroid hormone-related protein an autocrine regulatory factor in alveolar epithelial cells. Am J Physiol 1996;270:L353–L361.

130. Speziale MV, Manning FL, Hastings RH, Deftos LJ. Parathyroid hormone-related protein in tracheal aspirates of newborn infants. Pediatr Res 1998;43:660–665.

131. Shannon JM, Detering RR. Epithelial–mesenchymal interactions in lung development. In: McDonald JA. ed. Lung growth and development. New York: Marcel Dekker,1998: 81–118.

132. Beck F, Tucci J, Russell A, Senior PV, Ferguson MW. The expression of the gene coding for parathyroid hormone-related protein (PTHrP) during tooth development in the rat. Cell Tissue Res 1995; 280:283–290.

133. Gillespie MT, Martin TJ. The parathyroid hormone-related protein gene and its expression. Mol Cell Endocrinol 1994;100:143–147.

134. Rodan SB, Wesolowski G, Ianacone J, Thiede MA, Rodan GA. Production of parathyroid hormone-like peptide in a human osteosarcoma cell line: stimulation by phorbol esters and epidermal growth factor. J Endocrinol 1989;122:219–227.

135. Liu B, Goltzman D, Rabbani SA. Regulation of parathyroid hormone-related peptide production in vitro by the rat hypercalcemic Leydig cell tumor H-500. Endocrinology 1993;132:1658–1664.

136. Sebag M, Henderson J, Goltzman D, Kremer R. Regulation of parathyroid hormone-related peptide production in normal human mammary epithelial cells in vitro. Am J Physiol 1994;267:C723–730.

137. Rizzoli R, Feyen JH, Grau G, Wohlwend A, Sappino AP, Bonjour JP. Regulation of parathyroid hormone-related protein production in a human lung squamous cell carcinoma line. J Endocrinol 1994;143:333–341.

138. Dvir R, Golander A, Jaccard N, Yedwab, G, Otremski I, Spirer AZ, Weisman Y. Amniotic fluid and plasma levels of parathyroid hormone-related protein and hormonal modulation of its secretion by amniotic fluid cells. Eur J Endocrinol 1995;133:277–282.

139. Mitchell MD, Hunter C, Dudley DJ, Varner MW. Significant decrease in parathyroid hormone-related protein concentrations in amniotic fluid with labour at term but not preterm. Reprod Fertil Dev 1996;8:231–234.

140. Grone A, Weckmann MT, Capen CC, Rosol TJ. Regulation of parathyroid hormone-related protein expression in a canine squamous carcinoma cell line by colchicine. Exp Toxicol Pathol 1998;50:365–370.

141. Southby J, Murphy LM, Martin TJ, Gillespie MT. Cell-specific and regulator-induced promoter usage and messenger ribonucleic acid splicing for parathyroid hormone-related protein. Endocrinology 1996;137:1349–1357.

142. Casey ML, Mibe M, MacDonald PC. Transforming growth factor-β1 stimulation of parathyroid hormone-related protein expression in human uterine cells in culture: mRNA levels and protein secretion. J Clin Endocrinol Metab 1992;74:950–952.

143. Kiriyama T, Gillespie MT, Glatz JA, Fukumoto S, Moseley JM, Martin TJ. Transforming growth factor beta stimulation of parathyroid hormone-related protein (PTHrP): a paracrine regulator? Mol Cell Endocrinol 1993;92:55–92.

144. Merryman JI, DeWille JW, Werkmeister JR, Capen CC, Rosol TJ. Effects of transforming growth factor-beta on parathyroid hormone-related protein production and ribonucleic acid expression by a squamous carcinoma cell line in vitro. Endocrinology 1994;134:2424–2430.

145. Werkmeister JR, Blomme EA, Weckmann MT, Grone A, McCauley LK, Wade AB, O'Rourke J, Capen CC, Rosol TJ. Effect of transforming growth factor-beta1 on parathyroid hormone-related protein secretion and mRNA expression by normal human keratinocytes in vitro. Endocrine 1998;8:291–299.

146. Emly JF, Hughes S, Green E, Ratcliffe WA. Expression and secretion of parathyroid hormone-related protein by a human cancer cell line. Biochim Biophys Acta 1994;1220:193–198.

147. Zeimer HJ, Greenaway TM, Slavin J, Jards DK, Zhou H, Doery JCG, Hunter AN, Duffield A, Martin TJ, Grill V. Parathyroid hormone-related protein in sarcoidosis. Am J Pathol 1998;152:17–21.

148. Glatz JA, Heath JK, Southby J, O'Keeffe LM, Kiriyama T, Moseley JM, Martin TJ, Gillespie MT. Dexamethasone regulation of parathyroid horrmone-related protein (PTHrP) expression in a squamous cancer cell line. Mol Cell Endocrinol 1994;101:295–306.

149. Walsh CA, Birch MA, Fraser WD, Lawton R, Dorgan J, Walsh S, Sansom D, Beresford JN, Gallagher JA. Expression and secretion of parathyroid hormone-related protein by human bone-derived cells in vitro: effects of glucocorticoids. J Bone Miner Res 1995;10:17–25.

150. Kremer R, Sebag M, Champigny C, Meerovitch K, Hendy GN, White J, Goltzman D. Identification and characterization of 1,25-dihydroxyvitamin D3-responsive repressor sequences in the rat parathyroid hormone-related peptide gene. J Biol Chem 1996;271:16,310–16,316.

151. Lu C, Ikeda K, Deftos LJ, Gazdar AF, Mangin M, Broadus AE. Glucocorticoid regulation of parathyroid hormone-related peptide gene expression in a human neuroendocrine cell line. Mol Endocrinol 1989;3:2034–2040.

152. Falzon M, Zong J. The noncalcemic vitamin D analogs EB1089 and 22-oxacalcitriol suppress serum-induced parathyroid hormone-related peptide gene expression in a lung cancer cell line. Endocrinology 1998;139:1046–1053.

153. Law F, Bonjour JP, Rizzoli R. Transforming growth factor-beta: a down-regulator of the parathyroid hormone-related protein receptor in renal epithelial cells. Endocrinology 1994;134:2037–2043.

154. Jongen JW, Willemstein-van Hove EC, Van der Meer JM, Bos MP, Juppner H, Segre GV, Abou-Samra AB, Feyen JH, Herrmann-Erlee MP. Down-regulation of the receptor for parathyroid hormone (PTH) and PTH-related peptide by transforming growth factor-beta in primary fetal rat osteoblasts. Endocrinology 1995;136:3260–3266.

155. Schneider HG, Allan EH, Moseley JM, Martin TJ, Findlay DM. Specific down-regulation of parathyroid hormone (PTH) receptors and responses to PTH by tumour necrosis factor alpha and retinoic acid in UMR 106–06 osteoblast-like osteosarcoma cells. Biochem J 1991;280:451–457.

156. Brody JS, Williams MC. Pulmonary alveolar epithelial cell differentiation. Annu Rev Physiol 1992;54:351–371.

156. Urena P, Iida-Klein A, Kong XF, Juppner H, Kronenberg HM, Abou-Samra AB, Segre GV. Regulation of parathyroid hormone (PTH)/PTH-related peptide receptor messenger ribonucleic acid by glucocorticoids and PTH in ROS 17/2.8 and OK cells. Endocrinology 1994;134:451–456.

157 Adamson IY. Relationship of mesenchymal changes to alveolar epithelial cell differentiation in fetal rat lung. Anat Embryol 1992;185:275–280.

158. Shannon JM. Induction of alveolar type II cell differentiation in fetal tracheal epithelium by grafted distal lung mesenchyme. Dev Biol 1994;166:600–614.

159. Shin JH, Ji C, Casinghino S, McCarthy TL, Centrella M. Parathyroid hormone-related protein enhances insulin-like growth factor-I expression by rat fetal dermal fibroblasts. J Biol Chem 1997; 272:23,498–23,502.

160. Torday JS, Sanchez-Esteban J, Rubin LP. The role of keratinocyte growth factor in stretch-activated fetal lung development. Pediatr Res 1998;42:300A.

161. Elias JA, Tang W, Horowitz MC. Cytokine and hormonal stimulation of human osteosarcoma interleukin-11 production. Endocrinology 1995;136:489–498.

162. Hepworth WB, Seegmiller RE. A stereoscopic scanning microscopic study of pulmonary hypoplasia in chondrodystrophic mice. Scan Microsc 1989;3:1117–1134.

163. Foster MJ, Caldwell AP, Staheli J, Smith DH, Gardner JS, Seegmiller RE. Pulmonary hypoplasia associated with reduced thoracic space in mice with disproportionate micromelia (DMM) Anat Rec 1994;238:454–462.

164. Slavkin HC, Johnson R, Oliver P, Bringas P Jr, Don-Wheeler G, Mayo M, Whitsett JA. Lamellar body formation precedes pulmonary surfactant apoprotein expression during mouse lung development in vivo and in vitro. Differentiation 1989;41:223–236.

165. Wright JR, Dobbs LG. Regulation of surfactant secretion and clearance. Annu Rev Physiol 1991;53: 395–414.

166. Grant MM, Cutts NR, Brody JS. Alterations in lung basement membrane during fetal growth and type 2 cell development. Dev Biol 1983;97:173–183.

167. Adamson IY, Hedgecock C, Bowden DH. Epithelial–fibroblast interactions in lung injry and repair. Am J Pathol 1990;137:385–392.

168. Hu YS, Zhou H, Kartsogiannis V, Eisman JA, Martin TJ, Ng KW. Expression of rat homeobox gene, rHOX, in developing and adult tissues in mice and regulation of its mRNA expression in osteoblasts by bone morphogenetic protein 2 and parathyroid hormone-related protein. Mol Endocrinol 1998;12:1721–1732.

169. Pepicelli CV, Lewis PM, McMahon AP. Sonic hedgehog regulates branching morphogenesis in the mammalian lung. Curr Biol 1998;24:1083–1086.

170. Schipani E, Lanske B, Hunzelman J, Luz A, Kovacs CS, Lee K, Pirro A, Kronenberg HM, Juppner H. Targeted expression of constitutively active receptors for parathyroid hormone and parathyroid hormone-related peptide delays endochondral bone formation and rescues mice that lack parathyroid hormone-related peptide. Proc Natl Acad Sci USA 1997;94:13,689–13,694.

171. Torday JS, Londos C, Schultz CJ, Rubin LP. Distension of the developing lung triggers coordinate growth factor-mediated cell–cell signal transduction. Pediatr Res 1999;45:322A.

172. Kaplan NB, Grant MM, Brody JS. The lipid interstitial cell of the pulmonary alveolusAge and species differences. Am Rev Respir Dis 1985;132:1307–1312.

173. Penney DP, Keng PC, Derdak S, Phipps RP. Morphologic and functional characteristics of subpopulations of murine lung fibroblasts grown in vitro. Anat Rec 1992;232:432–443.

174. McGowan SE, Torday JS. The pulmonary lipofibroblast (lipid interstitial cell) and its contributions to alveolar development. Annu Rev Physiol 1997;59:43–62.

175. Maksvytis HJ, Vaccaro C, Brody JS. Isolation and characterization of the lipid-containing interstitial cell from the developing rat lung. Lab Invest 1981;45:248–259.

176. Torday JS, Hua J, Slavin R. Metabolism and fate of neutral lipids of fetal lung fibroblast origin. Biochim Biophys Acta 1995;1254:198–206.

177. Nunez JS, Torday JS. Fetal rat lung type II cells and fibroblasts actively recruit surfactant substrate. J Nutr 1995;125:S1639–S1644.

178. Wu TL, Insogna KL, Milstone L, Stewart AF. Skin-derived fibroblasts respond to human PTH-like adenylate cyclase-stimulating proteins. J Clin Endocrinol Metab 1987;65:105–109.

179. Insogna KL, Stewart AF, Morris CF, Hough LM, Milstone LM, Centrella M. Native and synthetic analogue of the malignancy-associated parathyroid hormone-like protein have in vivo transforming growth factor-like properties. J Clin Invest 1989;83:1057–1089.

180. Ni Z, Smogorzewski M, Massry SG. Effects of parathyroid hormone on cytosolic calcium of rat adipocytes. Endocrinology 1994;135:1837–1844.

181. Torday JS. Cellular timing of development. Semin Perinatol 1992;16:130–139.

182. Garite TJ, Rumney PJ, Briggs CG, Harding JA, Nageotte MP, Towers CV, Freeman R.K. A randomized placebo-controlled trial of betamethasone for the prevention of respiratory distress syndrome at 24 to 28 weeks' gestation. Am J Obstet Gynecol 1992;166:646–651.

183. Jiang HP, Serrero G. Isolation and characterization of a full-length cDNA coding for an adipose differentiation-related protein. Proc Natl Acad Sci USA 1992;89:7856–7860.

184. Brasaemle DL, Barber T, Wolins NE, Serrero G, Blanchette-Mackie EJ, Londos C. Adipose differentiation-related protein is an ubiquitously expressed lipid storage droplet-associated protein. J Lipid Res 1997;38:2249–2263.

185. Alcorn D, Adamson TM, Lambert TF, Maloney JE, Ritchie BC, Robinson PM. Morphological effects of chronic tracheal ligation and drainage in the fetal lamb lung. J Anat 1977;123:649–660.

186. Moessinger AC, Harding R, Adamson TM, Singh M, Kiu GT. Role of lung fluid volume in growth and maturation of the fetal sheep lung. J Clin Invest 1990;86:1270–1277.

187. Sanchez-Esteban J, Cicchiello L, Tsai SW, Williams LK, Rehan VK, Torday JS, Rubin LP. Mechanical stretch-activated type II cell-fibroblast interactions regulate surfactant protein gene expression and alveolar remodeling. Pediatr Res 1999;45:319A.

188. Yamamoto M, Harm SC, Grasser WA, Thiede MA. Parathyroid hormone-related protein in the rat urinary bladder: a smooth muscle relaxant produced locally in response to mechanical stretch. Proc Natl Acad Sci USA 1992;89:5326–5330.

189. Steers WD, Broder SR, Persson K, Bruns DE, Ferguson JE2d Bruns ME, Tuttle JB. Mechanical stretch increases secretion of parathyroid hormone-related protein by cultured bladder smooth muscle cells. J Urol 1998;160:908–912.

190. Thiede MA, Harm SC, McKee RL, Grasser WA, Duong LJ, Leach RM Jr. Expression of parathyroid hormone-related protein gene in the avian oviduct: potential role as a local modulator of vascular smooth muscle tension and shell gland motility during the egg-laying cycle. Endocrinology 1991;129:1958–1965.

191. Pirola CJ, Wang HM, Strgacich MI, Kamyar A, Cercek B, Forrester JS, Clemens TL, Fagin JA. Mechanical stimuli induce vascular parathyroid hormone-related protein gene expression in vivo and in votro. Endocrinology 1994;134:2230–2236.

192. Ito M, Ohtsuru A, Enomoto H, Ozeki S, Nakashima M, Nakayama T, Shichijo K, Sekine I, Yamashita S. Expression of parathyroid hormone-related peptide in relation to perturbations of gastric motility in the rat. Endocrinology 1994;134:1936–1942.

193. Torday JS, Sunday ME, Londos C, Schultz CJ Sanchez-Esteban J, Rubin LP. Mechanomolecular-disregulation of cell–cell signalling pathways bronchopulmonary dysplasia/chronic lung disease. Pediatr Res 1999;45:323A.

194. Turing AM. The chemical theory of morphogenesis. Phil Trans R Soc Lond B 1952;237:32–72.

195. Bard J, Lauder I. How well does Turing's theory of morphogenesis work? J Theor Biol 1974;45:501–531.

196. Harrison LG. What is the status of reaction–diffusion theory thirty-four years after Turing? J Theor Biol 1987;125:369–384.

197. Koch AJ, Meinhardt H. Biological pattern formation: from basic mechanisms to complex reactions. Rev Mod Phys 1994;66:1481–1507.

198. Cummings FW. A model of growth and form based on adhesion molecules. J Theor Biol 1996;178:229–238.

199. Dulos E, Boissonade J, Perraud J J, Rudovics B, De Kepper P. Chemical morphogenesis: Turing patterns in an experimental chemical system. Acta Biotheor 1996;44:249–261.

200. Odell G, Oster G, Alberch P, Burnside B. The mechanical basis of morphogenesis I: epithelial folding and invagination. Dev Biol 1981;85:44–52.

201. Oster GF, Murray JD, Harris AK. Mechanical aspects of mesenchymal morphogenesis. J Embryol Exp Morphol 1984;78:83–125.

202. Harris AK, Stopak D, Warner P. Generation of spatially periodic patterns by a mechanical instability: a mechanical alternative to the Turing model. J Embryol Exp Morphol 1984;80:1–20.

203. Schiffmann Y. An hypothesis: phosphorylation fields as the source of positional information and cell differentiation – (cAMP, ATP) as the universal morphogenetic Turing couple. Prog Biophys Mol Biol 1991;56:79–105.

204. Mok LLS, Nickols GA, Thompson JC, Cooper CW. Parathyroid hormone as a smooth muscle relaxant. Endocr Rev 1989;10:420–436.

205. Takahashi K, Inoue D,o K, Matsumoto T, Ikeda K, Fujita T. Parathyroid hormone-related peptide as a locally produced vasorelaxant: regulation of its mRNA by hypertension in rats. Biochem Biophys Res Commun 1995;208:447–455.

206. Schluter KD, Piper HM. Cardiovascular actions of parathyroid hormone and parathyroid hormone-related peptide. Cardiovasc Res 1998;37:34–41.

207. Okano K, Wu S, Huang X, Pirola CJ, Juppner H, Abou–Samra AB, Segre GV, Iwasaki K, Fagin JA, Clemens TL. Parathyroid hormone (PTH)/PTH-related protein (PTHrP) receptor and its messenger ribonucleic acid in rat aortic vascular smooth muscle cells and UMR osteoblast-like cells: cell–specific regulation of angiotensin-II and PTHrP. Endocrinology 1994;135:2093–2099.

208. Wang X, Briner VA, Schrier RW. Parathyroid hormone inhibition of vasopressin-induced vascular smooth muscle contraction. Am J Physiol 1993;264:F453–F457.

209. Maeda S, Wu S, Juppner H, Green J, Aragay AM, Fagin JA, Clemens TJ. Cell-specific signal transduction of parathyroid hormone (PTH)-related protein through stably expressed recombinant PTH/PTHrP receptors in vascular smooth muscle cells. Endocrinology 1996;137:3154–3162.

210. Chakraborty M, Chatterjee D, Kellokumpu S, Rasmussen H, Baron R. Cell cycle-dependent coupling of the calcitonin receptor to different G proteins. Science 1991;251:1078–1082.

211. Burton DW, Brandt DW, Deftos LJ. Parathyroid hormone-related protein in the cardiovascular system. Endocrinology 1994;135:253–261.

212. Vasavada RC, Garcia-Ocana A, Massfelder T, Dann P, Stewart AF. Parathyroid hormone-related protein in the pancreatic islet and the cardiovascular system. Recent Prog Horm Res 1998;53:305–338.

213. Jiang B, Morimoto S, Yang J, Niinoabu T, Fukuo K, Ogihara T. Expression of parathyroid hormone-related receptor in vascular endothelial cells. J Cardiovasc Pharmacol 1998;31:S142–S144.

214. Nagao S, Seto S, Kitamura S, Akahoshi M, Kiriyama T, Yano K. 1998; Central pressor effect of parathyroid hormone-related protein in conscious rats. Brain 785: 75–79.

215. Roca-Cusachs A, Dipette DJ, Nickols GA. Regional and systemic hemodynamic effects of parathyroid hormone related protein: preservation of cardiac function and coronary and renal flow with reduced blood pressure. J Pharmacol Exp Ther 1991;256:110–118.

216. Crass MF 3d, Scarpace PJ. Vasoactive properties of a parathyroid hormone-related protein in the rat aorta. Peptides 1993;14:179–183.

217. Macgill K, Moseley JM, Martin TJ, Brennecke SP, Rice GE, Wlodek ME. Vascular effects of PTHrP (1–34) and PTH (1–34) in the human fetal–placental circulation. Placenta 1997;18:587–592.

218. Garcia SI, Clemens TL, Fagin JA, Finbkielman S, Pirola CJ. Parathyroid hormone-related protein expression in vascular smooth muscle of spontaneously hypertensive rats: evidence for lack of response to angiotensin II. J Hypertens 1998;16:1467–1474.

219. Gao Y, Raj JU. Parathyroid hormone-related protein (PTHrP): a new role as a pulmonary vasodilator at birth. Pediatr Res 1999;45:302A.

220. Ishikawa M, Akishita M, Kozaki K, Toba K, Namiki A, Yamaguchi T, Orimo H, Ouchi Y. Amino-terminal fragment (1–34) of parathyroid hormone-related protein inhibits migration and proliferation of cultured vascular smooth muscle cells. Atherosclerosis 1998;136: 59–66.

221. Iwamura M, Abrahamsson PA, Foss KA, Wu G, Cockett AT, Deftos LJ. Parathyroid hormone-related protein: a potential autocrine growth regulator in human prostate cancer cell lines. Urology 1994;43:675–679.

222. Lam MH, Olsen SL, Rankin WA, Ho PW, Martin TJ, Gillespie MT, Moseley JM. PTHrP and cell division: expression and localization of PTHrP in a keratinocyte cell line (HaCaT) during the cell cycle. J Cell Physiol 1997;173:433–446.

222a. Holick MF, Ray S, Chen TC, Tian X, Persons KS. A parathyroid hormone antagonist stimulates epidermal proliferation and hair growth in mice. Proc Natl Acad Sci USA 1994;91:8014–8016.

223. Whitfield JF, Isaacs RJ, Jouishomme H, MacLean S, Chakravarthy BR, Morley P, Barison D, Regalia E, Armato U. C-terminal fragment of parathyroid hormone-related protein PTHrP-(107–111) stimulates membrane-associated protein kinase C activity and modulates the proliferation of human and murine skin keratinocytes. J Cell Physiol 1996;166:1–11.

224. Hastings RH, Summers-Torres D, Yaszay B, LeSueur J, Burton DW, Deftos LJ. Parathyroid hormone-related protein an autocrine growth inhibitor of alveolar type II cells. Am J Physiol 1997;272:L394–L399.

225. Ono T, Inokuchi K, Ogura A, Ikawa Y, Kudo Y, Kawashima S. Activity-dependent expression of parathyroid hormone-related protein (PTHrP) in rat cerebellar granule neurons: requirement of PTHrP for the activity-dependent survival of granule neurons. J Biol Chem 1997;272: 14,404–14,411.

226. Amling M, Neff L, Tanaka S, Inoue D, Kuida K, Weir E, Philbrick WM, Broadus AE, Baron R. Bcl-2 lies downstream of parathyroid hormone-related peptide in a signaling pathway that regulates chondro-cyte maturation during skeletal development. J Cell Biol 1997;136:205–213.

227. Hastings RH, Summers–Torres D, Burton DW, Deftos LJ. PTHrP alveolar pneumocyte apoptosis in vivo. Bone 1998;23:S359.

228. Lee K, Lanske B, Karaplis AC, Deeds JD, Kohno H, Nissenson RA, Kronenberg HM, Segre GV. Parathyroid hormone-related peptide delays terminal differentiation of chondrocytes during endochondral bone development. Endocrinology 1996;137:5109–5118.

229. Amizuka N, Henderson JE, Hoshi K, Warshawsky H, Ozawa H, Goltzman D, Karaplis AC. Programmed cell death of chondrocytes and aberrant chondrogenesis in mice homozygous for parathyroid hormone-related peptide gene deletion. Endocrinology 1996; 137:5055–5067.

230. Eckenhoff RG. Perinatal changes in lung surfactant calcium measured in situ. J Clin Invest 1989;84:1295–1301.

231. Nielsen PK, Rasmussen AK, Feldt-Rasmussen U, Brandt M, Christensen L, Olgaard K. Ectopic production of intact parathyroid hormone by a squamous cell lung carcinoma in vivo and in vitro. J Clin Endocrinol Metab 1996;81:3793–3796.

232. Li X, Drucker DJ. Parathyroid hormone-related peptide is a downstream target for ras and src activation. J Biol Chem 1994;269:6263–6266.

233. Kremer R, Goltzman D, Amizuka N, Webber MM, Rhim JS. Ras activation of human prostate epithelial cells induces overexpression of parathyroid hormone-related peptide. ClinCancer Res 1997;3:855–859.

234. Rudduck C, Duncan L, Center R, Garson OM. Co–amplification of the gene for parathyroid hormone-related protein (PTHrP) and KRAS2 in a human lung cancer cell line. Genes Chrom Cancer 1993;7:213–218.

235. Okano K, Pirola CJ, Wang HM, Forrester JS, Fagin JA, Clemens TL. Involvement of cell cycle and mitogen-activated pathways in induction of parathyroid hormone-related protein gene expression in rat aortic smooth muscle cells. Endocrinology 1995;136:1782–1789.

236. Ganderton RH, Briggs RS. CpG island methylation and promotor usage in the parathyroid hormone-related protein gene of cultured lung cells. Biochim Biophys Acta 1997;1352:303–310.

237. Burton PB, Knight DE. Parathyroid hormone-related peptide can regulate the growth of human lung cancer cells and may form part of an autocrine TGF-alpha loop. FEBS Lett 1992;305:228–232.

238. Hidaka N, Nishimura M, Nagao K. Establishment of two human small cell lung cancer cell lines: the evidence of accelerated production of parathyroid hormone-related protein with tumor progression. Cancer Lett 1998;125:149–155.

239. Liu JG, Tabata MJ, Yamashita K, Matsumura T, Iwamoto M, Kurisu K. Developmental role of PTHrP in murine molars. Eur J Oral Sci 1998;106:143–146.

# 16 Role of Neuroendocrine Cells in Fetal and Postnatal Lung

*Mary E. Sunday, MD, PHD, and
Ernest Cutz, MD*

## INTRODUCTION

Pulmonary neuroendocrine cells (PNECs) occur at peak relative numbers during fetal development and are phylogenetically highly conserved. In spite of these intriguing observations suggesting an important physiologic role for PNECs, these remain an enigmatic pulmonary epithelial cell type. The high abundance of PNECs at midgestation, immediately preceding lung organ maturation with type II cell differentiation, led to our first hypothesis that PNECs might play a fundamental role in promoting lung growth and development during the pseudoglandular to canalicular periods. The first section of this chapter addresses the ontogeny and function of PNECs during fetal lung development, with our focus on the PNEC-derived growth factor, bombesin-like peptide (BLP). The second section provides a comprehensive overview of our current thinking about the possible role of innervated PNEC clusters (neuroepithelial bodies [NEB]) as airway oxygen sensors as well as the cellular and molecular mechanisms involved in $O_2$ sensing. The third section reviews data on PNEC/NEB alterations in neonatal and pediatric lung diseases, with emphasis on the potential role of these cells and their peptide mediators in pulmonary pathophysiology.

From: *Contemporary Endocrinology: Endocrinology of the Lung: Development and Surfactant Synthesis*
Edited by: C. R. Mendelson © Humana Press Inc., Totowa, NJ

## ROLE OF PULMONARY NEUROENDOCRINE CELLS
## IN DEVELOPING LUNG

### Morphology of Normal Fetal Lung Development

Lung development is classically divided into five major stages in mammals:

Embryonic phase: 3–7 wk in humans versus gestational day 9.5 (e9.5)–e12 in mice
Pseudoglandular phase: 7–16 wk in humans versus e12-e16 in mice
Canalicular phase:16–24 wk in humans versus e16–e18 in mice
Saccular phase: 25–36 wk in humans and e18.5 to postnatal day 5 (P5) in mice
Alveolar phase: begins *in utero* in term human infants then continues until approx 18 mo
of age; in mice, the alveolar phase is entirely postnatal.

Details about the morphology of lung development are given elsewhere *(1)*. In brief, lung embryogenesis begins around week 3 in humans with outpouching of the primitive foregut endoderm into the surrounding mesenchyme *(2)*. All major bronchopulmonary segments are started by gestational week 7 *(2)*. During the pseudoglandular phase, branching of the conducting airways is completed and epithelial cell differentiation begins. During the canalicular phase, surfactant production begins, with detection of lamellar bodies by electron microscopy at approx 20–24 wk. Simultaneously, alveolar capillary development begins as a mesenchymal process close to the future airspace lumen *(3)*. The saccular and alveolar phases of lung development occur during the last half of human fetal gestation through the first year of postnatal life, and together comprise the process of "alveolarization." By contrast, the saccular phase begins about a day before birth in rodents, in which most of alveolarization occurs postnatally *(4)*. During alveolarization, the distal lung parenchyma undergoes extensive remodeling, with alveolar septation, increased capillary bed formation, and further mesenchymal thinning, which appears to reflect interstitial cell apoptosis *(5)*.

### Ontogeny of Neuroendocrine Cell Differentiation

Undifferentiated airway epithelium expresses a subset of epithelial markers during the pseudoglandular period of lung development. Protein gene product (PGP) 9.5, but not chromogranin A, is present in all of the primitive epithelium in human fetal lung *(6)*. The neuroendocrine marker, calcitonin gene-related peptide (CGRP), type II cell marker (SP-A), and clara cell marker (CC10) are similarly detected in the same primitive epithelial cells in murine fetal lung at e11–e15 *(7)*. Gene-related protein (GRP) mRNA was detected in distal airway epithelium of midgestation fetal rhesus monkeys using *in situ* hybridization *(8)*, but without associated immunostaining for GRP/proGRP. We hypothesized that this trilineage gene expression by undifferentiated epithelium reflects the phenotype of a pluripotent precursor cell.

The first epithelial cells to differentiate in human and murine fetal airways are the neuroendocrine cells *(4,9,10)* (Fig. 1). Isolated neuroendocrine cells (Fig. 1A) are demonstrated by electron microscopy *(11)*, immunohistochemistry and *in situ* hybridization *(12)* at week 8–9 in humans versus e14–e15 in mice *(10)*. It is not until approx 11 weeks in humans versus e16 in mice that presecretory and preciliated cells are detectable by immunostaining and/or morphology *(9)*. This suggested to us that PNECs could promote differentiation of other pulmonary epithelial cell types, potentially via dendritic processes emanating from the neuroendocrine cell body and extending along the base-

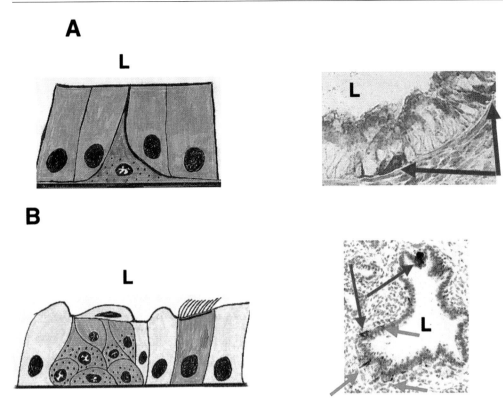

Fig. 1. Isolated PNECs and NEBs in human fetal lung. Diagrammatic representation (left) and photomicrographs of BLP-immunostaining (right). **(A)** In 9 wk gestation human fetal lung, isolated PNECs are observed in the proximal airway epithelium, which is otherwise undifferentiated at this stage of development (L, airway lumen; PNEC, magenta in diagram on left; PNECs indicated by red arrows in photograph, ×200). **(B)** By 20 wk gestation, PNEC clusters represent the majority of PNECs in the lung parenchyma, which eventually become innervated, termed NEBs. NEBs are scattered throughout the bronchiolar epithelium (given in magenta in diagram on left, and indicated by red arrows in photograph on right, ×50). NEBs are usually surrounded by Clara cells (given in yellow in diagram) and may also be seen in the vicinity of ciliated cells (shown in green in diagram) in more proximal airways. BLP-immunopositive dendritic processes emanate from the NEB cells along the airway basement membrane, as indicated by blue arrows in photomicrograph in B.

ment membrane between adjacent epithelial cells (photograph in Fig. 1B, blue arrows) *(13,14)*. We have observed such dendritic neuroendocrine cells in fetal airways, but not in adult lung *(4,14)*.

Similar to the hematopoietic cell lineages, neuroendocrine cells express their own developmental program, with distinct differentiation markers appearing at different times in ontogeny (Table 1). At 8 wk, PNECs immunostain for the neuroendocrine cell markers bombesin-like peptide (BLP), serotonin (5-HT), chromogranin A, neuron-specific enolase (NSE), and protein gene product 9.5 (PGP 9.5); gastrin-releasing peptide (GRP) mRNA occurs in a similar distribution by *in situ* hybridization *(15)*. Peak NSE and PGP 9.5 immunostaining occurs at 12–14 wk gestation *(6)*. By contrast, chromogranin A peaks later, at 18–22 wk, similar to calcitonin gene-related peptide (CGRP), serotonin, BLP, and other early neurosecretory granule markers. Calcitonin immuno-

Table 1
Biochemical Markers of Pulmonary Neuroendocrine Cells

Cytoplasmic markers
   Early (pseudoglandular phase)
      Neuron-specific enolase (NSE)
      Protein gene product 9.5 (PGP 9.5)
Neurosecretory granule markers
   Early (pseudoglandular phase)
      Chromogranin A
      Serotonin
      Bombesin-like peptide (BLP)/Gastrin-releasing peptide (GRP)
   Intermediate (canalicular phase)
      Calcitonin gene-related peptide (CGRP)
      Cholecystokinin (CCK)
   Late (saccular phase)a
      Adrenocorticotropin (ACTH)
      Human chorionic gonadotropin (hCG)
      Leu-enkephalin
      Calcitonin
   Cell surface markers (ontogeny unknown)
      Neural cell adhesion molecule (N-CAM)
      Leu7
      CD10/neutral endopeptidase 24.11 (CD10/NEP)

a Observed only in lungs of infants with chronic respirator-associated lung disease.

staining is not apparent until late in the second trimester *(12)*. There are single reports demonstrating cholecystokinin *(16)* and endothelin *(17,18)* in PNECs of normal human fetal lung. Endothelin, however, is not a PNEC-specific marker, being expressed also in nonneuroendocrine type II epithelial cells, endothelial cells, and alveolar macrophages *(19)*. Leu-enkephalin, hCG, and ACTH have only been observed in PNECs of infants with chronic lung disease *(12,20,21)*.

The formation of NEB begins with an increase in numbers of PNECs per cluster *(4,22)*. At 8 wk, most PNECs occur as isolated cells within the epithelial basement membrane (Fig. 1A). In human fetal lung, NEB begin to form at 9–10 wk of gestation and by 20 wk of gestation, NEB account for the majority of PNECs within the lung (Fig. 1B) *(4,23)*. These clusters of PNECs are often surrounded by Clara cells (indicated in yellow in diagram on the lefthand side of Fig. 1B) *(24)*. Subsequently, these clusters become innervated by both sympathetic and sensory (nonadrenergic, noncholinergic) nerve fibers *(11,25–29)*. Furthermore, about half of serotonin-positive NEBs in fetal rabbit lung occur in small distal airways, mostly at branchpoints *(30)*.

## *Molecular Mechanisms of Neuroendocrine Cell Differentiation*

Molecular mechanisms for PNEC differentiation have been explored using undifferentiated small cell lung carcinoma (SCLC) cell lines and murine lung buds in culture, and appear to be similar in many ways to neuronal differentiation. Understanding of genetics of neuronal differentiation is derived mostly from work in *Drosophila (31)*, in which neurons in the central nervous system (CNS) arise from neuroblasts in the neuroecto-

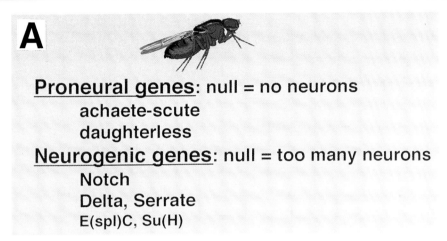

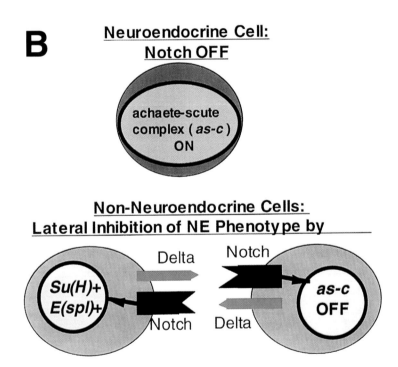

Fig. 2. Genetic regulation of neurogenesis in *Drosophila*. (**A**) The two major groups of genes involved in *Drosophila* neurogenesis are: the *proneural* genes, including *achaete–scute* and *daughterless*, for which the null mutation yields a phenotype lacking neurons; and the neurogenic genes, including Notch, Delta, Serrate, Enhancer of Split (E(Spl)), and Suppressor of Hairless (Su(H)), for which the null mutation yields an excess of neurons. (**B**) A simplified diagram of Notch signaling is shown here with nonneuronal cells (in green) expressing Notch and its ligand (Delta or Serrate): this is a system of "lateral inhibition" whereby Notch leads to positive feedback with activation of other neurogenic genes such as the transcription factors Su(H) and E(Spl), and inhibition of proneural gene expression, as exemplified by turning off achaete–scute. Cells committed to the neural/neuroendocrine fate, by contrast, do not express Notch and express achaete–scute as if by default.

derm, and neighboring cells become epidermoblasts. Similarly, the peripheral nervous system (PNS) develops from progenitor cells in the epidermis, which choose between neural and nonneural fates. Molecular mechanisms involved in cell fate choices for the CNS and PNS involve two major groups of genes (Fig. 2A):

1. "Proneural" genes lead to the commitment of cells to become neuronal precursors, namely, the *achaete–scute* complex, including *achaete*, *scute*, and *daughterless (da)*, which are transcription factors, the lack of which leads to a hypoplastic CNS and PNS.
2. Neurogenic genes, required for proper segregation of neural and epidermal lineages in both the CNS and PNS, include *Notch, Delta, Serrate, Enhancer of split complex (E(spl)C)*, and *Suppressor of Hairless (Su(H)) (31,32)*.

The complete loss of function of a neurogenic gene such as Notch causes presumptive epidermoblasts in the neuroectoderm to become neuroblasts, leading to massive neuronal hyperplasia. *Notch, Delta*, and *Serrate* encode transmembrane molecules with EGF-like repeats *(32)*; *Delta* and *Serrate* act as *Notch* ligands to activate a common intracellular signaling pathway *(32–34)* (Fig. 2B). *E(spl)C* and *Su(H)*, encode transcription factors required for interaction with the cytoplasmic domain of Notch, regulating responsiveness to epidermalizing signals *(35–37)*. These neurogenic genes all interact functionally in the same developmental pathway *(38)*.

The observation that neuroblasts rapidly decrease Notch expression as they begin to differentiate is consistent with the hypothesis that Notch functions as a cell surface receptor to inhibit the neuronal phenotype *(39)*. Decreased *Notch* gene expression in neuronal precursor cells would preserve neuronal phenotype during lateral inhibition, which suppresses neighboring cells from adopting a similar fate. However, the broad tissue distribution of Notch *(32,40)* suggests a greater developmental role of Notch than simply the control of epidermal vs neural lineages. Notch protein could act to mediate cell–cell adhesion with cells expressing Notch ligands, such as Delta or Serrate *(32)*. Upon binding of Notch to its ligand, the cytoplasmic domain of Notch can interact with the DNA-binding protein Su(H), which then translocates to the nucleus (Fig. 2B) *(36,37)*. The neurogenic pathway initiated by Notch appears to be critical for posttranscriptional activation of achaete–scute gene products *(34)*.

Mammalian homologs have been identified for several *Drosophila* proneural/neurogenic genes *(41–44)*. Of these, the human/mammalian *achaete–scute* homolog (hASH/MASH) has been best characterized as a functional proneural gene *(45,46)*. hASH is expressed in SCLCs only with NE features *(47)*; hASH gene transfer into SCLC cell lines leads to *trans*-activation of the calcitonin promoter *(47)*. hASH-knockout mice have widespread neuronal deficits and also total absence of pulmonary PNECs, implicating hASH as a key player in PNEC differentiation *(48)*. In spite of the total absence of PNECs, fetal lung development, including cell differentiation, appear to be normal, but these mice have wisespread CNS defects and die of respiratory failure shortly after birth *(48)* (R.I. Linnoila, *personal communication*, 1997). These observations suggest that nonneuroendocrine cells can compensate for the total absence of PNECs to ensure that normal fetal lung development, essential for life, is preserved.

The function of *Notch* is just beginning to be explored *(49)*. Using antisense oligonucleotides to diminish *Notch* activity or a retrovirally transduced constitutively active allele of *Notch*, Cepko et al. *(49)* demonstrated that the number of retinal ganglion cells produced was inversely related to the level of *Notch* activity. The Notch ligand

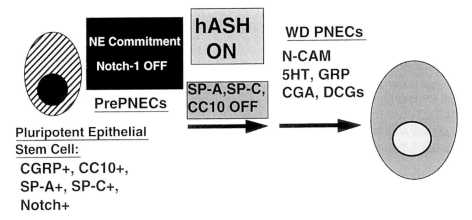

Fig. 3. Working hypothesis for PNEC differentiation. Pluripotent epithelial stem cells express Notch together with low levels of markers for multiple different cell lineages, including CGRP (neuroendocrine (NE) cell marker), CC10 (Clara cell marker), SP-A (type II and Clara cell marker), and SP-C (type II cell marker). NE cell commitment coincides with suppression of Notch gene expression. The resulting pre-PNECs begin to express the differentiated NE pheno-type following induction of the human achaete-scute homologue (hASH) and suppression of SP-A, SP-C, and CC-10. Full acquisition of the well-differentiated PNEC phenotype follows expression of other structural genes including N-CAM, 5-HT, GRP, and CGA, and the appear-ance of dense-core granules.

Delta also inhibited retinal progenitors from differentiating as ganglion cells to the same degree as did activated Notch. This is a versatile system for examining the Notch path-way in a specific cell fate decision. We have extended experiments with Notch antisense oligonucleotides to e11.5 murine lung buds, in which downregulation of Notch protein levels over 7 days of culture results in markedly increased numbers of CGRP-positive PNECs (M.E. Sunday and K. Avadhanam, *unpublished data*, 1998). We hypothesize that Notch gene downregulation is one of the earliest molecular events leading to com-mitment of undifferentiated pulmonary epithelial cells to the neuroendocrine cell lin-eage (Fig. 3). Similar to signaling events in *Drosophila* (Fig. 2), the proneural genes such as achaete–scute would then be turned on, and the PNEC differentiation program would unfold over time (Fig. 3). Experiments are in progress to test this hypothesis in our laboratory.

Cell differentiation can be modified by a variety of growth factors or cytokines, including tumor necrosis factor-alpha (TNFα) *(50)*, BLP *(51)*, basic fibroblast growth factor (FGF) *(52)*, glucocorticoids *(52)*, interferons *(53)*, and retinoic acid *(54–58)*. The observation of PNEC hyperplasia in association with inflammatory lung diseases or systemic immunization suggested to us that cytokines might mediate PNEC differenti-ation in vivo. Increased numbers of PNECs, commonly referred to as PNEC hyperplasia, represents predominantly a differentiation response *(59,60)*, and occurs in patients with chronic inflammatory lung diseases, including BPD *(61–63)*, bronchiectasis, asbestosis, and eosinophilic granuloma *(64–66)*.

We have recently observed that TNF treatment can induce phenotypic features of PNEC differentiation in undifferentiated SCLC cell lines *(67)*. TNF mRNA expression precedes the onset of PNEC hyperplasia in a hamster model of chronic lung injury *(59,60)*, in which increased numbers of PNECs was found to be predominantly due to

PNEC differentiation *(61)*. When either of two different SCLC cell lines are treated with TNF, there is rapid induction of GRP and/or DOPA decarboxylase (DDC) mRNAs (<5 min), through a mechanism apparently involving nuclear factor-kappa B (NF-κB). However, it takes 7–14 d before there is induction of positive immunostaining for NCAM and proGRP and ultrastructural evidence of dense core neurosecretory granules. The precise molecular mechanism for this TNF effect, in particular the events occurring during the lag period before phenotypic induction occurs, remain to be determined. We are beginning to explore the possible involvement of Notch-mediated signaling in these events.

### Role of Secreted Products of Neuroendocrine Cells in Lung Development During the Canalicular Phase

Multiple growth factors have been implicated in branching morphogenesis, cell proliferation, and cell differentiation in normal lung development *(52)*. Growth factors produced by the nonneuroendocrine epithelial cells include epidermal growth factor (EGF) *(68–70)*, parathyroid hormone-related protein (PTHrp) *(73)*, basic FGF *(72)*, and platelet-derived growth factor (PDGF) *(73)*, all of which appear to promote type II cell differentiation in a mesenchymal cell-dependent fashion *(74–79)*.

Much of our research has focused on the role of neuropeptides in developing fetal lung, especially the bombesin-like peptide (BLP) family *(80)*. Bombesin is an amphibian peptide originally isolated from the skin of the frog *Bombina bombina* in 1971 by Erspamer and coworkers, reviewed in ref. *80*, (Table 2). Using antibodies to amphibian bombesin, mammalian BLP was identified in 1978 as the first neuropeptide hormone localized to PNECs, with highest levels in human fetal lung *(81)*. BLP appears together with serotonin in PNECs as soon as the cells are detectable at approx 8 wk gestation *(63)*. A 27-aa mammalian homolog of the 14-aa frog skin peptide bombesin was identified by McDonald as "gastrin-releasing peptide" (GRP) (Table 2) (reviewed in ref. *80*). GRP is not exclusively a mammalian peptide, however, having been identified also in amphibian brain *(82)*. GRP and bombesin share a highly conserved amidated 7-aa C-terminus, which is required for immunogenicity and for high-affinity binding to bombesin-preferring receptors. GRP cDNAs have been cloned from a human pulmonary carcinoid tumor *(83)*, SCLCs *(84)*, and rat brain *(85)*, demonstrating high conservation of the critical 10 amino acid sequence at the C-terminus. Thus, BLP (GRP and/or bombesin) have essentially identical physiologic effects *(80)*, acting both as neuroregulatory peptides and as growth factors *(80)*. BLP stimulates proliferation of normal adult bronchial epithelial cells, fibroblasts, and several SCLC cell lines *(86–89)*, where growth of the latter was blocked either in culture or in nude mice by mAbs to bombesin (2A11) *(89)*. Because many SCLC lines both secrete BLP and bear BLP receptors, an autocrine feedback loop was implicated in tumor progression of SCLC *(90)*.

The second group of bombesin-related peptides includes neuromedin B (NMB), the 11-amino acid mammalian homolog of amphibian ranatensin, which was first identified in spinal cord *(91,92)*. NMB is structurally and functionally similar to BLP, but there are three amino acid differences between NMB and GRP in the bioactive C-terminus: the penultimate Phe is conserved in both amphibian ranatensin and NMB (Table 2). NMB is antigenically distinct from bombesin and GRP: antibodies to BLP do not cross-react with NMB or ranatensin *(93)*. NMB will trigger physiologic responses at BLP-preferring receptors, but require approx 50-fold higher concentrations than BLP (GRP or bombesin)

Table 2
The Three Major Groups of Bombesin-Related Peptides

1. BOMBESIN FAMILY (BLP)

|  | 1 | 14 |
|---|---|---|
| BOMBESIN | pGlu-Gln-Arg-Leu-Gly-Asn-Gln-Trp-Ala-Val-Gly-His-Leu-Met-NH2 | |
| GRP 14-27 | -Met-Tyr-Pro-Arg-Gly-Asn-His-Trp-Ala-Val-Gly-His-Leu-Met-NH2 | |

2. RANATENSIN (RN) FAMILY

|  | 1 | 11 |
|---|---|---|
| RN-C | pGlu-Val-Pro-Gln-Trp-Ala-Val-Gly-His-Phe-Met-NH2 | |
| NMB | Gly-Asn-Leu-Trp-Ala-Thr-Gly-His-Phe-Met-NH2 | |

3. PHYLLOLITORIN (PL) FAMILY

|  | 1 | 9 |
|---|---|---|
| $\text{Leu}^8$-PL (L8PL) | pGlu-Leu-Trp-Ala-Val-Gly-Ser-Leu-Met-NH2 | |
| $\text{Phe}^8$-PL (P8PL) | pGlu-Leu-Trp-Ala-Val-Gly-Ser-Phe-Met-NH2 | |

*a* Key C-terminal amino acid differences between the three groups are underlined.

to elicit an equivalent effect *(94,95)*, and vice versa. NMB was cloned from human hypothalamus *(93)* and found to represent a new gene distinct from GRP. We have been unable to detect NMB gene expression in primate fetal lung, even using the highly sensitive reverse transcriptase-polymerase chain reaction (RT-PCR) approach for mRNA detection (R.L. Emanuel, J.S. Torday, N. Asokananthan, Q. Mu, and M.E. Sunday, *unpublished data*, 1998).

The third group of bombesin-related peptides includes the amphibian phyllolitorins (Table 2), which are immunologically and functionally similar to bombesin *(96,97)*, having the third last amino acid as Ser instead of His. Originally characterized as potent smooth muscle constrictor peptides *(98)*, putative mammalian phyllolitorin(s) became of major interest when their potential clinical relevance emerged. By amino acid content analysis, BLP immunoreactivity present at high levels in bronchioloalveolar lavage fluid from asymptomatic human smokers was found to be most consistent with a phyllolitorin, containing Ser but no His *(66)*. Phyllolitorins can elicit the same panel of effects as BLP, including CNS effects and growth stimulation *(99–100)*. We have studied effects of leu[8]-phyllolitorin in mammalian lung organ cultures *(see below)*. Although cDNAs for the amphibian phyllolitorins have been identified *(101)*, the putative mammalian phyllolitorin has not yet been found.

Multiple BLP receptors have been identified, three of which are known to be present in mammals *(102,103)*. The two mammalian bombesin-preferring receptors are the bombesin/GRP-preferring receptor (GRP-R), cloned from murine fibroblasts *(104)*, and the orphan receptor bombesin receptor subtype-3 (BRS-3), cloned from uterus and testis *(104–106)*, both of which are G protein-coupled seven transmembrane-spanning receptors. One similar mammalian NMB-preferring receptor (NMB-R) *(107)* has been cloned thus far, for which the ligand specificity was mapped to a small segment of the fifth transmembrane domain *(108)*. In addition, a fourth amphibian receptor (BB4) specific for [Phe13]bombesin has been cloned from frog brain *(109)*. We are able to detect mRNAs encoding all three identified mammalian BLP receptors in murine fetal lung using RT-PCR. GRP-R is detected consistently and BRS-3 only occasionally in fetal nonhuman primate lung *(98)*. By *in situ* hybridization, GRP-R mRNA is primarily localized to the mesenchyme surrounding developing airways and blood vessels in rodents, humans, and nonhuman primates *(8,100,110–112)*, with some studies also detecting epithelial expression *(111)*.

In early studies, we found the GRP gene to be expressed in a proximal-to-distal pattern in human fetal lung in parallel with the growth of the developing airways, suggesting a role in development *(15)*. In a large body of subsequent work involving human, baboon, murine, and rat fetal lung, we have identified several major developmental effects of BLP and related peptides. Both bombesin and L8PL increase branching morphogenesis and cell proliferation in cultured embryonic mouse lung buds *(100)*.

During the canalicular phase of fetal lung development, endogenous GRP gene expression attains peak levels *(15,51)*. We have used three general approaches to investigate physiologic roles of BLP (either exogenous or endogenous) during this time period. First, exogenous bombesin was demonstrated to act as a potent growth and differentiation factor for fetal murine lung *in utero* and for human, baboon, and murine fetal lung in organ culture. In the initial functional investigations, BLP promoted widespread proliferation of mesenchymal and epithelial cells (in conducting airways and in primitive alveoli). BLP also induced differentiation of type II pneumocytes, as assessed biochemically using $^3$H-choline incorporation into surfactant phospholipids as a measure of the rate of surfactant phospholipid synthesis. Using electron microscopy, we observed a higher proportion of differentiated type II cells in lungs of mice treated with BLP in utero *(51)*. Other laboratories have confirmed these observations in primary cultures of rat type II cells *(113,114)*, in some of which BLP promotes surfactant phospholipid secretion via a mechanism involving protein kinase C *(114)*. However, it is unclear how many fibroblasts might have been present in the primary type II cell isolates in those studies *(113,114)*.

We have recently demonstrated that the BLP effect on e18 rat type II cell differentiation requires the presence of fetal mesenchymal cells *(115)*. In addition, BLP can promote differentiation of mesenchymal cells, leading to augmentation of triglyceride trafficking, suggesting that the effect of BLP on type II cells might be secondary to increased mesenchymal cell secretory processes *(115)*. In the course of investigating mechanisms by which BLP might stimulate surfactant synthesis and secretion *(116)*, we cloned several synaptic vesicle proteins from fetal rat lung, including rab-26, syntaxin-2 (epimorphin), munc-18, and syntaxin-1A. Of these, syntaxin-1A demonstrated the most profound developmental regulation, with peak mRNA levels occurring at e19, in parallel with induction of GRP-R gene expression. By immunostaining, syntaxin-1A was expressed in nerve fibers and neuroendocrine cells, as expected. However, surprisingly, the strongest expression of syntaxin-1A occurs in lipid-rich fibroblasts surrounding developing airways and blood vessels in fetal lung, which are believed to play a role in the induction of type II pneumocyte differentiation *(52,117,118)*. These are the same cells that bear GRP-R. Using a blocking monoclonal antibody to syntaxin-1A, we are able to completely inhibit bombesin-induced choline uptake; antisyntaxin antibodies also inhibit baseline choline uptake in a dose-dependent fashion and block most of the choline uptake stimulated by dexamethasone *(115)*. These observations suggest that syntaxin-1A and possibly other synaptic vesicle proteins function to promote secretion of biologically active molecules by fetal fibroblasts, and that this cellular mechanism is critical for effects of bombesin-like peptide on pulmonary epithelial cell differentiation.

GRP-R, NMB-R, and BRS-3 knockout mice have been developed independently in two different laboratories *(119,120)*. Although GRP-R knockout mice demonstrate a variety of behavioral abnormalities and lose bombesin-induced feeding suppression, there are no obvious structural or functional abnormalities of the lung on routine histopathologic examination. NMB-R knockout mice have normal lungs, whereas BRS-3 knockout mice are obese *(121)* and have generalized epithelial cell dysplasia in the bronchiolar epithelium (M.E. Sunday, K. Wada, and E. Wada, *manuscript in preparation*, 1998). Three mice have been generated lacking all three cloned mammalian BLP receptors: one of these mice had a lung adenocarcinoma (M.E. Sunday, K. Wada, and E. Wada, *manuscript in preparation*, 1998). These observations suggest that BRS-3 might play a role in lung epithelial cell proliferation, but do not rule out a role for any of the BLP receptors in lung development. In mice developing in the total absence of an important gene product, compensatory upregulation of genes leading to similar functions can occur. In retrospect, the earlier experiments using anti-BLP blocking antibodies and bombesin receptor specific antagonists gave more insight into developmental physiology, which is not apparent using a noninducible knockout system.

## THE ROLE OF NEUROEPITHELIAL BODIES AS AIRWAY SENSORS

### *Neuroepithelial Bodies as Oxygen Sensors: Historical Evidence*

In addition to solitary pulmonary neuroendocrine cells (PNEC) the existence of distinct organoid-like neuroepithelial bodies (NEB) within the airway mucosa of mammalian lungs (Fig. 4) was recognized at the turn of the century *(4)*. However, the progress in our knowledge as to the precise function of NEB in the lung has been relatively slow and still remains incomplete. Early morphologic studies recognized clusters of argyrophilic cells within the airway epithelium of human and animal lungs *(122)*. The suggestion for a possible sensory role for these intrapulmonary neuroepithelial clusters, including that of a chemoreceptor monitoring airway gas composition, stems from the early neuroanatomic studies *(4)*. This idea, however, was not explored further until early 1970s. At that time Lauweryns and colleagues *(123,124)*, based on morphologic and experimental studies, suggested that these intraepithelial corpuscles, which they termed NEB, may function as hypoxia sensitive airway chemoreceptors modulated by the central nervous system.

The morphologic features of NEB suggestive of a chemoreceptor included:

1. Preferential location of NEB at airway branching points
2. Cytoplasmic neurosecretory granules containing amine and peptide substances acting as neurotransmitter or neuromodulators
3. Apical microvilli in contact with the airway lumen
4. Sensory innervation derived from the vagus nerve *(125)*.

Some of the morphologic features of NEB are remarkably similar to those of well-defined arterial chemoreceptors, carotid bodies, monitoring the levels of $Po_2$, $Pco_2$, and pH in the blood *(126)*.

The first line of experimental evidence supporting a role for NEB as an airway sensor was provided by Lauweryns et al. *(124)*, who showed that in NEB cells of rabbit neonates exposed to short-term hypoxia (10% $O_2$ in $N_2$ for 20 min) there was increased exocytosis of neurosecretory granules and decreased amine fluorescence, implying amine (seroto-

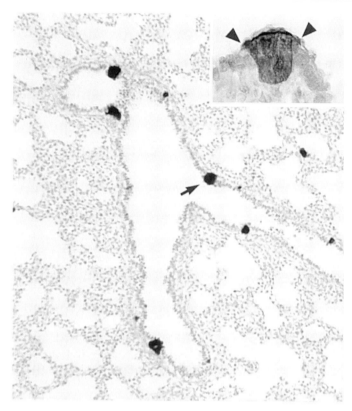

Fig. 4. Serotonin immunoreactive NEB in rabbit fetal lung (26-d gestation). NEBs are located within airway mucosa, particularly near bifurcations *(arrow)*. Immunoperoxidase method for serotonin (×100). **Insert:** At higher magnification, NEB's apical cytoplasm is exposed to airway lumen *(arrowheads)* (×250). (From ref. *145*, with permission.)

nin, 5-HT) release in response to acute hypoxia. In cross-circulation studies these authors have further shown that it was airway hypoxia specifically, but not hypoxemia that stimulated the release of amine from NEB cells *(127)*. The effects of high inspired $CO_2$ levels in the initial studies has been reported as similar to hypoxia, but in more recent and better controlled experiments these effects could not be replicated *(128)*. Similarly, hyperoxia had no apparent effect on NEB neurosecretory granule structure *(124)*.

The micro-anatomy of NEB innervation and its effects on modulation of hypoxia response was explored in experiments using various vagotomy procedures *(125,129, 130)*. Infranodose vagotomy resulted in degeneration of NEB nerve terminals indicating that the nerve cell bodies reside in the nodose ganglion. Based on ultrastructural findings of afferent and efferentlike nerve endings, it has been proposed that an axonlike reflex could modulate NEB responses *(129,131)*. Indirect evidence for hypoxia signaling via the afferent nerve fibers of NEB was obtained in experiments where unilateral hypoxia produced ultrastructural changes known to be associated with hypoxia stimulation (i.e., decreased synaptic vesicles and increase in membrane-bound cisternae and multivesicular bodies) *(132)*.

Developmental and morphometric studies indicate that NEB are more prominent in fetal/neonatal lungs and their numbers appear to decline postnatally *(30)*. This could indicate that the function of NEB may be more important during the perinatal period and in neonatal adaptation *(133)*. It should be pointed out, however, that NEB persist into adulthood and have been identified at all ages *(134)*. Based on ultrastructural observations of the site(s) and direction of stimulated neurosecretory granule discharge from NEB cells, several possible functions have been postulated *(135)*. The neurosecretory granule release at the basal membrane of NEB cells, in close proximity to fenestrated capillaries, suggested possible release into the bloodstream affecting local ventilation/perfusion ratio in the alveolus *(123,124)*. Local effects on airway smooth muscle has also been postulated *(125)*. The discharge at the nerve endings could initiate the transmission of hypoxia stimulus to the central nervous system, possibly affecting the control of respiration *(136)*. These function(s) may be particularly relevant during the transition from fetal to postnatal life. For example, NEB could be auxiliary chemoreceptors involved in the resetting of carotid bodies after birth when their function is not yet fully developed. Alternatively, NEB and their amine and peptide modulators could act directly or indirectly on the pulmonary vascular bed regulating the pulmonary vascular tone during the transition of pulmonary circulation from fetal to adult-type.

A second line of evidence supporting the role of NEB as hypoxia sensitive airway sensors stems from studies on the effects of chronic hypoxia. These findings, however, are contradictory due to experimental variables such as the duration and degree of hypoxia as well as the age and species of animals studied *(137)*. Nevertheless, the overall consensus is that chronic hypoxia is an appropriate "natural" stimulus for activation of NEB cells. Such an activation has been shown to cause alteration in neurotransmitter content and/or increase in the size and number of NEB cells. For example, adult Sprague-Dawley rats (but not Wistar rats) show striking hyperplasia and hypertrophy of NEB after 2 wk exposure to normobaric hypoxia *(138)*. An increased number of solitary NE cells and NEB has been described in rabbits kept in hypobaric chamber or raised at high altitude *(139,140)*. On the other hand, Wistar rats maintained in hypoxia between 1 and 3 wk showed elevated levels of intracellular CGRP without a change in NEB cell numbers *(141)*. Although not yet directly tested on pulmonary NEB, these changes are likely to involve the activation of hypoxia inducible genes via expression of transcription factors (NF-κB, c-fos/Jun) as has been recently suggested for carotid bodies' chief cells *(142)*.

## Cellular and Molecular Mechanism of Oxygen Sensing in NEB Cells

The studies discussed in the previous section solidified the view that NEB may indeed be hypoxia sensitive airway chemoreceptors and set the stage for exploration of $O_2$ sensing properties of NEBs at the cellular and molecular level. A critical first step was the development of an isolated NEB cell culture system, since these cells are sparse and are widely distributed within a spongelike lung parenchyma. To this end a technique to isolate and culture NEB cells from fetal rabbit lung using enzymatic dissociation and gradient centrifugation methods was developed *(143,144)*. This technique provided enriched fractions of NEB cells suitable for in vitro experimentation. In cultures exposed to moderate hypoxia ($Po_2 < 50$ torr) there was between 15% and 20% reduction in intracellular 5-HT content, whereas with severe hypoxia ($Po_2 < 20$ torr) up to 80% reduction was observed *(144)*. In a recycling experiment where cultures were first exposed to severe hypoxia and then left to recover in normoxia, the 5-HT levels returned to control levels, indicating modulation of 5-HT content by ambient oxygen concentration. Experiments using calcium ionophore confirmed that the intracellular signaling pathway for hypoxia is $Ca^{2+}$-dependent.

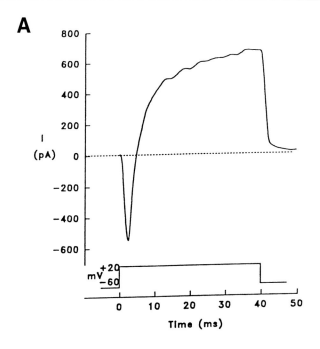

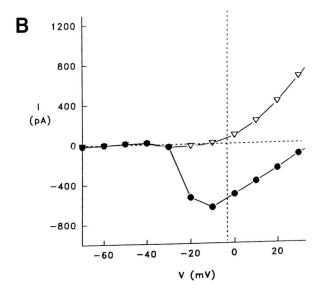

Fig. 5. Patch-clamp analyses of rabbit fetal NEB cells in culture. (**A**) Whole-cell voltage-acti
vated currents recorded from a rabbit fetal NEB cell in culture. Under voltage clamp conditions
with a holding potential of –60 mV and pulse duration of 40 ms, a voltage step to +20 mV showed
the presence of both an inward and outward current. Although the inward current was transient,
the outward current lasted for the entire duration of 40 ms pulse. (**B**) Current–voltage relation for
a cultured NEB cell. Voltage clamp currents were measured from a holding potential of -60 mV
to various test potentials. The outward (open triangles) and inward (closed circles) currents were
activated between –20 and –30 mV and peaked at approximately –10 MV. (**C**) Effects of hypoxia

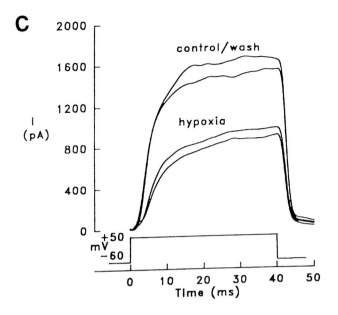

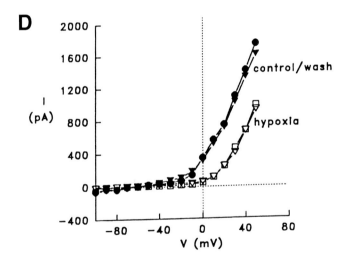

on outward potassium current from rabbit fetal NEB cell in culture. Potassium currents recorded by voltage steps to +50 mV from a holding potential of –60 mV. The same cell was repeatedly cycled between normoxic ($Po_2$:150 mmHg; control/wash) and hypoxic stimulus ($Po_2$:25–30 mm Hg). About 43% reduction in $K^+$ current was observed when the cell was first exposed to hypoxia; following recovery in normoxia (wash), a second exposure produced a similar reduction in $K^+$ current. **(D)** Current–voltage relationship in of cell in Fig. C. (Figs. A and D from ref. *145*, with permission; Fig. B from ref. *146*, with permission.)

These findings provided strong evidence indicating that NEB cells are the transducer of hypoxia stimulus and express an $O_2$ sensor that is coupled to an intracellular stimulus-secretion mechanism.

## IONIC CURRENTS IN NEB CELLS

The study of the membrane properties of NEB cells using electrophysiologic approaches became feasible once a method to visualize these cells in a living state was developed. A basic dye, neutral red (which is pH-sensitive and concentrates in acidic compartments of cells such as neurosecretory granules) was found to selectively stain NEB cells particularly in the lungs of species with high endogenous serotonin content. Subsequent whole cell patch-clamp studies using cultures of NEB isolated from rabbit fetal lung demonstrated the presence of voltage activated $Na^+$, $Ca^{2+}$, and $K^+$ currents — a key feature of excitable cells (145). Under voltage clamp, depolarizing voltage steps from a holding potential of –60 mV to +20 mV activated both a fast transient inward current and a prolonged outward current in NEB cells (Fig. 5A and B). Further pharmacologic dissection of the inward current indicated that it was carried by $Na^+$ and $Ca^{2+}$ ions, respectively (145,146). The outward current was carried by $K^+$ ions, since it was considerably reduced when $K^+$ channel blockers tetraethylammonium (TEA) and 4-aminopyridine (4-AP) were added to the bathing medium (145–147). Under current clamp mode, overshooting action potentials were generated after a short pulse of depolarizing current was applied to NEB cells.

## $O_2$ SENSITIVE $K^+$ CHANNELS AND THEIR MODULATION BY HYPOXIA

In order to test the effects of hypoxia on ionic currents, NEB cells bathed in a normoxic solution ($Po_2$ 150 mmHg) were exposed to hypoxia by switching to a hypoxic solution ($Po_2$ 25–30 mmHg). Hypoxia reversibly suppressed the outward $K^+$ current (25–35%) in NEB cells without affecting the inward $Na^+$ and $Ca^{2+}$ currents (Fig. 5C,D) (145–147). Under current clamp conditions, hypoxia caused an increase in the slope and frequency of the depolarizing pacemaker potentials in some NEB cells (Fig. 6) (145,146). Hence it was confirmed that NEB cells express hypoxia-sensitive $K^+(O_2)$ current similar to that identified in other $O_2$ sensing cells, namely, CB chief cells (148–150) pulmonary artery myocytes (151), and certain neurons in the brain (152). Further analysis of these whole-cell $K^+$ currents in $O_2$ sensitive cells revealed a $Ca^{2+}$-dependent $[I_K(C_a)]$ and $Ca^{2+}$-independent components with both currents inhibited by low $Po_2$ (153). Using a newly developed lung slice technique (which allows the study of NEB in their natural setting, without potential effects induced by cell isolation and culture), we have recently identified in NEB of rabbit neonates both types of voltage activated $K^+$ currents, one with properties $I_K(C_a)$ and the other $Ca_{2+}$ independent $K^+$ current (147). We have also found both types of $K^+$ currents to be hypoxia-sensitive in NEB cells. The role of $Ca^{2+}$ dependent $K^+$ current in $O_2$ chemotransduction has not yet been fully defined. More is known about $Ca^{2+}$ independent $K^+$ channels whose kinetic and pharmacologic properties resemble delayed rectifier or slow-inactivating $K^+$ channels found in different $O_2$-sensing cells as well as in neurons (154).

## MOLECULAR BIOLOGY AND STRUCTURE OF $O_2$-SENSITIVE $K^+$ CHANNELS

Molecular-genetic studies on voltage-gated $K^+$ channels revealed a great diversity of genes coding for the various channel proteins. The native voltage-activated $K^+$ channels

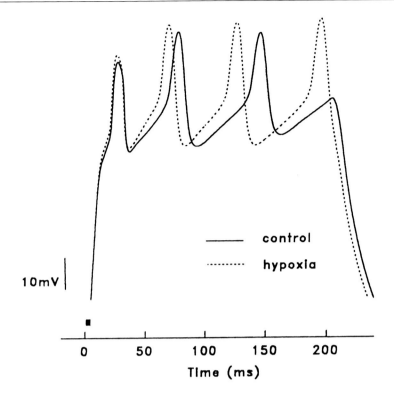

Fig. 6. Current clamp recordings from an NEB cell. Repetitive firing was triggered by a brief (5-ms) suprathreshold depolarizing stimulus applied during the period indicated (horizontal bar). After termination of the stimulus, the spontaneous firing frequency and slope of the depolarizing pacemaker potentials were increased with exposure to hypoxia (dashed line) compared with normoxic control (full line). (From ref. *145*, with permission.)

are composed of four membrane-bound, pore-forming $\alpha$-subunits and four auxiliary $\beta$-subunits *(155)*. The $\alpha$-subunits form functional tetramers with each subunit encoded by a unique gene. There are four main subfamilies of genes encoding $\alpha$-subunits (Shaker, Shal, Shab, and Shaw) with more than 20 transcripts identified in mammals *(156)*. The molecular-genetic identity of $O_2$-sensitive $K^+$ channels has not yet been fully character-ized. Using *in situ* hybridization and Northern blot we have identified expression of mRNA for Shaw related KV3.3a in NEB cells of fetal rabbit and human neonatal lungs as well as in several small cell lung carcinoma cell lines related to NEB *(157)*. Other investigators have reported expression of Shaker gene related mRNA's in PC-12 cell line (used as a model for CB chief cells) and in pulmonary artery myocytes. Transcripts of Shaker $KV_{1.2}$ mRNA were selectively increased by prolonged hypoxia in PC-12 cells *(158)*, but a decrease was reported in rat pulmonary artery myocytes *(159)*. These studies suggest much diversity of $O_2$-sensitive $K^+$ channel expression at the molecular level, which could be the basis of their functional versatility. The common molecular feature of $O_2$-sensitive $K^+$ channels appears to be a shared cysteine residue in the $\alpha$-subunit close to the N-terminus, critical for channel gating mechanism *(160)*. The cysteine residue is known to be affected by the redox status of channel proteins and is sensitive to oxygen free radicals, including $H_2O_2$ *(161)*.

## O$_2$ SENSING PROTEIN AND ITS ROLE IN O$_2$ CHEMOTRANSDUCTION BY NEB CELLS

The membrane model proposed to explain the modulation of ion channels by O$_2$ tension includes three possible mechanisms: (i) The ion channel itself constitutes the O$_2$ sensor; (ii) the channel is modulated by an independent O$_2$ sensor; or (iii) via a closely associated O$_2$ sensing protein *(149,150,162)*. At present the most convincing evidence points to a direct O$_2$ sensor–K$^+$ channel interaction within the plasma membrane, as O$_2$ sensitivity has been demonstrated in excised membrane patches devoid of cytoplasmic mediators *(163)*. Acker and colleagues *(164)* proposed a heme-linked NADPH oxidase as a candidate for an O$_2$-sensing protein in CB glomus cells. Using a highly sensitive absorption spectrophotometry Cross et al. *(165)* identified b-type cytochrome in the plasma membrane of rat CB glomus cells. This heme protein can generate H$_2$O$_2$ and is similar to NADPH oxidase of neutrophils and phagocytes *(166)*. Molecular studies of NADPH oxidase in neutrophils have identified a membrane-bound cytochrome b$_{558}$ consisting of a 91-kDa (gp91 phox) and 22-kDa (p 22 phox) subunits localized in the plasma membrane and the membrane of neutrophil-specific granules where it serves as the terminal electron carrier of the oxidase *(167)*. Additional cytosolic cofactors p 47 phox, p 67 phox and rac$_2$ are required for activation of the oxidase *(166,167)*. Using immunohistochemistry with specific antibodies, the expression of various components of both membrane bound (gp91 phox, p 22 phox) and cytosolic components of neutrophil NADPH oxidase has been identified in NEB cells of rabbit fetal lung as well as in rat CB glomus cells *(168,169)*. Furthermore, expression of mRNAs encoding gp 91 phox and p 22 subunits of the oxidase have been demonstrated in NEB cells of rabbit fetal and human neonatal lungs *(157)*.

Histochemical evidence for a functional oxidase in NEB cells was obtained using dyhydrorhodamine (DHR 123) used as a fluorescence probe for H$_2$O$_2$ generation *(145, 157)*. Using this assay, increased oxidase activity was observed after simulation with phorbol ester and inhibition of oxidase activity by diphenenyleniodonium (DPI) a blocker of the flavoprotein within the oxidase complex *(157)*. It is of interest to note that the oxidase in NEB cells exhibits "basal" activity without prior stimulation in contrast to neutrophil oxidase, which requires activation via assembly of cytoplasmic and membrane components *(166,167)*. This finding also suggests that the oxidase in NEB cells may not be identical to the one in neutrophils and may exist in a preassembled form *(169)*.

The membrane model of O$_2$ sensing proposes that H$_2$O$_2$ produced by the oxidase acts as a second messenger modulating the O$_2$-sensitive K$^+$ channel *(150,157,162)* (Fig. 7). The evidence of such an interaction includes the effects of NADPH inhibitor DPI causing O$_2$ sensitive K$^+$ channel closure as with hypoxia *(145,147)*. In addition, direct application of H$_2$O$_2$ on the surface of NEB cells increases the open probability of O$_2$-sensitive K$^+$ channels *(147,157)*. Also of interest are recent electrophysiologic studies on NEBs in oxidase deficient (gp 91 knockout) mouse *(170)*. In this model, voltage activated K$^+$ channels in NEB cells exhibit appropriate pharmacologic and electrophysiologic properties including responses to external application of H$_2$O$_2$, but fail to respond to hypoxia stimulus or DPI application *(171)*.

## Model of O$_2$ Sensing and Signal Transduction in NEB Cells

The general model of O$_2$ sensing by NEB cells (Fig. 8) is based on that proposed for CB glomus cells *(149,150,162)*. The central event in this model is hypoxia-induced

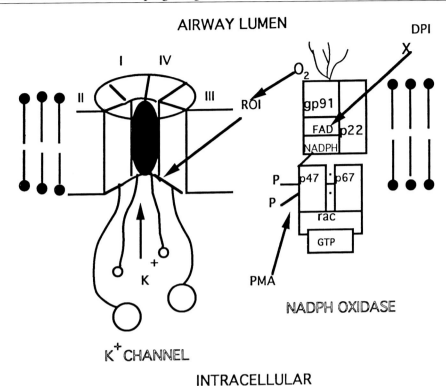

AIRWAY LUMEN

DPI

$K^+$ CHANNEL

NADPH OXIDASE

INTRACELLULAR

Fig. 7. Association of NADPH oxidase complex with the specific $K^+$ channel protein. In this simplified mode, the NADPH oxidase complex is shown to associate with the specific $K^+$ channel protein. In one scenario, signaling of the ion channel response may be mediated via reactive oxygen intermediates (ROI) generated by the oxidase. Another scenario may involve signaling via metabolites at the cytoplasmic aspect of the complex (i.e., reductive events). We also indicate that DPI can inhibit oxidase function through inhibition of the flavoprotein activity (FAD) while PMA can stimulate phosphorylation (i.e., activation) of the cytoplasmic components of the oxidase complex. Our immunohistochemical and electrophysiological data support functional cooperation between the oxidase and $K^+$ channel during $O_2$ sensing. (From ref. *157*, with permission.)

increase in intracellular $Ca^{2+}$, which in turn activates the exocytosis machinery, resulting in neurotransmitter release. The first step in the detection of low-$Po_2$ is postulated to occur at the level of $O_2$ sensor (NADPH oxidase). The reduced availability of $O_2$-substrate could result in decreased $H_2O_2$ production. This, in turn, could alter the redox status of specific residues in $O_2$-sensitive $K^+$ channel proteins leading to channel closure. The closure or inactivation of $O_2$ sensitive $K^+$ channel would initiate depolarization of NEB cell membrane and opening of voltage-sensitive $Ca^{2+}$ channels. The influx of extracellular $Ca^{2+}$ would trigger neurotransmitter release with relay of information via afferent nerve fibers to the brain stem *(131,136)*.

The above model of $O_2$ sensing has been further expanded by Acker *(172,173)* and includes additional cellular functions. Central to this proposal is the role of $H_2O_2$ as a second messenger system, which may influence not only the open-probability of $K^+$ channels but also regulate gene expression *(172,173)*. This scenario is more relevant to the effects of prolonged or chronic hypoxia where levels of $H_2O_2$ could be modulated by

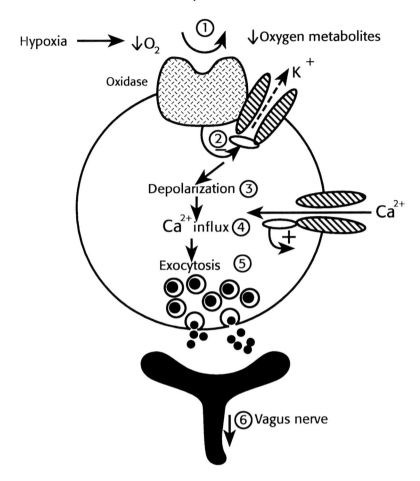

Fig. 8. Proposed mechanism of chemotransduction in NEB cells. The reduced availability of $O_2$ substrate with hypoxia causes a reduction in the level of byproducts of $O_2$ reduction by the oxidase (i.e., $H_2O_2$) (1). This, in turn, alters the redox potential of the cell, causing a change in the protein conformation of a particular subset of the $K^+$ channel proteins, specifically the $O_2$-sensitive $K^+$ channel (2). The result is a closure of these channels preventing the outward flux of $K^+$ ions. The closure or inactivation of the $K^+$ channel effectively leads to depolarization allowing the NEB to reach threshold faster and thus increasing its spiking frequency (3). The increase in spike activity causes waves of depolarization to spread over the cell leading to calcium influx and neurotransmitter release (4,5). The binding of neurotransmitter to sensory afferent terminals causes a relay of information to the breathing centers in the brainstem (6). In response to sensory input, classic homeostatic mechanisms come into play (i.e., alteration in ventilation and/or pulmonary blood vessel diameter) to compensate for the reduced $O_2$ levels in the airway. (Modified from ref. 149.)

the glutathione system, activate the guanylate cyclase and/or transcription factors. These signal transduction systems could, in turn, stimulate DNA synthesis and gene expression of $O_2$-sensitive elements (142). These pathways could constitute a link between the plasma membrane bound $O_2$ sensor and other cellular functions involved in the maintenance of optimal $Po_2$.

# PULMONARY NEUROENDOCRINE CELL–NEUROEPITHELIAL BODY ALTERATIONS IN NEONATAL AND PEDIATRIC LUNG DISEASE

## PNEC Changes in Pulmonary Hypoplasia and Other Congenital Lesions With Abnormal Lung Growth and Development

Because of known effects of bombesin as a growth factor involved in lung morphogenesis, its expression in pulmonary hypoplasia and various congenital lung malformations has been examined in several studies. However, the reported findings on quantitation of PNEC in *pulmonary hypoplasia* are variable ranging from marked decrease, no difference or an increase compared to age-matched controls *(174,175)*. Such variability, however, is not surprising, since the pathogenesis of pulmonary hypoplasia involves diverse mechanisms. For example, a study on the distribution and frequency of bombesin and calcitonin immunoreactive PNEC in cases of pulmonary hypoplasia secondary to anencephaly, showed no significant differences when compared to controls *(176)*. This study concluded that the PNEC developmental program is probably independent of CNS development. On the other hand, in cases of pulmonary hypoplasia, secondary to omphalocele or diaphragmatic hernia, hyperplasia of bombesin immunoreactive PNECs has been reported *(175,177)*. Interpretation of these changes is complicated because of clinical and treatment variables as well as paucity of suitable cases for study. Possible mechanisms proposed include compensatory increases in PNEC numbers related to impaired lung development and/or failure of neuropeptide release during neonatal adaptation *(174,175)*. In a rat model of congenital diaphragmatic hernia (CDH) which results in pulmonary hypoplasia, PNEC changes similar to those described in human cases have been reported *(178)*. These studies used CGRP as a marker of PNEC and showed increased number of these cells in term rat pups with CDH compared to normal control pups. In a follow-up study focusing on PNEC changes during different stages of lung development, decreased numbers of PNEC were found in lungs of rat fetuses with CDH on day 18 but an increase on day 22 when compared to normal controls *(179)*. This suggested that, since CGRP exhibits growth factor-like properties acting on both endothelial and epithelial cells, the lack of this morphogenic factor during the critical stage of lung development (i.e., canalicular stage) may contribute to the pathogenesis of pulmonary hypoplasia associated with CDH. By contrast, the increased number of PNEC observed in neonates with CDH may result in an imbalance of vasoactive mediators necessary for successful neonatal pulmonary adaptation.

Among congenital lung malformations, *congenital cystic adenomatoid malformation* (CCAM) and *pulmonary sequestration* (PS) have been examined for expression of amine and peptides produced by PNEC *(174)*. While CCAM is considered to be a hamartomalike lesion with several subtypes recognized, PS arises as a separate segment of lung tissue supplied by systemic arteries. In both CCAM and PS, the immunostaining pattern within the lesional epithelium resembled that of early fetal lung with up to a fivefold increase in serotonin immunoreactive PNECs, sparse bombesin immunoreactivity and negative immunostaining for calcitonin and CGRP. In addition, there was a predominance of solitary PNECs with decrease in NEB formation. While the significance of these findings is at present unknown, a possibility exists that lack of peptide growth factor(s) during a critical developmental period may lead to abnormal growth and differentiation of airway epithelium associated with these lesions.

## PNEC Changes in Acute and Chronic Lung Disease
## of Prematurity: Human Studies

Since PNEC and NEB appear most prominent during the fetal/neonatal period, initial studies on alterations of these cells in pathologic conditions focused on pulmonary disorders affecting the newborn infants. The chronic lung disease in premature infants (bronchopulmonary dysplasia, BPD) usually evolves from acute lung injury characterized by diffuse alveolar damage with hyaline membrane formation and airway epithelial injury as a consequence of surfactant deficiency. The pathophysiology of BPD is believed to be multifactorial, with factors contributing to lung injury include mechanical trauma, oxygen toxicity, inflammation and immaturity (180).

The initial studies on *hyaline membrane disease* (HMD) of prematurity have shown a marked decrease in the number of bombesin immunoreactive PNEC/NEB compared to control infants (61). This was confirmed by RIA for bombesin in lung tissue extracts as well as by finding of decreased expression of GRP (181,182). Other studies demonstrated a generalized decrease in bombesin, calcitonin, and serotonin-immunoreactive PNEC/NEB in lungs of infants dying of HMD (183). The possible explanations for these findings include degranulation of PNEC/NEB cells in response to hypoxia related to respiratory distress, widespread necrosis and injury of the airway epithelium with loss of PNEC/NEB or a combination of the above.

The chronic progression of HMD into *bronchopulmonary dysplasia* (BPD) is characterized by ongoing airway epithelial cell injury accompanied simultaneously with repair and scarring of the lung tissue. The healing response involves both fibrosis and epithelial regeneration, which seems to affect the state of PNEC system. Increased numbers of PNEC/NEB immunoreactive for bombesin, calcitonin, and serotonin have been reported in infants dying of BPD (61,62). The degree of PNEC hyperplasia in BPD peaks between 2- to 3-mo of postnatal age after which it appears to decline (61). These changes are most likely due to variables in clinical and treatment modalities as well as to local pathologic processes. For example, the number PNEC/NEB tend to be lower or absent in areas of epithelial squamous metaplasia and obliterative bronchiolitis, whereas more prominent PNEC/NEB are found in small peripheral airways with better preserved epithelium (184). The precise mechanism for PNEC/NEB hyperplasia in BPD is not known. Since these cells are terminally differentiated with low mitotic potential, increased recruitment from precursor cells stimulated by chronic local hypoxia may be one of the potential factors. The functional consequences of PNEC/NEB hyperplasia in infants with BPD are unknown. It is postulated that these cells and their amine/peptide mediators may be directly or indirectly involved in the pathogenesis of BPD-associated pulmonary functional abnormalities including pulmonary hypertension and airway hyperreactivity (185).

At present, BPD remains a major problem in perinatal medicine, paradoxically due to the success in improving survival of preterm infants now that respiratory distress syndrome is routinely treated with surfactant replacement therapy (186). Improvements in medical management have reduced the severity of BPD occurring in human infants over the past decade (180,187,188). Prenatal therapy with dexamethasone and postnatal treatment with vitamin A have reduced the severity of BPD, but exogenous surfactant therapy has not reduced the incidence of BPD, suggesting that type II cell immaturity is not the cause of this disease (188,189). In spite of many medical advances, there is no biologic marker for identifying which very low birth weight infants will go on to develop chronic lung disease (190).

## PNEC and Bombesin-like Peptide
## in a Baboon Model of Bronchopulmonary Dysplasia

Although there are several animal models for HMD *(191–197)* and some for chronic lung disease similar to BPD *(198–200)*, preterm baboons represent the best nonhuman animal model for both HMD and its chronic sequelae, which clinically and pathologically most closely approximates human BPD *(201–206)*. The increasing incidence of BPD as one of the major unsolved problems in perinatal medicine resulted in the initiation of a collaborative program by the National Institutes of Health whereby the baboon model of BPD established by Coalson, Seidner, and coworkers *(204–206)* in San Antonio, Texas has been designated as a key tool in investigating this illness. Preterm animals delivered by caesarean section at 140 d gestation (term = 185 d) and maintained on 100% $O_2$ (140 d/100%$O_2$) for 10 d develop clinical and pathologic features typical of moderate to severe BPD ("old BPD") similar to those described by Northway in 1967 *(207)*. By contrast, control 140 d gestation preterm baboons maintained for 10 d on $O_2$ PRN (to keep arterial blood hemoglobin above 90% $O_2$ saturation) [140 d/PRN] do develop acute respiratory distress syndrome (RDS) with HMD between 1 and 48 h after delivery, but recover from the acute injury and do not develop subsequent clinical or pathologic changes reminiscent of BPD. Coalson et al. *(205,206)* have developed another model of mild BPD in extremely premature baboons (125 d gestation) receiving $O_2$ PRN and requiring exogenous surfactant to survive, which is much more similar to the version of BPD currently seen in human infants *(208)*. In this model of "new BPD," over 90% of 125 d/PRN animals develop characteristic clinical and pathologic features of chronic lung disease found in ventilated extremely low birth weight human infants, including reactive airways disease and arrested alveolar septation *(206)*.

Because infants with BPD have increased PNECs containing BLP, a growth factor and bronchoconstrictor *(209)*, we hypothesized that BLP mediates lung injury in BPD *(63)*. The kinetics of BLP mRNA and peptide levels in normal baboon lung are similar to those in humans *(112)*. Control animals (140 d/PRN), which do not develop BPD have no significant change in mean urine BLP levels between 24 and 72 h after delivery. By contrast, 140 d/100% $O_2$ baboons developing severe BPD have a significant doubling in mean urine BLP levels between 24 and 48 h [ΔurBLP (24–48)] *(63)*. All of these animals manifest moderate to severe oxygenation impairment (OI > 2.5) and chest X-ray changes after 8 to 10 d, where OI is defined as ($Fio_2$ × mean airway pressure) × 100/$Pao_2$. A small percentage (approx 15%) of 140 d/100% $O_2$ animals do not develop significant chronic lung disease. Urine BLP levels from two such animals declined rather than increased. In animals treated with 100% $O_2$, there was a direct correlation between ΔurBLP (24–48) and OI at 10 d ($R$ = .93, $p$ = .022) *(63)*.

To provide assessment of changes in urine BLP and BPD independently of therapy with 100% $O_2$, we also measured urine BLP levels in the second baboon model of "new BPD" (125 d gestation baboons treated with $O_2$ PRN and exogenous surfactant therapy) *(145)*. In these animals, there was a significant (approx 30%) increase in urine BLP between 24 and 48 h after birth, with doubling occurring at 72 h *(63)*. We observed a significant correlation between urine BLP levels at 72 h and OI at 14 d in this model (M. Sunday and B. Yoder, *unpublished data*). Therefore, elevated urine BLP levels might be associated with chronic lung disease occurring in diverse clinical settings.

To test whether BLP might play a causative role in the pathophysiology of BPD, we administered the well-characterized murine monoclonal anti-BLP blocking antibody

2A11 to five 140 d/100% $O_2$ baboons beginning 2 h after birth. The most striking immediate effect of 2A11 given 2 h after birth is marked improvement in mean OI between birth and 12 h of age, which occurs between 4 and 6 h after beginning 2A11 and is sustained for at least 3 d (63). None of the 2A11 animals developed a pneumothorax or required high-frequency ventilation, in contrast to 31–54% of the 140 d/100% $O_2$ and 140 d/PRN controls. Two of the 2A11-treated animals developed late septicemia with acute pneumonia (63). When we analyzed animals without clinical evidence of septicemia, these three 2A11-treated animals had improved OI compared to 140 d/100%$O_2$ animals not receiving the antibody ($p < .001$). Histopathologically, after 10 d of 100% $O_2$ treatment, the five animals receiving 2A11 had only mild disruption of alveolar architecture, with some mild saccular overdistension and minimal interstitial thickening, but no evidence of peribronchiolar fibrosis.

It appears therefore, that postnatal administration of blocking anti-BLP antibody protects against the development of clinical and pathologic features of BPD. Although the precise mechanism is unknown, multiple molecular interactions underlying the anti-BLP antibody effect are likely including decreased macrophage activation and blockade of direct effects of BLP as a bronchoconstrictor. It is unlikely that the late beneficial effect on the course of BPD is simply due to the early improvement in OI of anti-BLP antibody (2A11)-treated animals as compared to both the untreated 100% $O_2$ and $O_2$ PRN animals: one male 2A11-treated animal did develop severe RDS, but had minimal evidence of chronic lung disease after 10 d of 100% $O_2$.

These studies also support the interesting concept of PNECs modulating inflammatory responses. It has been demonstrated that cytokines such as tumor necrosis factor-alpha can induce neuroendocrine cell differentiation in human small cell lung cancer cell lines (67), which could explain the increased number of these cells in the lungs of guinea pigs immunized systemically with ovalbumin (210). Similarly, BPD might be viewed as an inflammatory response gone awry. This concept suggests possible clinical usefulness of BLP blocking agents such as 2A11 or BLP receptor-specific antagonists (211–213) to prevent lung injury.

## PNEC/NEB Changes in Disorders of Respiratory Control

Hyperplasia of PNEC/NEB linked to the dysfunction of peripheral chemoreceptors has been recently proposed as a potential mechanism for *congenital central hypoventilation syndrome* (CCHS) (218) and for *sudden infant death syndrome* (SIDS) (215,216). While both CCHS and SIDS are heterogeneous disorders with different pathogenic mechanisms involved, they include significant subgroups with alterations in PNEC system. We have reported two cases of CCHS with marked hypoplasia of carotid body glomus cells accompanied by twofold increase in PNEC/NEB size and number (214). It is postulated that in CCHS, PNEC hyperplasia may be compensatory and could indicate interaction between arterial and airway $O_2$ sensors. In cases of SIDS where metabolic, environmental, infectious, and unnatural causes of death have been excluded, the PNEC system shows consistent hyperplasia compared to age-matched control infants (215,216). The hyperplasia and hypertrophy of NEB is particularly striking in small peripheral airways and at bronchiole–alveolar junctions. The increased number and size of bombesin immunoreactive PNEC/NEB determined by morphometric analysis of SIDS lungs compared to controls, correlates well with concentrations of bombesin-like peptide detected by RIA (216). The etiology or mechanisms of PNEC/NEB hyperplasia in lungs of SIDS victims remains unknown. Effects of chronic hypoxia and/or developmental delay have been postulated as possible factors. An additional mechanism may involve maternal smoking, especially during pregnancy, known to be a significant risk factor for SIDS. A recent study on PNEC in relation to SIDS reported potentiation of PNEC/NEB hyperplasia in lungs of SIDS infants whose mothers smoked during pregnancy *(217)*. Mild airway inflammation documented in up to 30% of SIDS cases could be another potential mechanism affecting the function of PNEC/NEB and represent another potential triggering factor for SIDS. In particular, local production of inflammatory cytokines and reactive oxygen intermediates including $H_2O_2$ may alter $O_2$ sensor on NEB cell membrane (see the subsection "Cellular and Molecular Mechanism of Oxygen Sensing in NE Cells"). The failure to signal airway hypoxia could in turn initiate a chain of events leading by SIDS. In this context, a recent report by Southall and colleagues *(218)* on effects of mild airway hypoxia (as may occur at high altitude or during airflights) triggering apnea in a proportion of "normal" infants would support this hypothesis. Both BPD and Wilson–Mikity syndrome, a rare chronic lung disease of premature infants, are associated with increased incidence of sudden unexpected death *(184,219)*. In both of these conditions, marked hyperplasia of PNEC/NEB has been documented *(184,220)*.

## *Effects of Nicotine and Maternal Smoking on PNEC*

A number of epidemiologic and experimental studies have provided evidence linking cigarette smoking with a variety of pulmonary diseases, including chronic obstructive lung disease and lung cancer. There is increasing evidence that some of the effects of cigarette smoke and its main ingredient nicotine, may involve alterations in PNEC function. It has been previously documented that cigarette smoking or exposure to nicotine is associated with increased numbers of PNECs in lungs of experimental animals as well as in humans *(221,222)*. Smoking during pregnancy has been recognized as a significant risk factor for SIDS as well as a predisposing factor for the development of chronic lung disease in offspring *(223,224)*. For these reasons, the effects of cigarette smoke or nicotine on PNEC has been investigated in a number of experimental studies using both in vivo and in vitro approaches. For example, hamsters exposed to cigarette smoke for 90 days have shown an increased number of PNEC with concomitant increase in the concentration of bombesin and calcitonin in the serum and lung tissue extracts *(221)*. Transplacental administration of nicotine to pregnant mice or hamsters induced significant increase in PNEC in the lungs of offspring *(225)*. In addition, the lungs of these newborn animals showed abnormal airway structure when examined by scanning electron microscopy *(226)*. Chen et al. *(227)* reported increased size and number of NEB in lungs of human fetuses and newborns born to mothers who smoked during pregnancy.

In vitro experiments on the effects of nicotine, using dissociated PNECs from newborn hamster lungs replicated an apparent proliferative response and increased peptide synthesis observed in vivo *(228)*. Since these effects could be blocked by specific antagonists and mimicked by cholinergic/nicotinic agonists, these findings indicated that the PNEC responses are mediated via a nicotinic acetylcholine receptor (nAChR) *(228)*. There is recent electrophysiologic, molecular, and immunohistochemical evidence confirming the expression of nAChR on NEB cells in hamster fetal and neonatal lungs (E. Cutz, *unpublished observations*). Therefore, it is reasonable to postulate that the effects of nicotine on PNEC in fetal/neonatal lung involves activation of nAChR. Since this receptor is a prototype of a receptor directly linked to an ion channel, its activation can induce changes in a variety of cellular functions via different intracellular signal transduction pathways *(229)*. In addition, the effects of nicotine are multisystemic and may involve different mechanisms. Maternal smoking, for example, has been shown to cause fetal hypoxia via direct vasoconstrictive effects of nicotine on the placenta *(230)*, and nicotine has been identified in the placenta, amniotic fluid, and fetal blood *(231)*. However, given the selective uptake of nicotine by the lung tissue *(232)*, and an apparent expression of nAChR on PNEC/NEB, these cells may be particularly vulnerable. Therefore, in the setting of fetal exposure to nicotine there are potential interaction(s) with other factors (i.e., hypoxia via $O_2$ sensor) which could affect PNEC function in developing lung.

### *Possible Role of PNEC in the Pathogenesis of Pediatric Asthma*

At present, there is only limited information available on the possible involvement of PNEC in the pathogenesis of pediatric asthma. A single report described hyperplasia of PNEC in airways of patients with "intrinsic" nonallergic asthma *(233)*. An ultrastructural study of lung biopsy tissue from two children with asthma revealed no apparent abnormalities in PNEC structure *(234)*. In theory, the involvement of PNEC in the pathogenesis of "hypereactive" airway disease can be anticipated, given the strategic location of these cells widely distributed within the airway epithelium; the synthesis and release of potent amine and peptide mediators with effects on airway smooth muscle; potential direct or indirect interaction with mast cells and other inflammatory cells in the airways *(235)*. In animal studies, close topographical association of immune cells with PNEC/NEB has been reported in lungs of neonatal dogs, cats and hamsters *(236)*. Since some of the substances produced by PNEC (i.e., bombesin) exhibit chemotactic properties, an interaction of these cells during local inflammatory and immune responses has been proposed *(237)*. Furthermore, changes in PNEC have been reported after antigen sensitization and challenge in a guinea pig model *(210)*. In this context, the concept of airway epithelium-derived factors modulating the contractility of airway smooth muscle may be of particular interest *(135,238)*. The removal of airway epithelium resulted in altered responses of airway smooth muscle to such agents as acetylcholine, serotonin, or histamine which could not be attributed to local trauma with consequent increased production of eicosanoids or to nitric oxide *(238)*. Whether PNEC are the source of this inhibitory influence is at present unknown. By analogy with vascular endothelium and its effects on vascular smooth muscle contraction, this area of investigation of PNEC function may provide new insight into understanding bronchial asthma and related disorders.

## CONCLUSIONS, UNIFYING OVERALL HYPOTHESIS, AND FUTURE DIRECTIONS

Over the past two decades, the *raison d'etre* of PNECs has begun to be elucidated at the physiologic and molecular levels. Figure 9 presents a summary diagram of several major pulmonary cell types including PNECs and secreted factors capable of mediating lung growth and maturation. During the pseudoglandular and canalicular phases of fetal lung development, PNECs promote cell proliferation and type II pneumocyte differentiation via BLP. These cellular events appear to be mediated via GRP receptors on fibroblasts, which secrete other growth factors (including KGF and CRH) which, in turn, are believed to induce type II cell differentiation. To date, our studies of PNEC

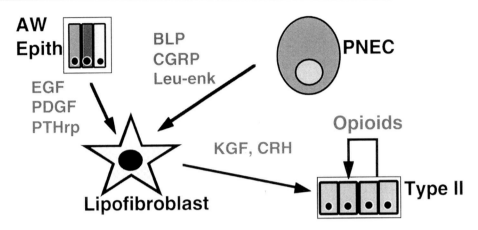

Fig. 9. Summary of hormonal interactions occurring in the fetal pulmonary neurosecretory system. Neuropeptide growth factors, derived from PNECs (both isolated PNECs and NEBs), include BLP, CGRP, and possibly leu-enkephalin. Additional growth factors derived from non-NE airway (AW) epithelium include EGF, PDGF, and PTHrp. These growth factors converge in their action by triggering growth and differentiation of undifferentiated mesenchymal cells into the neurosecretory mesenchymal cells known as lipofibroblasts or lipocytes. In turn, the mesenchymal cells secrete additional growth factors capable of acting directly on type II pneumocytes to induce alveolar epithelial growth and differentiation. New observations suggest that novel opioid-like peptides produced by the alveolar lining cells can modulate type II cell development as well.

function have focused on BLP as a paradigm of a developmentally expressed neuropeptide. However, it is likely that other PNEC-derived peptides, such as CGRP and leu-enkephalin, also function in lung development, either autonomously and/or by modulating the effects of other peptides. The observation of apparently normal lung development in hASH knockout mice which appear to lack PNECs suggests that other cell types can compensate effectively for the absence of PNECs. Candidate compensatory peptides produced by non-neuroendocrine epithelial cells include EGF, PDGF, and PTHrp, all of which appear to act via a mesenchymal intermediary to induce type II cell differentiation, similar to BLP. We have recently identified Ala-deltorphin, an endogenous opioid peptide, in alveolar lining cells in fetal murine lung; this peptide also functions as a potent inducer of type II cell differentiation and growth arrest *(239)*. Thus, multiple cellular and molecular checkpoints can act to promote normal lung maturation, which is essential for postnatal survival.

Several observations are now beginning to suggest why neuroendocrine cells are phylogenetically so strongly conserved in lungs and gills of vertebrates consistent with an important function in the respiratory system. In fact, the phylogenetic origin of PNEC can be traced back some 450 million years. The gills and airways of air-breathing fishes contain solitary PNEC, which express a whole range of peptides, amine (5-HT), and other neuroendocrine markers found in mammalian lungs *(240)*. Innervated PNEC clusters, the NEB, first appear in terrestrial vertebrates (i.e., amphibia) perhaps as a reflection of adaptation to air breathing and a shift from gill to pulmonary respiration. This may be analogous to neonatal pulmonary adaptation with a switch from aqueous environment of fetal lung to extrauterine air breathing. The phylogeny of $O_2$ sensor proteins is also of interest since the candidate for the $O_2$ sensitive $K^+$ channel in NEB cells is related to the *Drosophila* Shaker K$^+$ channel gene family *(156)*. Furthermore, there is evidence that the Shaker K$^+$ channel β subunit belongs to an NAD(P)H-dependent oxidoreductase family with homology found in bacteria and plants *(241)*.

The expression by PNEC/NEB cells of specialized cell membrane proteins involved in O$_2$ signaling together with amine and peptide neurotransmitter/neuromodulation or growth factors has been conserved during evolution since it provides the versatility required for multifunctional role(s). Our unifying hypothesis links the expression of the pulmonary O$_2$ sensor with a developmental program of PNECs. According to this hypothesis, the relative hypoxic microenvironment of fetal lung could represent a natural driving force directing the expression of the PNEC phenotype and thus play a crucial role in paracrine interactions via peptides and growth factors of epithelial and/or mesenchymal origin (Fig. 9). Downregulation of neuropeptide-initiated signalling can occur at the level of peptide gene expression by PNECs, as occurs late in gestation and in the early neonatal period for GRP, and also at the level of peptide receptor gene expression, which in the case of the GRP receptor appears to be completely suppressed immediately after birth. When genes normally restricted to *in utero* expression are abnormally over-expressed in the postnatal period, as might occur with hyperoxic lung injury and barotrauma, chronic lung disease can result, as exemplified by BPD, which is mediated at least in part by BLP. Cumulatively, these observations suggest that the relatively hypoxic environment *in utero* is actually required for gene expression of specific developmentally important genes. Therefore, lung development could provide yet another example of complex interaction between hypoxic gene regulation and environmental cues as recently described for vascular and other developmental programs *(242)*.

# REFERENCES

1. Snyder JM, Mendelson CR, Johnston JM. The morphology of lung development in the human fetus. In: Nelson GH, ed. Pulmonary development: transition from intrauterine to extrauterine life. New York: Marcel Dekker, 1985:19–46.
2. O'Rahilly R. The early prenatal development of the human respiratory system. In: Nelson GH, ed. Pulmonary development: transition from intrauterine to extrauterine life. New York: Marcel Dekker, 1985:3–18.
3. deMello DE, Sawyer D, Galvin N, Reid LM. Early fetal development of lung vasculature. Am J Respir Cell Mol Biol 1997;16:568–581.
4. Sorokin SP, Hoyt RF. Neuroepithelial bodies and solitary small–granule cells. Lung Cell Biol 1989;41:191–344.
5. Scavo LS, Ertsey R, Chapin CJ, Allen L, Kitterman JA. Apoptosis in the development of rat and human fetal lungs. Am J Respir Crit Care Med 1998;18:21–31.
6. Haley K, Drazen J, Osathanondh R, Sunday ME. Comparison of the ontogeny of protein gene product 9.5, chromogranin A and proliferating cell nuclear antigen in human fetal lung. Microsc Res Tech 1997;37:62–681.
7. Wuenschell CW, Sunday ME, Singh G, Minoo P, Slavkin HC, Warburton D. Embryonic mouse lung epithelial progenitor cells co–express immunohistochemical markers of diverse mature cell lineages. J Histochem Cytochem 1996;44:113–123.
8. Li K, Nagalla SR, Spindel ER. A rhesus monkey model to characterize the role of gastrin–releasing peptide (GRP) in lung development. J Clin Invest 1994;94:1605–1615.
9. Cutz E. Cytomorphology and differentiation of airway epithelium in developing human lung. In: McDowell EM, ed.Lung carcinomas: current problems in tumor pathology. Edinburgh: Churchill Livingstone, 1987:1–41.
10. Ten Have-Opbroek AAW. Lung development in the mouse embryo. Exp Lung Res 1991;17:111–130.
11. Stahlman MT, Gray ME. Ontogeny of neuroendocrine cells in human fetal lung. I. An electron microscopic study. Lab Invest 1984;51:449–463.

12. Stahlman MT, Kasselberg AG, Orth DN, Gray ME. Ontogeny of neuroendocrine cells in human fetal lung: II. An immunohistochemical study. Lab Invest 1985;52:52–60.

13. Hage E. Morphology and histochemistry of the normal and abnormal pulmonary endocrine cell. Endocr Lung Health Dis 1984;10:193–209.

14. Johnson DE. Pulmonary neuroendocrine cells. In: The airway epithelium. Farmer SG, Hay DWP, ed. New York: Marcel Dekker, 1991:335–381.

15. Spindel ER, Sunday ME, Hofler H, Wolfe HJ, Habener JF, Chin WW. Transient elevation of mRNAs encoding gastrin–releasing peptide (GRP), a putative pulmonary growth factor, in human fetal lung. J Clin Invest 1987;80:1172–1179.

16. Wang YY, Cutz E. Localization of cholecystokinin–like peptide in neuroendocrine cells of mammalian lungs: A light and electron microscopic immunohistochemical study. Anat Rec 1993;236:198–205.

17. Giaid A, Polak JM, Gaitonde V, Hamid QA, Moscoso G, Legon S, Uwanogho D, Roncalli M, Shinmi O, Sawamura T, Kimura S, Yanagisawa M, Masaki T, Springall DR. Distribution of endothelin-like immunoreactivity and mRNA in the developing and adult human lung. Am J Respir Cell Mol Biol 1991;4:50–58.

18. Seldeslagh KA, Lauweryns JM. Endothelin in normal lung tissue of newborn mammals: immunocytochemical distribution and colocalization with serotonin and calcitonin gene-related peptide. J Histochem Cytochem 1993;41:1495–1502.

19. Michael JR, Markewitz BA. Endothelins and the lung. Am J Respir Crit Care Med 1996;154:555–581.

20. Tsutsumi Y, Osamura Y, Watanabe K, Yanaihara N. Immunohistochemical studies on gastrin-releasing peptide- and adrenocorticotropic hormone-containing cells in the human lung. Lab Invest 1983;48:623–632.

21. Osamura RY, Tsutsumi Y, Watanabe K. Light and electron microscopic localization of ACTH and proopiomelanocortin-derived peptides in human development and neoplastic cells. J Histochem Cytochem 1984;32:885–893.

22. Sorokin SP, Hoyt RF, Pearsall AD. Comparative biology of small granule cells and neuroepithelial bodies in the respiratory system. Am Rev Respir Dis 1983;128:S26–S31.

23. Watanabe H. Pathological studies of neuroendocrine cells in human embryonic and fetal lung. Acta Pathol Jpn 1988;38:59–74.

24. Khoor A, Gray ME, Singh G, Stahlman MT. Ontogeny of Clara cell–specific protein and its mRNA: their association with neuroepithelial bodies in human fetal lung and in bronchopulmonary dysplasia. J Histochem Cytochem 1998;44:1429–1438.

25. Barnes PJ, Baraniuk JN, Belvisi MG. State of the art: neuropeptides in the respiratory tract. Part I. Am Rev Respir Dis 1991;144:1187–1198.

26. Barnes PJ, Baraniuk JN, Belvisi MG. State of the art: neuropeptides in the respiratory tract. Part II. Am Rev Respir Dis 1991;144:1391–1399.

27. Springall DR, Bloom SR, Polak JM. Neural, endocrine, and endothelial regulatory peptides. In: Crystal RG, West JB, Barnes PJ, Cherniak NS, Weibel ER, ed. The lung: scientific foundations. New York: Lippincott-Raven, 1991:69–90.

28. Van Lommel ATL, Lauweryns JM. Ultrastructure and innervation of neuroepithelial bodies in the lungs of newborn cats. Anat Rec 1993;236:181–190.

29. Lauweryns JM, Van Lommel A. The intrapulmonary neuroepithelial bodies after vagotomy: demonstration of their sensory neuroreceptor-like innervation. Experientia 1983;39:1123–1124.

30. Cho T, Chan W, Cutz E. Distribution and frequency of neuroepithelial bodies in post-natal rabbit lung: quantitative study with monoclonal antibody against serotonin. Cell Tissue Res 1989;255:353–362.

31. Campos-Ortega JA, Jan YN. Genetic and molecular bases of neurogenesis in Drosophila melanogaster. Annu Rev Neurosci 1991;14:399–420.

32. Artavanis-Tsakonas S, Delidakis C, Fehon RG. The notch locus and the cell biology of neuroblast segregation. Annu Rev Cell Biol 1991;7:427–452.

33. De Celis JF, Marí-Beffa M, García-Bellido A. Cell-autonomous role of Notch, an epidermal growth factor homologue, in sensory organ differentiation in Drosophila. Proc Natl Acad Sci USA 1991;88:632–636.

34. Cabrera C. Lateral inhibition and cell fate during neurogenesis in Drosophila: the interactions between scute, notch and delta. Development 1990;109:733–742.

35. Enust E, Tietze K, Campos-Ortega JA. Molecular analysis of the neurogenic locus enhancer of split of Drosophila melanogaster. Embo J 1987;6:4113–4123.

36. Lyman D, Young M. Further evidence for function of the Drosophila notch protein as a transmembrane receptor. Proc Natl Acad Sci 1993;USA 90:10395–10399.

37. Fortini M, Artavanis-Tsakonas S. The suppressor of hairless protein participates in Notch receptor signaling. Cell 1994;79:273–282.

38. Jan YN, Jan LY. HLH proteins, fly neurogenesis, and vertebrate myogenesis. Cell 1993;75:827–830.

39. Fehon RG, Johansen K, Rebay I, Artavanis-Tsakonas S. Complex cellular and subcellular regulation of Notch expression during embryonic and imaginal development of Drosophila : implications for notch function. J Cell Biol 1991;113:657–669.

40. Ellisen LW, Bird J, West DC, Soreng AL, Reynolds TC, Smith SD, Sklar J. TAN-1, the human homolog of the Drosophila Notch gene, is broken by chromosomal translocations in T lymphoblastic neoplasms. Cell 1991;66:649–661.

41. Sasai Y, Kageyama R, Tagawa Y, Shigemoto R, Nakanishi S. Two mammalian helix-loop-helix factors structurally related to Drosophila hairy and Enhancer of split. Genes Dev 1992;6:2620–2634.

42. Akazawa C, Sasai Y, Nakanishi S, Kageyama R. Molecular characterization of a rat negative regulator with a basic helix-loop-helix structure predominantly expressed in the development nervous system. J Biol Chem 1992;267:21879–21885.

43. Dou S, Zeng X, Cortes P, Erdjument-Bromage H, Tempst P, Honjo T, Vales LD. The recombination signal sequence-binding protein RBP-2N functions as a transcriptional repressor. Mol Cell Biol 1994;14:3310–3319.

44. Brou C, Logeat F, Lecourtois M, Vandekerckhove J, Kourilsky P, Schweisguth F, Israel A. Inhibition of the DNA-binding activity of Drosophila suppressor of hairless and of its human homolog, KBF2/RBP-Jk, by direct protein-protein interaction with Drosophila hairless. Genes Dev 1994;8:2491–2503.

45. Kageyama R, Sasai Y, Akazawa C, Ishibashi M, Takebayashi K, Shimizu C, Tomita K, Nakanishi S. Regulation of mammalian neural development by helix-loop-helix transcription factors. [Review]. Crit Rev Neurobiol 1995;9:177–188.

46. Guillemot F. Analysis of the role of helix–loop–helix transcription factors in the development of neural lineages in the mouse. Biol Cell 1995;84:3–6.

47. Ball DW, Azzoli CG, Baylin SB, Chi D, Dou S, Donis-Keller H, Cumaraswamy A, Borges M, Nelkin BD. Identification of a human achaete-scute homolog highly expressed in neuroendocrine tumors. Proc Natl Acad Sci USA 1993;90:5648–5652.

48. Borges M, Linnoila RI, van de Velde HJ, Chen H, Nelkin BD, Mabry M, Baylin SB, Ball DW. An achaete-scute homologue essential for neuroendocrine differentiation in the lung. Nature 1997; 386:852–855.

49. Austin CP, Feldman DE, Ida Jr JA, Cepko CL. Vertebrate retinal ganglion cells are selected from competent progenitors by the action of Notch. Development 1995;121:3637–3650.

50. Takeda K, Iwamaot S, Sugimoto H, Takuma T, Kawatani N, Noda M, Masaki A, Morise H, Arimura H, Konno K. Identity of differentiation inducing factor and tumor necrosis factor. Nature 1986;323:338–340.

51. Sunday ME, Hua J, Dai HB, Nusrat A, Torday JS. Bombesin increases fetal lung growth and maturation in utero and in organ culture. Am J Respir Cell Mol Biol 1990;3:199–205.

52. Smith BT, Post M. The influence of hormones on fetal lung development. In: Tulchinsky D, Little AB, eds. Maternal–fetal endocrinology. Philadelphia: WB Saunders, 1994:365–378.

53. Clemens MJ, McNurlan MA. Regulation of cell proliferation and differentiation by interferons. Biochem J 1985;226:345–360.

54. Doyle LA, Giangiulo D, Hussain A, Park HJ, Yen RWC, Borges M. Differentiation of human variant small cell lung cancer cell lines to a classic morphology by retinoic acid. Cancer Res 1989; 49:6745–6751.

55. Wu R, Nolan E, Turner C. Expression of tracheal differentiated functions in serum-free hormone-supplemented medium. J Cell Physiol 1985;125:167–181.

56. Ochiai A, Emura M, Mohr U, Tahara E, Dungworth DL. Induction and characterization of secretory differentiation in human fetal bronchial epithelial cell line (HFBE) cultured on collagen gel in growth hormone and vitamin A-supplemented medium. Exp Pathol 1991;41:157–168.

57. Feyles V, Sikora LKJ, McGarry RC, Jerry LM. Effects of retinoic acid and bromodeoxyuridine on human melanoma-associated antigen expression in small cell lung carcinoma cells. Oncology 1991;48:58–64.

58. Nervi C, Vollberg TM, George MD, Zelent A, Chambon P, Jetten AM. Expression of nuclear retinoic acid receptors in normal tracheobronchial cells and in lung carcinoma cells. Exp Cell Res 1991;195:163–170.

59. Sunday ME, Willett CG, Patidar K, Graham SA. Modulation of oncogene and tumor suppressor gene expression in a hamster model of chronic lung injury with varying degrees of pulmonary neuroendocrine cell hyperplasia. Lab Invest 1994;70:875–888.

60. Sunday ME, Willett CG. Induction and spontaneous regression of intense pulmonary neuroendocrine cell differentiation in a model of preneoplastic lung injury. Cancer Res. 1992;52(Suppl):2677s–2686s.

61. Johnson DE, Lock JE, Elde RP, Thompson TR. Pulmonary neuroendocrine cells in hyaline membrane disease and bronchopulmonary dysplasia. Pediatr Res 1982;16:446–454.

62. Johnson DE, Anderson WR, Burke BA. Pulmonary neuroendocrine cells in pediatric lung disease: alterations in airway structure in infants with bronchopulmonary dysplasia. Anat Rec 1993;236:115–119.

63. Sunday E, Yoder BA, Cuttitta F, Haley KJ, Emanuel, RL. Bombesin-like peptide mediates lung injury in a baboon model of bronchopulmonary dysplasia. J Clin Invest 1998;102:584–594.

64. Gould VE, Linnoila RI, Memoli VA, Warren WH. Biology of disease: neuroendocrine components of the bronchopulmonary tract: hyperplasias, dysplasias, and neoplasms. Lab Invest 1983;49:519–537.

65. Chejfec G, Capella C, Solcia E, Jao W, Gould VE. Amphicrine cells, dysplasias, and neoplasias. Cancer 1985;56:2683–2690.

66. Aguayo SM, Kane MA, King TE, Schwarz MI, Grauer L, Miller YE. Increased levels of bombesin-like peptides in the lower respiratory tract of asymptomatic cigarette smokers. J Clin Invest 1989;84:1105–1113.

67. Haley KJ, Patidar K, Zhang F, Emanuel RL, Sunday ME. Tumor necrosis factor induces neuroendocrine cell differentiation in small cell lung cancer cell lines. Am J Physiol 1998;275:L311–L321.

68. Warburton D, Seth R, Shum L, Horcher PG, Hall FL, Werb Z, Slavkin HC. Epigenetic role of epidermal growth factor expression and signalling in embryonic mouse lung morphogenesis. Dev Biol 1992;149:123–133.

69. Nielsen HC, Martin A, Volpe MV, Hatzis D, Vosatka RJ. Growth factor control of growth and epithelial differentiation in embryonic lungs. Biochem Mol Med 1997;60:38–48.

70. Ruocco S, Lallemand A, Tournier JM, Gaillard D. Expression and localization of epidermal growth factor, transforming growth factor-alpha, and localization of their common receptor in fetal human lung development. Pediatr Res 1996;39:448–455.

71. Lee K, Deeds JD, Segre GV. Expression of parathyroid hormone-related peptide and its receptor messenger ribonucleic acids during fetal development of rats. Endocrinology 1995;136:453–463.

72. Han RNN, Liu J, Tanswell AK, Post M. Expression of basic fibroblast growth factor and receptor: immunolocalization studies in developing rat fetal lung. Pediatr Res 1992;31:435–440.

73. Han RNN, Mawdsley C, Souza P, Tanswell AK, Post M. Platelet-derived growth factors and growth-related genes in rat lung. III. Immunolocalization during fetal development. Pediatr Res 1992;31:323–329.

74. Sen N, Cake MH. Enhancement of disaturated phosphatidylcholine synthesis by epidermal growth factor in cultured fetal lung cells involves a fibroblast-epithelial cell interaction. Am J Respir Cell Mol Biol 1991;5:337–343.

75. Rubin L, Kifor O, Hua J, Brown EM, Torday JS. Parathyroid hormone (PTH) and PTH-related protein stimulate surfactant phospholipid synthesis in fetal rat lung, apparently by a mesenchymal-epithelial mechanism. Biochim Biophys Acta 1994;1223:91–100.

76. Karaplis AC, Luz A, Glowacki J, Bronson RT, Tybulewicz VLJ, Kronenberg HM, Mulligan RC. Lethal skeletal dysplasia from targeted disruption of the parathyroid hormone-related peptide gene. Genes Dev. 1994;8:277–289.

77. Ganser G, Stricklin G, Matrisian L. EGF and TGFα influence in vitro lung development by the induction of matrix-degrading metalloproteinases. Int J Dev Biol 1991;35:453–461.

78. Miettinen PJ, Warburton D, Bu D, Zhao JS, Berger JE, Minoo P, Koivisto T, Allen L, Dobbs L, Werb Z, Derynck R. Impaired lung branching morphogenesis in the absence of functional EGF receptor. Dev Biol 1997;186:224–236.

79. Lee M, Hwang C, Lee J, Slavkin H, Warburton D. TGF–beta isoforms differentially attenuate EGF mitogenicity and receptor activity in fetal lung mesenchymal cells. Am J Physiol 1997;273:L374–L381.

80. Sunday ME, Kaplan LM, Motoyama E, Chin, WW, Spindel ER. Biology of disease: gastrin-releasing peptide (mammalian bombesin) gene expression in health and disease. Lab Invest 1988;59:5–24.

81. Wharton J, Polak JM, Bloom SR, Ghatei MA, Solcia E, Brown MR, Pearse AGE. Bombesin-like immunoreactivity in the lung. Nature 1978;273:769–770.

82. Nagalla SR, Gibson BW, Tanf D, Reeve JR Jr, Spindel ER. Gastrin-releasing peptide (GRP) is not mammalian bombesin: identification and molecular cloning of a true amphibian GRP distinct from amphibian bombesin in Bombina orientalis. J Biol Chem 1992;267:6916–6922.

83. Spindel ER, Chin WW, Price J, Rees LH, Besser GM, Habener JF. Cloning and characterization of cDNAs encoding human gastrin–releasing peptide. Proc Natl Acad Sci USA 1984;81:5699–5703.
84. Sausville EA, Lebacq-Verheyden AM, Spindel ER, Cuttitta F, Gazdar AF, Battey JF. Expression of the gastrin-releasing peptide gene in human small cell lung cancer: evidence for alternative processing resulting in three distinct mRNAs. J Biol Chem 1986;261:2451–2457.
85. Lebacq-Verheyden AM, Krystal G, Sartor O, Way J, Battey JF. The prepro gastrin releasing peptide gene is transcribed from two initiation sites in the brain. Mol Endocrinol 1988;2:556–563.
86. Willey JC, Lechner JF, Harris CC. Bombesin and the C-terminal tetradecapeptide of gastrin-releasing peptide are growth factors for normal human bronchial epithelial cells. Exp Cell Res 1984;153:245–248.
87. Siegfried JM, Guentert PJ, Gaither AL. Effects of bombesin and gastrin–releasing peptide on human bronchial epithelial cells from a series of donors: individual variation and modulation by bombesin analogs. Anat Rec 1993;236:241–247.
88. Rozengurt E, Sinnett-Smith J. Early signals underlying the induction of the c–fos and c–myc genes in quiescent fibroblasts: studies with bombesin and other growth factors. Prog Nucleic Acid Res Mol Biol 1988;35:261–295.
89. Cuttitta F, Carney DN, Mulshine J, Moody TW, Fedorko J, Fischler A, Minna JD. Bombesin-like peptides can function as autocrine growth factors in human small cell cancer. Nature 1985;316:823–826.
90. Minna JD, Cuttitta F, Battey JF, Mulshine JL, Linnoila I, Gazdar AF, Trepel J, Sausville EA. Gastrin–releasing peptide and other autocrine growth factors in lung cancer: pathogenetic and treatment implications. In: DeVita, VT, Hellman S, Rosenberg SA, eds. Important advances in oncology. Philadelphia: Lippincott,1988:55–64.
91. Minamino N, Kangawa K, Matsuo H. Neuromedin B: a novel bombesin-like peptide identified in porcine spinal cord. Biochem Biophys Res Commun 1983;114:541–548.
92. Minamino N, Kangawa K, Matsuo H. Neuromedin B is a major bombesin-like peptide in rat brain: regional distribution of neuromedin B and neuromedin C in rat brain, pituitary and spinal cord. Biochem Biophys Res Commun 1984;124:925–932.
93. Krane IM, Naylor SL, Helin-Davis D, Chin WW, Spindel ER. Molecular cloning of cDNAs encoding the human bombesin–like peptide neuromedin B. J Biol Chem. 1988;263:13317–13323.
94. Severi C, Jensen RT, Erspamer V, D'Arpino L, Coy DH, Torsoli A, Delle Fave G. Different receptors mediate the action of bombesin-related peptides on gastric smooth muscle cells. Am J Physiol Gastrointest Liver Physiol 1991;260:G683–G690.
95. Moody T, Staley J, Zia F, Coy D, Jensen R. Neuromedin B binds with high affinity, elevates cytosolic calcium and stimulates the growth of small-cell lung cancer cell lines. J Pharmacol Exp Ther 1992;263:311–317.
96. Yasuhara T, Nakajima T, Nokihara K, Yanaihara C, Yanaihara N, Erspamer V, Erspamer GF. Two new frog skin peptides, phyllolitorins, of the bombesin-ranatensin family from Phyllomedusa sauvagei. Biomed Res 1983;4:407–412.
97. Lazarus LH, Wilson WE, Gaudino G, Irons BJ, Guglietta A. Evolutionary relationship between nonmammalian and mammalian peptides. Peptides 1985;6:295–307.
98. Erspamer GF, Mazzanti G, Farruggia G, Nakajima T, Yanaihara N. Parallel bioassay of litorin and phyllolitorins on smooth muscle preparations. Peptides 1984;5:765–768.
99. Masui A, Kato N, Itoshima T, Tsunashima K, Nakajima T, Yanaihara N. Scratching behavior induced by bombesin-related peptides: comparison of bombesin, gastrin-releasing peptide and phyllolitorins. Eur J Pharmacol 1993;238:297–301.
100. King KA, Torday JS, Sunday ME. Bombesin and [leu8]phyllolitorin promote fetal mouse lung branching morphogenesis via a specific receptor-mediated mechanism. Proc Natl Acad Sci USA 1995;92:4357–4361.
101. Nagalla SR, Barry BJ, Spindel ER. Cloning of complementary DNAs encoding the amphibian bombesin-like peptides Phe8 and Leu8 phyllolitorin from Phyllomedusa sauvagei: potential role of U to C RNA editing in generating neuropeptide diversity. Mol Endocrinol 1994;8:943–951.
102. Minna J. Bombesin receptor gene cloned. Science 1990;249:1377.
103. Battey J, Wada E. Two distinct receptor subtypes for mammalian bombesin-like peptides. Trends Neurosci 1991;14:524–528.
104. Battey JF, Way JM, Corjay MH, Shapira H, Kusano K, Harkins R, Wu JM, Slattery T, Mann E, Feldman RI. Molecular cloning of the bombesin/gastrin-releasing peptide receptor from Swiss 3T3 cells. Proc Natl Acad Sci USA 1991;88:395–399.
105. Gorbulev V, Akhundova A, Buchner H, Farenholz F. Molecular cloning of a new bombesin receptor subtype expressed in uterus during pregnancy. Eur J Biochem 1992;208:405–410.

106.Fathi Z, Corjay MH, Shapira H, Wada E, Benya R, Jensen R, Viallet J, Sausville EA, Battey JF. BRS-3: a novel bombesin receptor subtype selectively expressed in testis and lung carcinoma cells. J Biol Chem 1993;268:5979–5984.

107.Wada E, Way J, Shapira H, Kusano K, Lebacq-Verheyden AM, Coy D, Jensen R, Battey J. cDNA cloning, characterization, and brain region-specific expression of a neuromedin-B-preferring bombesin receptor. Neuron 1991;6:421–430.

108.Fathi Z, Benya RV, Shapira H, Jensen RT, Battey JF. The fifth transmembrane segment of the neuromedin B receptor is critical for high affinity neuromedin B binding. J Biol Chem 1993;268:14622–14626.

109.Nagalla S, Barry B, Creswick K, Eden P, Taylor J, Spindel E. Cloning of a receptor for amphibian (Phe13) bombesin distinct from the receptor for gastrin-releasing peptide: identification of a fourth bombesin receptor subtype (BB4). Proc Natl Acad Sci USA 1995; 92:6205–6209.

110.Wada E, Battey J, Wray S. Bombesin receptor gene expression in rat embryos: transient GRP-R gene expression in the posterior pituitary. Mol Cell Neurosci 1993;4:13–24.

111.Wang D, Yeger H, Cutz E. Expression of gastrin releasing peptide receptor gene in developing lung. Am J Respir Cell Mol Biol 1996;14:409–416.

112.Emanuel RL, Torday JS, Mu Q, Asokananthan N, Sikorski KA, Sunday ME. Bombesin-like peptides and receptors in normal fetal baboon lung: roles in lung growth and maturation. Am J Physiol 1999.

113.Fraslon C, Bourbon JR. Comparison of effects of epidermal and insulin-like growth factors, gastrin releasing peptide and retinoic acid on fetal lung cell growth and maturation in vitro. Biochim Biophysica Acta 1992;1123:65–75.

114.Asokananthan N, Cake MH. Stimulation of surfactant lipid secretion from fetal type II pneumocytes by gastrin-releasing peptide. Am J Physiol 1996;270:L331–L337.

115.Brimhall BB, Sikorski KA, Haley KJ, Torday JS, Sunday ME. Syntaxin 1A is expressed in fetal lung mesenchymal cells and regulates cell growth and differentiation. 2000, in press.

116.Asokananthan N, Cake MH. Stimulation of surfactant lipid secretion from fetal type II pneumocytes by gastrin-releasing peptide. Am J Physiol 1996;270:L331–L337.

117.Post M, Barsoumian A, Smith BT. The cellular mechanism of glucocorticoid acceleration of fetal lung maturation: fibroblast-pneumonocyte factor stimulates choline-phosphate cytidylyltransferase activity. J Biol Chem 1986;261:2179–2184.

118.Torday J, Hua J, Slavin R. Metabolism and fate of neutral lipids of fetal lung fibroblast origin. Biochim Biophys Acta 1995;1254:198–206.

119. Wada E, Watase K, Yamada K, Ogura H, Yamano M, Inomata Y, Eguchi J, Yamamoto K, Sunday ME, Maeno H, Mikoshiba K, Ohki-Hamazaki H, Wada K. Generation and characterization of mice lacking gastrin-releasing peptide receptor. Biochem Biophys Res Commun 1997;239:28–33.

120.Hampton LL, Ladenheim EE, Akeson M, Way JM, Weber HC, Sutliff VE, Jensen RT, Wine LJ, Arnheiter H, Battey JF. Loss of bombesin-induced feeding suppression in gastrin-releasing peptide receptor-deficient mice. Proc Natl Acad Sci USA 1998;95:3188–3192.

121.Ohki-Hamazaki H, Watase K, Yamamoto K, Ogura H, Yamano M, Yamada K, Maeno H, Imaki J, Kikuyama S, Wada E, Wada K. Mice lacking bombesin receptor subtype-3 develop metabolic defects and obesity. Nature 1997;390:165–169.

122.Feyerter F. In: über diffuse endocrine epitheliale Organe. Leipzig: JA Barth, 1938.

123.Lauweryns JM, Cokelaere M. Hypoxia sensitive neuropeithelial bodies intrapulmonary secretory neuroreceptors modulated by the CNS. Z Zellforsh 1973;145:521–540.

124.Lauweryns JM, Cokelaere M, Delesnyder M. Intrapulmonary neuroepithelial bodies in newborn rabbits: influence of hypoxia, hyperoxia, hypercapnia, nicotine, reserpine, L-DOPA and 5-HTP. Cell Tissue Res 1977;182:425–440.

125.Lauweryns JM, Van Lommel A, Dom RJ. Innervation of rabbit intrapulmonary neuroepithelial bodies: quantitative and qualitative ultrastructural study after vagotomy. J Neurol Sci 1985;67:81–92.

126.McDonald DM. Peripheral chemoreceptors: structure-function relationships of the carotid body. In: Hornbein TF, ed. Regulation of breathing. New York: Marcel Dekker, 1981;105–319.

127.Lauweryns JM, Cokelaere M, Lerut T. Cross–circulation studies on the influence of hypoxia and hypoxaemia on neuroepithelial bodies in your rabbits. Cell Tissue Res 1978;193:373–386.

128.Lauweryns JM, Tierens SA, Decramer M. Influence of hypercapnia on rabbit intrapulmonary neuroepithelial bodies: microfluorimetric and morphometric study. Eur Respir J 1990;3:182–186.

129.Lauweryns JM, Van Lommel A. Effects of various vagotomy procedures on the reaction to hypoxia of rabbit neuroepithelial bodies: modulation by intrapulmonary axon reflexes? Exp Lung Res 1986; 11:319–339.

130. Van Lommel A, Lauweryns JM. Ultrastructure and innervation of neuroepithelial bodies in the lungs of newborn cats. Anat Rec 1993;236:181–190.

131. Adriaensen D, Sheuermann DW. Neuroendocrine cells and nerves of the lung. Anat Rec 1993;236:70–85.

132. Lauweryns JM, Van Lommel A. Morphometric analysis of hypoxia induced synaptic activity in intrapulmonary neuroepithelial bodies. Cell Tissue Res 1982;226:201–214.

133. Cutz E, Gillan JE, Bryan AC. Neuroendocrine cells in the developing human lung: morphologic and functional considerations. Ped Pulmonol 1985;1:S21–S29.

134. Gosney JR. Neuroendocrine cell populations in postnatal human lungs: minimal variations from childhood to old age. Anat Rec 1993;236:177–180.

135. Sorokin SP, Hoyt RF Jr. On supposed function of neuroepithelial bodies in adult mammalian lungs. News Physiol Sci 1990;5:89–95.

136. Donnelly DF, Haddad GG. The possible role of neuroepithelial bodies as airway chemoreceptors. In: Cutz E, ed. Cellular and molecular biology of airway chemoreceptors. Austin, TX: Landes Bioscience, 1997;35–45.

137. Gosney JR. Pulmonary neuroendocrine cells in species at high altitude. Ant Rec 1993;236:105–107.

138. Pack RJ, Barker S, Howe A. The effects of hypoxia on the number of amine–containing cells in the lung of the adult rat. Eur J Respir Dis 1986;68:121–130.

139. Keith IM, Will JA. Hypoxia and the neonatal lung: neuroendocrine cell numbers, 5-HT fluorescence intensity and the relationship to arterial thickness. Thorax 1981;36:767–773.

140. Taylor W. Pulmonary argyrophil cells at high altitude. J Pathol 1977;122:137–144.

141. Montuenga LM, Springall DR, Gaer J. CGRP–immunoreactive endocrine cell proliferation in normal and hypoxic rat lung studied by immunocytochemical detection of incorporation of 5'-bromodeoxyuridine. Cell Tissue Res 1992;268:9–15.

142. Beitner–Johanson D, Shull GE, Dedman JR, Milhorn DE. Regulation of gene expression by hypoxia: a molecular approach. Respir Physiol 1997;110:87–97.

143. Cutz E, Yeger H, Wong V. In vitro characteristics of pulmonary neuroendocrine cells from rabbit fetal lung. I. Effects of culture media and nerve growth factor. Lab Invest 1985;53:672–683.

144. Cutz E, Speirs V, Yeger H. Cell biology of pulmonary neuroepithelial bodies: validation of an in vitro model. Anat Rec 1993;236:41–52.

145. Youngson C, Nurse C, Yeger H, Cutz E. Oxygen–sensing in airway chemoreceptors. Nature 1993;365:153–155

146. Youngson C, Nurse C, Wang D, Cutz E: Ionic currents and oxygen–sensing mechanism in neuroepithelial body cells. I: Cutz E, ed. Cellular and molecular biology of airway chemoreceptors. Austin, TX: Landes Bioscience, 1997:71–108.

147. Fu XW, Nurse C, Wang YT, Cutz E. Selective modulation of membrane currents by hypoxia in intact airway chemoreceptors from neonatal rabbit. J Physiol 1998;514:139–150.

148. Lopez-Barneo J, Lopez-Lopez J, Urena J, Gonzalez C. Chemotransduction in the carotid body: $K^+$ current modulated by $PO_2$ in type 1 chemoreceptor cells. Science 1988;241:586–582.

149. Gonzalez C, Almaraz L, Obeso A, Rigual R. Oxygen and acid chemoreception in the carotid body chemoreceptors. Trends Neurosci 1992;15:146–153.

150. Lopez-Barneo J, Benot AR, Urena J. Oxygen-sensing and the electrophysiology of arterial chemoreceptor cells. News Physiol Sci 1993;8:191–195.

151. Yuan XJ, Goldman WF, Tod ML, Rubin LJ. Hypoxia induces potassium currents in cultured rat pulmonary myocytes but not mesenteric arterial myocytes. Am J Physiol 1993;264:L116–L123.

152. Jiang C, Haddad GG. A direct mechanism for sensing low oxygen levels by central neurons. Proc. Natl Acad Sci USA 1994;91:7198–7201.

153. Peers C. Hypoxic suppression of $K^+$ current in type I carotid body cells: selective effect on the $Ca^{2+}$ activated $K^+$ current. Neurosci Lett 1990;119:253–256.

154. Cobbert P, Legrende P, Mason WT. Characterization of three types of potassium currents in cultured neurons of rat supraoptic nucleus area. J Physiol 1989;410:443–462.

155. Rettig J, Helnemann SH, Wunder F, Lorra C, Parcej DN, Dolly JO, Pongs O. Inactivation properties of voltage–gated $K^+$ channels altered by presence of $\beta$ subunits. Nature 1994;369:289–294.

156. Rudy B, Kentros C, Vega–Saenz de Meira E. Families of potassium channel genes in mammals: toward an understanding of the molecular basis of potassium channel diversity. Mol Cell Neurosci 1991;2:89–102.

157. Wang D, Youngson C, Wong V, Yeger H, Dinauer MC, Vega–Saenz de Meira E, Rudy B, Cutz E. NADPH–oxidase and hydrogen peroxide–sensitive $K^+$ channel may function as an oxygen sensor complex in airway chemoreceptors and small cell lung carcinoma cell lines. Proc Natl Acad Sci USA 1996;93:13182–13187.

158. Conforti L, Milhorn DE. Selective inhibition of a slow-inactivating voltage-dependent K⁺ channel in rat PC-12 cells by hypoxia. J Physiol 1997;502:293–305.

159. Wang J, Juhasz M, Rubin LJ. Hypoxia inhibits gene expression of voltage–gated K⁺ channel α–subunits in pulmonary artery smooth muscle cells. J Clin Invest 1997;100:2347–2353.

160. Ruppersberg JP, Stocker M, Pongs O, Heinemann SH, Frank R, Koenen M. Regulation of fast inactivation of cloned $I_K(A)$ channels by cysteinee oxidation. Nature 1991;352:711–714.

161. Vega–Saenz de Miera E, Rudy B. Modulation of K⁺ channels by hydrogen peroxide. Biochem Biophys Res Commun 1992;186:1681–1687.

162. Lopez–Barneo J. Oxygen-sensing by ion channels and the regulation of cellular functions. Trends Neurosci 1996;19:435–440.

163. Ganfornina MD, Lopez-Barneo J. Single K⁺ channels in membrane patches of arterial chemoreceptor cells are modulated by $O_2$ tension. Proc Natl Acad Sci USA 1991;88:2927–2930.

164. Acker H, Dufau E, Huber J, Sylvester D. Indications to an NAD(P)H oxidase as a possible $PO_2$ sensor in the rat carotid body. FEBS Lett 1989;256:75–78.

165. Cross AR, Henderson L, Jones O, Delpiano M. Involvement of an NAD(P)H oxidase as a $PO_2$ sensor protein in the rat carotid body. Biochem J 1990;272:743–747.

166. Babior BM. The respiratory burst oxidase. Adv Enzymol Relat Areas Mol Biol 1992;65:49–95.

167. Parkos CA, Allen RA, Cochrane CG, Jesiatis AJ. The quantenary structure of the plasma membrane b–type cytochrome of human granulocytes. Biochem Biophys Acta 1988;932:71–83.

168. Youngson C, Nurse C, Yeger H, Curnutte JT. Immunohistochemical localization of $O_2$ sensing protein (NADPH oxidase) in chemoreceptor cells. Microsc Res Tech 1997;37:101–106.

169. Kummer W, Acker H. Immunohistochemical demonstration of four subunits of neutrophil NAD(P)H oxidase in type I cells of carotid body. J Appl Physiol 1995;78:1904–1909.

170. Pollock JD, Williams DA, Gifford AC, Li LL, Du X, Fisherman J, Orkin SH, Doerschuk CM, Dinauer MC. Mouse model of X-linked chronic granulomatous disease, an inherited defect in phagocyte superoxide production. Nat Genet 1995;9:202–209.

171. Fu XW, Wang YT, Dinauer MC, Cutz E. Hypoxia sensitive K⁺ currents in pulmonary airway sensors show altered responses in mice with NADPH oxidase deficiency. [Abstract] Arch Anat Cytol Pathol Clin Exp Path 1998;46:558.

172. Acker H. Mechanisms and meaning of cellular oxygen sensing in the organism. Respir Physiol 1994;95:1–10.

173. Acker H, Xue D. Mechanism of $O_2$ sensing in the carotid body in comparison with other $O_2$–sensing cells. News Physiol Sci 1995;10:211–216.

174. Cutz E, Gillan Je, Perrin DG. Pulmonary neuroendocrine system: an overview of cell biology and pathology with emphasis on pediatric lung disease. Perspect Pediatr Pathol 1995;18:32–70.

175. Durbin J, Thomas P, Langston C, Goswami S, Greco A. Gastrin-releasing peptide in hypoplastic lungs. Pediatr Pathol Lab Med 1996;6:927–934.

176. Ito T, Nakatani Y, Nagahara N, Ogawa T, Shibagaki T, Kanisawa M. Quantitative study of pulmonary endocrine cells in anencephaly. Lung 1987;165:297–704.

177. Ijsselstijn H, Gaillard JLJ, de Jongste JC, Tibboel D, Cutz E. Abnormal expression of pulmonary bombesin–like peptide immunostaining cells in infants with congenital diaphragmatic hernia. Pediatr Res 1997;42:712–720.

178. Ijsselstijn H, Perrin DG, de Jongste JC, Cutz E, Tibboel D. Pulmonary neuroendocrine cells in neonatal rats with congenital diaphragmatic hernia. J Pediatr Surg 1995;30:413–415.

179. Ijsselstijn H, Hung N, de Jongste JC, Tibboel D, Cutz E. Calcitonin gene-related peptide expression is altered in pulmonary neuroendocrine cells in developing lungs of rats with congenital diaphragmatic hernia. Am J Respir Cell Mol Biol 1998;19:278–285.

180. Hansen T, Corbet A. Chronic lung disease - Bronchopulmonary dysplasia. In: Taeusch HW, Ballard RA, Avery ME, eds. Diseases of the newborn. Toronto: WB. Saunders, 1991:519–526.

181. Ghatei MA, Sheppard MN, Henzen-Logman S, Blank MA, Polak JM, Bloom SR. Bombesin and vasoactive intestinal polypeptide in the developing lung: marked changes in acute respiratory distress syndrome. J Clin Endocrinol Metab 1983;57:1226–1232.

182. Sunday ME, Kaplan LM, Motoyama E, Chin WW, Spindel ER. Gastin releasing peptide (mammalian bombesin) gene expressionin health and disease. Lab Invest 1988;59:5–24.

183. Johnson DE, Georgieff MK. Pulmonary neuroendocrine cells, their secretory products and their potential roles in health and chronic lung disease in infancy.

184. Cutz E, Gillan JE, Track NS. Pulmonary endocrine cells in developing human lung and during neonatal adaptation. In: Becker KL, Gazdar AF, eds. Endocrine lung in health and disease. Philadelphia: Saunders, 1984:210–231.

185. Johnson DE, Gregorieff K. Pulmonary endocrine cells: their secretory products and their potential roles in health and chronic lung disease of infancy. Am Rev Respir Dir 1989;143:815–819.

186. Parker RA, Lindstrom DP, Cotton RB. Improved survival accounts for most, but not all of the increase in bronchopulmonary dysplasia. Pediatrics 1992;90:663–668.

187. Avery ME, Tooley WH, Keller JB, Hurd SS, Bryan MH, Cotton RB, Epstein MF, Fitzhardinge PM, Hansen CB, Hansen TN, Hodson WA, James LS, Kitterman JA, Nielsen HC, Poirier TA, Truog WE, Wung J-T. Is chronic lung disease in low birth weight infants preventable?: a survey of eight centers. Pediatrics 1987;79:26–30.

188. Jobe AH. Pulmonary surfactant therapy. N Engl J Med 1993;328:861–868.

189. Jobe AH, Mitchell BR, Gunkel H. Beneficial effects of the combined use of prenatal corticosteroids and postnatal surfactant on preterm infants. Am J Obstet Gynecol 1993;168:508–513.

190. Feinberg E, Richardson DK, Als H, Sell E, Parad RB. Late pulmonary outcomes poorly predicted by early risk factors in very low birth weight infants. Pediatr Res 1997;39:263A.

191. Tanswell AK, Wong L, Possmayer F, Freeman BA. The preterm rat: a model for studies of acute and chronic neonatal lung disease. Pediatr Res 1989;25:525–529.

192. Kessler DL, Truog WE, Murphy JH, Palmer S, Standaert TA, Woodrum DE, Hodson WA. Experimental hyaline membrane disease in the premature monkey: Effects of antenatal dexamethasone. Am Rev Respir Dis 1982;126:62–69.

193. Goetzman B, Read L, Plopper C, Tarantal A, George-Nascimento C, Merrit T, Whitsett J, Styne D. Prenatal exposure to epidermal growth factor attenuates respiratory distress syndrome in rhesus infants. Pediatr Res 1994;35:30–36.

194. Meredith KS, Delemos RA, Coalson JJ, King RJ, Gerstmann DR, Kumar R, Kuehl TJ, Winter DC, Taylor A, Clark RH, Null DM. Role of lung injury in the pathogenesis of hyaline membrane disease in premature baboons. J Appl Physiol 1989;66:2150–2158.

195. deLemos R, Wolfsdorf J, Nachman R, Block AJ, Leiby G, Wilkinson HA, Allen T, Haller JA, Morgan W, Avery ME. Lung injury from oxygen in lambs: the role of artificial ventilation. Anesthesiology 1969;30:610–618.

196. Nilsson R. The artificially ventilated preterm rabbit neonate as experimental model of hyaline membrane disease. Acta Anaesth Scand 1982;26:89–103.

197. Lorenzo AV. The preterm rabbit: A model for the study of acute and chronic effects of premature birth. Pediatr Res 1985;19:201–205.

198. Han RN, Buch S, Tseu I, Young J, Christie NA, Frndova H, Lye SJ, Post M, Tanswell AK. Changes in structure, mechanics, and insulin-like growth factor-related gene expression in the lungs of newborn rats exposed to air or 60% oxygen. Pediatr Res 1996;39:921–929.

199. Veness-Meehan KA, Moats-Staats BM, Price WA, Stiles AD. Re-emergence of a fetal pattern of insulin-like growth factor expression during hyperoxic rat lung injury. Am J Respir Cell Mol Biol 1997;16:538–548.

200. Pierce RA, Albertine KH, Starcher BC, Bohnsack JF, Carlton DP, Bland RD. Chronic lung injury in preterm lambs: disordered pulmonary elastin deposition. Am J Physiol 1997;272:L452–L460.

201. Escobedo MB, Hilliard JL, Smith F, Meredith K, Walsh W, Johnson D, Coalson JJ, Kuehl TJ, Null DM, Robotham JL. A baboon model of bronchopulmonary dysplasia: I. Clinical features. Exp Mol Pathol 1982;37:323–334.

202. Coalson JJ, Kuehl TJ, Escobedo MB, Hilliard JL, Smith F, Meredith K, Null DM, Walsh W, Johnson D, Robotham JL. A baboon model of bronchopulmonary dysplasia: II. Pathologic features. Exp Mol Pathol 1982;37:335–350.

203. Delemos RA, Coalson JJ. The contribution of experimental models to our understanding of the pathogenesis and treatment of bronchopulmonary dysplasia. Clin Perinatol 1992;19:521–539.

204. Coalson JJ, Winter VT, Gerstmann DR, Idell S, King RJ, Delemos RA. Pathophysiologic, morphometric, and biochemical studies of the premature baboon with bronchopulmonary dysplasia. Am Rev Respir Dis 1992;145:872–881.

205. Seidner S, Curnin P, Coalson JJ, Cornell D, Castro R. A new model of chronic lung injury in surfactant treated baboons. Pediatr Res 1993;33:344A.

206. Coalson JJ, Winter V, Yoder B. Dysmorphic vascular development in premature baboons with bronchopulmonary dysplasia (BPD). Am J Respir Crit Care Med 1997;155:A262.

207. Northway WH, Rosan RC, Porter DY. Pulmonary disease following respirator therapy of hyaline membrane disease. N Engl J Med 1967;276:357–368.

208. Northway WH. Bronchopulmonary dysplasia: twenty-five years later. Pediatrics 1992;89:969–973.
209. Sunday ME. Neuropeptides and lung development. In: McDonald JA, ed. Growth and development of the lung. New York:Marcel Dekker, 1996:401–494.
210. Bousbaa H, Poron F, Fleury-Feith J. Changes in chromogranin A-immunoreactive guinea-pig pulmonary neuroendocrine cells after sensitization and challenge with ovalbumin. Cell Tissue Res 1994;275:195–199.
211. Coy DH, Heinz-Erian P, Jiang N-Y, Sasaki Y, Taylor J, Moreau JP, Wolfrey WT, Gardner JD, Jensen RT. Probing peptide backbone function in bombesin: a reduced peptide bond analogue with potent and specific receptor antagonist activity. J Biol Chem 1988;263:5056–5060.
212. Wang LH, Coy DH, Taylor JE, Jiang NY, Kim SH, Moreau JP, Huang SC, Mantey SA, Frucht H, Jensen RT. Desmethionine alkylamide bombesin analogues: a new class of bombesin receptor antagonists with potent antisecretory activity in pancreatic acini and antimitotic activity in Swiss 3T3 cells. Biochemistry 1990;29:616–622.
213. Jensen RT, Coy DH. Progress in the development of potent bombesin receptor antagonists. TIPS 1991;12:13–19.
214. Cutz E, Ma TKF, Perrin DG, Moore AM, Becker LE. Peripheral chemoreceptors in congenital central hypoventilation syndrome. Am J Respir Crit Care Med 1997; 155:358–363.
215. Gillan GE, Curran E, O'Reilly Cahalane SF, Unwin AR. Abnormal pattern of pulmonary neuroendocrine cells in victims of sudden infant death syndrome. Pediatrics 1989;84:828–834.
216. Perrin DG, MacDonald TJ, Cutz E. Hyperplasia of bombesin–immunoreactive pulmonary neuroendocrine cells and neuroepithelial bodies in sudden infant death syndrome. Pediatr Pathol 1991;11:431–447.
217. Cutz E, Perrin DG, Hackman R, Czegledy-Nagy N. Maternal smoking and pulmonary neuroendocrine cells in sudden infant death syndrome. Pediatrics 1996;98:668–672.
218. Parkins KJ, Poets CF, O'Brien LM, Stebben SVA, Southall DP. Effects of exposure to 15% oxygen on breathing patterns of oxygen saturation in infants: interventional study. Br M J 1998;316:887–891.
219. Werthammer J, Brown ER, Neff RF, Taeusch HW. Sudden infant death syndrome in infants with bronchopulmonary dysplasia. Pediatrics 1982;69:301–304.
220. Gillan JE, Cutz E. Abnormal pulmonary bombesin immunoreactive cells in Wilson-Mikity syndrome (pulmonary dysmaturity) and bronchopulmonary dysplasia. Pediatr Pathol 1993;13:165–180.
221. Tabassian AR, Nylen ES, Linnoila RI, Sinder RH, Cassidy MM, Becker KL. Stimulation of hamster pulmonary neuroendocrine cells and associated peptides by repeated exposure to cigarette smoke. Am Rev Respir Dis 1989;140:436–440.
222. Aguayo SM, Kane MA, King TE, Schwartz MI, Graner L, Miller YE. Increased levels of bombesin-like peptides in the lower respiratory tract of asymptomatic cigarette smokers. J Clin Invest 1989;84:1105–1113.
223. Haglund B, Cnattingius. Cigarette smoking as a risk factor for sudden infant death syndrome: a population based study. Am J Public Health 1990;80:29–32.
224. Cunningham J, Dockery DW, Speizer FE. Maternal smoking during pregnancy as a predictor of lung function in children. Am J Epidemiol 1994;139:1139–1152.
225. Nylen ES, Linnoila RI, Becker KL. Prenatal cholinergic stimulation of pulmonary endocrine cells by nicotine. Acta Physiol. Scand. 1988; 132:117–118.
226. Wang NS, Chen MF, Schraufnagel DE, Yao YT: The cumulative scanning electron microscopic changes in mouse lungs following prenatal and post natal exposure to nicotine. J Pathol 1984;144:89–100.
227. Chen MF, Kimizuka G, Wang NS. Human fetal lung changes associated with maternal smoking during pregnancy. Pediatr Pulmonol 1987;3:51–58.
228. Nylen ES, Becker KL, Snider RM, Tabassian AR, Cassidy MM, Linnoila RI. Cholinergic-nicotinic control of growth and secretion of cultured pulmonary neuroendocrine cells. Anat Rec 1993;236:129–135.
229. Lindstrom J, Anand V, Gerzanich V, Peng X, Wang F, Wells G Structure and function of neuronal nicotinic acetylcholine receptors. Prog. Brain Res. 1996;109:125–137.
230. Mochizuki M, Maruo T, Masuko K, Ohtsu T. Effects of smoking on fetoplacental-maternal systems during pregnancy. Am J Obstet Gynaecol 1984;149:413–420.
231. Luck W, Nan H. Exposure of the fetus, neonate and nursed infant to nicotine and cotinine from maternal smoking. N Engl J Med 1984;311:672.
232. Lindquist NG, Ullberg S. Autoradiography of intravenously injected $^{14}$C–nicotine indicates long term retention in the respiratory tract. Nature 1973;248:600–601.
233. Stanislawski EC, Hernandez–Garcia J, de la Mora–Torres MC, Abranjan–Polanco E. Lung neuroendocrine structures: topography, morphology, composition and relation with intrinsic asthma (nonimmune). Arch Invest Med (Mex) 1981;12:559–577.

234.Cutz E, Levison M, Cooper DM. Ultrastructure of airways in children with asthma. Histopathology 1978;2:407–421.

235.Cutz E, Orange RP. Mast cells and endocrine (APUD) cells of the lung. In: Lichtenstein LM, Austen KF, eds. Asthma: physiology, immunopharmacology, and treatment. New York: Academic Press,1977:51–76.

236.Van Lommel A, Van den Steen P, Lauweryns JM. Association of immune cells with neuroepithelial bodies in the lungs of neonatal dogs, cats and hamsters. Cell Tissue Res 1995;282:519–522.

237.Del Rio M, de la Fuente M. Chemo-attractant capacity of bombesin, gastrin-relating peptide and neuromedium C is mediated through PKC activation in murine peritoneal macrophages. Reg Peptides 1994;49:185–193.

238.Morrison KJ, Gao Y, Vanhoutte PM. Epithelial modulation of airway smooth muscle. Am J Physiol 1990;258:L254–L262.

239.Sunday ME, Haley KJ, Emanuel RL, Asokananthan N, Sikorski K, Kong YP, Torday JS, Mu Q, Erspamer V. Fetal alveolar epithelial cells contain [D-Ala2] and opiate receptors mediate. Am J Respir Cell Mol Biol 2000, in press.

240.Faccone G, Fasulo S, Ainis L, Licata A. Paraneurons in the gills and airways of fisher. Micr Res Tech 1997;37:4–12.

241.McCormack T, McCormack K. Shaker K$^+$ channel β subunits belong to a NAD(P)H–dependent oxidoreductase superfamily. Cell 1994;79:1133–1135.

242.Maltepe E, Simon MC. Oxygen, genes, and development: an analysis of the hypoxic gene regulation during murine vascular development. J Mol Med 1998;76:391–401.

# INDEX